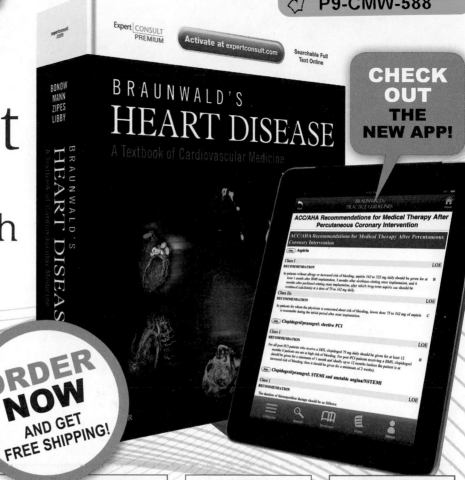
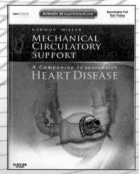
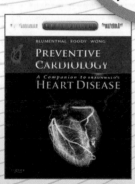
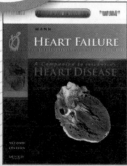
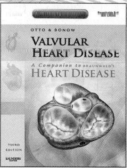
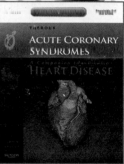
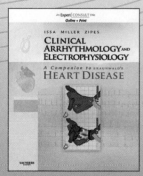
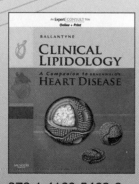
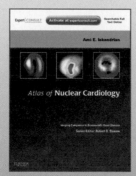
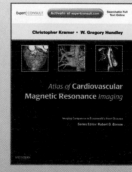
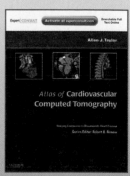

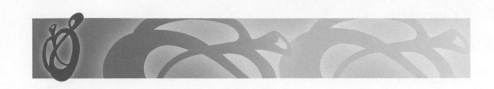

BRAUNWALD'S
HEART DISEASE

REVIEW AND ASSESSMENT

NINTH EDITION

LEONARD S. LILLY, MD
PROFESSOR OF MEDICINE
HARVARD MEDICAL SCHOOL
CHIEF, BRIGHAM AND WOMEN'S/FAULKNER CARDIOLOGY
BRIGHAM AND WOMEN'S HOSPITAL
BOSTON, MASSACHUSETTS

ELSEVIER
SAUNDERS

ELSEVIER
SAUNDERS

1600 John F. Kennedy Blvd.
Ste. 1800
Philadelphia, PA 19103-2899

BRAUNWALD'S HEART DISEASE: REVIEW AND ASSESSMENT,
NINTH EDITION

ISBN: 978-1-4557-1147-5

Copyright © 2012, 2008, 2006, 2001, 1997, 1992, 1989 by Saunders, an imprint of Elsevier Inc.

Notice

Knowledge and best practice in this field are constantly changing. As new research and experience broaden our knowledge, changes in practice, treatment and drug therapy may become necessary or appropriate. Readers are advised to check the most current information provided (i) on procedures featured or (ii) by the manufacturer of each product to be administered, to verify the recommended dose or formula, the method and duration of administration, and contraindications. It is the responsibility of the practitioner, relying on their own experience and knowledge of the patient, to make diagnoses, to determine dosages and the best treatment for each individual patient, and to take all appropriate safety precautions. To the fullest extent of the law, neither the Publisher nor the Authors assume any liability for any injury and/or damage to persons or property arising out of or related to any use of the material contained in this book.

The Publisher

ISBN: 978-1-4557-1147-5

Executive Content Strategist: Dolores Meloni
Content Development Specialist: Angela Rufino
Publishing Services Manager: Patricia Tannian
Senior Project Manager: John Casey
Design Manager: Steven Stave

Printed in the United States of America

Last digit is the print number: 10 9 8 7 6 5 4 3 2

CONTRIBUTORS

Marc P. Bonaca, MD, MPH
Instructor in Medicine, Harvard Medical School
Cardiovascular Division, Brigham and Women's
  Hospital
Boston, Massachusetts

Akshay S. Desai, MD, MPH
Assistant Professor of Medicine, Harvard Medical School
Advanced Heart Disease Section, Cardiovascular Division,
  Brigham and Women's Hospital
Boston, Massachusetts

Swathy Kolli, MD, MSPH
Cardiovascular Imaging Fellow, Brigham and Women's
  Hospital
Boston, Massachusetts

Neal K. Lakdawala, MD, MSc
Instructor in Medicine, Harvard Medical School
Advanced Heart Disease Section, Cardiovascular
  Division, Brigham and Women's Hospital
Boston, Massachusetts

Leonard S. Lilly, MD
Professor of Medicine, Harvard Medical School
Chief, Brigham and Women's/Faulkner Cardiology
Brigham and Women's Hospital
Boston, Massachusetts

Amy Leigh Miller, MD, PhD
Instructor in Medicine, Harvard Medical School
Cardiovascular Division, Brigham and Women's Hospital
Boston, Massachusetts

Sara L. Partington, MD
Cardiovascular Imaging Fellow, Brigham and Women's
  Hospital
Boston, Massachusetts

Fidencio Saldaña, MD
Instructor in Medicine
Faculty Assistant Dean for Student Affairs
Office of Recruitment and Multicultural Affairs,
  Harvard Medical School
Cardiovascular Division
Brigham and Women's Hospital
Boston, Massachusetts

Garrick C. Stewart, MD
Instructor in Medicine, Harvard Medical School
Advanced Heart Disease Section, Cardiovascular Division,
  Brigham and Women's Hospital
Boston, Massachusetts

Neil J. Wimmer, MD
Fellow in Cardiovascular Medicine
Brigham and Women's Hospital
Harvard Medical School
Boston, Massachusetts

PREFACE

Review and Assessment is a comprehensive study guide designed to accompany the ninth edition of *Braunwald's Heart Disease: A Textbook of Cardiovascular Medicine*, edited by Dr. Robert O. Bonow, Dr. Douglas L. Mann, Dr. Douglas P. Zipes, and Dr. Peter Libby. It consists of 706 questions that address key topics in the broad field of cardiovascular disease. A detailed answer is provided for each question, often comprising a "mini-review" of the subject matter. Each answer refers to specific pages, tables, and figures in *Braunwald's Heart Disease* and in most cases to additional pertinent citations. Topics of greatest clinical relevance are emphasized, and subjects of particular importance are intentionally reiterated in subsequent questions for reinforcement.

Review and Assessment is intended primarily for cardiology fellows, practicing cardiologists, internists, advanced medical residents, and other professionals wishing to review contemporary cardiovascular medicine in detail. The subject matter and structure are suitable to help prepare for the Subspecialty Examination in Cardiovascular Disease offered by the American Board of Internal Medicine.

All questions and answers in this book were designed specifically for this edition of *Review and Assessment*. I am grateful for the contributions by my colleagues at Brigham and Women's Hospital who expertly authored new questions and updated material carried forward from the previous edition: Dr. Marc Bonaca, Dr. Akshay Desai, Dr. Neal Lakdawala, Dr. Amy Miller, Dr. Fidencio Saldaña, Dr. Garrick Stewart, and Dr. Neil Wimmer. We are very appreciative to Dr. Sara Partington and Dr. Swathy Kolli for submitting many of the new noninvasive images and to the following colleagues who provided additional graphics or support to this edition: Dr. Ron Blankstein, Dr. Sharmila Dorbala, Dr. Eric Green, Dr. Raymond Kwong, and Dr. Saurabh Rohatgi. We also acknowledge and thank the Brigham and Women's Hospital team of cardiac ultrasonographers, led by Jose Rivero, who expertly obtained and alerted us to many of the images that appear in this book.

It has been a pleasure to work with the editorial and production departments of our publisher, Elsevier, Inc. Specifically, I thank Ms. Natasha Andjelkovic, Ms. Dolores Meloni, Ms. Angela Rufino, and Mr. John Casey for their expertise and professionalism in the preparation of this edition of *Review and Assessment*.

Finally, and as always, I am very grateful to each member of my family for their support and patience during the often-long hours required to prepare this text.

On behalf of the contributors, I hope that you find this book a useful guide in your review of cardiovascular medicine.

Leonard S. Lilly, MD
Boston, Massachusetts

CONTENTS

FUNDAMENTALS OF CARDIOVASCULAR DISEASE; MOLECULAR BIOLOGY AND GENETICS; EVALUATION OF THE PATIENT

DIRECTIONS: For each question below, select the ONE BEST response.

QUESTION 1

A 54-year-old African-American man with a history of hypertension and hypercholesterolemia undergoes a treadmill exercise test using the standard Bruce protocol. He stops at 11 minutes 14 seconds because of fatigue, at a peak heart rate of 152 beats/min and peak systolic blood pressure of 200 mm Hg. The diastolic blood pressure declines by 5 mm Hg during exercise. During recovery, the systolic blood pressure decreases to 15 mm Hg below his pre-exercise pressure. There are no ischemic changes on the ECG during or after exercise. Which of the following is correct?

A. His peak systolic blood pressure during exercise exceeds that normally observed
B. The change in diastolic blood pressure during exercise is indicative of significant coronary artery disease
C. This test is nondiagnostic owing to an inadequate peak heart rate
D. These results are consistent with a low prognostic risk of a coronary event
E. The postexercise reduction in systolic blood pressure is suggestive of severe coronary artery disease

QUESTION 2

When present, each of the following heart sounds occurs shortly after S_2 EXCEPT:
A. Opening snap
B. Third heart sound
C. Ejection click
D. Tumor plop
E. Pericardial knock

QUESTION 3

A state-of-the-art blood test has been developed for the rapid, noninvasive diagnosis of coronary artery disease. The assay has a sensitivity of 90% and a specificity of 90% for the detection of at least one coronary stenosis of > 70%. In which of the following scenarios is the blood test likely to be of most value to the clinician?
A. A 29-year-old man with exertional chest pain who has no cardiac risk factors
B. A 41-year-old asymptomatic premenopausal woman
C. A 78-year-old diabetic woman with exertional chest pain who underwent two-vessel coronary stenting 6 weeks ago
D. A 62-year-old man with exertional chest pain who has hypertension, dyslipidemia, and a 2 pack-per-day smoking history
E. A 68-year-old man with chest discomfort at rest accompanied by 2 mm of ST-segment depression in the inferior leads on the ECG

QUESTION 4

A murmur is auscultated during routine examination of an 18-year-old asymptomatic college student, at the second left intercostal space, close to the sternum. The murmur is crescendo-decrescendo, is present throughout systole and diastole, and peaks simultaneously with S_2. It does not change with position or rotation of the head. Which of the following best describes this murmur?
A. This is a continuous murmur, most likely a venous hum commonly heard in adolescents
B. This is a continuous murmur resulting from mixed aortic valve disease
C. This is a continuous murmur due to a congenital shunt, likely a patent ductus arteriosus
D. Continuous murmurs of this type can only be congenital; murmurs due to acquired arteriovenous connections are purely systolic
E. This murmur, the result of left subclavian artery stenosis, is not considered continuous, because a continuous murmur can result only from an arteriovenous communication

QUESTION 5

Unequal upper extremity arterial pulsations commonly are found in each of the following disorders EXCEPT:
A. Aortic dissection
B. Takayasu disease

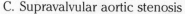

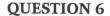

C. Supravalvular aortic stenosis
D. Subclavian artery atherosclerosis
E. Subvalvular aortic stenosis

QUESTION 6

A 58-year-old woman with metastatic breast cancer presents with exertional dyspnea and is found to have a large circumferential pericardial effusion, jugular venous distention, and hypotension. Which of the following echocardiographic signs is likely present?
A. Collapse of the right ventricle throughout systole
B. Exaggerated decrease in tricuspid inflow velocity during inspiration
C. Exaggerated decrease in mitral inflow velocity during inspiration
D. Exaggerated increase in left ventricular outflow tract velocity during inspiration
E. Markedly increased E/A ratio of the transmitral Doppler velocity profile

QUESTION 7

Which of the following statements about pulsus paradoxus is correct?
A. Inspiration in normal individuals results in a decline of systolic arterial pressure of up to 15 mm Hg
B. Accurate determination of pulsus paradoxus requires intra-arterial pressure measurement
C. Pulsus paradoxus in tamponade is typically accompanied by the Kussmaul sign
D. Pulsus paradoxus is unlikely to be present in patients with significant aortic regurgitation, even in the presence of tamponade
E. Pulsus paradoxus is common in patients with hypertrophic cardiomyopathy

QUESTION 8

Which of the following electrocardiographic features is typical of left anterior fascicular block?
A. Q waves in the inferior leads
B. Mean QRS axis between 0 and −30 degrees
C. QRS duration >0.12 millisecond
D. rS pattern in the inferior leads and qR pattern in lateral leads
E. Marked right-axis deviation

QUESTION 9

Each of the following combinations has the potential for significant pharmacologic interaction and drug toxicity EXCEPT:
A. Simvastatin and erythromycin
B. Sildenafil and nitroglycerin
C. Pravastatin and ketoconazole
D. Cyclosporine and St. John's wort
E. Digoxin and verapamil

QUESTION 10

Each of the following conditions is a contraindication to exercise stress testing EXCEPT:
A. Symptomatic hypertrophic obstructive cardiomyopathy
B. Advanced aortic stenosis
C. Acute myocarditis
D. Abdominal aortic aneurysm with transverse diameter of 5.5 cm
E. Unstable angina

QUESTION 11

A 42-year-old woman with hypertension and dyslipidemia underwent a 1-day rest-stress exercise myocardial perfusion single-photon emission computed tomography (SPECT) study with technetium-99m imaging to evaluate symptoms of "atypical" chest pain. Her resting ECG showed left ventricular hypertrophy. She exercised for 12 minutes 30 seconds on the standard Bruce protocol and attained a peak heart rate of 155 beats/min. She developed a brief sharp parasternal chest pain during the test that resolved quickly during recovery. Based on the images in Figure 1-1, which of the following statements is correct?
A. The SPECT myocardial perfusion images are diagnostic of transmural myocardial scar in the distribution of the mid-left anterior descending coronary artery
B. The anterior wall defect on the SPECT images is likely an artifact due to breast tissue attenuation
C. Thallium-201 would have been a better choice of radiotracer to image this patient
D. Gated SPECT imaging cannot differentiate attenuation artifacts from a true perfusion defect
E. A transmural scar is associated with reduced wall motion but normal wall thickening on gated SPECT imaging

QUESTION 12

Which of the following statements regarding the second heart sound (S_2) is TRUE?
A. Earlier closure of the pulmonic valve with inspiration results in physiologic splitting of S_2
B. Right bundle branch block results in widened splitting of S_2
C. Paradoxical splitting of S_2 is the auscultatory hallmark of an ostium secundum atrial septal defect
D. Fixed splitting of S_2 is expected in patients with a right ventricular electronically paced rhythm
E. Severe pulmonic valvular stenosis is associated with a loud P_2

QUESTION 13

A 56-year-old asymptomatic man with a history of hypertension and cigarette smoking is referred for a screening exercise treadmill test. After 7 minutes on the standard Bruce protocol, he is noted to have 1 mm

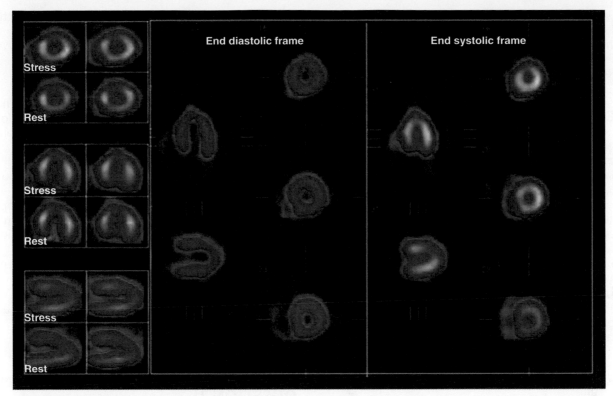

End diastolic frame

End systolic frame

Stress

Rest

Stress

Rest

Stress

Rest

FIGURE 1-1

of flat ST-segment depression in leads II, III, and aVF. He stops exercising at 9 minutes because of leg fatigue and breathlessness. The peak heart rate is 85% of the maximum predicted for his age. The ST segments return to baseline by 1 minute into recovery. Which of the following statements is correct?

A. This test is conclusive for severe stenosis of the proximal right coronary artery
B. His risk of death due to an acute myocardial infarction during the next year is >50%
C. He should proceed directly to coronary angiography
D. The test predicts a 25% risk of cardiac events over the next 5 years, most likely the development of angina
E. This is likely a false-positive test

QUESTION 14

In which of the following clinical scenarios do ST-segment depressions during standard exercise testing increase the diagnostic probability of significant coronary artery disease?

A. A 56-year-old man with left bundle branch block and a family history of premature coronary disease
B. A 45-year-old woman with diabetes and hypertension, with left ventricular hypertrophy on her baseline ECG
C. A 76-year-old woman with new exertional dyspnea, a history of cigarette smoking, and a normal baseline ECG
D. A 28-year-old woman with pleuritic left-sided chest pain after a gymnastics class
E. A 63-year-old man with exertional dyspnea on beta-blocker, digoxin, and nitrate therapies

QUESTION 15

Which of the following statements regarding cardiac catheterization is TRUE?

A. The risk of a major complication from cardiac catheterization is 2.0% to 2.5%
B. The incidence of contrast-induced nephrotoxicity in patients with renal dysfunction is decreased with intravenous administration of mannitol before and after the procedure
C. High osmolar nonionic contrast agents demonstrate a reduced incidence of adverse hemodynamic reactions compared with low osmolar ionic contrast agents
D. One French unit (F) is equivalent to 0.33 mm
E. Retrograde left-sided heart catheterization is generally a safe procedure in patients with tilting-disc prosthetic aortic valves

QUESTION 16

A 75-year-old woman was brought to the cardiac catheterization laboratory in the setting of an acute myocardial infarction. She had presented with chest pain, epigastric discomfort, and nausea. Physical examination was pertinent for diaphoresis, heart rate 52 beats/min, blood pressure 85/50 mm Hg, jugular venous distention, and slight bilateral pulmonary rales. Coronary angiography demonstrated ostial occlusion of a dominant right coronary artery, without significant left-sided coronary artery disease. The presenting ECG likely showed all of the following features EXCEPT:

A. ST-segment elevation in leads II, III, and aVF
B. ST-segment depression in leads V_1 and V_2
C. Sinus bradycardia
D. ST-segment elevation in lead V_4R
E. PR-segment depression

QUESTION 17

Using Doppler echocardiography methods, the following values are obtained in a patient with a restrictive ventricular septal defect (VSD) and mitral regurgitation: systolic transmitral flow velocity = 5.8 m/sec and systolic flow velocity at the site of the VSD = 5.1 m/sec. The patient's blood pressure is 144/78 mm Hg. The estimated right ventricular systolic pressure is (choose the single best answer):
A. 35 mm Hg
B. 40 mm Hg
C. 45 mm Hg
D. 50 mm Hg
E. Not able to be determined from the provided information

QUESTION 18

Which of the following statements regarding left bundle branch block (LBBB) is TRUE?
A. The majority of patients with LBBB do not have structural heart disease
B. In LBBB, the S_2 is widely split with normal respiratory variation
C. The presence of LBBB is associated with significantly reduced long-term survival
D. In LBBB, the T wave vectors are oriented in the same direction as the QRS complex
E. LBBB does not impair myocardial performance

QUESTION 19

Which of the following statements regarding altered electrolytes and electrocardiographic abnormalities is TRUE?
A. Hypocalcemia causes prolongation of the QT interval
B. Hyperkalemia causes QRS narrowing and increased P wave amplitude
C. Hypomagnesemia is associated with monomorphic ventricular tachycardia
D. Hypokalemia causes peaked T waves

E. Severe hypocalcemia has been associated with the presence of a J wave (Osborn wave)

QUESTION 20

For which of the following scenarios is the diagnostic sensitivity of standard exercise testing sufficient to forego additional imaging with either nuclear scintigraphy or echocardiography?
A. A 53-year-old woman with hypertension and left ventricular hypertrophy by echocardiography who has developed exertional chest pressure
B. A 74-year-old man with a history of cardiomyopathy with a normal baseline electrocardiogram on angiotensin-converting enzyme inhibitor, beta-blocker, and digoxin therapies
C. A 37-year-old asymptomatic woman with incidentally detected left bundle branch block
D. A 44-year-old male smoker with Wolff-Parkinson-White syndrome and a family history of coronary artery disease with new exertional chest discomfort
E. A 53-year-old man with hyperlipidemia, a normal baseline ECG, and sharp, fleeting chest pains

QUESTION 21

All of the following statements about the ECG depicted in Figure 1-2 are correct EXCEPT:
A. The basic rhythm is atrial fibrillation
B. The fifth QRS complex on the tracing is likely an example of aberrant conduction
C. The Ashman phenomenon is based on the fact that the refractory period is directly related to the length of the preceding RR interval
D. Right bundle branch block morphology is commonly present in Ashman beats
E. The bundle of His is the likely anatomic location of the conduction delay because it has the longest refractory period

QUESTION 22

The timing of an "innocent" murmur is usually:
A. Early systolic
B. Presystolic
C. Midsystolic
D. Holosystolic
E. Early diastolic

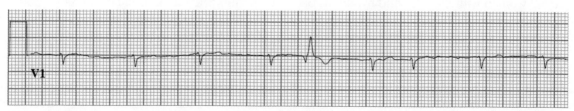

FIGURE 1-2 From Marriott HJL: Rhythm Quizlets: Self Assessment. Philadelphia, Lea & Febiger, 1987, p 14.

QUESTION 23

Which of the following statements about the jugular venous waveform is TRUE?
A. Kussmaul's sign is pathognomonic for constrictive pericarditis
B. The *c* wave is a reflection of ventricular diastole and becomes visible in patients with diastolic dysfunction
C. The *x* descent is less prominent than the *y* descent in cardiac tamponade
D. Phasic declines in venous pressure (the *x* and *y* descents) are typically more prominent to the eye than the positive pressure waves (the *a*, *c*, and *v* waves)
E. Cannon *a* waves indicate interventricular conduction delay

QUESTION 24

Which of the following statements regarding the measurement of cardiac output is correct?
A. In the thermodilution method, cardiac output is directly related to the area under the thermodilution curve
B. The thermodilution method tends to underestimate cardiac output in low-output states
C. In the presence of tricuspid regurgitation, the thermodilution method is preferred over the Fick technique for measuring cardiac output
D. A limitation of the Fick method is the necessity of measuring oxygen consumption in a steady state
E. Cardiac output is directly proportional to systemic vascular resistance

QUESTION 25

Which of the following conditions is associated with the Doppler transmitral inflow pattern shown in Figure 1-3?

A. Gastrointestinal hemorrhage
B. Constrictive pericarditis
C. Normal aging
D. Restrictive cardiomyopathy
E. Hyperthyroidism

QUESTION 26

A 32-year-old woman, a native of India, is referred by her primary care physician for further evaluation for dyspnea on exertion. On examination, both an opening snap and mid-diastolic rumble are appreciated at the apex. An echocardiogram is obtained. The transmitral Doppler tracing shown in Figure 1-4 permits accurate assessment of each of the following EXCEPT:
A. The presence of mitral stenosis
B. The presence, but not the severity, of mitral regurgitation
C. The transmitral diastolic pressure gradient
D. The etiology of the valvular lesion
E. The mitral valve area

QUESTION 27

A patient with a history of pulmonary embolism undergoes evaluation including noninvasive assessment by Doppler echocardiography. The following values are determined:
    Right atrial pressure = 9 mm Hg
    Peak systolic velocity across the tricuspid valve = 4 m/sec
What is this patient's right ventricular systolic pressure?
A. 64 mm Hg
B. 73 mm Hg
C. 50 mm Hg
D. 20 mm Hg
E. The information given is insufficient to determine the value

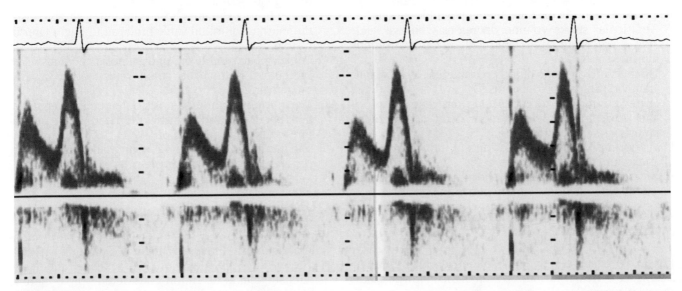

FIGURE 1-3

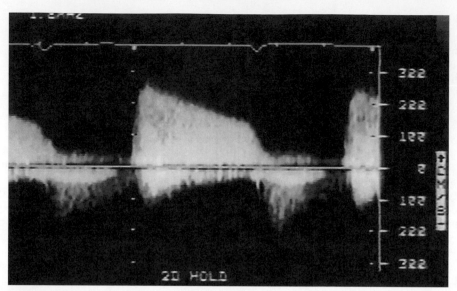

FIGURE 1-4

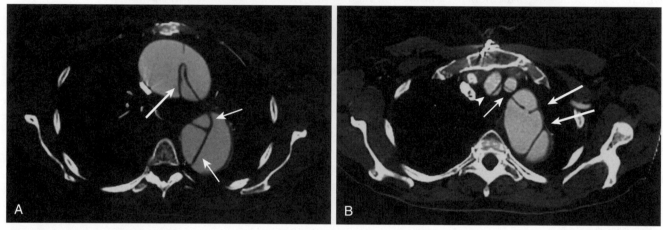

FIGURE 1-5 Courtesy of R. C. Gilkeson, MD, Case Western Reserve University, Cleveland, Ohio.

QUESTION 28

Which of the following statements is TRUE regarding the response to aerobic exercise by healthy older adults?
A. Ventricular stroke volume decreases with age such that there is an age-related fall in cardiac output during exercise
B. Systolic and diastolic blood pressures each rise significantly during aerobic exercise
C. A decline in beta-adrenergic responsiveness contributes to a fall in the maximum heart rate in older individuals
D. A normal adult's cardiac output doubles during maximum aerobic exercise
E. Maximum aerobic capacity does not change significantly with age in sedentary individuals

QUESTION 29

Physiologic states and dynamic maneuvers alter the characteristics of heart murmurs. Which of the following statements is correct?

A. In acute mitral regurgitation, the left atrial pressure rises dramatically so that the murmur is heard only during late systole
B. Rising from a squatting to a standing position causes the murmur of mitral valve prolapse to begin later in systole
C. The diastolic rumble of mitral stenosis becomes more prominent during the strain phase of a Valsalva maneuver
D. The murmur of aortic stenosis, but not mitral regurgitation, becomes louder during the beat after a premature ventricular contraction
E. The murmur of acute aortic regurgitation can usually be heard throughout diastole

QUESTION 30

Which of the following statements regarding the computed tomograms of the chest shown in Figure 1-5 is TRUE?
A. The patient's disorder should be managed medically, with surgical intervention considered only if there is evidence of secondary organ involvement

B. The left common carotid artery is spared by this process
C. The sensitivity of computed tomography for the diagnosis of this condition is >95%
D. Fewer than 50% of patients with this condition will report chest pain
E. Transesophageal echocardiography is necessary to confirm the diagnosis

QUESTION 31

Which of the following statements regarding ST-segment changes during exercise testing is TRUE?
A. The electrocardiographic localization of ST-segment depression predicts the anatomic territory of coronary obstructive disease
B. The J point is the proper isoelectric reference point on the ECG
C. J point depression during exercise is diagnostic for significant cardiac ischemia
D. Persistence of ST-segment depression for 60 to 80 milliseconds after the J point is necessary to interpret the electrocardiographic response as abnormal
E. ST-segment depression must be present both during exercise and in recovery to be interpreted as abnormal

QUESTION 32

An ECG is obtained as part of the routine preoperative evaluation of an asymptomatic 45-year-old man scheduled to undergo wrist surgery. The tracing is shown in Figure 1-6 and is consistent with:
A. Right ventricular hypertrophy
B. Left posterior fascicular block
C. Reversal of limb lead placement
D. Left anterior fascicular block and counterclockwise rotation
E. Dextrocardia with situs inversus

QUESTION 33

Which of the following statements is TRUE regarding exercise test protocols?
A. Regardless of the exercise protocol, the heart rate and systolic and diastolic blood pressures all must increase substantially to achieve a valid test
B. Bicycle, treadmill, and arm ergometry protocols all produce approximately equal heart rate and blood pressure responses
C. The standard Bruce protocol is characterized by only small increases in oxygen consumption between stages
D. A fall in systolic blood pressure during exercise is associated with severe coronary artery disease
E. An optimal graded treadmill exercise test rarely requires more than 5 minutes of exercise on the Bruce protocol

QUESTION 34

Which of the following patients is LEAST likely to have a cardiac cause of his/her recent onset of dyspnea?
A. An active 54-year-old man with a congenitally bicuspid aortic valve who has recently noticed shortness of breath walking his usual 18 holes of golf
B. A 70-year-old woman who sustained an anterior myocardial infarction 1 year ago with a left ventricular ejection fraction of 50% at that time. She has not had recurrent angina but has noted dyspnea during her usual housework over the past 2 months
C. A 46-year-old woman with a history of asymptomatic rheumatic mitral stenosis who recently noticed irregular palpitations and shortness of breath while climbing stairs
D. A 38-year-old woman with a previously asymptomatic ostium secundum atrial septal defect, now 8 months pregnant, who has noted shortness of breath during her usual weekly low-impact aerobics class

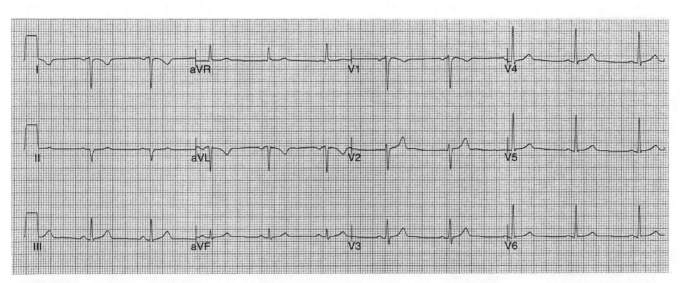

FIGURE 1-6

E. A 22-year-old man with trisomy 21 and a heart murmur who has described shortness of breath carrying grocery bundles over the past 3 months

QUESTION 35

A 68-year-old man with a history of diabetes, hypertension, and hyperlipidemia presents to the emergency department via ambulance, complaining of crushing substernal chest pain. Emergency Medical Services personnel report that anterior ST segments were elevated on the ECG en route. Which of the following electrocardiographic findings is LEAST likely in this patient experiencing an acute anterior ST-segment elevation myocardial infarction?
A. ST-segment elevation in leads V_2 to V_5
B. Shortened QT interval
C. New right bundle branch block
D. ST-segment depression in leads III and aVF
E. Hyperacute T waves in the precordial leads

QUESTION 36

All of the following statements regarding nuclear imaging and acute myocardial infarction (MI) are true EXCEPT:
A. The size of the resting myocardial perfusion defect after acute MI correlates with the patient's prognosis
B. Increased lung uptake of thallium-201 at rest correlates with an unfavorable prognosis
C. Submaximal exercise imaging soon after MI is a better predictor of late complications than adenosine myocardial perfusion imaging
D. Technetium-99m sestamibi imaging can be used to assess the effectiveness of thrombolytic therapy
E. Measuring infarct size by technetium-99m sestamibi imaging before discharge from the hospital is a reliable way to predict subsequent ventricular remodeling

QUESTION 37

Which of the following statements regarding ST-segment elevation during exercise testing is TRUE?
A. ST-segment elevation during exercise testing is a common finding in patients with coronary artery disease
B. ST-segment elevation in a lead that contains a pathologic Q wave at baseline indicates severe myocardial ischemia
C. The electrocardiographic leads that manifest ST-segment elevation during exercise localize the anatomic regions of ischemia
D. ST-segment elevation that develops during exercise is usually a manifestation of benign early repolarization
E. ST-segment elevation during exercise is commonly associated with the development of complete heart block

QUESTION 38

Which of the following statements regarding coronary calcium assessment by electron beam tomography (EBT) is TRUE?
A. The amount of calcium on EBT strongly correlates with the severity of coronary disease detected by angiography
B. Patients who benefit most from screening with EBT are those at a high risk for coronary events based on traditional risk factors
C. The absence of coronary calcium completely excludes the presence of severe obstructive coronary artery stenosis
D. Interpretation of the calcium score is independent of the patient's age and gender
E. A coronary calcium score higher than the median confers an increased risk of myocardial infarction and death

QUESTION 39

Which of the following statements is TRUE regarding prognosis as determined by myocardial perfusion imaging?
A. Patients with normal perfusion in the presence of angiographically documented coronary artery disease have very low rates of cardiac events (<1% per year).
B. Thallium is the preferred isotope for myocardial perfusion imaging in women
C. Transient ischemic dilatation of the left ventricle and lung uptake of the nuclear tracer imply the presence of minor coronary artery disease
D. The combination of clinical and cardiac catheterization data is more predictive of subsequent cardiac events than the combination of clinical and myocardial perfusion data
E. The risk of future cardiac events is unrelated to the number or extent of myocardial perfusion defects

QUESTION 40

A previously healthy 28-year-old man presented to the hospital because of 1 month of progressive exertional dyspnea, weakness, and weight loss. One day before hospitalization he was unable to climb one flight of stairs because of shortness of breath. On examination, he appeared fatigued with mild respiratory distress. His blood pressure was 110/70 mm Hg without pulsus paradoxus. His heart rate was 110 beats/min and regular. The jugular veins were distended without the Kussmaul sign. Pulmonary auscultation revealed scant bibasilar rales. The heart sounds were distant. There was mild bilateral ankle edema. As part of the evaluation during hospitalization, he underwent cardiac magnetic resonance imaging. A short-axis view at the midventricular level is shown in Figure 1-7. Which of the following is the most likely diagnosis?

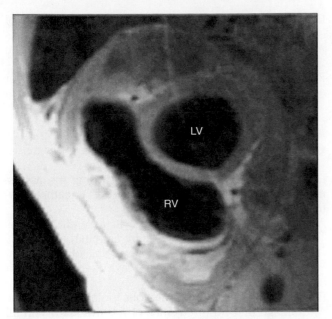

FIGURE 1-7

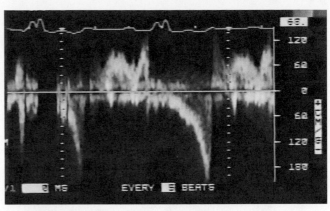

FIGURE 1-8

A. Pericardial malignancy
B. Chronic organized pericardial hematoma
C. Constrictive pericarditis
D. Extracardiac tumor compression of the heart
E. Congenital partial absence of the pericardium with cardiac herniation

QUESTION 41

Each of the following statements regarding intracardiac shunts is true EXCEPT:
A. A left-to-right shunt should be suspected if the difference in oxygen saturation between the superior vena cava (SVC) and the pulmonary artery is 8% or more
B. Oxygen saturation in the inferior vena cava is normally higher than that in the SVC
C. In a suspected atrial septal defect with left-to-right flow, mixed venous O_2 content should be measured at the level of the pulmonary artery
D. A pulmonic-to-systemic blood flow ratio of <1 indicates a net right-to-left shunt
E. Pulmonary artery oxygen saturation exceeding 80% should raise the suspicion of a left-to-right shunt

QUESTION 42

A 46-year-old man with dyspnea on exertion is noted to have a systolic ejection murmur along the left sternal border. An echocardiogram is obtained. Figure 1-8 shows Doppler pulsed-wave interrogation of the left ventricular outflow tract, recorded from the apex. Which of the following initial recommendations would be appropriate?
A. Strict fluid restriction
B. Compression stockings
C. Avoid volume depletion
D. Aortic valve replacement
E. Bed rest

QUESTION 43

Each of the following statements regarding echocardiography in pericardial disease is true EXCEPT:
A. Small pericardial effusions tend to accumulate anterior to the heart
B. Up to 50 mL of pericardial fluid is present in normal individuals
C. In cardiac tamponade, right ventricular diastolic collapse may not occur if pulmonary hypertension is present
D. In the presence of a pericardial effusion, right atrial diastolic indentation is a less specific sign of cardiac tamponade than early diastolic collapse of the right ventricle
E. Chest computed tomography is superior to transthoracic echocardiography as a means to accurately measure pericardial thickness

QUESTION 44

Which of the following statements regarding nuclear imaging in cardiac disease is TRUE?
A. The use of single-photon emission computed tomography (SPECT) with electrocardiographic gating has no impact on the specificity of nuclear testing in women with attenuation artifacts
B. Exercise nuclear stress imaging, rather than pharmacologic stress testing, is the preferred diagnostic modality for patients with left bundle branch block
C. The presence of reversible defects on pharmacologic stress perfusion imaging before noncardiac surgery predicts an increased risk of perioperative cardiac events, but the magnitude of risk is not related to the extent of ischemia
D. Cardiovascular event rates are similar in diabetics compared with nondiabetics for any given myocardial perfusion abnormality
E. Viability of noncontracting myocardium can be accurately evaluated by thallium-201 imaging

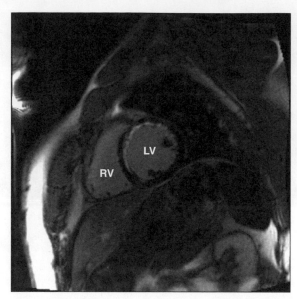

FIGURE 1-9

QUESTION 45

A 45-year-old woman was referred for exercise echocardiography because of a history of intermittent chest pain. She has a strong family history of premature coronary artery disease but no other atherosclerotic risk factors. The exercise echocardiogram achieved the desired heart rate goal and demonstrated a focal wall motion abnormality of the left ventricular anterior wall at rest, which was unchanged at maximum exercise. A subsequent cardiac magnetic resonance study was performed to characterize the myocardial tissue in that region. A delayed image taken after intravenous administration of gadolinium is shown in Figure 1-9. What is the most likely cause of the anterior wall motion abnormality?

A. Transient myocardial ischemia due to a significant coronary artery stenosis
B. Prior myocardial infarction
C. Myocarditis
D. Infiltrative cardiomyopathy
E. Breast attenuation artifact

QUESTION 46

Which of the following statements concerning the echocardiographic evaluation of aortic stenosis is TRUE?

A. The peak-to-peak gradient measured at cardiac catheterization routinely exceeds the peak instantaneous aortic valve pressure gradient assessed by Doppler echocardiography
B. Patients with impaired left ventricular function may have severe aortic stenosis, as determined by the continuity equation, despite a peak outflow velocity between 2 and 3 m/sec
C. Among echocardiographic-Doppler techniques, the most accurate transaortic valve flow velocity in aortic stenosis is determined by pulse-wave Doppler imaging

D. The greatest degree of error in the calculation of aortic valve area using the continuity equation resides in inaccurate measurement of the transaortic valve flow velocity
E. The mean aortic valve gradient measured by Doppler echocardiography is invariably higher than the mean gradient measured by cardiac catheterization

QUESTION 47

Each of the following statements regarding the assessment for intracardiac shunts during cardiac catheterization is true EXCEPT:

A. In normal subjects, O_2 content in different portions of the right atrium may vary by as much as 2 vol % (20 mL O_2/L), reflecting the streaming of blood that forms from the superior vena cava, the inferior vena cava, and the coronary sinus
B. Atrial septal defect, anomalous pulmonary venous drainage, and ruptured sinus of Valsalva aneurysm all are associated with a significant step-up in O_2 saturation between the venae cavae and the right atrium
C. Because of the normal variability in O_2 saturation, shunts with pulmonary-to-systemic flow ratios (Qp/Qs) ≤ 1.3 at the level of the pulmonary artery or right ventricle may escape detection by oximetry run analyses
D. When a shunt is unidirectional (e.g., left-to-right only), its magnitude can be calculated as the difference between the pulmonary and systemic blood flows (Qp – Qs) as determined using the Fick equations
E. In patients with a pure right-to-left shunt, the Qp/Qs ratio should be >1.0

QUESTION 48

Each of the following findings during an exercise test is associated with multivessel (or left main) coronary artery disease EXCEPT:

A. Early onset of ST-segment depression
B. Persistence of ST-segment changes late into the recovery phase
C. ST-segment elevation in lead aVR
D. Sustained ventricular tachycardia
E. Failure to increase systolic blood pressure by at least 10 mm Hg

QUESTION 49

Which of the following statements regarding the auscultatory findings in aortic stenosis is TRUE?

A. Initial squatting decreases the intensity of the murmur
B. The murmur is increased in intensity during the strain phase of the Valsalva maneuver
C. The murmur would be diminished by inhalation of amyl nitrite
D. In patients with premature ventricular contractions, aortic stenosis can be differentiated from mitral regurgitation because there is beat-to-beat variation in the

intensity of the aortic stenosis murmur while the intensity of the mitral regurgitation remains constant

E. Respiration typically has a prominent effect on the intensity of the murmur

QUESTION 50

A 59-year-old business executive presents because of episodes of retrosternal chest discomfort. It is an aching, burning sensation, occurring most frequently at night, occasionally awakening the patient shortly after he has fallen asleep. It does not occur while walking or climbing stairs. His internist prescribed nitroglycerin, which he has taken infrequently. However, it does relieve his pain, usually within 10 to 20 minutes. The previous day during a luncheon meeting he had a severe episode while presenting a new financial plan; the discomfort seemed to lessen when he sat down and finished lunch. The most likely explanation for his chest discomfort is:

A. Prinzmetal angina

B. Esophageal reflux and spasm

C. Pericarditis

D. Unstable angina pectoris

E. Biliary colic

QUESTION 51

A 44-year-old man with diabetes and a strong family history of premature coronary artery disease underwent cardiac evaluation because of episodes of exertional substernal chest pressure. His resting ECG demonstrated normal sinus rhythm and borderline left ventricular hypertrophy. During exercise myocardial perfusion imaging, he developed his typical chest discomfort and stopped at 03:20 minutes of the standard Bruce protocol, at a peak heart rate of 105 beats/min (60% of his age-predicted maximal heart rate). The systolic blood pressure decreased by 20 mm Hg at peak exercise. Based on the myocardial perfusion images in Figure 1-10, each of the following statements is true EXCEPT:

A. There is evidence of reversible ischemia in the territory of the left anterior descending coronary artery

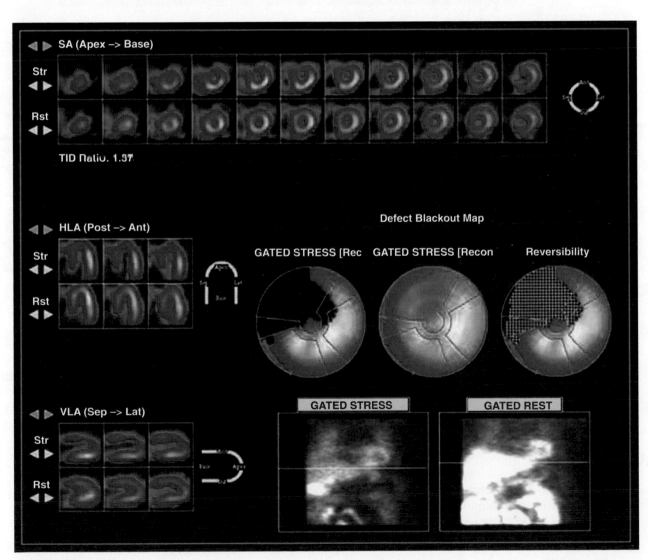

FIGURE 1-10

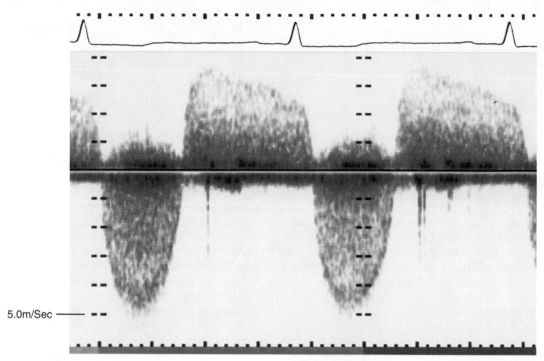

5.0m/Sec

FIGURE 1-11

B. There is transient dilatation of the left ventricle after exercise stress, and this finding is a marker of extensive and severe coronary artery disease
C. The increased lung uptake of the radiotracer evident on stress imaging is indicative of elevated left ventricular filling pressure
D. There is increased right ventricular tracer uptake on the post-stress images, which is a specific marker of multivessel or left main coronary disease
E. The test results are inconclusive owing to failure to achieve the target heart rate

QUESTION 52

Which of the following statements about the transaortic valve Doppler flow tracing shown in Figure 1-11 is TRUE?
A. The probability of critical aortic stenosis in this patient is very low
B. The estimated peak transaortic valvular gradient is 90 to 100 mm Hg
C. Aortic insufficiency is severe
D. Based on the Doppler findings, premature closure of the mitral valve is likely
E. The echocardiogram likely reveals normal left ventricular wall thickness

QUESTION 53

Each of the following statements regarding abnormalities of the extremities in cardiac conditions is true EXCEPT:
A. Arachnodactyly is associated with Marfan syndrome
B. A thumb with an extra phalanx commonly occurs in Turner syndrome
C. Quincke sign is typical of chronic aortic regurgitation

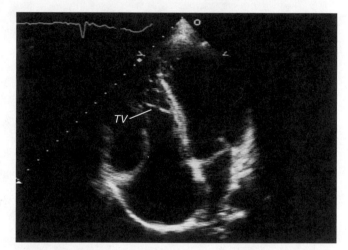

FIGURE 1-12 From De Freitas RAO, Marx GR, Landzberg MJ: In St. John Sutton MG, Rutherford JD (eds): Clinical Cardiovascular Imaging. Philadelphia, Elsevier, 2004, p 387.

D. Osler nodes are tender, erythematous lesions of the fingers and toes in patients with infective endocarditis
E. Differential cyanosis is typical of patent ductus arteriosus with a reversed shunt

QUESTION 54

Each of the following is commonly associated with the disorder illustrated in Figure 1-12 EXCEPT:
A. Tricuspid regurgitation
B. Patent foramen ovale
C. Wolff-Parkinson-White syndrome
D. Systemic hypertension
E. Atrial fibrillation

QUESTION 55

Which of the following statements is TRUE regarding the echocardiographic evaluation of suspected infective endocarditis?
A. After successful antibiotic therapy, previously detected vegetations should not be visible by echocardiography
B. Bacterial vegetations are most commonly located on the downstream, lower-pressure side of a valve
C. Serial echocardiograms should be obtained during antibiotic therapy, even if clinical improvement is evident
D. Functional and structural consequences of valvular infection are rarely observed by transthoracic echocardiographic evaluation, such that a transesophageal study is always mandatory
E. When endocarditis is suspected, the absence of vegetations on a transthoracic echocardiogram is reassuring and should turn the diagnostic evaluation elsewhere

QUESTION 56

Which of the following statements is TRUE regarding examination of the arterial pulse?
A. A reduced-volume brachial pulse with a late systolic peak is the most characteristic arterial finding on physical examination in patients with severe aortic stenosis
B. A bisferious pulse is characterized by a systolic and then a diastolic peak and is typical of mixed mitral valve disease
C. The carotid artery is the blood vessel used to best appreciate the contour, volume, and consistency of the peripheral vessels
D. In coarctation of the aorta, the femoral pulse demonstrates a later peak than the brachial pulse
E. The abdominal aorta is normally palpable both above and below the umbilicus

QUESTION 57

Each of the following statements regarding cardiac catheterization is true EXCEPT:
A. The risk of retroperitoneal hemorrhage is decreased when the femoral artery puncture is made below the inguinal ligament
B. Protamine can be administered to reverse the anticoagulation effect of unfractionated heparin
C. A history of shellfish allergy predisposes to reactions to contrast media
D. Pseudoaneurysm formation is more likely to occur if the femoral artery puncture is made below the bifurcation of the common femoral artery
E. Coronary arteriography was first performed in 1959

QUESTION 58

Which of the following statements regarding the use of cardiopulmonary exercise testing in patients with congestive heart failure is TRUE?

A. A peak oxygen consumption <14 mL/kg/min identifies patients who would benefit from cardiac transplantation
B. Patients with ejection fractions <20% consistently have peak oxygen consumptions <10 mL/kg/min, and exercise testing is of little utility in this population
C. The exercise limitation in severe heart failure is due primarily to an inability to raise the heart rate
D. Exercise training in congestive heart failure patients improves functional capacity but has no effect on abnormalities of autonomic and ventilatory responsiveness or increased lactate production
E. Results of exercise testing are rarely useful when making clinical decisions about heart failure patients, such as timing of cardiac transplantation

QUESTION 59

Magnetic resonance imaging is a superior imaging modality in the assessment of each of the following clinical scenarios EXCEPT:
A. Diagnosis of iron overload cardiomyopathy in a pediatric patient with beta-thalassemia major and congestive heart failure
B. Diagnosis of arrhythmogenic right ventricular cardiomyopathy in a 24-year-old man who recently survived a cardiac arrest
C. Diagnosis of aortic coarctation in a 17-year-old girl with hypertension and radial-femoral artery delay on physical examination
D. Serial evaluation of left ventricular function in a 54-year-old woman with metastatic breast cancer receiving doxorubicin chemotherapy
E. Diagnosis of renal artery stenosis in a 78-year-old man with chronic renal insufficiency and refractory hypertension

QUESTION 60

A 45-year-old man with a history of recurrent supraventricular tachycardia was recently found to have oral squamous cell carcinoma. He underwent chest magnetic resonance imaging as part of the evaluation for intrathoracic metastases. That study identified a cardiac abnormality, and a representative image is shown in Figure 1-13. Which of the following is the most likely diagnosis?
A. Cardiac amyloidosis
B. Pericardial tumor
C. Right atrial myxoma
D. Lipomatous hypertrophy of the interatrial septum and right atrial wall
E. Metastatic squamous cell carcinoma

QUESTION 61

Each of the following statements concerning the echocardiographic findings in hypertrophic cardiomyopathy (HCM) is true EXCEPT:

A. The presence of systolic anterior motion of the mitral valve is consistent with dynamic outflow tract obstruction

B. Systolic notching of the aortic valve on M-mode examination is typical in patients with outflow tract obstruction

C. Cardiac magnetic resonance imaging is greatly superior to echocardiography in identifying the presence of asymmetric septal hypertrophy

D. Normal septal thickness can be present in patients with HCM

E. Myocardial relaxation velocities measured by tissue Doppler imaging are typically reduced

QUESTION 62

Each of the following statements regarding cardiac hemodynamics is true EXCEPT:

A. The x descent of the right atrial pressure waveform represents relaxation of the atrium and downward pulling of the tricuspid annulus by right ventricular contraction

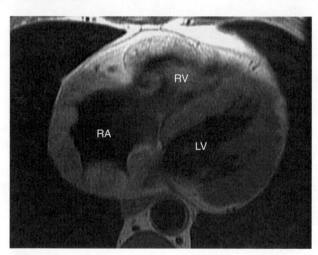

FIGURE 1-13

B. In the left atrium, in contrast to the right atrium, the v wave is more prominent than the a wave

C. A prominent y descent is typical of constrictive pericarditis

D. Atrial ischemia can result in blunting of the x descent

E. Tricuspid stenosis results in a prominent y descent

QUESTION 63

Which of the following statements regarding the effects of maneuvers on the auscultation of cardiac murmurs is TRUE?

A. In patent ductus arteriosus, the diastolic phase of the murmur is softened by isometric handgrip

B. The murmur of hypertrophic obstructive cardiomyopathy becomes softer with standing or during a Valsalva strain maneuver

C. The murmur of a ventricular septal defect decreases with isometric handgrip

D. Isometric handgrip decreases the diastolic murmur of aortic regurgitation

E. The diastolic murmur of mitral stenosis becomes louder with exercise

QUESTION 64

A 62-year-old previously healthy man is brought to the emergency department because of severe headache and dizziness. He has no chest pain or dyspnea. He takes no medications. His blood pressure is 186/98 mm Hg; his heart rate is 56 beats/min and regular. The presenting ECG is shown in Figure 1-14. Which of the following actions is appropriate?

A. Initiate antiplatelet therapy with aspirin and clopidogrel

B. Initiate antithrombotic therapy with heparin

C. Initiate anti-ischemic therapy with intravenous nitroglycerin and a beta blocker

D. Obtain a head computed tomographic scan

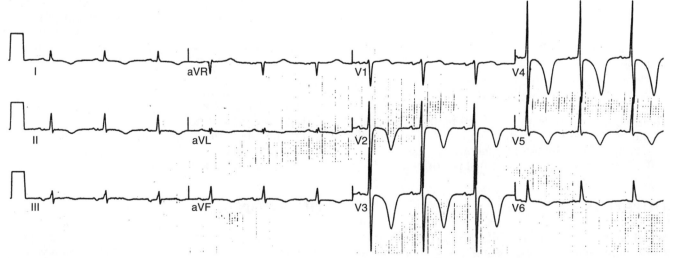

FIGURE 1-14

E. Proceed directly to cardiac catheterization if ST-segment/T wave abnormalities fail to quickly normalize with anti-ischemic therapy

QUESTION 65

Each of the following statements about diastolic murmurs is true EXCEPT:
A. Diastolic murmurs are classified according to their time of onset as early diastolic, mid-diastolic, or late diastolic
B. In aortic regurgitation due to aortic root dilatation, the murmur typically radiates to the right sternal border
C. It is possible to differentiate the murmur of acute severe aortic regurgitation from that of chronic aortic regurgitation at the bedside
D. Late diastolic (presystolic) accentuation of the murmur indicates that the patient is in atrial fibrillation
E. The Graham Steell murmur begins in early diastole after a loud P_2

QUESTION 66

Each of the following statements regarding coronary artery anatomy is true EXCEPT:
A. At cardiac catheterization, the left main coronary artery is best visualized in the anteroposterior projection with slight caudal angulation
B. A ramus intermedius branch is present in more than 25% of people
C. The left circumflex artery is the dominant vessel in 45% of people
D. The most densely vascularized area of the heart is the interventricular septum
E. The abnormality shown in Figure 1-15 is the most common type of coronary congenital abnormality that is hemodynamically significant

QUESTION 67

Each of the following statements regarding continuous murmurs is true EXCEPT:
A. Continuous murmurs and holosystolic murmurs are synonymous
B. By definition, a continuous murmur must continue without interruption through S_2
C. Patent ductus arteriosus causes a continuous murmur
D. A continuous cervical venous hum is commonly found in healthy children
E. Arterial continuous murmurs occur in both constricted and nonconstricted arteries

QUESTION 68

Which one of the following echocardiographic findings suggests that aortic regurgitation is severe?
A. Diastolic flow reversal in the descending thoracic aorta
B. Premature closure of the aortic valve
C. Pressure half-time of the aortic regurgitation Doppler spectrum of 500 milliseconds
D. A color Doppler regurgitant jet that extends to the tips of the papillary muscles
E. The left ventricular outflow tract systolic gradient is 64 mm Hg

QUESTION 69

Each of the following statements regarding pharmacologic agents used in myocardial perfusion stress testing is true EXCEPT:
A. Patients who cannot perform exercise can be adequately evaluated for coronary artery disease (CAD) using vasodilating medications and nuclear scintigraphy
B. Dipyridamole blocks the cellular uptake of adenosine, an endogenous vasodilator

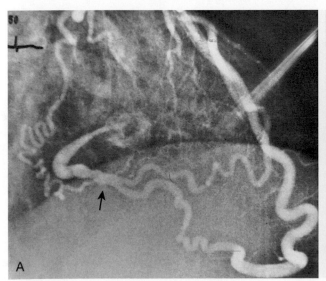
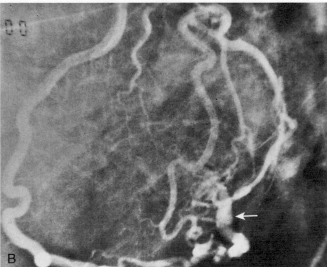

FIGURE 1-15

C. During perfusion stress testing, administration of adenosine or dipyridamole commonly provokes myocardial ischemia in patients with CAD

D. Radiopharmaceutical agents should be injected 1 to 2 minutes before the end of exercise

E. Dobutamine is an alternative pharmacologic agent for stress testing of patients with contraindications to adenosine and dipyridamole

QUESTION 70

Each of the following statements regarding the auscultatory findings of mitral stenosis is correct EXCEPT:

A. The opening snap (OS) is an early diastolic sound

B. A long A_2-OS interval implies severe mitral stenosis

C. In atrial fibrillation, the A_2-OS interval varies with cycle length

D. The "snap" is generated by rapid reversal of the position of the anterior mitral leaflet

E. The presence of an opening snap implies a mobile body of the anterior mitral leaflet

QUESTION 71

True statements about digitalis-induced arrhythmias include all of the following EXCEPT:

A. Ventricular bigeminy with varying morphology and regular coupling is a sign of digitalis toxicity

B. Nonparoxysmal junctional tachycardia is a common digitalis-induced arrhythmia

C. Atrial tachycardia with block is diagnostic of digitalis toxicity

D. The development of atrioventricular dissociation in a patient taking digitalis is a likely indication of digitalis toxicity

E. Ventricular premature beats are common but are not highly specific for the presence of digitalis toxicity

QUESTION 72

An 82-year-old man presents after a recent non–ST-elevation myocardial infarction. Coronary angiography had revealed severe three-vessel disease with 100% occlusion of the proximal left anterior descending (LAD) coronary artery, 100% mid-right coronary artery occlusion, and a 70% stenosis of the proximal left circumflex coronary artery. Echocardiography demonstrated akinesis of the entire anterior wall, septum, and mid- and apical anterolateral wall, with an estimated left ventricular ejection fraction of 20%. Myocardial viability was evaluated using cardiac positron emission tomography (PET) with rest rubidium-82 (^{82}Rb flow tracer) and ^{18}F-labeled fluorodeoxyglucose (^{18}FDG glucose metabolism tracer) as shown in Figure 1-16. The images show a large region of PET perfusion metabolism mismatch in the mid-LAD distribution. Each of the following statements about myocardial viability is true EXCEPT:

A. This finding is consistent with the presence of hibernating (viable) myocardium

B. Radionuclide techniques are more sensitive than measurement of inotropic contractile reserve by dobutamine echocardiography for the detection of viable myocardium

C. Inotropic contractile reserve measured by dobutamine echocardiography is more specific than radionuclide techniques for predicting functional recovery after revascularization

D. Survival benefit associated with revascularization of hibernating myocardium has been demonstrated in randomized clinical trials

E. The transmural extent of myocardial scar can be assessed accurately using gadolinium-enhanced cardiac magnetic resonance imaging

QUESTION 73

Which of the following statements regarding physical findings that distinguish the murmur of aortic stenosis (AS) from the murmur of hypertrophic cardiomyopathy (HCM) is TRUE?

A. The strain phase of the Valsalva maneuver decreases the intensity of the murmurs of both AS and HCM

B. The carotid upstroke in HCM is more brisk than in AS

C. The murmurs of AS and HCM both radiate to the carotid arteries

D. If a systolic thrill is present, it is most often located in the second right intercostal space in HCM and at the apex in AS

E. Squatting increases the intensity of the murmur of HCM

QUESTION 74

A 42-year-old man presents to the emergency department complaining of chest pain. In addition to myocardial ischemia, each of the following is a potential cause of chest discomfort EXCEPT:

A. Esophageal spasm

B. Aortic dissection

C. Herpes zoster

D. Bronchiectasis

E. Costochondritis

QUESTION 75

A 73-year-old woman with exertional angina is referred for a standard Bruce protocol exercise tolerance test with thallium-201 single-photon emission computed tomography. Her nuclear images are shown in the Figure 1-17. What is the likely diagnosis?

A. Dilated cardiomyopathy

B. Single-vessel coronary artery disease involving the left circumflex artery

C. Prior inferior myocardial infarction with high-grade stenosis of the right coronary artery

D. Left main or severe multivessel coronary artery disease

E. Normal coronary arteries; the images demonstrate breast attenuation artifact

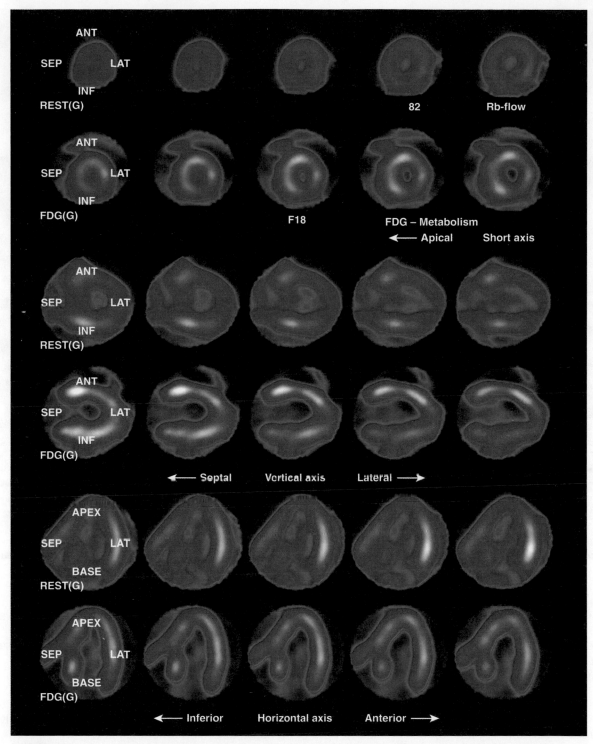

FIGURE 1-16

QUESTION 76

Each of the following statements regarding pulsus alternans in patients with marked LV dysfunction is true EXCEPT:

A. It is usually associated with electrical alternans of the QRS complex
B. It is more readily detected in the femoral as compared with radial arteries
C. It can be detected by sphygmomanometry
D. It can be elicited by the assumption of erect posture
E. It is common for patients with pulsus alternans also to have an S_3 gallop

QUESTION 77

Which of the following statements regarding exercise testing is TRUE?

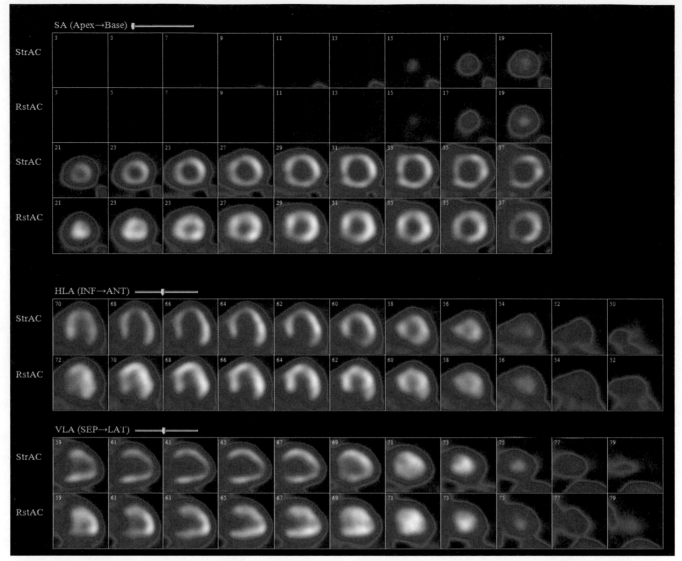

FIGURE 1-17

A. Frequent ventricular ectopy in the early postexercise phase predicts a worse long-term prognosis than ectopy that occurs only during exercise

B. Patients who develop QT interval prolongation during exercise testing are good candidates for Class IA antiarrhythmic drugs

C. The appearance of sustained supraventricular tachycardia during exercise testing is diagnostic of underlying myocardial ischemia

D. Exercise-induced left bundle branch block is not predictive of subsequent cardiac morbidity and mortality

E. Tachyarrhythmias are commonly precipitated during exercise testing in patients with Wolff-Parkinson-White syndrome

QUESTION 78

Each of the following statements regarding systolic ejection sounds is true EXCEPT:

A. Ejection sounds are high-frequency "clicks" that occur early in systole

B. Ejection sounds due to a dilated aortic root have a similar timing as those associated with aortic valvular disease

C. The ejection sound associated with pulmonic stenosis decreases in intensity during inspiration

D. Aortic ejection sounds vary with respiration, occurring later in systole during inspiration

E. The bedside maneuver of standing from a squatting position causes the ejection click of mitral valve prolapse to occur earlier in systole

QUESTION 79

Which of the following statements regarding the ECG in chronic obstructive lung disease with secondary right ventricular hypertrophy is correct?:

A. The mean QRS axis is typically <15 degrees

B. The amplitude of the QRS complex is abnormally high in the precordial leads

C. Even mild right ventricular hypertrophy produces diagnostic electrocardiographic abnormalities

D. A deep S wave in V_6 is typical
E. Precordial lead transition is typically rotated in a counterclockwise fashion (early transition)

QUESTION 80

Each of the following statements regarding shunt detection is true EXCEPT:
A. When a "physiologic" shunt is present, arterial oxygen saturation normalizes with administration of 100% oxygen
B. Methods of shunt detection include oximetry, echocardiography, radionuclide imaging, and magnetic resonance imaging
C. Among the sources of right atrial venous blood, the inferior vena cava has the lowest oxygen saturation
D. Although the sensitivity of oximetry for shunt detection is low, most clinically relevant left-to-right shunts can be detected using this method
E. The Flamm formula is used to estimate mixed venous oxygen saturation

QUESTION 81

Each of the following conditions is often associated with a prominent R wave in electrocardiographic lead V_1 EXCEPT:
A. Right ventricular hypertrophy
B. Wolff-Parkinson-White syndrome
C. Duchenne muscular dystrophy
D. Left anterior fascicular block
E. Misplacement of the chest leads

QUESTION 82

The hemodynamic tracing illustrated in Figure 1-18 is associated with each of the following features EXCEPT:
A. A large systolic pressure gradient between the left ventricular midcavity and aorta
B. A bifid aortic pulse contour
C. Increased ventricular stiffness resulting in an elevated left ventricular end-diastolic pressure
D. A slow and delayed rise in the aortic pressure as compared with that of the left ventricle
E. No clinical improvement with aortic valve replacement

QUESTION 83

Each of the following statements regarding axis positions of the heart and findings on the ECG is correct EXCEPT:
A. A "horizontal" heart results in a tall R wave in lead aVL
B. "Clockwise rotation" refers to a delayed transition zone in the precordial leads
C. In patients with a "vertical" heart, the QRS complex is isoelectric in lead I
D. "Counterclockwise rotation" mimics left ventricular hypertrophy

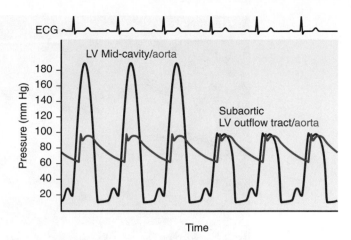

FIGURE 1-18 From Doshi SN, Kim MC, Sharma SK, et al: Images in cardiovascular medicine: Circulation 106:E3, 2002. Copyright 2002, American Heart Association.

E. When all six limb leads show isoelectric complexes, it is not possible to calculate the axis in the frontal plane

QUESTION 84

Which of the following statements concerning the cardiac catheterization laboratory evaluation of valve orifice areas is TRUE?
A. Valve area as calculated by the Gorlin formula is inversely proportional to the flow across the valve
B. The presence of valvular regurgitation will result in a falsely high calculated valve area because actual flow across the valve is less than the flow calculated from the systemic cardiac output
C. Calculation of mitral valve area typically relies on substitution of a confirmed pulmonary capillary wedge pressure for left atrial pressure
D. Valve area calculation is more strongly influenced by errors in the pressure gradient measurement than by errors in cardiac output measurement

QUESTION 85

A 56-year-old man who underwent coronary artery bypass graft surgery 6 years ago has experienced exertional chest discomfort in recent months. He is not able to perform an exercise test because of chronic hip pain. He undergoes an adenosine PET vasodilator stress test, images from which are shown in Figure 1-19. What is the correct interpretation of this study?
A. No perfusion defects
B. A partially reversible defect of the entire inferior wall
C. A severe predominantly reversible defect of the anterior wall
D. A fixed defect of the anterior wall without reversibility
E. Fixed defects of the apex and lateral walls

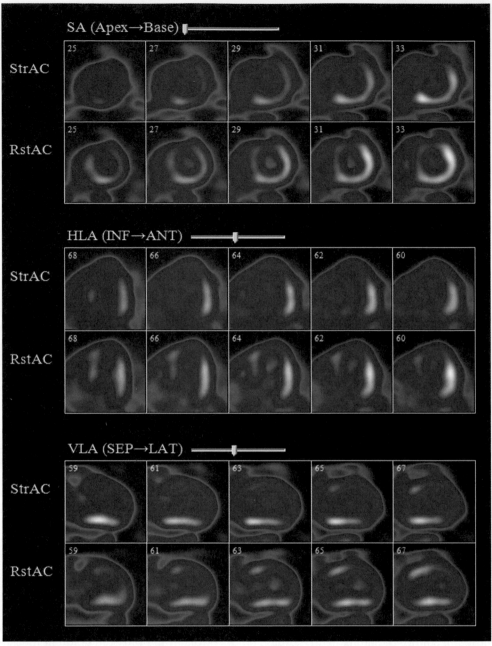

FIGURE 1-19

QUESTION 86

A 40-year-old man presents to the office with shortness of breath on exertion, peripheral edema, and arthritis of his hands. On examination, his vital signs are normal. His sclerae are icteric and his skin has a bronzed hue. Lung examination demonstrates rales at the bases; the carotids are of normal upstroke. The cardiac impulse is displaced laterally and there is an audible S_3. His abdomen is distended, with evidence of hepatospleno-megaly and ascites. There is peripheral pitting edema. Laboratory studies reveal a serum glucose level of 225 mg/dL and a transferrin saturation of 70%. Which of the following statements about this condition is TRUE?

A. It is inherited as an autosomal dominant condition
B. Cardiac involvement results in a mixed dilated and restrictive cardiomyopathy
C. Early cardiac death is common, due primarily to accelerated atherosclerosis
D. Ventricular hypertrophy with increased QRS voltages is the most common electrocardiographic finding
E. Echocardiography often shows a thickened ventricle with a "granular sparkling" appearance

QUESTION 87

A 56-year-old woman presents for routine evaluation. On examination, a systolic murmur is noted. Which of the following responses to maneuvers would be suggestive of mitral valve prolapse as the cause of the murmur?

A. With isometric handgrip, the murmur starts earlier in systole and becomes louder
B. With standing from a supine position, the murmur begins later in systole
C. Carotid sinus massage increases the intensity of the murmur
D. Valsalva maneuver causes the murmur to arise earlier in systole
E. Squatting from a standing position moves the onset of the murmur earlier in systole

QUESTION 88

Which of the following statements regarding the effect of the potassium concentration on the ECG is TRUE?

A. The earliest electrocardiographic sign of hyperkalemia is a reduction in P wave amplitude
B. Deep symmetric T wave inversions are characteristic of early hyperkalemia
C. Hyperkalemia predisposes to digitalis-induced tachyarrhythmias
D. Prominent U waves are a characteristic feature of hyperkalemia
E. QRS complex widening is common in severe hyperkalemia

QUESTION 89

Each of the following conditions can result in significant electrocardiographic Q waves in the absence of infarction EXCEPT:

A. Left bundle branch block
B. Left ventricular dilatation with posterior rotation of the heart
C. Electrocardiographic lead misplacement
D. Acidosis
E. Wolff-Parkinson-White syndrome

QUESTION 90

Each of the following statements regarding the interpretation of exercise electrocardiography is true EXCEPT:

A. The presence of right bundle branch block decreases the sensitivity of exercise electrocardiography for the diagnosis of myocardial ischemia
B. ST-segment depressions in the inferior leads during exercise testing are specific for significant right coronary artery disease
C. The location of ST-segment elevations during exercise testing predicts the anatomic site of clinically advanced coronary stenosis
D. Features that predict high-risk coronary disease include 2-mm ST-segment depressions during exercise or ST-segment depressions that persist >5 minutes during the recovery phase
E. Digoxin therapy is associated with false-positive findings of exercise electrocardiography even if the baseline ST segments are normal

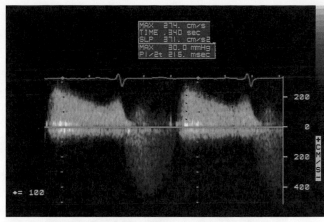

FIGURE 1-20

QUESTION 91

A patient underwent echocardiography as part of the evaluation of exertional dyspnea. Figure 1-20 displays an image from the continuous-wave Doppler interrogation across the mitral valve, obtained from the apical long-axis view. Each of the statements below is true EXCEPT:

A. The early diastolic peak velocity of 2.7 m/sec is within the normal range
B. There is an abnormally delayed decline of the transmitral velocity signal during diastole
C. Significant mitral stenosis is present
D. Abnormal transmitral systolic blood flow is demonstrated
E. With color Doppler imaging, the extent of mitral regurgitation can be underestimated if the regurgitant jet is directed along the left atrial wall

QUESTION 92

A 25-year-old asymptomatic man presents for routine physical examination with his new primary care physician. The physician notes that the patient is tall with unusually long limbs and pectus excavatum. There is no known family history of Marfan syndrome. Which of the following is among the "major criteria" for the diagnosis of Marfan syndrome?

A. Mitral valve prolapse
B. Mild pectus excavatum
C. Joint hypermobility
D. Descending aortic aneurysm
E. Ectopia lentis

QUESTION 93

A 25-year-old man died suddenly while jogging, and a postmortem examination was performed. A histologic section of left ventricular myocardium is shown in Figure 1-21. Which of the following statements is TRUE?

A. The histologic findings are of normal myocardium subjected to chronic vigorous exercise
B. This condition is inherited as an autosomal dominant trait
C. This is a disease of plasma membrane protein synthesis

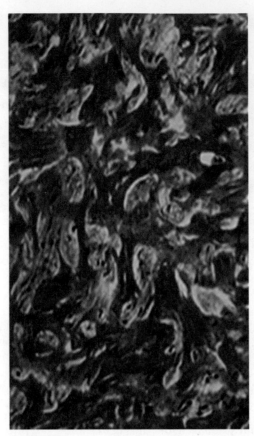

FIGURE 1-21

D. The greatest risk to affected patients is the development of complete heart block
E. One specific mutation has been identified that accurately predicts sudden cardiac death in the majority of patients with this disorder

QUESTION 94

A 28-year-old woman presents for evaluation after a syncopal episode. Her family history is notable for sudden death in an older sibling. Physical examination reveals woolly hair and palmar keratosis. Electrocardiography demonstrates T wave inversions in leads V_1 to V_3. An ambulatory (Holter) electrocardiographic monitor captures runs of ventricular tachycardia with a left bundle morphology and superior axis. A signal-averaged ECG demonstrates late potentials. Echocardiography demonstrates a mildly dilated right ventricle with reduced systolic function; the left ventricle appears structurally normal. Which of the following statements is TRUE about this condition?
A. The majority of patients with this disorder have an abnormality of the ryanodine receptor
B. Endomyocardial biopsy establishes the diagnosis with high sensitivity
C. This patient likely has a mutation in the plakoglobin gene
D. This condition is transmitted in an autosomal dominant fashion
E. Noncaseating granulomas are likely present in the right ventricular myocardium

QUESTION 95

Each of the following statements regarding mitochondrial chromosomal disorders is correct EXCEPT:
A. MELAS (mitochondrial myopathy, encephalopathy, lactic acidosis, and stroke-like episodes), the most common of the mitochondrial inherited disorders, is associated with both hypertrophic and dilated cardiomyopathies
B. Males are affected more frequently than females
C. Only maternal transmission occurs; offspring of affected men do not inherit these conditions
D. Great variability of phenotypic expression within a family is common
E. All offspring of an affected woman may inherit the condition

DIRECTIONS: Each group of questions below consists of lettered headings followed by a set of numbered questions. For each question, select the ONE lettered heading with which it is most closely associated. Each lettered heading may be used once, more than once, or not at all.

QUESTIONS 96 TO 100

Match each of the following clinical scenarios to the most likely cause of syncope:
A. Ventricular tachycardia
B. High-degree atrioventricular block
C. Epilepsy
D. Neurocardiogenic syncope
E. Hysterical fainting

96. A 73-year-old man with a remote history of myocardial infarction feels the onset of palpitations while driving, then awakens having driven his car into a ditch, unaware of what has transpired
97. A 25-year-old woman on chronic antiseizure medication becomes warm, diaphoretic, and very pale after donating blood, then suffers frank syncope while seated upright in a chair. After being helped to the floor, she awakens embarrassed and alert
98. A 73-year-old woman with recent episodes of dizziness begins to feel lightheaded while seated at church, then within seconds turns pale and slumps to the floor with a few clonic jerks. She regains consciousness 1 minute later, completely aware of where she is and asks what has happened. When an ambulance arrives, her blood pressure is 108/70 mm Hg and the heart rate is 60 beats/min
99. A 32-year-old man with a history of prior syncope notices an odd odor, after which he falls to the ground. He awakens 3 minutes later confused and disoriented and is found to be incontinent of urine
100. An 18-year-old Army recruit falls to the ground while standing at attention for 20 minutes during his first week of basic training. He immediately awakens, feels a bit groggy, but quickly is able to rejoin his squad

QUESTIONS 101 TO 104

For each clinical scenario, select the most likely ECG from the four tracings shown in Figure 1-22:

101. A 19-year-old male college student with exertional lightheadedness and a harsh systolic murmur that intensifies after standing from a squatting position

102. A 56-year-old woman with sudden onset of pleuritic chest discomfort and dyspnea

103. A 36-year-old man with sharp inspiratory precordial chest discomfort that radiates to the left shoulder

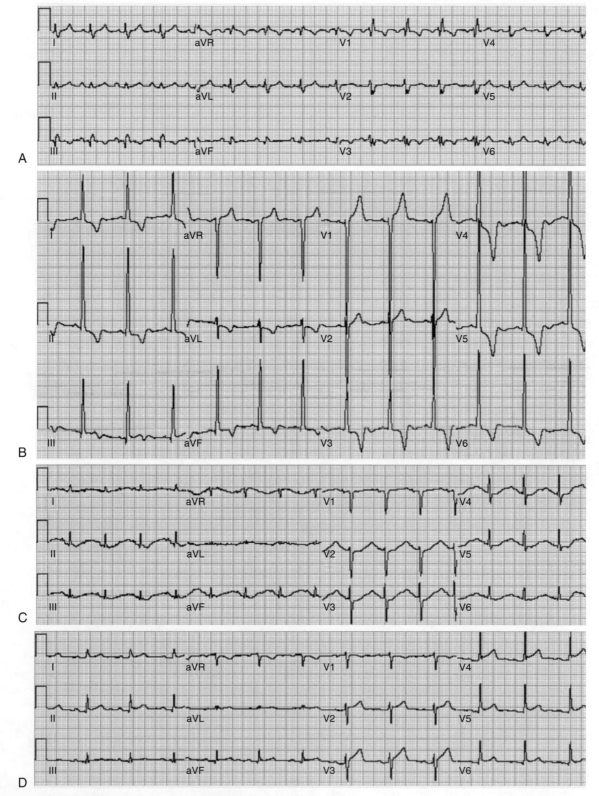

FIGURE 1-22

104. A 71-year-old alcoholic man with epigastric discomfort after 18 hours of intermittent vomiting

QUESTIONS 105 TO 109

Match the most appropriate descriptive phrase to each angiogram shown in Figure 1-23:

105. Right anterior oblique (RAO) projection: left anterior descending (LAD) artery, demonstrating myocardial bridging with narrowing in systole and near-normal caliber in diastole

106. Left anterior oblique (LAO) projection: right coronary arteriogram demonstrating anomalous origin of the left circumflex artery from the right coronary sinus

107. Collateral vessels arising from the distal RCA and supplying an occluded LAD artery

108. Right coronary arteriogram demonstrating diffuse coronary spasm and restoration of normal caliber with introduction of nitroglycerin

109. A dilated left circumflex artery and subsequent coronary sinus opacification due to a congenital coronary fistula

QUESTIONS 110 TO 113

For each clinical scenario, match the most likely computed tomogram in Figure 1-24:

110. A 53-year-old woman with exertional dyspnea, recurrent transient ischemic attacks, lightheadedness

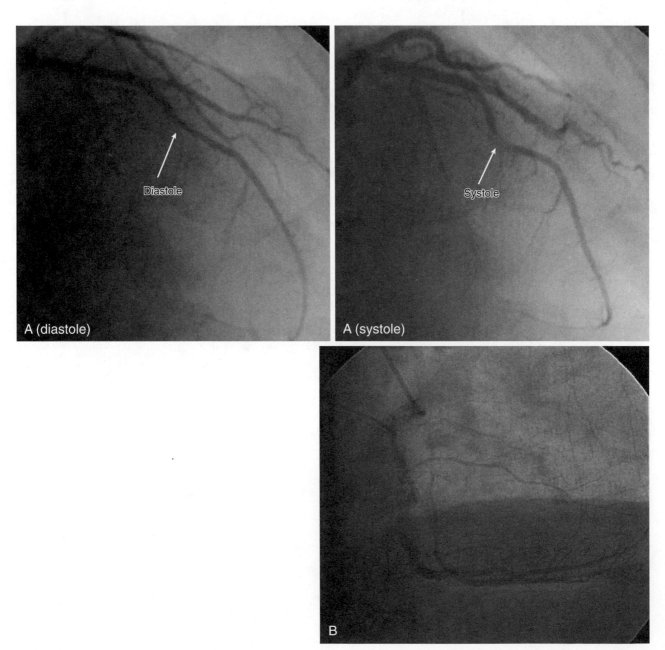

FIGURE 1-23

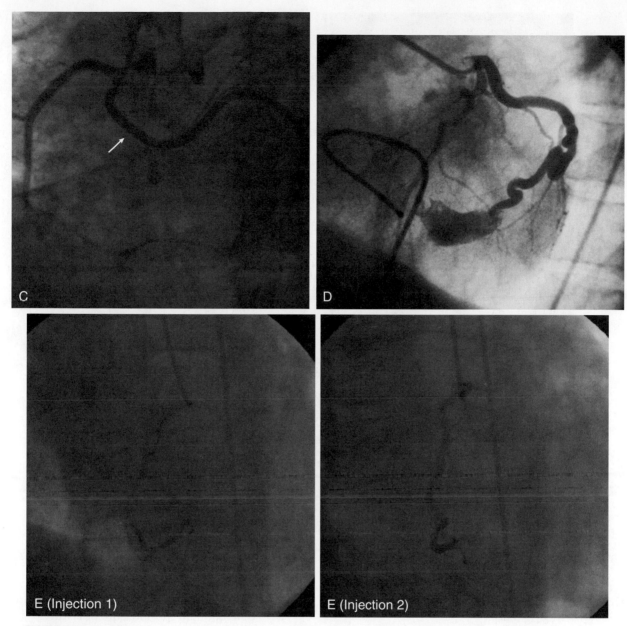

FIGURE 1-23, cont'd

with sudden changes in position, and a 15-pound weight loss over the past 6 months

111. A 21-year-old man with recurrent syncope
112. A 69-year-old woman with recent myocardial infarction and subsequent stroke
113. A 71-year-old man with jugular venous distention, ascites, and marked peripheral edema

QUESTIONS 114 TO 117

For each condition, match the appropriate pattern of left ventricular (LV) filling as recorded by Doppler of diastolic mitral flow velocities (E wave = early diastolic filling; A wave = period of atrial contraction; normal LV deceleration time in early diastole is >190 milliseconds):

A. E wave > A wave, LV deceleration time >190 milliseconds
B. E wave > A wave, LV deceleration time <190 milliseconds
C. E wave < A wave, LV deceleration time >200 milliseconds
D. E wave >> A wave, LV deceleration time <150 milliseconds

114. Restrictive cardiomyopathy
115. Normal pattern
116. Pseudonormalized pattern
117. Impaired LV diastolic relaxation

QUESTIONS 118 TO 121

For each of the chest radiographs shown in Figure 1-25, match the most appropriate cardiac diagnosis:

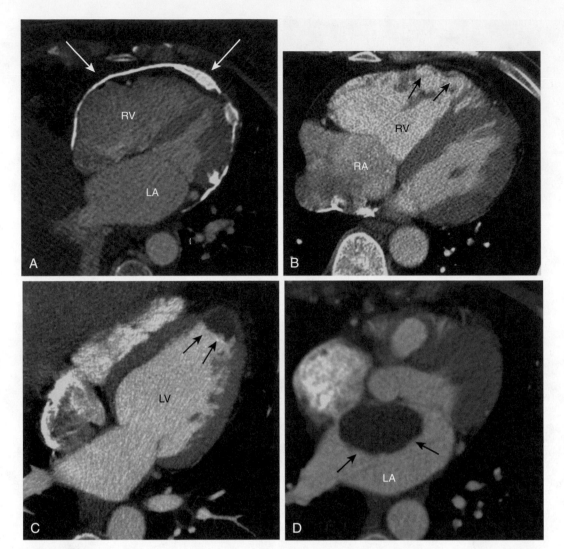

FIGURE 1-24

118. Mitral stenosis
119. Aortic regurgitation
120. Atrial septal defect
121. Pericardial effusion

QUESTIONS 122 TO 125

Match each description below to the most appropriate cardiac rhythm:
A. Atrial tachycardia
B. Atrial flutter
C. Sinus rhythm
D. Atrioventricular nodal reentrant tachycardia
E. Atrial fibrillation

122. P waves are negative in lead aVR and upright in leads I, II, and aVF
123. Rhythm can be due to automaticity, reentry, or triggered mechanisms
124. Macroreentrant mechanism in the right atrium

125. The initial P wave of the tachycardia is usually different than the subsequent P waves

QUESTIONS 126 TO 129

For the receiver-operating curve (ROC) for two diagnostic tests shown in Figure 1-26, please match the following:
A. 11%
B. 40%
C. 59%
D. 47%
E. Test A
F. Test B

126. The false-positive rate of Test A at a sensitivity of 98%
127. The sensitivity of Test A at a specificity of 98%
128. The positive predictive value of Test A with a sensitivity of 98%, for a population with disease prevalence of 50/1000.
129. The superior screening test

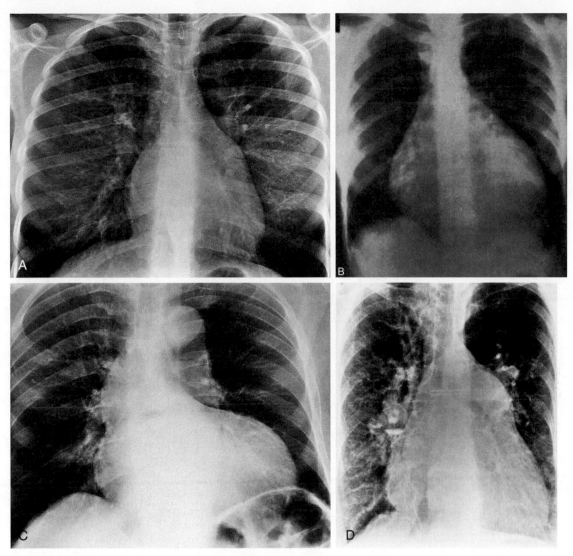

FIGURE 1-25 **A, C,** and **D** from Miller SW: Cardiac Imaging: The Requisites. 2nd ed. Philadelphia, Elsevier, 2005. **B,** from Daves ML: Cardiac Roentgenology. Chicago, Year Book Publishers, 1981, p 470.

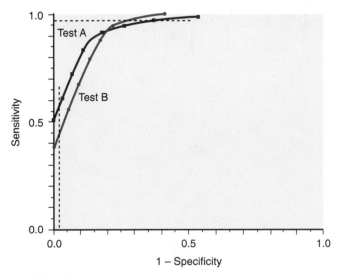

FIGURE 1-26 From McPherson RA, Pincus MR (eds): Henry's Clinical Diagnosis and Management by Laboratory Methods. 21st ed. Philadelphia, Elsevier, 2006, p 73.

QUESTIONS 130 TO 133

For each clinical scenario, select the appropriate ECG from those provided in Figure 1-27:

130. A 49-year-old man with chronic renal failure and progressive fatigue
131. A 37-year-old man with a recent viral syndrome and sharp anterior chest pain that worsens when he changes position
132. A 59-year-old man with severe lightheadedness
133. A 38-year-old woman with perioral and peripheral cyanosis, digital clubbing, and a history of cardiac surgery as a child

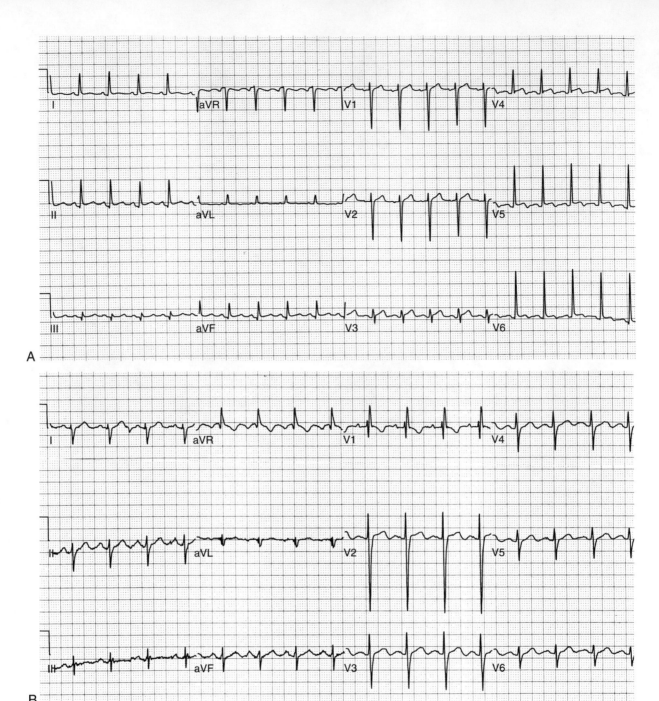

FIGURE 1-27

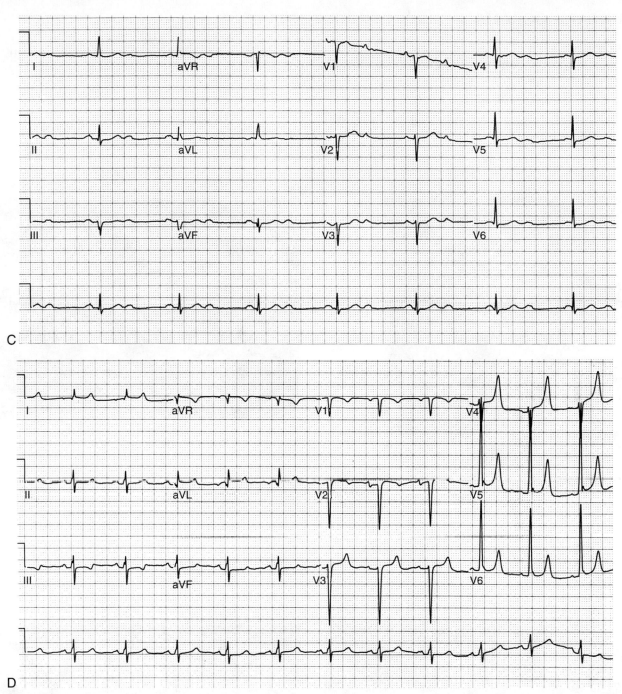

C

D

FIGURE 1-27, cont'd

ECHOCARDIOGRAMS

DIRECTIONS: Each of the still-frame echocardiographic images below is introduced by a brief clinical scenario. For each image, comment on the major abnormal findings:

134. A 62-year-old man who sustained a myocardial infarction 1 month ago (Fig. 1-28)

135. A 33-year-old woman with an early systolic click (Fig. 1-29)

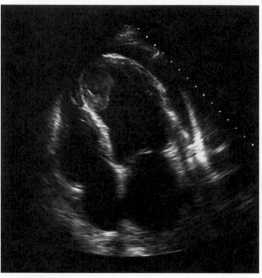

FIGURE 1-28

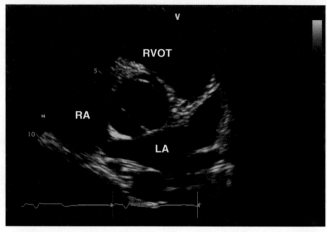

FIGURE 1-29

136. A 26-year-old man with a loud asymptomatic systolic murmur (Fig. 1-30)

137. A tall, thin 31-year-old woman with a diastolic murmur (Fig. 1-31)

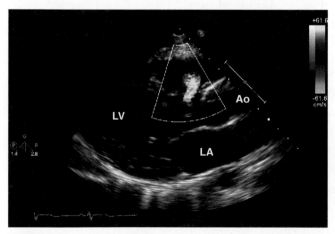

FIGURE 1-30

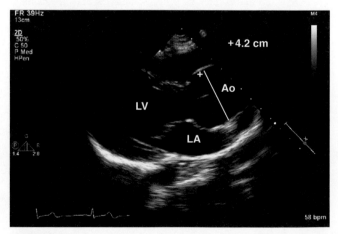

FIGURE 1-31

138. A 59-year-old woman with a systolic murmur
    (Fig. 1-32)

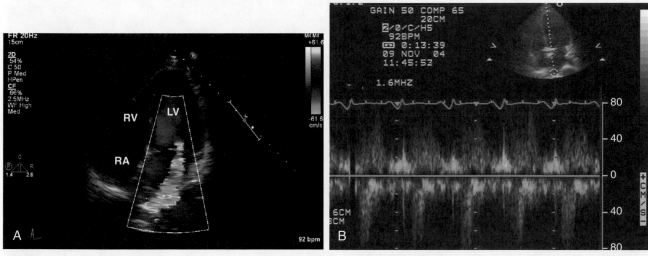

FIGURE 1-32

139. Doppler tissue imaging in a 54-year-old man with
    multiple myeloma, exertional dyspnea, and periph-
    eral edema (Fig. 1-33)

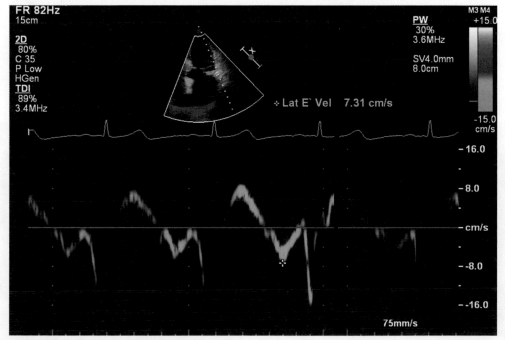

FIGURE 1-33

140. A 44-year-old woman with an acute stroke (Fig. 1-34)

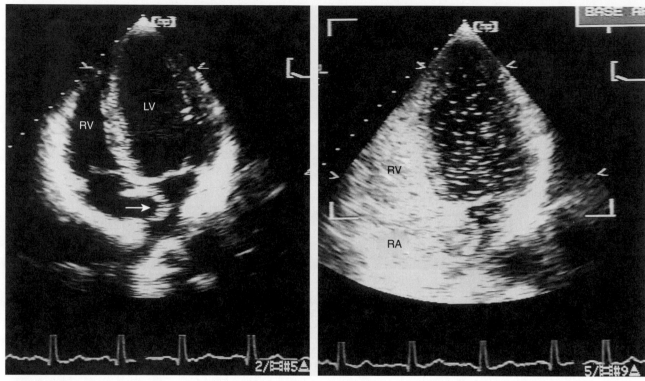

FIGURE 1-34

141. A 78-year-old woman with atrial fibrillation (Fig. 1-35)

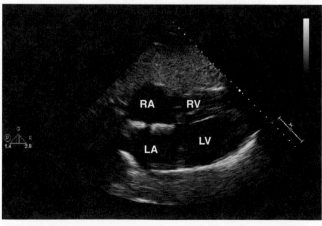

FIGURE 1-35

142. A 66-year-old man with dyspnea (Fig. 1-36)

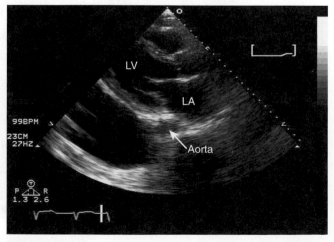

FIGURE 1-36

ELECTROCARDIOGRAMS

DIRECTIONS: Each of the 12-lead ECGs below is introduced by a brief clinical description of the patient. For each ECG, perform a systematic reading. Consider the rhythm, rate, axis, and intervals and whether atrioventricular conduction disturbances are present. Then determine if criteria are met for atrial or ventricular hypertrophy, intraventricular conduction disturbances, or prior myocardial infarction. Continue by noting abnormalities of the ST segment and T waves. Conclude by suggesting a clinical diagnosis compatible with each tracing. You may use the electrocardiographic response form and numerical codes on page 46, representative of that used by the American Board of Internal Medicine Certification Examination, as a framework.

143. A 72-year-old man presents to the cardiology clinic with a history of remote chest pain and more recent dyspnea on exertion (Fig. 1-37)

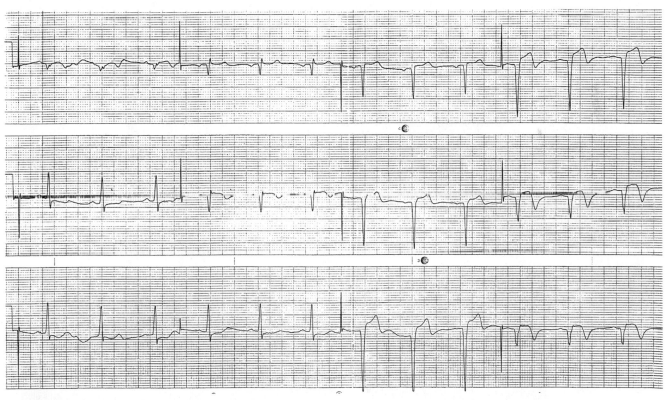

FIGURE 1-37

144. An 86-year-old woman with an extensive history of cigarette smoking presents to the emergency department with shortness of breath (Fig. 1-38)

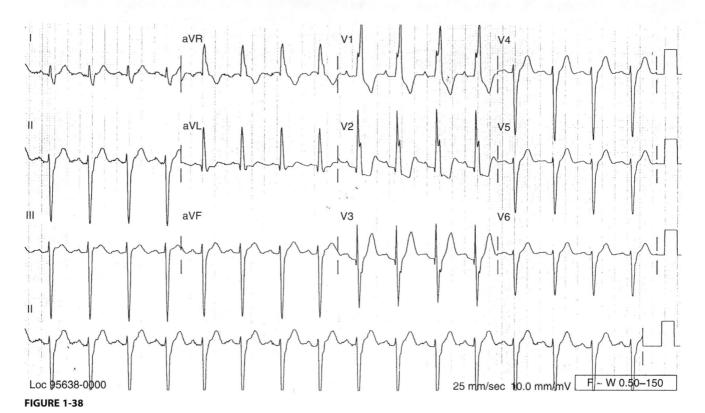

FIGURE 1-38

145. An 18-year-old woman with a history of exertional syncope (Fig. 1-39)

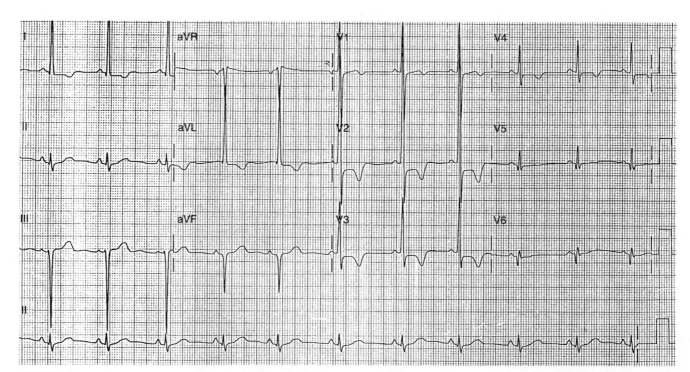

FIGURE 1-39

146. An 85-year-old woman who comes for a routine appointment with her cardiologist (Fig. 1-40)

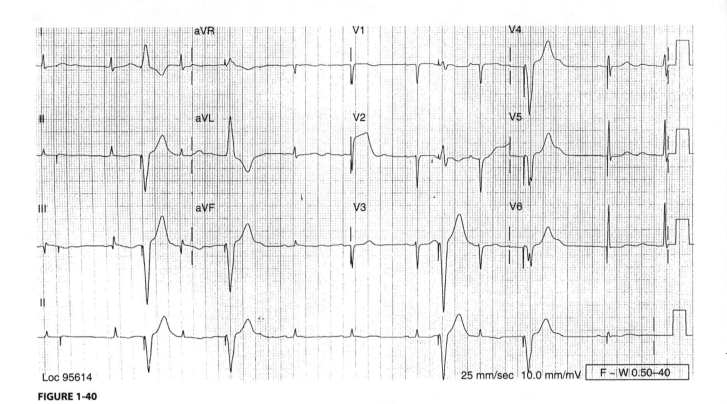

FIGURE 1-40

147. A 15-year-old boy with episodes of palpitations (Fig. 1-41)

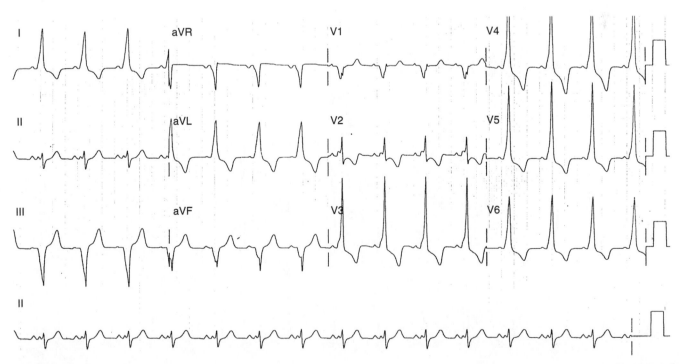

FIGURE 1-41

148. A 63-year-old man with a rapid heart rate (Fig. 1-42)

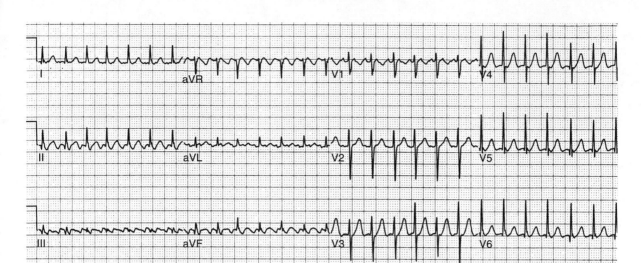

FIGURE 1-42

149. A 35-year-old woman with a history of a heart murmur who presents with shortness of breath (Fig. 1-43)

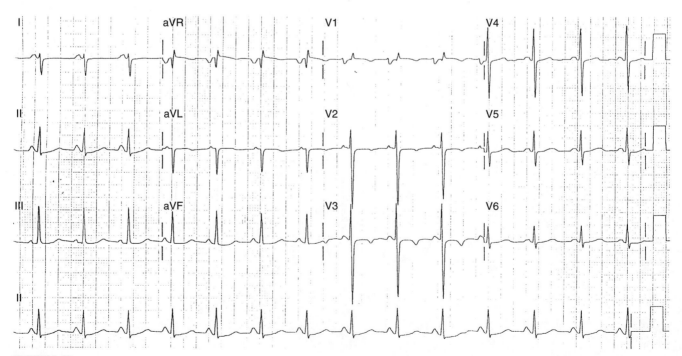

FIGURE 1-43

150. A 21-year-old woman with palpitations and presyncope (Fig. 1-44)

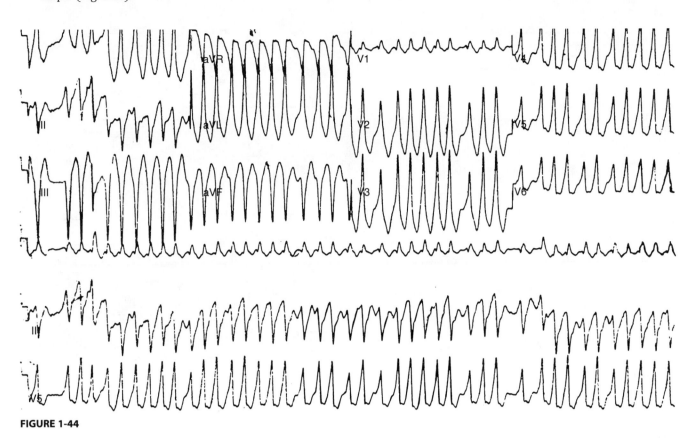

FIGURE 1-44

151. A 48-year-old woman with nausea (Fig. 1-45)

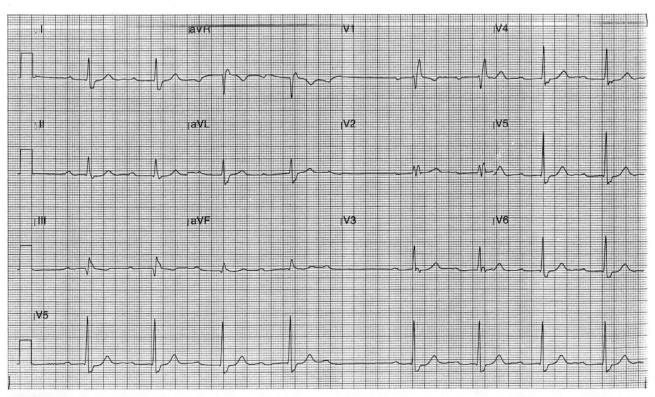

FIGURE 1-45

152. A 75-year-old man with exertional dizziness (Fig. 1-46)

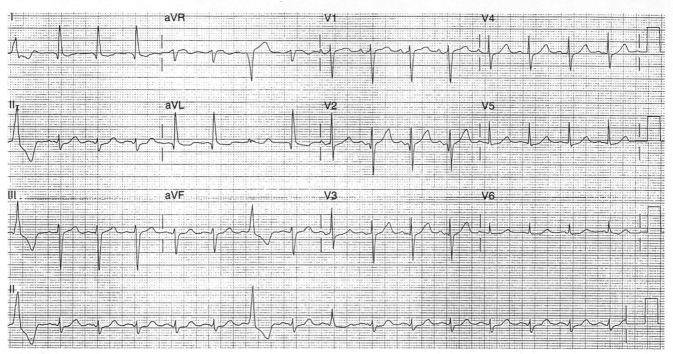

FIGURE 1-46

153. A 43-year-old woman presents to the emergency department with rapid palpitations and lightheadedness (Fig. 1-47)

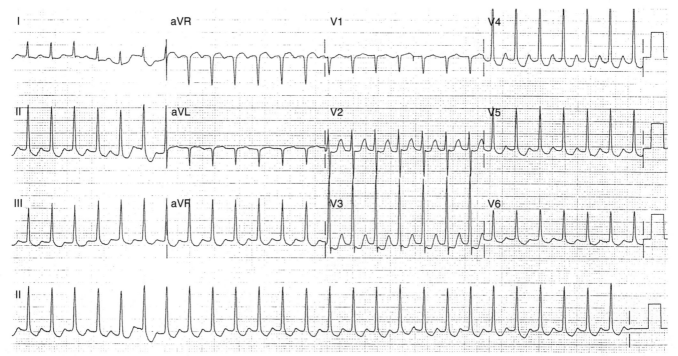

FIGURE 1-47

154. A 74-year-old man with an irregular pulse (Fig. 1-48)

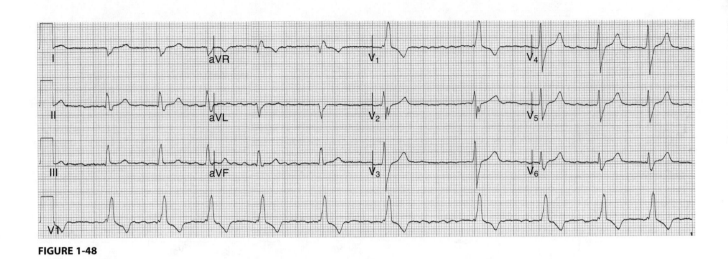

FIGURE 1-48

155. A 28-year-old man presents for a pre-employment physical examination (Fig. 1-49)

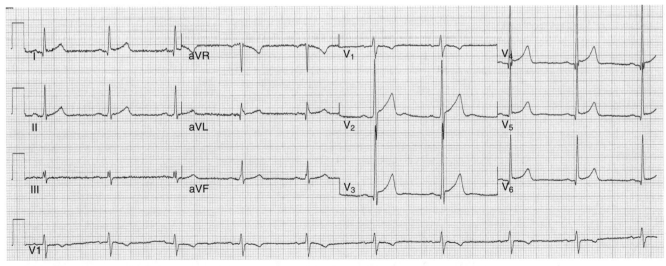

FIGURE 1-49

156. A 66-year-old woman with renal failure, palpitations, and lightheadedness (Fig. 1-50)

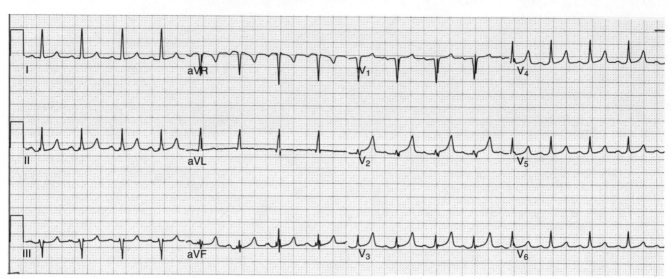

FIGURE 1-50

157. A 68-year-old man with an episode of prolonged chest pain and dyspnea 6 months earlier (Fig. 1-51)

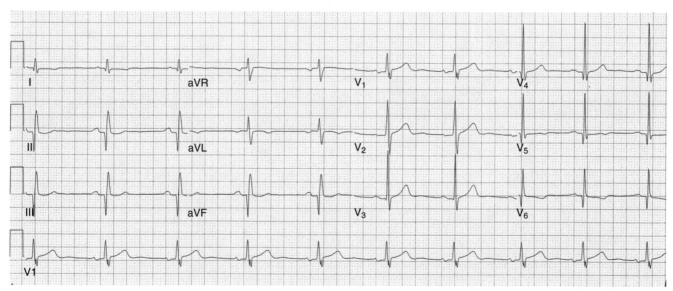

FIGURE 1-51

158. A 54-year-old man with sudden lightheadedness
(Fig. 1-52)

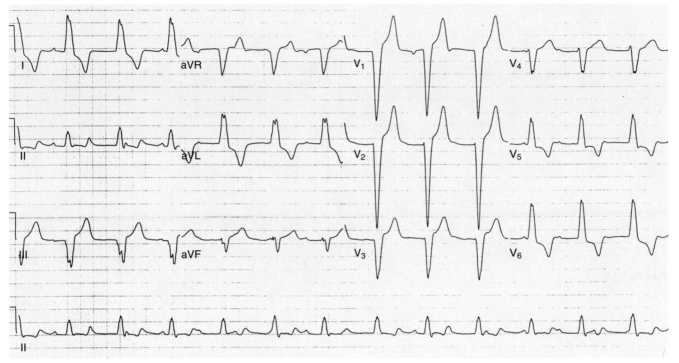

FIGURE 1-52

159. A 64-year-old woman with profound nausea and
diaphoresis (Fig. 1-53)

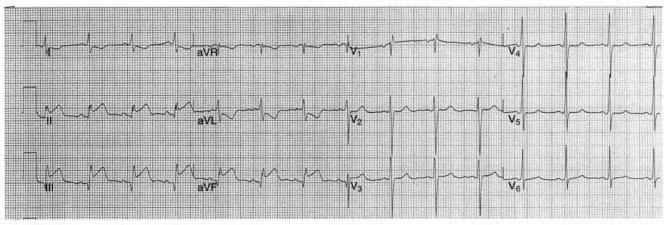

FIGURE 1-53

160. A 55-year-old man with long-standing hypertension (Fig. 1-54)

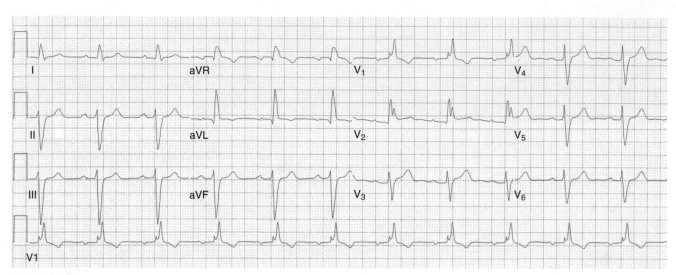

FIGURE 1-54

161. An asymptomatic 36-year-old man presents for an insurance physical examination (Fig. 1-55)

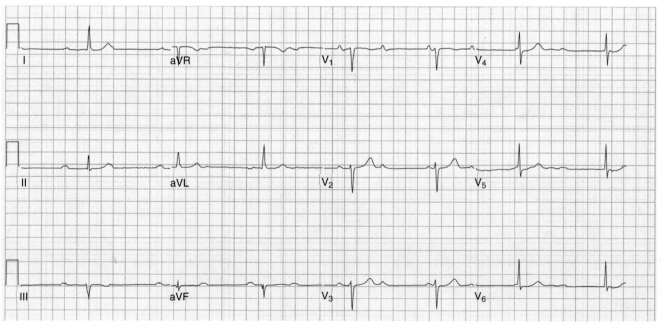

FIGURE 1-55

162. A 23-year-old woman referred to the cardiology
    clinic because of a murmur and abnormal ECG
    (Fig. 1-56)

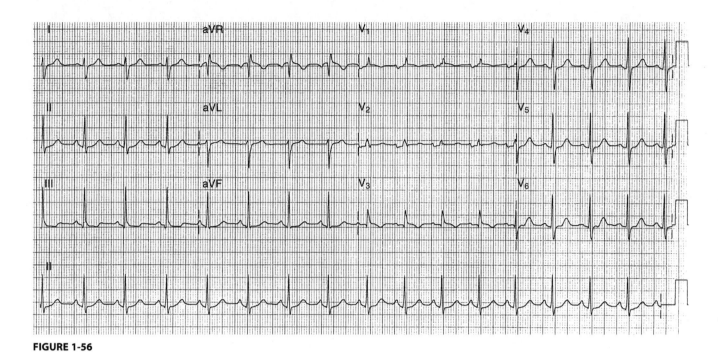

FIGURE 1-56

163. A 51-year-old woman with discrete episodes of pre-
    syncope (Fig. 1-57)

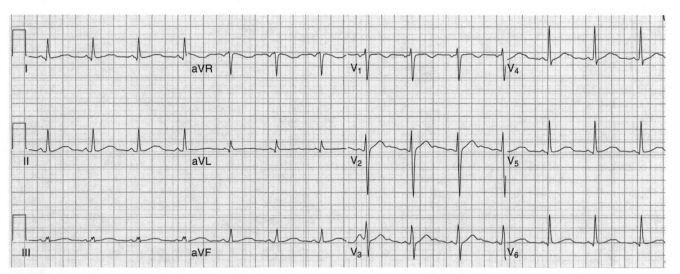

FIGURE 1-57

164. A 72-year-old man with palpitations after coronary artery bypass surgery (Fig. 1-58)

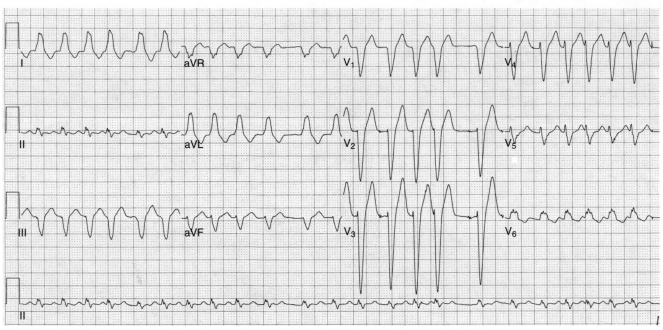

FIGURE 1-58

165. A 71-year-old man who presents to the emergency department with dizziness and shortness of breath (note that this tracing was obtained using right-sided chest leads) (Fig. 1-59)

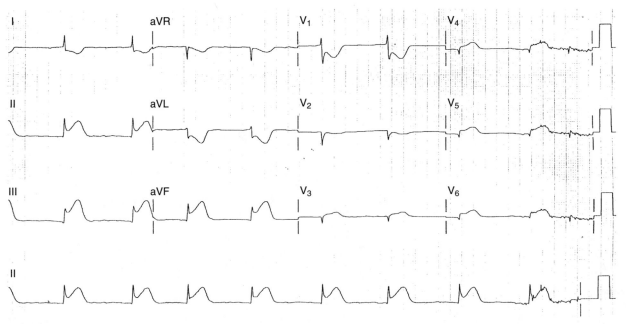

FIGURE 1-59

166. A 38-year-old man with syncope after vigorous physical activity (Fig. 1-60)

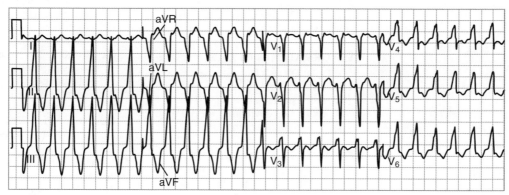

FIGURE 1-60

167. An elderly nursing home resident with occasional dizziness (Fig. 1-61)

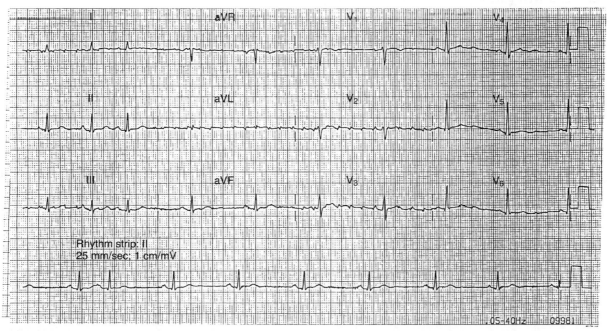

FIGURE 1-61

ECG SCORING SHEET

GENERAL FEATURES

☐ 1. Normal ECG
☐ 2. Borderline normal ECG or normal variant
☐ 3. Incorrect electrode placement
☐ 4. Artifact

P WAVE ABNORMALITIES

☐ 5. Right atrial abnormality/ enlargement
☐ 6. Left atrial abnormality/ enlargement

ATRIAL RHYTHMS

☐ 7. Sinus rhythm
☐ 8. Sinus arrhythmia
☐ 9. Sinus bradycardia (<60)
☐ 10. Sinus tachycardia (>100)
☐ 11. Sinus pause or arrest
☐ 12. Sinoatrial exit block
☐ 13. Atrial premature complexes
☐ 14. Atrial parasystole
☐ 15. Atrial tachycardia
☐ 16. Atrial tachycardia, multifocal
☐ 17. Supraventricular tachycardia
☐ 18. Atrial flutter
☐ 19. Atrial fibrillation

AV JUNCTIONAL RHYTHMS

☐ 20. AV junctional premature complexes
☐ 21. AV junctional escape complexes
☐ 22. AV junctional rhythm/tachycardia

VENTRICULAR RHYTHMS

☐ 23. Ventricular premature complex(es)
☐ 24. Ventricular parasystole
☐ 25. Ventricular tachycardia (3 or more consecutive complexes)
☐ 26. Accelerated idioventricular rhythm
☐ 27. Ventricular escape complexes or rhythm
☐ 28. Ventricular fibrillation

AV CONDUCTION

☐ 29. AV block, 1°
☐ 30. AV block, 2°— Mobitz type I (Wenckebach)
☐ 31. AV block, 2°— Mobitz type II
☐ 32. AV block, 2:1
☐ 33. AV block, 3°
☐ 34. Wolff-Parkinson-White pattern
☐ 35. AV dissociation

ABNORMALITIES OF QRS VOLTAGE OR AXIS

☐ 36. Low voltage
☐ 37. Left axis deviation (> −30°)
☐ 38. Right axis deviation (> +100°)
☐ 39. Electrical alternans

VENTRICULAR HYPERTROPHY

☐ 40. Left ventricular hypertrophy
☐ 41. Right ventricular hypertrophy
☐ 42. Combined ventricular hypertrophy

INTRAVENTRICULAR CONDUCTION

☐ 43. RBBB, complete
☐ 44. RBBB, incomplete
☐ 45. Left anterior fascicular block
☐ 46. Left posterior fascicular block
☐ 47. LBBB, complete
☐ 48. LBBB, incomplete
☐ 49. Intraventricular conduction disturbance, nonspecific type
☐ 50. Functional (rate-related) aberrancy

Q WAVE MYOCARDIAL INFARCTION

	AGE RECENT, OR PROBABLY ACUTE	AGE INDETERMINATE, OR PROBABLY OLD
Anterolateral	☐ 51.	☐ 52.
Anterior or anteroseptal	☐ 53.	☐ 54.
Lateral	☐ 55.	☐ 56.
Inferior	☐ 57.	☐ 58.
Posterior	☐ 59.	☐ 60.

ST, T, U WAVE ABNORMALITIES

☐ 61. Normal variant, early repolarization
☐ 62. Normal variant, juvenile T waves
☐ 63. Nonspecific ST and/or T wave abnormalities
☐ 64. ST and/or T wave abnormalities suggesting myocardial ischemia
☐ 65. ST and/or T wave abnormalities suggesting myocardial injury
☐ 66. ST and/or T wave abnormalities suggesting electrolyte disturbances
☐ 67. ST and/or T wave abnormalities secondary to hypertrophy
☐ 68. Prolonged Q-T interval
☐ 69. Prominent U waves

CLINICAL DISORDERS

☐ 70. Digitalis effect
☐ 71. Digitalis toxicity
☐ 72. Antiarrhythmic drug effect
☐ 73. Antiarrhythmic drug toxicity
☐ 74. Hyperkalemia
☐ 75. Hypokalemia
☐ 76. Hypercalcemia
☐ 77. Hypocalcemia
☐ 78. Atrial septal defect, secundum
☐ 79. Atrial septal defect, primum
☐ 80. Dextrocardia, mirror image
☐ 81. Chronic lung disease
☐ 82. Acute cor pulmonale including pulmonary embolus
☐ 83. Pericardial effusion
☐ 84. Acute pericarditis
☐ 85. Hypertrophic cardiomyopathy
☐ 86. Central nervous system disorder
☐ 87. Myxedema
☐ 88. Hypothermia
☐ 89. Sick sinus syndrome

PACEMAKER FUNCTION

☐ 90. Atrial or coronary sinus pacing
☐ 91. Ventricular demand pacemaker (VVI), normally functioning
☐ 92. Dual-chamber pacemaker (DDD), normally functioning
☐ 93. Pacemaker malfunction, not constantly capturing (atrium or ventricle)
☐ 94. Pacemaker malfunction, not constantly sensing (atrium or ventricle)

FUNDAMENTALS OF CARDIOVASCULAR DISEASE; MOLECULAR BIOLOGY AND GENETICS; EVALUATION OF THE PATIENT

ANSWER TO QUESTION 1

D (Braunwald, pp. 168, 177-178)

The normal systolic blood pressure response during exercise is a progressive increase to a peak value between 160 and 200 mm Hg. The higher end of this range is more commonly observed in older patients; in general, black patients tend to have a higher systolic blood pressure response to exercise than white patients. A failure to increase systolic blood pressure to at least 120 mm Hg, or a decline in systolic blood pressure during exercise, is abnormal. Such exertional hypotension occurs in 3% to 9% of patients and is suggestive of underlying multivessel or left main coronary artery disease. Other causes of a decline in systolic blood pressure, or a failure to increase systolic blood pressure with exercise, include cardiomyopathy, vasovagal reactions, ventricular outflow obstruction, hypovolemia, arrhythmias, and prolonged vigorous exercise. Subjects who demonstrate hypotension in the *postexercise* period are much less likely to have advanced underlying coronary artery disease; about 3% of normal subjects younger than 55 years of age demonstrate such a response.

In normal subjects, diastolic blood pressure does not change significantly during exercise. A large change in diastolic blood pressure is uncommon and has not been shown to correlate with underlying coronary artery disease.

The age-related maximum predicted heart rate (MPHR) is estimated from the formula:

$$MPHR = 220 - age \, (in \, years)$$

which in this patient would be 166 beats/min. The peak heart rate he achieved during the test was 152 beats/min, or 92% of the MPHR (i.e., 152/166 beats/min). An achieved heart rate of ≥85% MPHR is indicative of an adequate diagnostic workload.

Predictors of low prognostic coronary risk in his case include his very good functional capacity (having achieved stage IV of the Bruce protocol) and lack of cardiopulmonary symptoms or ST-segment changes during the test.

REFERENCE

Froelicher VF, Myers J: Exercise and the Heart. 5th ed. Philadelphia, WB Saunders, 2006.

ANSWER TO QUESTION 2

C (Braunwald, pp. 114-117; Fig. 12-8)

S_2 coincides with closure of the aortic and pulmonic valves and marks the onset of diastole at the bedside. Several abnormal heart sounds may follow S_2. The opening snap of mitral stenosis is a high-frequency sound that occurs shortly after S_2. It is generated when the superior bowing of the anterior mitral leaflet during systole rapidly reverses direction toward the left ventricle in early diastole, owing to the high left atrial (LA) pressure. The delay between the aortic component of S_2 and the opening snap corresponds to the left ventricular (LV) isovolumic relaxation time. As mitral stenosis becomes more severe, this phase shortens because of the greater LA pressure, and the interval between S_2 and the opening snap becomes less. Other sounds that occur shortly after S_2 are associated with the rapid filling phase of diastole. These include the third heart sound (S_3), which is a low-frequency sound that is thought to be caused by sudden limitation of LV expansion during brisk early diastolic filling. An S_3 is normal in children and young adults, but the presence of this sound beyond age 40 is abnormal and reflects flow into a dilated ventricle or an increased volume of flow in early diastole, as may occur in mitral regurgitation. A tumor "plop" may be auscultated when an atrial myxoma, attached to the interatrial septum by a long stalk, moves into and obstructs the mitral or tricuspid valve orifice during early diastole. In constrictive pericarditis, a pericardial "knock" may be heard during the rapid filling phase of early diastole as the high-pressure atria rapidly decompress into relatively noncompliant ventricles.

An ejection click is an early systolic sound that represents opening of an abnormal semilunar valve, characteristically a bicuspid aortic valve.

ANSWER TO QUESTION 3

D (Braunwald, pp. 35-36, 178-179; Table 14-3)

In addition to accuracy and reliability, the performance of a diagnostic test depends on its ability to distinguish between the presence and absence of disease. Test performance depends on its sensitivity and specificity, as well as the prevalence of disease in the population of patients to be studied or the pretest probability of disease in a particular patient. Sensitivity and specificity are characteristics of the diagnostic test that are not altered by disease prevalence or pretest probability. Sensitivity is the percentage of patients with disease who will be correctly identified by the test. Specificity is the percentage of patients without disease who will be correctly identified as disease free by the test. Positive predictive value is the probability that a positive test correctly identifies the presence of disease. Negative predictive value is the probability that a negative test correctly identifies the absence of disease. A perfect diagnostic test has a positive predictive value of 100% (no false-negative results) and a negative predictive value of 100% (no false-positive results).

For a diagnostic test with moderately high sensitivity and specificity, the test will perform best in a population of patients with an intermediate pretest probability of disease (patient D). In patients with a low pretest probability of disease (patients A and B), the positive predictive value of the test is low and there will be a large number of false-positive tests that may prompt unnecessary testing and procedures. In patients with an extremely high pretest probability of disease (patients C and E), the negative predictive value of the test is low and the possibility that a negative result represents a false negative is unacceptably high.

ANSWER TO QUESTION 4

C (Braunwald, pp. 115-118; Table 12-5; Fig. 12-8)

The term *continuous* applies to murmurs that begin in systole and continue without interruption into part or all of diastole. The murmur described here, that of a patent ductus arteriosus, is the classic continuous murmur, peaking in intensity just before or after S_2 then decreasing in intensity during diastole, sometimes disappearing before the subsequent first heart sound. Continuous murmurs may be congenital or acquired and can be caused by (1) an aortopulmonary shunt, such as patent ductus arteriosus; (2) an arteriovenous shunt, including arteriovenous fistulas, coronary artery fistulas, or rupture of an aortic sinus of Valsalva aneurysm into a right heart chamber; (3) constricted arterial vessels (e.g., a femoral arterial atherosclerotic stenosis); (4) turbulence in nonconstricted arteries (e.g., the "mammary souffle," an innocent flow murmur heard during late pregnancy and the puerperium over the lactating breast and augmented by light pressure with the stethoscope); or (5) venous murmurs, such as a cervical venous hum, an often "rough" sounding murmur present in healthy children and young adults. The cervical hum may be accentuated by deforming the internal jugular vein with rotation of the head. It is augmented during pregnancy and in disease states in which there is increased venous flow, such as thyrotoxicosis.

The combined murmurs of aortic stenosis and regurgitation have distinct systolic and diastolic components and do not constitute a continuous murmur.

ANSWER TO QUESTION 5

E (Braunwald, pp. 111-114)

Reduced or unequal arterial pulsations may occur in the arms of patients with atherosclerosis affecting the subclavian arteries, aortic dissection, and unusual arteritides such as Takayasu disease. In supravalvular aortic stenosis there may be selective streaming of the arterial jet toward the innominate artery and right arm, leading to higher pressures in that extremity. This is not the case, however, with subvalvular or valvular aortic stenosis. Valvular aortic stenosis leads to pulsus parvus et tardus, a slowly rising and weak pulse best appreciated by palpation of the carotid arteries. Coarctation of the aorta in adults usually involves the aorta distal to the origin of the left subclavian artery and leads to higher blood pressure in the upper extremities compared with the legs; the arm pulses and pressures are typically equal.

REFERENCE

Lane D, et al: Inter-arm differences in blood pressure: When are they clinically significant? J Hypertens 20:1089, 2002.

ANSWER TO QUESTION 6

C (Braunwald, pp. 252-254, 1655-1665, 1893-1894; Figs. 15-73 and 75-8)

This patient with metastatic breast cancer and a large pericardial effusion has clinical findings consistent with cardiac tamponade.[1] Tamponade physiology results when an accumulation of pericardial effusion causes equilibration of intrapericardial and intracardiac pressures.[2,3] In addition to the presence of an echo-free space surrounding the heart, characteristic echocardiographic and Doppler findings reflect the aberrant pathophysiology of this disorder. Collapse of the right ventricle during early *diastole* occurs because the abnormally elevated pericardial pressure transiently exceeds right ventricular (RV) pressure at that phase of the cardiac cycle. Indentation of the right atrial wall during diastole is a more sensitive marker of increased pericardial pressure but is less specific for tamponade physiology than RV collapse and tends to occur earlier in the course of hemodynamically significant pericardial effusion. Cardiac tamponade is associated with exaggerated ventricular interdependence, a phenomenon manifested at the bedside by pulsus paradoxus. The Doppler correlate of pulsus paradoxus is amplified respirophasic variation of flow across the right- and left-sided cardiac valves. This includes a prominent inspiratory decrease in flow velocity across the mitral and aortic valves (see the transmitral tracing in Figure 1-62), whereas inspiration causes a prominent reciprocal *increase* in flow velocity across the tricuspid and pulmonic valves.

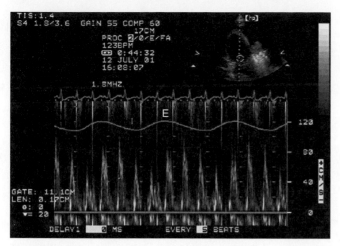

FIGURE 1-62

A marked increase of the E/A ratio of the mitral valve inflow velocity is a finding typical of constrictive pericarditis, not cardiac tamponade.

REFERENCES

1. Chiles C, Woodard PK, Gutierrez FR, Link KM: Metastatic involvement of the heart and pericardium: CT and MRI imaging. RadioGraphics 21:439, 2001.
2. Spodick DH: Acute cardiac tamponade. N Engl J Med 349:684, 2003.
3. Roy CL, Minor MA, Brookheart MA, et al: Does this patient with a pericardial effusion have cardiac tamponade? JAMA 297:1810, 2007.

ANSWER TO QUESTION 7

D (Braunwald, pp. 111-113, 124, 1656)

Pulsus paradoxus is an exaggeration of the normal tendency for arterial pulse strength to fall with inspiration and can be measured easily and accurately at the bedside with a sphygmomanometer. A decline of more than 8 to 10 mm Hg with inspiration is considered abnormal and can be observed in a variety of conditions. Pulsus paradoxus is characteristic of patients with cardiac tamponade, is seen in approximately one third of patients with chronic constrictive pericarditis, and is noted as well in patients with wide intrapleural pressure swings (e.g., bronchial asthma and emphysema), pulmonary embolism, pregnancy, extreme obesity, and hypovolemic shock.

Notably, aortic regurgitation augments left ventricular diastolic pressure and tends to prevent pulsus paradoxus even in the presence of tamponade.

Kussmaul's sign manifests as inappropriate augmentation of the jugular venous pressure during inspiration and implies the presence of constrictive pericarditis, not isolated cardiac tamponade.

ANSWER TO QUESTION 8

D (Braunwald, pp. 144-145; Fig. 13-27; Table 13-6)

Left anterior fascicular block (LAFB) is a common abnormality that can develop in healthy people or in patients with a wide variety of cardiac diseases, including prior anterior myocardial infarction, left ventricular hypertrophy, cardiomyopathies, and degenerative diseases of the conduction system. It results in an alteration of the ventricular activation sequence without prolongation of the QRS complex duration. The characteristic electrocardiographic finding is marked left-axis deviation (−45 to −90 degrees) because of delayed activation of the anterosuperior left ventricular wall. Because inferior and posterior forces are unopposed during early ventricular activation, and anterosuperior forces are unopposed at the termination of activation, the ECG records characteristic rS complexes in the inferior leads and qR complexes in the anterolateral leads. The precordial leads may demonstrate deep S waves in the lateral territory (leads V_4 to V_6), reflecting the late anterosuperior forces.

The development of LAFB can mask the Q waves of a prior inferior myocardial infarction.

REFERENCE

Surawicz B, et al: Recommendations for the standardization and interpretation of the electrocardiogram: III. Intraventricular conduction disturbances. Circulation 119:e235, 2009.

ANSWER TO QUESTION 9

C (Braunwald, pp. 93-94; Tables 10-1 and 10-2)

All drugs prescribed to achieve a particular clinical benefit also have the potential for toxicity. Many factors determine the likelihood of drug toxicity, including the pharmacokinetic and pharmacodynamic properties of the drug and its target, genetic variability in the patient's response to the drug, and drug–drug interactions.

Many medications are metabolized by isoforms of the cytochrome P-450 (CYP) enzyme system, which are expressed in the liver and other tissues. Ketoconazole, erythromycin, and clarithromycin (but not azithromycin) are examples of drugs that inhibit CYP3A4 and 3A5. Because these P-450 isoforms are responsible for metabolism of simvastatin, atorvastatin, and lovastatin, combined therapy with such inhibitors may increase the likelihood of myopathy due to these statins.[1] Pravastatin is not metabolized by the CYP3A system, and thus the risk of myopathy is not increased in the presence of CYP3A inhibitors.

St. John's wort induces activity of CYP3A and results in decreased cyclosporine levels.[2]

Sildenafil, a selective inhibitor of phosphodiesterase type 5 prescribed to treat erectile dysfunction, potentiates the vasodilatory effect of nitrates. Administration of nitrates within 24 hours of sildenafil use has been associated with profound hypotension.

Verapamil inhibits the P-glycoprotein–mediated efflux of digoxin into bile and urine and may contribute to digoxin toxicity.

REFERENCES

1. Thompson PD, Clarkson P, Karas RH: Statin-associated myopathy. JAMA 289:1681, 2003.

2. Zhou S, Gao Y, Jiang W, et al: Interactions of herbs with cytochrome P450. Drug Metab Rev 35:35, 2003.

ANSWER TO QUESTION 10

D (Braunwald, pp. 189-190, 1476; Table 14-5)

Treadmill exercise testing is a safe procedure with an associated mortality of <0.01% and risk of myocardial infarction of 0.04%.[1] The risk of a procedure-related complication is determined by the clinical characteristics of the patient to be studied. Patients with high-grade obstruction of the left ventricular outflow tract, such as those with hypertrophic obstructive cardiomyopathy or critical aortic stenosis, are at an increased risk of a procedural complication owing to the inability of cardiac output to compensate for peripheral vasodilatation during exercise. Patients with unstable angina should not be subjected to the high myocardial oxygen demands of exercise and generally should be referred for coronary angiography instead. Acute myocarditis is associated with an increased risk of exercise-associated sudden death.

Despite the theoretical risk of aortic rupture due to increased wall stress, treadmill exercise testing may be safely performed in patients with an abdominal aortic aneurysm.[2] In contrast, aortic dissection is a contraindication to the stress of exercise testing.

REFERENCES

1. Myers J, Arena R, Franklin B, et al: Recommendations for clinical exercise laboratories: A scientific statement from the American Heart Association. Circulation 119:3144, 2009.
2. Best PJ, Tajik AJ, Gibbons RJ, Pellikka PA: The safety of treadmill exercise stress testing in patients with abdominal aortic aneurysms. Ann Intern Med 129:628, 1998.

ANSWER TO QUESTION 11

B (Braunwald, pp. 302-303, 325, 326; Fig. 17-12)

The images show a fixed defect in the mid and apical anterior wall segments with preserved wall motion and thickening as evident from the end-diastolic and end-systolic frames. These findings are most consistent with imaging artifact due to breast tissue attenuation.

Attenuation artifacts are a common source of error in single-photon emission computed tomography (SPECT). Regional wall motion and wall thickening should be assessed on the electrocardiographic gated SPECT data in any region that shows a fixed perfusion defect. Although a transmural myocardial scar would be associated with reduced wall motion and wall thickening, attenuation artifact is more likely where there is a fixed perfusion defect with normal regional wall motion and wall thickening.

Thallium-201 is a lower-energy radiotracer that results in more attenuation artifacts than technetium-99m imaging, and hence would be an inferior choice in this case.

REFERENCE

Garcia EV, Galt JR, Faber TL, et al: Principles of nuclear cardiology imaging. In Dilsizian V, Narula J, Braunwald E (eds): Atlas of Nuclear Cardiology. 3rd ed. Philadelphia, Current Medicine Group, 2009, pp 1-36.

ANSWER TO QUESTION 12

B (Braunwald, pp. 114-117, 121-124)

The normal second heart sound (S_2) consists of two parts, an earlier aortic component and a later pulmonic component. During inspiration, the increased filling of the right ventricle prolongs the ejection phase of the right side of the heart leading to *delayed* closure of the pulmonic valve. This is the predominant factor in normal inspiratory splitting of the S_2. Right bundle branch block delays right ventricular activation and ejection and is therefore associated with *widened* splitting of S_2. Conditions in which left ventricular activation is late, such as left bundle branch block or right ventricular pacing, cause closure of the aortic valve to be delayed. In that setting, the pulmonic valve closure sound actually precedes that of the aortic valve. Then, during inspiration (and prolongation of right ventricular ejection), the delayed closure of the pulmonic valve narrows the timing between the two sounds, a situation known as *paradoxical* splitting.

Fixed splitting of the S_2 is typical of an uncomplicated ostium secundum atrial septal defect. In this condition, closure of the pulmonic valve is delayed because of the increased flow through the right-sided cardiac chambers and an increase in pulmonary vascular capacitance, contributing to a widened split of S_2. On inspiration, augmentation of the systemic venous return is counterbalanced by a reciprocal decrease in the volume of the left-to-right shunt, such that right ventricular filling and the timing of P_2 relative to A_2 do not change, resulting in the fixed splitting.

When valvular stenosis restricts opening of a cardiac valve, the decreased excursion of the leaflets *reduces* the intensity of the closure sound. Thus, in pulmonic stenosis, the pulmonic component of S_2 becomes softer.

ANSWER TO QUESTION 13

D (Braunwald, pp. 172-175, 180)

Electrocardiographic changes during exertion in an asymptomatic patient must be interpreted in light of the pretest likelihood of coronary disease. An exercise-induced ST-segment abnormality is an independent predictor of future cardiac events in men with and without conventional risk factors for coronary disease, although the risk is greatest among the former. However, over 5 years of follow-up, only one in four such patients will actually develop symptoms of cardiac disease, most commonly angina. Because the patient described in this question is asymptomatic and demonstrates good exercise capacity, there is no need for immediate aggressive intervention such as cardiac catheterization. Appropriate recommendations for this patient with asymptomatic coronary artery disease would include aggressive risk factor modification: smoking cessation, control of hypertension, the addition of aspirin, 81 to 325 mg/d, and treatment of dyslipidemia (e.g., statin therapy to achieve low-density lipoprotein <100 mg/dL).

The distribution of ST-segment depressions during exercise testing correlates poorly with the location of coronary stenoses. Conversely, the location of ST-segment *elevations*, when present, does correlate well with the anatomic lesion causing ischemia.

REFERENCES

Greenland P, Alpert JS, Beller GA, et al: 2010 ACCF/AHA guideline for the assessment of cardiovascular risk in asymptomatic adults: Executive summary. A report of the American College of Cardiology Foundation/American Heart Association Task Force on Practice Guidelines. Circulation 122:2748, 2010.
Lauer M, Freolicher ES, Williams M, et al: Exercise testing in asymptomatic adults: A statement from professionals from the American Heart Association Council on Clinical Cardiology, Subcommittee on Exercise, Cardiac Rehabilitation, and Prevention. Circulation 112:771, 2005.

ANSWER TO QUESTION 14

C (Braunwald, pp. 179, 185, 324; Tables 14-3 and 14G-4)

Several clinical situations affect the ST segment and impair the diagnostic utility of the standard exercise ECG. These include the presence of left bundle branch block (LBBB), left ventricular hypertrophy, ventricular preexcitation (Wolff-Parkinson-White syndrome), and digitalis therapy. In these situations, other aspects of the exercise test, such as exercise duration, presence or absence of symptoms, and abnormal blood pressure or heart rate responses, may still provide useful diagnostic information. However, in the presence of these baseline electrocardiographic abnormalities, concurrent imaging (nuclear scintigraphy or echocardiography) is frequently required when more specific diagnostic information is needed. In the case of LBBB, a pharmacologic adenosine stress test with myocardial perfusion imaging helps to avoid artifactual septal perfusion defects compared with exercise protocols.

In patients with a low prior probability of significant coronary artery disease, such as a young woman without significant cardiac risk factors, the development of ST segment depression on exercise testing is more often a nonspecific false-positive result than an indicator of previously undetected coronary artery disease.

REFERENCE

Gibbons RJ, Balady GJ, Bricker JT, et al: ACC/AHA 2002 guideline update for exercise testing: Summary article. A report of the American College of Cardiology/American Heart Association Task Force on Practice Guidelines (Committee to Update the 1997 Exercise Testing Guidelines). J Am Coll Cardiol 40:1531, 2002.

ANSWER TO QUESTION 15

D (Braunwald, pp. 383-385, 390, 404, 1937-1940)

Diagnostic cardiac catheterization is a relatively safe procedure, with an overall risk of a major complication of <1%. Mortality rates related to the procedure depend on the population studied and range from 0.08% to 0.75%. The risk of myocardial infarction is approximately 0.05%, and neurologic complications occur in 0.03% to 0.2% of patients. The incidence of acute renal dysfunction in patients with baseline renal insufficiency can be most effectively decreased with intravenous saline administration before and after the procedure. The addition of mannitol or furosemide to saline infusion has been shown to *worsen* renal outcomes in patients receiving an intravenous contrast agent.

Nonionic low osmolar contrast agents reduce the likelihood of adverse hemodynamic and electrophysiologic reactions during angiography. They also reduce the incidence of contrast-induced nephropathy in patients with baseline renal insufficiency, with or without diabetes. Of note, in patients with normal renal function, there is no advantage of low osmolar agents over ionic agents in the prevention of nephrotoxicity.

Cardiac catheters are available in many sizes, shapes, and lengths. The outer diameter of the catheter is specified using French units (F), where 1 F is equal to 0.33 mm.

Patients with tilting-disc prosthetic aortic valves should not undergo retrograde left-sided heart catheterization because of the risk of catheter entrapment, occlusion of the valve, or possible dislodgment of the disc with embolization.

REFERENCE

Smith SC, Feldman TE, Hirshfeld JW, et al: ACC/AHA/SCAI 2005 guideline update for percutaneous coronary intervention: A report of the American College of Cardiology/American Heart Association Task Force on Practice Guidelines (ACC/AHA/SCAI Writing Committee to update the 2001 Guidelines for Percutaneous Coronary Intervention). Circulation 113:e166, 2006.

ANSWER TO QUESTION 16

E (Braunwald, pp. 149-156, 1093, 1101, 1153-1156; Figs. 13-35 and 54-4)

Proximal occlusion of a dominant right coronary artery (RCA) leads to infarction of the left ventricular (LV) inferior wall but often also involves the posterior wall, the right ventricle, and portions of the conduction system, which are all supplied by branches of the RCA. ST-segment elevation in leads II, III, and aVF is the sine qua non of transmural infarction of the inferior wall. If the posterior wall is involved, ST-segment depression is usually evident in V_1 and V_2, reflecting a current of injury on the side of the heart opposite those leads (if unipolar leads were placed on the patient's back overlying the posterior wall, ST-segment elevation would be observed instead). Very proximal occlusion of the RCA is often accompanied by right ventricular (RV) infarction because the RV

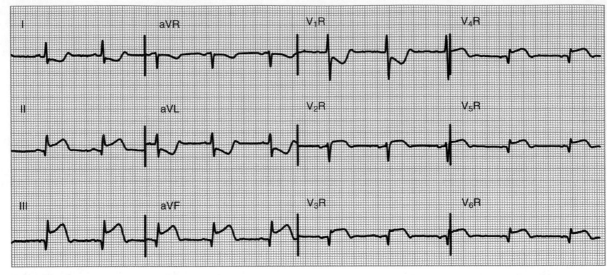

FIGURE 1-63

arterial branch arises near the origin of that vessel. If RV infarction is present, right-sided precordial electrocardiographic leads, particularly V_4R, often demonstrate ST-segment elevation as well (Fig. 1-63). Sinus bradycardia is common in the setting of acute myocardial infarction, especially in inferior or posterior infarction. This arrhythmia, particularly when accompanied by hypotension, may arise from stimulation of cardiac vagal afferent fibers, which are prominent in the inferoposterior left ventricle. Sinus bradycardia may also be a vasovagal response to the severe chest pain in acute myocardial infarction or reflect ischemia of the sinoatrial artery, which arises from the RCA in 60% of the population. Another potential cause of bradycardia in this patient is the development of atrioventricular (AV) block because of either vagal stimulation or ischemia of the AV node. The AV node is supplied by the AV nodal artery, which arises from the RCA 85% of the time.

PR-segment deviations are common in patients with acute pericarditis, not acute myocardial infarction.

ANSWER TO QUESTION 17

B (Braunwald, pp. 230-240)

One of the most clinically important applications of Doppler technology is the estimation of pressure gradients across stenotic orifices or septal defects in the cardiovascular system. The Bernoulli equation relates the pressure difference across a narrowed area to the convective acceleration, flow acceleration, and viscous friction. By modifying the Bernoulli equation, a more clinically useful simplified formula is derived. The simplified Bernoulli equation states that the pressure difference across a flow-limiting orifice = $4V^2$, where V is the peak velocity distal to the obstruction. In this question, we are given the information that the patient's systolic blood pressure is 144 mm Hg, which, in the absence of

left ventricular (LV) outflow obstruction, is also the LV systolic pressure. If the ventricular septal defect flow is 5.1 m/sec, then using the modified Bernoulli equation, the pressure gradient across the ventricular septal defect is $4 \times (5.1)^2 = 104$ mm Hg. The right ventricular systolic pressure can then be simply calculated by subtracting that gradient from the LV systolic pressure: $144 - 104$, or 40 mm Hg.

If the patient's blood pressure had not been given, it would still be possible to estimate the LV systolic pressure using the mitral regurgitation velocity. If the mitral regurgitation velocity is 5.8 m/sec, then we know, using the modified Bernoulli equation, that the pressure difference across the mitral valve in systole is 135 mm Hg. An estimate of the left atrial pressure is then made using two-dimensional and Doppler parameters, and this value is added to the transmitral systolic gradient to derive an estimate of LV systolic pressure. Thus, if the estimated left atrial pressure were 10 mm Hg, then the LV systolic pressure would be 145 mm Hg.

REFERENCE

Armstrong WF, Ryan T: Feigenbaum's Echocardiography. 7th ed. Philadelphia, Lippincott Williams & Wilkins, 2010, pp 217-240.

ANSWER TO QUESTION 18

C (Braunwald, pp. 145-146, 746-748)

Left bundle branch block (LBBB) most commonly develops in individuals with underlying structural heart disease. The presence of this conduction abnormality portends a reduced long-term survival, with 10-year mortality rates as high as 50%. In patients with known coronary atherosclerosis, the development of LBBB implies more extensive disease and is often associated with left ventricular (LV) dysfunction. If left-axis deviation accompanies LBBB, more severe clinical disease is likely. The delayed LV activation in LBBB leads to paradoxical splitting of the second heart sound because pulmonic valve closure abnormally precedes aortic valve closure (see Answer to Question 12).

In LBBB, repolarization of the left ventricle is typically altered, such that the ST segment and T waves are discordant with (i.e., directed opposite to) the QRS complex.

The abnormal ventricular activation in LBBB results in a dyssynchronous pattern of contraction that may impair stroke volume. The duration of the QRS complex in LBBB inversely correlates with the LV ejection fraction.[1] Cardiac resynchronization therapy with biventricular pacing was developed to improve LV function in patients with cardiomyopathy and LBBB and has been shown to improve outcomes in patients with advanced heart failure.[2]

REFERENCES

1. Das MK, Cheriparambil K, Bedi A, et al: Prolonged QRS duration and left-axis deviation in the presence of left bundle branch block: A marker for poor ventricular function? Am Heart J 142:756, 2001.
2. Epstein AE, et al: ACC/AHA/HRS 2008 guidelines for device-based therapy of cardiac rhythm abnormalities: A report of the ACC/AHA Task Force on Practice Guidelines. Circulation 117:e350, 2008.

ANSWER TO QUESTION 19

A (Braunwald, pp. 159-161)

Many electrolyte disturbances result in characteristic electrocardiographic manifestations. Decreased extracellular calcium in hypocalcemia prolongs phase 2 of the action potential (AP), thereby lengthening the AP duration and the QT interval. The long QT interval in hypocalcemia is characteristically flat (i.e., isoelectric), without the concave configuration of many drug-induced prolonged QT states. *Increased* extracellular calcium shortens the ventricular action potential and the duration of the QT interval. The appearance of a J wave (also known as an Osborn wave—see arrow in Figure 1-64), an extra deflection at the junction of the QRS complex, and the ST segment typically observed in cases of severe hypothermia has been reported with severe *hyper*calcemia.[1]

Hyperkalemia causes a specific sequence of electrocardiographic changes depending on its severity. The earliest manifestation is narrow, peaked T waves. The QT interval is usually decreased at that time because of shortened action potential duration. Progressive

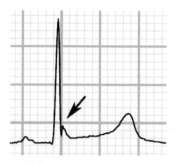

FIGURE 1-64

hyperkalemia reduces the resting membrane potentials in both the atria and ventricles, thus inactivating sodium channels. The net result is to slow depolarization and reduce action potential conduction velocity. The ECG shows widening of the QRS complex with a decrease in P wave amplitude. PR-segment prolongation may also occur. Very marked hyperkalemia leads to slow, undulating ventricular flutter (a "sine wave" appearance) followed by eventual asystole. Hypokalemia, in contrast, manifests primarily as ST-segment depressions with flattened T waves and U wave prominence. Because of prolongation of the QT interval there is a propensity for polymorphic ventricular tachycardia (torsades de pointes).

The effects of magnesium on the surface ECG are not as well characterized. Magnesium deficiency may predispose to prolongation of the QT interval, primarily as a result of a prolonged U wave (QU interval), and torsades de pointes.

REFERENCE

1. Otero J, Lenihan DJ: The "normothermic" Osborn wave induced by severe hypercalcemia. Tex Heart Inst J 27:316, 2000.

ANSWER TO QUESTION 20

E (Braunwald, pp. 178-179, 185-186, 193-194; Table 14-3; see also Answer to Question 14)

Meta-analyses show that the sensitivity and specificity of the exercise ECG for the detection of coronary artery disease (CAD) are 68% and 77%, respectively. The sensitivity for diagnosis is impaired by resting ST-segment depression or other repolarization abnormalities, including left ventricular hypertrophy, digitalis therapy (even if digitalis effect is not evident on the resting ECG), left bundle branch block, and preexcitation syndromes. In addition, severe hypertension, hyperventilation, and hypokalemia may distort the ST segment, leading to false-positive electrocardiographic interpretations. One of the main diagnostic values of the standard exercise test is to exclude CAD in patients with chest pain with a low pretest likelihood of disease based on age and gender who have a normal resting ECG. If such a patient achieves the maximum heart rate without ST-segment deviations and a normal blood pressure response, it is very unlikely that CAD is the cause of chest pain. For most other populations, the exercise ECG is limited by the suboptimal sensitivity and specificity. Both myocardial perfusion imaging and stress echocardiography increase the sensitivity and specificity of exercise testing in patients with resting electrocardiographic abnormalities. In particular, the negative predictive value of both of these techniques is excellent.

REFERENCE

Gibbons RJ, Balady GJ, Bricker JT, et al: ACC/AHA 2002 guideline update for exercise testing: Summary article. A report of the American College of Cardiology/American Heart Association Task Force on Practice Guidelines (Committee to Update the 1997 Exercise Testing Guidelines). J Am Coll Cardiol 40:1531, 2002.

ANSWER TO QUESTION 21

E (Braunwald, p. 148; Fig. 13-28)

The underlying rhythm is atrial fibrillation. The Ashman phenomenon (as exemplified by the fifth QRS complex in the tracing) represents conduction aberrancy caused by changes in the preceding cycle length. Because the duration of the refractory period is a function of the immediate preceding cycle length, the longer the preceding cycle, the longer the ensuing refractory period and the more likely that the next impulse will be conducted with delay. Normally the refractory periods of the conduction system components are right bundle branch > left bundle branch = atrioventricular node >> His bundle. Therefore, it would be unusual for the bundle of His to be the site of conduction delay and, as is commonly the case, the aberrant beat on this tracing demonstrates right bundle branch block morphology in lead V_1.

ANSWER TO QUESTION 22

C (Braunwald, pp. 115-117; Fig. 12-10)

Innocent (normal) systolic murmurs are related to intracardiac flow rates and are usually loudest in midsystole. They may be caused by normal vibrations of the pulmonary leaflets or exaggeration of normal ejection vibrations within the pulmonary artery or be associated with sclerosis at the base of the aortic valve leaflets in the absence of significant valvular stenosis. The normal mammary souffle, heard over the breasts of women in late pregnancy or during lactation, may be midsystolic in timing or continuous. Careful auscultation usually reveals a time delay between S_1 and onset of this murmur, which is the transit time of flow from the proximal aorta to the mammary arteries.

ANSWER TO QUESTION 23

D (Braunwald, pp. 110-111, 124; Figs. 12-2 and 12-3)

A great deal of information about right-sided heart hemodynamics can be ascertained from the jugular venous pressure waveforms. The a wave results from venous distention due to right atrial contraction; the x descent reflects atrial relaxation and downward descent of the base of the right atrium during right ventricular (RV) systole. The c wave is an inconstant positive deflection in the jugular venous pulse that interrupts the x descent and corresponds to ventricular contraction. The v wave results from right atrial filling during ventricular systole when the tricuspid valve is closed, and the y descent occurs after the tricuspid valve opens and right atrial pressure declines. It is easier for an observer to see the x and y descents than the positive pressure waves ($a, c,$ and v waves) in the neck because the former produce larger excursions. An elevated jugular venous pressure reflects increased right atrial pressure. During inspiration, the jugular venous pressure normally declines as intrathoracic pressure becomes more negative. Kussmaul's sign is a paradoxical rise in the height of the venous pressure during inspiration. It reflects an inability of the right-sided chambers to accept additional volume, typical of constrictive pericarditis, but may also be observed in patients with right-sided heart failure, severe cor pulmonale, or tricuspid stenosis.

The a wave becomes more prominent in conditions that increase the resistance to right atrial contraction, such as RV hypertrophy, pulmonary hypertension, or tricuspid stenosis. Amplified "cannon" a waves are evident during any situation that causes atrioventricular dissociation, because the right atrium contracts against a closed tricuspid valve at least intermittently.

In constrictive pericarditis, the y descent is rapid and deep because the earliest phase of diastolic RV filling is unimpeded. In contrast, in cardiac tamponade, the y descent is blunted and it is the x descent that is most prominent.

ANSWER TO QUESTION 24

D (Braunwald, pp. 396-398; Figs. 20-11 and 20-12)

There is no completely accurate method for measuring cardiac output in the cardiac catheterization laboratory. Two commonly used methods are the thermodilution and the Fick techniques. The former involves injection of a bolus of fluid (i.e., saline or dextrose) into the proximal port of a right-sided balloon flotation (e.g., Swan-Ganz) catheter, after which alterations in temperature are measured at the distal end of the catheter. The change in the temperature over time is then plotted to derive the cardiac output, which is *inversely* related to the area under the thermodilution curve (Fig. 1-65). In low cardiac output states there is a larger area under the curve owing to the longer time required for the temperature curve to return to its baseline. However, this technique tends to *overestimate* cardiac output in the setting of low output states, because the dissipation of the cooler temperature to the surrounding cardiac structures results in

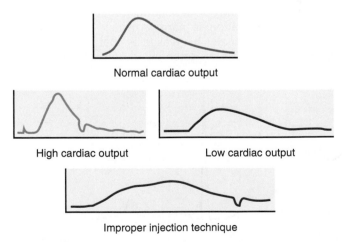

Normal cardiac output

High cardiac output

Low cardiac output

Improper injection technique

FIGURE 1-65

a reduction in the total area under the curve. In addition, the back and forth flow across the tricuspid valve in patients with severe tricuspid regurgitation also creates significant error in measurement, producing a falsely low cardiac output by this technique.

The Fick technique is based on the principle that cardiac output is equal to the oxygen consumption divided by the difference in oxygen content between arterial and mixed venous blood. That is:

$$\text{Cardiac output} = \frac{O_2 \text{ Consumption}}{\text{A-VO}_2 \text{ Difference}}$$

The Fick technique is more accurate than thermodilution in patients with low cardiac outputs; however, its main limitation is in measuring true oxygen consumption in a steady state. Many laboratories use an "assumed" oxygen consumption by considering the patient's age, gender, and body surface area. Inaccuracy in the oxygen consumption measurement can result in substantial variability in reported cardiac outputs.

Systemic vascular resistance (SVR) is derived by dividing the difference between the mean aortic and right atrial (RA) pressures by the systemic cardiac output (and then multiplying by a constant to convert to the commonly used units of dyne·sec·cm^{-5}):

$$SVR = 80 \times \frac{\text{Mean Aortic Pressure} - \text{Mean RA Pressure}}{\text{Systemic cardiac output}}$$

The pulmonary vascular resistance (PVR) is obtained by dividing the difference between the mean pulmonary artery (PA) and left atrial (LA) pressures by the pulmonic cardiac output (then multiplying by the same constant). The pulmonary capillary wedge (PCW) pressure is commonly used as a surrogate for left atrial pressure:

$$PVR = 80 \times \frac{\text{Mean PA Pressure} - \text{Mean LA (or PCW) Pressure}}{\text{Pulmonic cardiac output}}$$

In the absence of intracardiac shunts, the systemic and pulmonic cardiac outputs should be the same.

ANSWER TO QUESTION 25

C (Braunwald, pp. 220-223; Figs. 15-26 and 15-27)

Pulsed Doppler interrogation of mitral valve inflow is useful in identifying disorders of left ventricular (LV) diastolic function. In normal adults, the early (E wave) velocity exceeds the late (A wave) velocity such that the normal E/A ratio is >1.2. The figure accompanying this question illustrates an abnormal pattern of mitral inflow, with an E/A ratio >1.0. Although this pattern may be present in patients who have documented abnormalities of LV relaxation, it can also occur as a result of normal aging.[1] In fact, most people older than age 70 have an E/A ratio <1.0. In addition, the pattern of diastolic mitral

inflow is load dependent. If a patient with the illustrated pattern of impaired relaxation were administered intravenous volume, the mitral inflow pattern could change to the "pseudonormalized" form, with an E/A ratio >1.0, without any alteration in the intrinsic relaxation properties of the ventricle. Caution should thus be used when inferring a diastolic or relaxation abnormality from the mitral inflow pattern. Although none of the available echocardiographic indices of diastolic function is infallible, and even stepwise approaches using the mitral inflow pattern, Doppler tissue imaging, and assessment of pulmonary venous inflow can result in internally inconsistent results,[2] echocardiographic measures of diastolic function nonetheless provide clinically important diagnostic and prognostic information.[3]

Constrictive pericarditis and restrictive cardiomyopathy are clinical situations in which the bulk of ventricular filling occurs in early diastole. In these conditions there is a high E/A ratio, often >2.0. Hyperthyroidism and hemorrhage each result in hyperdynamic states in which diastolic relaxation is enhanced, such that reversal of the E/A ratio would be unusual.

REFERENCES

1. Paulus WJ, et al: How to diagnose diastolic heart failure: a consensus statement on the diagnosis of heart failure with normal left ventricular ejection fraction by the Heart Failure and Echocardiography Associations of the European Society of Cardiology. Eur Heart J 28:2539, 2007.
2. Tschope C, Paulus WJ: Doppler echocardiography yields dubious estimates of left ventricular diastolic pressures. Circulation 120:810, 2009.
3. Little WC, Ho JK: Echocardiographic evaluation of diastolic function can be used to guide care. Circulation 120:802, 2009.

ANSWER TO QUESTION 26

D (Braunwald, pp. 232-240, 1490-1491; Figs. 15-38, 15-39, 15-47, and 66-19)

The figure accompanying this question displays continuous Doppler interrogation of transmitral valvular flow obtained from the apical four-chamber transducer position. During diastole, the deceleration of transmitral inflow is prolonged, consistent with a persistent pressure gradient between the left atrium and left ventricle (i.e., mitral stenosis). In systole, a faint signal of mitral regurgitation (MR) is seen as a downward velocity spectrum. To determine the extent of MR noninvasively, simultaneous two-dimensional echocardiography and color Doppler interrogation would be required. However, the presented Doppler spectrum of mitral inflow is sufficient to determine the severity of mitral stenosis, including the transmitral pressure gradient and the valve area, as described below. The mitral valve area can be calculated noninvasively by three distinct noninvasive echo-Doppler methods. First, if an adequate two-dimensional short-axis image can be obtained in diastole, the valve orifice can be traced and the valve area measured directly using planimetry (see Braunwald, Fig. 66-19). The second method (which can be applied to the provided figure) utilizes the Doppler pressure half-time (PHT), which calculates the time in milliseconds required for the diastolic transmitral pressure gradient to decline to one half of its peak value (see Braunwald, Figs. 15-39 and 15-47). Because of the relationship between velocity and pressure, this requires determining the time it takes for the peak diastolic velocity to fall to the peak velocity divided by the square root of 2. Most modern echocardiographic machines calculate the PHT automatically once the Doppler profile is traced on the screen, using the equation:

$$\text{Mitral valve area} = 220 \div \text{PHT}$$

This relationship becomes less accurate when there is marked MR or aortic regurgitation, which interferes with the measured pressure gradient across the mitral valve. The third method to calculate the mitral valve area utilizes the continuity equation, which is based on the principle that the volume rate of flow through the heart is constant (see Braunwald, Fig. 15-38). The cause of mitral stenosis in the vast majority of adults is rheumatic heart disease. Occasionally, other causes can be identified, such as congenital abnormalities of the valve or heavy senile calcification that restricts transvalvular flow. The transvalvular Doppler pattern cannot distinguish the etiology of mitral stenosis, but two-dimensional echocardiographic imaging is usually diagnostic in this regard.

ANSWER TO QUESTION 27

B (Braunwald, p. 235)

The general calculation of the pressure gradient across a cardiac value is determined by the equation

$$\Delta \text{Pressure} = 4 \times \text{velocity}^2$$

In this instance, the pressure gradient is 64 mm Hg (4×4^2). With a right atrial pressure of 9 mm Hg and a pressure gradient of 64 mm Hg, the right ventricular pressure equals 73 mm Hg (64 + 9). Pressure gradients across other cardiac valves and across a ventricular septal defect can be calculated in a similar manner.

ANSWER TO QUESTION 28

C (Braunwald, pp. 168-170, 171, 177-178, 187)

With normal aerobic exercise, the heart rate and systolic blood pressure both rise. Diastolic blood pressure, however, typically does not change significantly. During *isometric* exercise, both systolic and diastolic blood pressures may increase. In normal individuals, the cardiac output rises fourfold to sixfold above basal levels during maximum exercise. The physiologic response to physical activity often becomes attenuated as an individual ages. The heart rate response to exercise is blunted in the elderly, and the predicted maximum heart rate decreases with age (estimated by 220 – age in years). This is due in part to decreased beta-adrenergic responsiveness in older individuals. The average stroke volume is preserved in normal older adults, and the observed decline in maximum cardiac output is due primarily to the blunted heart rate response. Maximal aerobic capacity ($\dot{V}_{O_2}$max) declines 8% to 10% per decade in sedentary individuals, such that there is a 50% fall between ages 30 and 80. Thus, the exercise protocol chosen to test elderly individuals should take into account predicted limitations in exertional capacity.

ANSWER TO QUESTION 29

D (Braunwald, pp. 115-118, 121-124, 1473-1474, 1490-1493, 1499-1504, 1520-1512; Table 12-6)

The intensity of a heart murmur is related to the pressure gradient and rate of flow across the responsible orifice. Physiologic changes or bedside maneuvers that alter the driving pressure gradient or the rate of flow lead to audible changes in murmur intensity. In acute mitral regurgitation (MR), flow is directed backward from the left ventricle into a relatively noncompliant left atrium, leading to a rapid increase in left atrial pressure during systole. Because this abolishes the pressure gradient between the left ventricle and left atrium in late systole, the murmur of acute MR is often present only in early systole. Similarly, in acute aortic regurgitation, the left ventricular (LV) diastolic pressure rises rapidly, leading to cessation of the diastolic murmur in mid to late diastole, as LV and aortic pressures equalize. In patients with mitral valve prolapse, the auscultatory findings vary prominently with physiologic alterations. The valve physically prolapses into the left atrium, and the associated click/murmur commences when the reduction of LV volume during contraction reaches the point at which the mitral leaflets fail to coapt. Maneuvers that decrease LV volume, such as standing from a squatting position, cause the valve prolapse, the click, and the murmur to all occur earlier in systole. In mitral stenosis, the diastolic rumbling murmur increases with any maneuver that augments transvalvular flow and decreases in situations that reduce transmitral flow, such as the strain phase of the Valsalva maneuver.

The systolic murmurs of aortic valvular stenosis and MR are sometimes difficult to distinguish. However, the intensity of aortic stenosis varies from beat to beat when the duration of diastole is not constant, as in atrial fibrillation or after a premature contraction. The murmur of MR is not affected in this manner, because the changes in driving pressure between the left ventricle and the left atrium are smaller.

ANSWER TO QUESTION 30

C (Braunwald, pp. 373, 1319-1335)

This computed tomogram demonstrates a type A aortic dissection involving the ascending (large arrow, A) and descending (small arrows, A) thoracic aorta. In addition, the dissection extends into the aortic arch vessels (large arrows, B), the left common carotid artery (small arrow, B), and the innominate artery (arrowhead, B). Dissection membranes are clearly visualized in the involved segments. Acute aortic dissection is a rare but often lethal illness. Survival depends on prompt clinical recognition and definitive imaging of the aorta. Stanford type A aortic dissections involve the ascending aorta. Type B aortic dissections do not involve the ascending aorta. The most common symptom of acute aortic dissection is chest or back pain, reported in up to 96% of patients. The pain is typically sudden in onset and severe, often with a "ripping" or "tearing" quality. The patient discussed in this question may have also presented with pulse deficits or neurologic symptoms, given the branch artery involvement demonstrated on the computed tomogram. Consensus guidelines regarding the diagnosis and management of thoracic aortic dissections were published in 2010.[1] Computed tomography (CT) and magnetic resonance imaging (MRI) have outstanding sensitivity for the diagnosis of aortic dissection, on the order of 96% to 100%. Transesophageal echocardiography (TEE) is unnecessary in this case, but it is also an excellent imaging modality for the diagnosis of aortic dissection (sensitivity of ~98% and specificity of 94% to 97%), with the caveat that visualization of the distal ascending aorta and proximal aortic arch may be limited by interference by the trachea and bronchus. Conversely, the sensitivity of standard transthoracic echocardiography for aortic dissection is relatively poor (59% to 85%). Aortography is rarely necessary and has inferior diagnostic capabilities for aortic dissection compared with CT and MRI. Because of its rapid availability in most emergency departments, CT is the initial diagnostic test of choice for suggested aortic dissection in many centers.

All patients with acute aortic dissection should receive immediate parenteral therapy for hypertension, such as intravenous beta blockers to provide rate control, after which vasodilators can be added as needed to control blood pressure. Patients with acute type A aortic dissection should be referred for emergent surgery. Surgery is also the treatment of choice for patients with acute type B aortic dissection complicated by vital organ compromise, rupture or impending aortic rupture, retrograde extension into the ascending aorta, or Marfan syndrome. Patients with uncomplicated acute type B aortic dissections can typically be managed initially with parenteral agents for blood pressure control, monitoring in the coronary care unit, and serial imaging of the aorta to exclude retrograde extension or other indications for surgery and then converted to therapy with oral antihypertensive agents.

REFERENCE

1. Hiratzka LF: 2010 ACCF/AHA/AATS/ACR/ASA/SCA/SCAI/SIR/STS/SVM Guidelines for the diagnosis and management of patients with thoracic aortic disease: Executive summary. J Am Coll Cardiol 55:1509, 2010.

ANSWER TO QUESTION 31

D (Braunwald, pp. 172-177)

ST-segment displacement is the primary means by which ischemia is detected during exercise testing. ST-segment depression is the most common form of abnormal response, whereas ST-segment elevation in a lead without pathologic Q waves is found only in about 1% of patients with obstructive coronary disease. J point depressions with upsloping ST segments are a normal finding during exercise. Patients with ischemic heart disease usually display true ST-segment depression with a horizontal or downsloping configuration. The correct isoelectric reference point for the ST segment is the TP segment. However, because this segment is shortened during exercise, the PQ junction is typically chosen as the reference point instead. In normal individuals who have an early repolarization pattern on the resting ECG, the chronically elevated J point usually returns to baseline during exercise. In this setting, any ST-segment deviations during exercise should be referenced to the PQ junction, not to the original J point position. Ischemic ST-segment depressions may develop only during exercise or may occur during exercise and persist into recovery. In 10% of patients, ischemic changes are observed only during the recovery phase. The onset of ST-segment changes during recovery occurs more commonly in asymptomatic individuals compared with those with symptomatic coronary artery disease. An abnormal ST-segment response is considered to be 0.10 mV (1 mm) or greater of J point depression, with a flat or downsloping ST segment that remains depressed to 0.10 mV or greater at 80 milliseconds after the J point.

Although ST-segment *elevation* is helpful to localize ischemia to particular coronary territories, the location of ST-segment *depression* during exercise does not accurately predict the responsible coronary anatomy.

ANSWER TO QUESTION 32

C (Braunwald, pp. 135, 141-145, 156, 162-163; Tables 13-5 and 13-6)

This ECG demonstrates extreme right-axis deviation of the QRS complex and an abnormally rightward P wave axis (the P waves are inverted in leads I and aVL). Although this pattern might suggest dextrocardia with situs inversus, the normal progression of the R waves in the precordial leads is not consistent with that diagnosis (in dextrocardia R wave progression would be reversed). Rather, the tracing is most consistent with right and left arm lead reversal, a common error of lead placement. In this situation, the recordings from leads aVL and aVR are interchanged and the complexes in lead I are the mirror image of what would be expected in that lead had the limb leads been placed correctly. Figure 1-66 here shows the ECG from the same patient with the leads placed correctly.

ANSWER TO QUESTION 33

D (Braunwald, pp. 168-172, 177-178)

An understanding of the differences between stress testing protocols is required to choose the appropriate study for a specific patient. Six to 12 minutes of progressive exercise, leading to a level of maximal oxygen consumption, provides the greatest diagnostic and prognostic information. An optimal exercise study is characterized by an appropriate rise in both heart rate and systolic

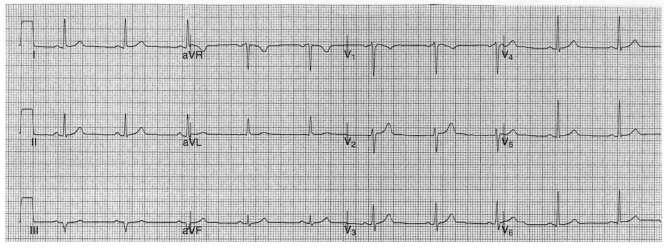

FIGURE 1-66

blood pressure. The diastolic blood pressure may fall, rise, or stay the same, depending on the protocol used and the workload achieved. When systolic blood pressure falls during exercise, it is often indicative of severe underlying coronary artery disease (typically three-vessel or left main disease) or severe left ventricular (LV) contractile dysfunction. Other potential causes include LV outflow obstruction (e.g., advanced aortic stenosis or hypertrophic obstructive cardiomyopathy) and hypovolemia.

Treadmill protocols are the most commonly used form of stress testing and are characterized by achievement of high maximum heart rates and oxygen consumption. Bicycle protocols are sometimes better tolerated by deconditioned patients because of the ramped nature of the test and achieve maximum heart rates similar to, but maximal oxygen consumption less than, treadmill tests. Arm crank ergometry can be useful for patients who cannot perform leg exercise, such as patients with severe peripheral arterial disease. Arm protocols typically produce a higher heart rate and blood pressure response for a given workload than leg exercise protocols; however, the maximum heart rate achieved during arm ergometry testing is typically only about 70% of that achieved during treadmill or bicycle tests. Maximal oxygen consumption and minute ventilation are also lower for arm cycling than for leg exercise. The standard treadmill Bruce protocol is the most commonly used, and a large diagnostic and prognostic database has been accumulated with this regimen. The primary limitation of the Bruce protocol is the large increase in oxygen consumption from one stage to the next, which limits the utility of this protocol in elderly, deconditioned, or ill individuals. In such patients a more gradual regimen, such as the Naughton or Weber protocol, using 1- to 2-minute stages with 1-MET increases per stage, or a ramped bicycle protocol with small increases in workload each minute, is typically better tolerated.

REFERENCE

Gibbons RJ, Balady GJ, Bricker JT, et al: ACC/AHA 2002 guideline update for exercise testing: Summary article. A report of the American College of Cardiology/American Heart Association Task Force on Practice Guidelines (Committee to Update the 1997 Exercise Testing Guidelines). J Am Coll Cardiol 40:1531, 2002.

ANSWER TO QUESTION 34

D (Braunwald, pp. 107-108, 121-124, 1420, 1426-1428, 1472-1473, 1494-1495)

The development of new exertional dyspnea in a patient with cardiac disease may herald progression or a change in the clinical syndrome. Each of the patients in this question has a known, previously asymptomatic cardiac lesion and has recently developed shortness of breath with physical activities. A congenitally bicuspid aortic valve often becomes progressively stenotic with age, and symptoms associated with aortic stenosis (angina, syncope, heart failure) frequently develop in mid to late adulthood. A patient with a history of myocardial infarction who presents with new dyspnea without recurrent angina is likely to have developed left ventricular (LV) dysfunction due to ventricular remodeling. Other potential contributing factors include dyspnea as an anginal equivalent or a superimposed arrhythmia. New irregular palpitations in a patient with a history of rheumatic heart disease may indicate superimposed atrial fibrillation. This is a poorly tolerated complication in patients with mitral stenosis because of the abbreviated LV diastolic filling period during rapid heart rates.

Most young adults with an uncomplicated ostium secundum atrial septal defect (ASD) have normal exercise tolerance. Previously asymptomatic ostium secundum ASDs, in the absence of pulmonary hypertension, are typically well tolerated during pregnancy. Although problems may arise because of paradoxical embolism in the setting of lower extremity venous thrombosis, symptoms of ventricular dysfunction or reversed shunting across the ASD are rare. Exertional dyspnea in the third trimester of pregnancy in such patients is more likely the result of impaired diaphragmatic excursion from the increasing size of the uterus.

The most common causes of morbidity and mortality in trisomy 21 (Down syndrome) are congenital heart defects, which are present in 40% to 50% of patients. The most characteristic abnormalities are endocardial cushion defects, such as ostium primum ASD and "cleft" mitral valve with mitral regurgitation. Approximately one third of the congenital heart lesions are complex defects that are detected early, but simpler cardiac anomalies may remain unnoticed into adulthood. The new onset of exertional dyspnea in a patient with trisomy 21 warrants a full cardiac evaluation, including careful echocardiographic study.

ANSWER TO QUESTION 35

B (Braunwald, pp. 149-159; Fig. 13-35)

Early recognition of myocardial infarction (MI) is critical to take full advantage of emergent percutaneous revascularization or fibrinolytic therapy. The earliest electrocardiographic finding in acute ST-elevation MI is ST-segment elevation and hyperacute (tall, positive) T waves overlying the affected region of myocardium. Reciprocal ST-segment depressions are often noted in leads overlying the opposite cardiac territories. In the absence of reperfusion therapy, T wave inversions become evident in the leads overlying the region of infarction over a matter of hours, accompanied by Q wave development. In the case of an anterior Q wave MI, the early ST- segment deflections become apparent in the anterior precordial leads, whereas ST-segment depressions are often present in the inferior leads. A normal ECG at the time of presentation does not exclude an acute infarction; however, it is unlikely that the ECG would remain normal over hours in the presence of ongoing transmural ischemia. Acute infarction affecting portions of the conduction system may produce a new bundle branch block. The presence of a new right bundle branch block (RBBB) does not obscure the diagnosis of an acute MI, because the ST-segment elevations in the precordium should remain interpretable. However, the ST-segment and T wave changes that accompany a new left bundle branch block (LBBB) typically mask the ST-segment and T wave changes of acute infarction, making the diagnosis more difficult. In a patient with a convincing history of prolonged ischemic chest discomfort, a new LBBB is an acceptable criterion of acute infarction. Interestingly, appearance of a new RBBB during an acute anterior MI has been shown to portend a worse prognosis than a new LBBB in fibrinolytic[1,2] and interventional studies.[3]

A shortened QT interval is typical of hypercalcemia, not acute MI.

REFERENCES

1. Go AS, Barron HV, Rundle AC, et al: Bundle-branch block and in-hospital mortality in acute myocardial infarction. National Registry of Myocardial Infarction 2 Investigators. Ann Intern Med 129:690, 1998.
2. Wong CK, Stewart RA, Gao W, et al: Prognostic differences between different types of bundle branch block during the early phase of acute myocardial infarction: Insights from the Hirulog and Early Reperfusion or Occlusion (HERO)-2 trial. Eur Heart J 27:21, 2006.
3. Kurisu S, Inoue I, Kawagoe T, et al: Right bundle-branch block in anterior acute myocardial infarction in the coronary intervention era: Acute angiographic findings and prognosis. Int J Cardiology 116:57, 2007.

ANSWER TO QUESTION 36

C (Braunwald, pp. 294, 305-306, 326-330)

Myocardial perfusion imaging with either thallium-201– or technetium-99m–labeled compounds (e.g., technetium-99m sestamibi) is useful for the detection of myocardial ischemia and infarction (MI), to characterize infarct size (which predicts future ventricular remodeling), and to determine the effectiveness of acute revascularization. Nuclear imaging is also useful for early risk stratification after an acute MI. The size of the resting myocardial perfusion defect correlates with prognosis: the larger the defect, the worse the outcome.

Certain resting image patterns seen after acute MI, such as increased lung uptake of thallium-201, have been associated with an unfavorable prognosis because they are indicative of impaired left ventricular function. Lastly, pharmacologic stress testing with nuclear imaging after an acute MI has been shown to be safe and to predict in-hospital and late cardiac complications better than submaximal exercise stress imaging. Gated single-photon emission computed tomography (SPECT) myocardial perfusion imaging allows for determination of left ventricular function, which adds additional prognostic information in the management of the postinfarction patient.

REFERENCE

Dilsizian V: SPECT and PET perfusion imaging: Tracers and techniques. In Dilsizian V, Narula J, Braunwald E (eds): Atlas of Nuclear Cardiology. 3rd ed. Philadelphia, Current Medicine, 2009, pp 37-60.

ANSWER TO QUESTION 37

C (Braunwald, p. 175; see also Answer to Question 31)

The development of ST-segment elevation during exercise testing is predictive of the presence of transmural ischemia owing to vasospasm or a high-grade coronary narrowing. It is quite uncommon, occurring in only about 1% of patients with obstructive coronary artery disease. In contrast to ST-segment depression, the development of ST-segment elevation is useful in localizing the anatomic site of ischemia and typically correlates with a perfusion defect on imaging studies. In patients with early repolarization, the normal response is for the elevated J points to return to baseline during exercise.

ST-segment elevation during exercise testing does not have predictive significance when it occurs in leads that contain pathologic Q waves. In that situation, it may represent a region of myocardial scar with a resting wall motion abnormality.

There is no direct association between exercise-induced ST-segment elevation and the development of conduction system abnormalities.

ANSWER TO QUESTION 38

E (Braunwald, pp. 365-368)

Assessment of coronary artery calcification by electron beam tomography (EBT) using electrocardiographic gating is a technique to screen for coronary artery disease (CAD). Although coronary artery calcification is a surrogate marker for coronary atherosclerotic plaque, the correlation between the amount of coronary calcium and the actual angiographic severity of the CAD is weak. The complete absence of coronary calcification on EBT has a strong negative predictive value for high-grade coronary stenosis but does not completely rule out the presence of significant CAD. The Agatston score is the most frequently used system for reporting the severity of coronary artery calcifications, and reference data sets for interpretation are stratified by age and gender. Annual rates of myocardial infarction or cardiovascular death rise with increasing Agatston scores, even in patients with similar Framingham risk scores. Coronary EBT is of most clinical value for patients who are at *intermediate* risk for coronary events based on traditional cardiovascular risk factors and for whom an abnormal scan will have an impact on clinical management. There is currently no role for serial assessment of coronary calcification with EBT in clinical practice.

REFERENCE

Greenland P, Bonow RO, Brundage BH, et al: ACC/AHA 2007 clinical expert consensus document on coronary artery calcium scoring by computer tomography in global cardiovascular risk assessment and in evaluation of patients with chest pain. J Am Coll Cardiol 49:378, 2007.

ANSWER TO QUESTION 39

A (Braunwald, pp. 294-302, 310-316, 320-329)

Myocardial perfusion imaging provides an important source of prognostic information in patients with coronary artery disease (CAD). Stress myocardial perfusion imaging has been shown to be a powerful predictor of subsequent cardiac events. The combination of clinical and myocardial perfusion data is more predictive than the combination of clinical and cardiac catheterization data. Indeed, even when angiographic CAD is present, a normal myocardial perfusion study confers a very low risk of a subsequent cardiovascular event (<1% per year).

Stress perfusion defects in multiple locations corresponding to multiple vascular territories are suggestive of left main or three-vessel coronary artery disease. Other indicators of high-risk coronary artery disease include large defects, transient pulmonary uptake of tracer, and left ventricular cavity dilatation with exercise. The severity of a myocardial perfusion defect can be assessed in terms of both its size and the extent of its reversibility. A severe defect is one that has little or no uptake with stress imaging, whereas a mild defect may have only a slight reduction in counts with stress. The severity of defects as well as their number and size are important indicators of prognosis. The predictive value of myocardial perfusion imaging is independent of the imaging technique (planar or single-photon emission computed tomography) and the imaging agent used (thallium-201 or technetium-99m sestamibi), with one important exception. There is a decreased likelihood of significant breast attenuation artifact with the use of technetium-99m sestamibi imaging in women, and this imaging agent is preferable in female patients.

REFERENCES

1. Klocke FJ, Baird MG, Lorell BH, et al: ACC/AHA/ASNC guidelines for the clinical use of cardiac radionuclide imaging: A report of the American College of Cardiology/American Heart Association Task Force on Practice Guidelines (ACC/AHA/ASNC Committee to Revise the 1995 Guidelines for the Clinical Use of Radionuclide Imaging). J Am Coll Cardiol 42:1318, 2003.
2. Dilsizian V: SPECT and PET perfusion imaging: Tracers and techniques. *In* Dilsizian V, Narula J, Braunwald E (eds): Atlas of Nuclear Cardiology. 3rd ed. Philadelphia, Current Medicine, 2009, pp 37-60.

ANSWER TO QUESTION 40

A (Braunwald, pp. 351-352)

Cardiac magnetic resonance (CMR) imaging is an excellent technique to define pericardial abnormalities. It is highly sensitive for the detection of pericardial fluid, masses, and pericardial thickening. The T1-weighted spin-echo CMR image in this case demonstrates diffuse encasement of the heart by a structure within the pericardium that has intermediate signal intensity resembling myocardial tissue (labeled with asterisks in Fig. 1-67). This abnormality is homogeneous in signal intensity such that organized hematoma is unlikely. The features are most consistent with pericardial malignancy.

Biopsy of the affected region demonstrated pericardial angiosarcoma. This is a rare primary pericardial

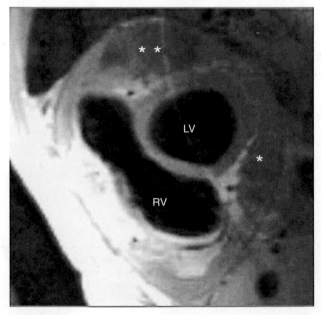

FIGURE 1-67

malignancy that arises from the pericardial vasculature and typically does not metastasize. However, it usually proliferates widely throughout the pericardial cavity and may invade the myocardium. This case was considered inoperable at surgery and the patient died 4 days after presentation.

REFERENCE

Hundley WG, et al: ACCF/SCCT/ACR/AHA/ASNC/NASCI/ SCMR 2010 Expert consensus document on cardiovascular magnetic resonance: A report of the American College of Cardiology Foundation Task Force on Expert Consensus Documents. J Am Coll Cardiol 56:2614, 2010.

ANSWER TO QUESTION 41

C (Braunwald, pp. 396-398, 400-401)

In a normal individual, systemic and pulmonary cardiac outputs are approximately equal. In the presence of an intracardiac shunt, blood flows abnormally between the pulmonary and systemic circulations. Although many shunts are suspected before cardiac catheterization, certain findings during the procedure may point to unexpected intracardiac communications. For example, suspicion for a left-to-right shunt should be raised if the pulmonary artery oxygen saturation exceeds 80% or if the difference in oxygen saturation between the superior vena cava (SVC) and the pulmonary artery is 8% or more. A right-to-left shunt should be considered if the systemic arterial saturation is < 93% without any other reason.

Normally, the oxygen saturation in the inferior vena cava (IVC) is higher than that in the SVC. Mixed venous saturation is most accurately determined in the pulmonary artery, because complete mixing of venous return has occurred at that level. However, if one is assessing a transatrial shunt with left-to-right flow, the mixed venous saturation must be determined proximal to the shunt and can be estimated by the Flamm formula, measuring oxygen content in the SVC and IVC:

$$\text{Mixed venous oxygen content} = \frac{3(\text{SVC O}_2 \text{ content}) + 1(\text{IVC O}_2 \text{ content})}{4}$$

The ratio of pulmonic to systemic blood flow (Qp/Qs) is used to determine the significance of an intracardiac shunt. A Qp/Qs of <1 indicates net right-to-left shunting. A Qp/Qs of 2.0 or more indicates a large left-to-right shunt that generally requires repair. A Qp/Qs of 1.0 to 1.5 indicates a small left-to-right shunt.

ANSWER TO QUESTION 42

C (Braunwald, pp. 247-250, 1582-1588; Fig. 15-66)

The pulsed-wave Doppler spectrum in the illustration demonstrates late systolic acceleration of flow characteristic of left ventricular outflow tract (LVOT) obstruction, typically seen in patients with hypertrophic cardiomyopathy. This abnormal Doppler signal ("dagger" pattern) is detected in the LVOT and peaks significantly later than that of valvular aortic stenosis, owing to the dynamic nature of the obstruction. Because the disorder is at the subvalvular level, there is no therapeutic role for aortic valve surgery.

The LVOT obstruction may be worsened by any action that decreases left ventricular volume and narrows the distance between the interventricular septum and the anterior mitral leaflet, including volume depletion. Although compression stockings may redistribute volume and increase venous return, such therapy is typically not sufficient to prevent or treat LVOT obstruction. Similarly, bed rest has no specific role in the management of hypertrophic cardiomyopathy.

ANSWER TO QUESTION 43

A (Braunwald, pp. 251-256, 351-352, 1655-1660; Figs. 75-8 and 75-9)

Echocardiography is an excellent technique to detect and grossly quantify the volume of pericardial effusions. The normal pericardial space contains 35 to 50 mL of serous fluid between the visceral and parietal pericardial layers. Small pathologic effusions tend to accumulate posteriorly, external to the left ventricular free wall, because of the effects of gravity. Larger effusions tend to circumscribe the heart. Certain echocardiographic features are good indicators of the presence of cardiac tamponade physiology in patients with pericardial effusion. These include early diastolic collapse of the right ventricle, which indicates the presence of elevated intrapericardial pressure (see Braunwald, Fig. 75-8). However, right ventricular (RV) diastolic collapse may be absent in clinical tamponade if pulmonary hypertension or RV hypertrophy is present, because these forces oppose RV indentation. Diastolic invagination of the right atrium (see Braunwald, Fig. 75-9) is a more sensitive, but less specific, marker of tamponade physiology. Doppler interrogation can also provide clues to the presence of tamponade, including exaggerated respiratory variation of transvalvular velocities (see Answer to Question 6).

Transthoracic echocardiographic imaging is often inadequate in direct assessment of the thickness of the pericardium; transesophageal echocardiography, computed tomography, and magnetic resonance imaging are more accurate techniques for this purpose.

ANSWER TO QUESTION 44

E (Braunwald, pp. 302, 310-311, 316-319, 320-325, 327, 334)

Although nuclear stress testing is commonly used in the evaluation of women with suspected coronary artery disease (CAD), there is the possibility of breast attenuation artifact in female patients. The use of technetium-99m–based agents with single-photon emission computer tomography imaging and electrocardiographic gating reduce the likelihood of a false-positive study due to such artifact, thereby increasing the specificity of nuclear testing in women. Breast attenuation artifact typically appears as a fixed defect of the anterior or anterolateral wall. If this defect is due to artifact rather than prior infarction, the involved segment(s) will demonstrate normal wall motion on the gated images (see Braunwald, Fig. 17-12, and Answer to Question 11).

Patients with left bundle branch block (LBBB) may demonstrate artifactual exercise-induced perfusion defects, especially in the septal and anteroapical regions. Pharmacologic stress testing with dipyridamole or adenosine minimizes the incidence of such artifacts. Thus it is recommended that patients with complete LBBB on the ECG be evaluated by vasodilatory agents, rather than an exercise protocol, to avoid false-positive results.

Nuclear imaging is a useful modality for preoperative risk stratification before noncardiac surgery, especially for patients at intermediate clinical risk.[1] For example, dipyridamole stress testing with perfusion imaging is predictive of perioperative cardiac events and the magnitude of risk correlates with the extent of ischemia. Patients with diabetes are at increased risk for CAD and its complications, and perfusion defects during testing predict higher event rates in diabetics compared with nondiabetics.[2]

In patients with CAD, assessment of myocardial viability is often of great importance in defining revascularization options. Modalities for the determination of myocardial viability include thallium-201 imaging, magnetic resonance imaging, dobutamine echocardiography, and positron emission tomography.[3]

REFERENCES

1. Fleisher LA, Beckman JA, Brown KA, et al: ACC/AHA 2007 guidelines on perioperative cardiovascular evaluation and care for noncardiac surgery. Circulation 116:e418, 2007.
2. Young LH, Wackers FJ, Chyun DA, et al: Cardiac outcomes after screening for asymptomatic coronary artery disease in patients with type 2 diabetes. JAMA 301:1547, 2009.
3. Partington SL, Kwong RY, Dorbala S: Multimodality imaging in the assessment of myocardial viability. Heart Fail Rev 16:381-395, 2011.

ANSWER TO QUESTION 45

B (Braunwald, pp. 343-346)

In this delayed cardiac magnetic resonance (CMR) image, the midseptum and midanterior segments of the left ventricle demonstrate subendocardial late enhancement (the bright area indicated by the white arrows in Fig. 1-68) that involves approximately half of the transmural thickness of the myocardium. This finding, as well as the matching wall motion abnormality by echocardiography, is most consistent with a prior nontransmural myocardial infarction (MI). The presence of MI (acute or old) can be determined accurately using the protocol of late enhancement, which involves injecting intravenous gadolinium and performing CMR after a delay. Gadolinium is an extracellular contrast agent that only minimally

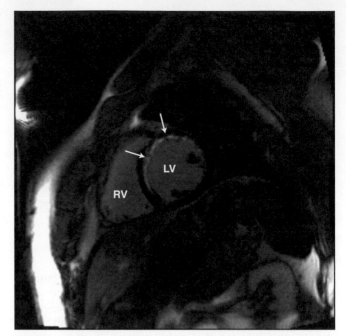

FIGURE 1-68

enters normal myocardial cells. However, disrupted myocardium after an MI allows expansion of the volume of distribution and delayed entry of the contrast agent into the affected region. A subendocardial distribution is indicative of myocardial infarction. Both conventional CMR and late gadolinium enhancement are useful in assessing myocardial viability, to help determine whether a segment of poorly contracting myocardium would benefit from mechanical revascularization. For example, improved wall thickening with low-dose dobutamine CMR correlates well with the presence of viable myocardium. With the late gadolinium enhancement technique, a transmural extent of MI (i.e., region of late enhancement) of <50% is also predictive of functional recovery after revascularization.

REFERENCE

Hundley WG, Bluemke DA, Finn JP, et al: ACCF/ACR/AHA/NASCI/SCMR 2010 Expert consensus document on cardiovascular magnetic resonance: A report of the American College of Cardiology Foundation Task Force on Expert Consensus Documents. J Am Coll Cardiol 55:2614, 2010.

ANSWER TO QUESTION 46

B (Braunwald, pp. 230-231, 234-236, 398, 1474)

As with most stenotic valvular lesions, echocardiographic evaluation of aortic stenosis is accurate and clinically useful. The morphology of the valve can be examined by two-dimensional imaging to assess for congenital or rheumatic abnormalities or age-related changes of valvular architecture. The peak outflow velocity is then measured using continuous-wave Doppler imaging. Important aortic stenosis usually results in outflow velocities of

3.5 m/sec or greater, which is out of the range for accurate quantification by pulsed-wave Doppler imaging. From the continuous-wave Doppler measurement, both the peak and mean gradients can be determined using the modified Bernoulli equation (see Braunwald, Figs. 15-36 and 15-44). The peak instantaneous gradient measured by Doppler imaging reflects the true maximum pressure difference between the left ventricle and aorta. The peak-to-peak gradient measured in the catheterization laboratory has no actual physiologic basis and does not directly correspond to the echocardiographically measured values—the peak instantaneous gradient routinely exceeds the peak-to-peak valve gradient. Conversely, the mean gradients measured noninvasively and in the catheterization laboratory show excellent agreement, because they both measure the difference in pressure between the left ventricular (LV) and aorta averaged throughout systole.

The aortic valve area can be calculated using the continuity equation (see Braunwald, Fig. 15-38), comparing the volume rate of flow across the left ventricular outflow tract (LVOT) with that through the aortic valve. The greatest potential error introduced into this calculation resides in inaccurate measurement of the LVOT diameter (see Braunwald, Fig. 15-37). In practice, a peak transaortic valvular gradient >50 mm Hg correlates with clinically significant aortic stenosis. Similarly, a patient with normal LV contractile function and a low gradient is unlikely to have significant stenosis. However, in the presence of impaired LV function, a more modest gradient (corresponding to transvalvular velocities of 2 to 3 m/sec) may be clinically important, and calculation of the aortic valve area by the continuity equation can be very helpful in this case.

REFERENCES

Bonow RO, Carabello BA, Chatterjee K, et al: 2008 focused update incorporated into the ACC/AHA 2006 guidelines for the management of patients with valvular heart disease. A report of the American College of Cardiology/American Heart Association Task Force on Practice Guidelines (writing committee to revise the 1998 guidelines for the management of patients with valvular heart disease) endorsed by the Society of Cardiovascular Anesthesiologists, Society for Cardiovascular Angiography and Interventions, and Society of Thoracic Surgeons. Circulation 118:e523, 2008.

Baumgartner H, Hung J, Bermejo J, et al: Echocardiographic assessment of valve stenosis: EAE/ASE recommendations for clinical practice. J Am Soc Echocardiogr 22:1, 2009.

ANSWER TO QUESTION 47

E (Braunwald, pp. 400-401)

Detection and localization of intracardiac shunts is possible at catheterization by a traditional oximetry run, in which samples are drawn at numerous sites in the right side of the heart and adjacent vessels. The technique involves measurement of O_2 saturations to identify a significant step-up between consecutive chambers. Using averaged samples, an O_2 saturation step-up of ≥7% is necessary to diagnose a left-to-right shunt at the atrial level, whereas one ≥5% suffices at the level of the right ventricle or pulmonary artery. The data obtained in the course of an oximetry run may be used to quantify shunt size. Pulmonary and systemic blood flows can be calculated using the standard Fick equation. The ratio of pulmonary to systemic blood flow (Qp/Qs) is used to determine the significance of a shunt. A Qp/Qs of <1.5 indicates a small left-to-right shunt. A Qp/Qs of 2.0 or more indicates a large left-to-right shunt that generally warrants percutaneous or surgical closure. Because of normal variability in O_2 saturation, left-to-right shunts with Qp/Qs ≤1.3 at the pulmonary artery or right ventricular levels and those with Qp/Qs <1.5 at the atrial level may not be detected. A QpQs of <1 indicates a net right-to-left shunt (e.g., as may be the case in tetralogy of Fallot). For unidirectional shunts, the magnitude of the shunt can also be expressed by the difference Qp − Qs. From this calculation, it can be deduced that a negative value will occur with pure right-to-left shunts.

REFERENCE

Baim DS (ed): Grossman's Cardiac Catheterization, Angiography, and Intervention. 7th ed. Baltimore, Lippincott Williams & Wilkins, 2006, pp 163-172.

ANSWER TO QUESTION 48

C (Braunwald, pp. 172-178, 184; Table 14-4)

The exercise ECG is very likely to be abnormal in patients with severe coronary artery disease (CAD). There are several abnormalities that are suggestive of multivessel CAD and an adverse prognosis. These include the early onset of ischemic ST-segment depression, such as that occurring during the first stage of a standard Bruce protocol. In addition, ST-segment depression of ≥2 mm (0.20 mV) involving five or more leads, or persisting ≥5 minutes into recovery, is suggestive of more severe underlying coronary atherosclerosis. Exercise-induced ST-segment elevation is also consistent with multivessel CAD, except in lead aVR, which may demonstrate ST-segment elevation in a variety of circumstances, including less severe coronary disease. A failure to increase systolic blood pressure by 10 mm Hg, or a sustained decrease in systolic blood pressure of 10 mm Hg or more, is suggestive of multivessel (or left main) CAD and an adverse prognosis. Multifocal premature ventricular contractions occurring during exercise in and of themselves are not correlated with extensive disease, but reproducible sustained or symptomatic ventricular tachycardia is highly suggestive of multivessel CAD.

ANSWER TO QUESTION 49

D (Braunwald, pp. 117-118, 123; Table 12-6)

Squatting increases venous return to the heart and ventricular stroke volume. The resultant augmented flow and turbulence across the stenotic aortic valve increase the intensity of the murmur. In distinction, during the early phase of the Valsalva maneuver, venous return (and therefore stroke volume) is decreased so that the intensity of the murmur of aortic stenosis (AS) lessens. Amyl nitrite causes vasodilatation followed by reflex tachycardia; the augmented cardiac output intensifies the murmur of AS.

The systolic murmur of AS can be confused with mitral regurgitation. However, if the patient has an irregular rhythm or premature ventricular contractions, beat-to-beat variations in diastolic filling of the left ventricle result in changes of the intensity of the AS murmur, whereas the murmur of MR does not demonstrate such variability. Respiration has little effect on the intensity of left-sided heart murmurs, including AS, but can accentuate most right-sided murmurs, including tricuspid regurgitation.

ANSWER TO QUESTION 50

B (Braunwald, pp. 107-108, 1076-1079; Table 53-1)

This man has classic findings of chest discomfort caused by esophageal reflux and spasm. Differentiation of esophageal disorders from ischemic heart disease can be difficult, because the sensations are often located in similar areas and both can be associated with emotional stress. However, although each condition may produce substernal burning, features in this case are more suggestive of an esophageal rather than cardiac origin. These include a prolonged continuous ache, a discomfort that is primarily retrosternal but does not radiate toward the arms, and the fact the symptom is not precipitated by exercise but occurs while recumbent. Classically, esophageal disease associated with regurgitation causes "water brash," a taste in the mouth consistent with regurgitation of gastric contents. Frequently, patients with esophageal spasm experience some relief with nitroglycerin. Unlike angina due to myocardial ischemia, however, esophageal pain is often relieved by milk, antacids, or food. Biliary colic also may be confused with angina pectoris. It is usually caused by a rapid rise in biliary pressure due to obstruction of the cystic or bile ducts. Thus, the pain is usually abrupt in onset and steady in nature and lasts from minutes to hours. In many cases, the discomfort is described as colicky. It should be suspected when a history of dyspepsia, fatty food intolerance, and indigestion is present.

The chest discomfort of pericarditis is typically described as sharp, stabbing, or knife like. Pain due to pericarditis is often localized in the substernal or apical areas and can radiate to the neck or left shoulder. The pain is often worsened by deep breathing or lying in a supine position. Patients may find relief from the chest discomfort of pericarditis by sitting up and leaning forward.

ANSWER TO QUESTION 51

E (Braunwald, pp. 177-178, 300-302)

The perfusion images display a large region of reversible ischemia in the anteroseptal territory, in the distribution of the left anterior descending coronary artery. In addition, compared with the rest images, there are additional postexercise abnormalities, including dilatation of the left ventricular (LV) cavity (best seen on the short-axis images), increased right ventricular tracer uptake (most evident in the horizontal long-axis images), and increased lung uptake. Transient dilatation of the LV cavity after stress is associated with extensive and severe coronary artery disease. It is thought to represent diffuse subendocardial ischemia resulting in an apparent LV dilatation, rather than true cavity enlargement. Increased pulmonary radiotracer uptake after stress is a marker of elevated LV end-diastolic pressure and is predictive of a poor prognosis. It is usually associated with multivessel coronary artery disease (CAD), depressed LV function, and extensive ischemia. Increased right ventricular tracer uptake on the post-stress images, compared with the rest images, is a specific marker of severe multivessel or left main disease. Finally, a fall in systolic blood pressure of 10 mm Hg or more during exercise is also predictive of left main or three-vessel CAD.

In this case, all of these findings are present, along with a large and severe reversible perfusion defect, indicative of severe CAD despite failure to achieve the target heart rate.

ANSWER TO QUESTION 52

B (Braunwald, pp. 234-236, 237-238)

The Doppler tracing was obtained across the left ventricular outflow tract of a patient with combined aortic stenosis and aortic insufficiency. The tracing shows a characteristic delayed onset of peak velocity, consistent with significant aortic stenosis. The pressure gradient across the aortic valve can be calculated using the modified Bernoulli equation (pressure gradient $= 4 \times V^2$). The peak velocity across the aortic valve of approximately 4.8 m/sec in the figure corresponds to an instantaneous peak systolic gradient of 92 mm Hg. In general, when the aortic flow velocity is more than 4 m/sec, the probability of critical aortic stenosis is high. Similarly, a normal or slightly elevated aortic flow velocity is usually associated with only mild aortic stenosis. For aortic flow velocities that are intermediate, echocardiographic calculation of the aortic valve area or additional hemodynamic data are often needed.

The diastolic flow on this tracing represents aortic insufficiency. Severe aortic insufficiency is associated with a rapidly declining flow velocity, whereas mild aortic insufficiency demonstrates a gradually declining velocity. In this case, the decline in diastolic velocity is gradual and the degree of aortic insufficiency is likely mild. Unlike in this patient, premature diastolic closure of the mitral valve may be observed in patients with severe, acute aortic insufficiency owing to the greatly elevated diastolic left ventricular (LV) pressure.

Additional findings on the echocardiogram that may help assess the severity of aortic valve disease include measurements of LV size and thickness. In this patient with severe aortic stenosis one would expect to find concentric LV hypertrophy.

ANSWER TO QUESTION 53

B (Braunwald, pp. 78-79, 109-110, 123, 1420, 1432-1433)

Many congenital and acquired cardiac diseases are associated with abnormalities of the extremities. Arachnodactyly—abnormally long and slender digits—is a manifestation of Marfan syndrome. A common finding in arachnodactyly is that when a clenched fist is made around the thumb the latter extends beyond the ulnar side of the hand (the "thumb sign"). The Holt-Oram syndrome consists of an atrial septal defect and skeletal abnormalities, including deformities of the radius and ulna, and a "fingerized" thumb (i.e., the thumb has an extra phalanx). Characteristic extremity abnormalities associated with Turner syndrome include short stature and bowed arms.

Quincke sign, systolic flushing of the nail beds, is common in chronic aortic regurgitation and other conditions with a widened pulse pressure. It can be readily detected by pressing a flashlight against the terminal digits.

Osler nodes are small, tender erythematous skin lesions observed primarily on the pads of the fingers and toes but also on the palms of the hands and soles of the feet. They result from infective microemboli in patients with endocarditis. In contrast, Janeway lesions are slightly raised, nontender, hemorrhagic lesions on the palms of the hands and soles of the feet that may also appear in patients with infective endocarditis. Both types of lesions were more common in the preantibiotic era.

Differential cyanosis is the condition in which the hands and fingers are pink but the feet and toes are cyanotic. It is typical of patent ductus arteriosus with pulmonary hypertension and a reversed shunt, in which case desaturated blood is directed to the lower body.

ANSWER TO QUESTION 54

D (Braunwald, pp. 794, 1450-1452)

The echocardiographic image demonstrates an apical four-chamber view of a patient with Ebstein anomaly. Ebstein anomaly is a congenital malformation of the tricuspid valve characterized by elongation and tethering of the anterior leaflet ("sail-like" appearance) and apical displacement of a diminutive septal leaflet. This anomaly results in conversion of a portion of the right ventricle into an "atrialized" right ventricle. There is typically severe right atrial enlargement. Because of the structural deformity of the tricuspid valve, varying degrees of tricuspid regurgitation, and occasionally tricuspid stenosis, are present. The symptomatic presentation of patients with Ebstein anomaly depends on the severity of the valvular regurgitation and the presence of additional congenital heart lesions.

Ebstein anomaly is associated with a number of other congenital heart defects, including patent foramen ovale or atrial septal defect in approximately 50% of patients.

Up to 25% of patients with Ebstein anomaly will have an accessory conduction pathway (Wolff-Parkinson-White pattern on the ECG), which is typically right sided. Atrial arrhythmias, particularly atrial fibrillation and atrial flutter, are common.

Although coarctation of the aorta can rarely be associated with Ebstein anomaly, systemic hypertension is not a common finding among patients with this disorder.

REFERENCE

Connolly HM: Ebstein's anomaly. *In* Warnes CA (ed): Adult Congenital Heart Disease. Oxford, Blackwell Publishing, 2009.

ANSWER TO QUESTION 55

B (Braunwald, pp. 244-245, 1546-1549, 1554-1556; Table 67G-3)

Echocardiography plays a key role in the diagnosis and evaluation of infective endocarditis. The echocardiographic hallmark is the presence of a valvular vegetation, which is a collection of thrombus, necrotic valvular debris, inflammatory material, and bacteria. Typically, vegetations are located on the downstream, lower pressure side of the valve; however, large and aggressive lesions may involve both surfaces of the valve. Transesophageal echocardiography (TEE) is more sensitive than standard transthoracic study for detection of small vegetations in endocarditis. However, there is little additional diagnostic yield of TEE when a high-quality transthoracic study is completely normal, without evidence of valve thickening or pathologic regurgitation. Echocardiography also plays a critical role in the identification of structural and functional impairments that result from endocarditis. The degree of valvular destruction and regurgitation can be assessed, particularly with TEE, although, again, TEE is not mandatory if a high-quality transthoracic study provides all relevant information. TEE is more sensitive than transthoracic echocardiography for identification of myocardial abscess formation, valvular perforation, chordal rupture, and endocarditis of prosthetic valves.

Echocardiography can assist in determining whether corrective surgical intervention is appropriate in endocarditis, but the decision to operate should be made primarily on clinical grounds. Factors that predict poor outcome and favor earlier surgical intervention include a perivalvular abscess, intractable heart failure due to valve dysfunction, very large (>1 cm) and hypermobile vegetations, recurrent embolic events despite antibiotic therapy, infection by aggressive organisms, or persistent bacteremia (see Braunwald, Table 67G-3).

It is not necessary to routinely repeat echocardiography in the presence of clinical improvement, nor is it cost effective to do so. Residual vegetation often is evident despite bacteriologic cure, and the patient's clinical status, as well as repeat blood cultures after completion of an appropriate antibiotic course, should dictate further clinical decision making.

REFERENCES

Baddour LM, Wilson WR, Bayer AS, et al: Infective endocarditis: diagnosis, antimicrobial therapy, and management of complications: A statement of healthcare professionals from the Committee on Rheumatic Fever, Endocarditis, and Kawasaki Disease, Council on Cardiovascular Disease in the Young, and the Councils on Clinical Cardiology, Stroke, and Cardiovascular Surgery and Anesthesia, American Heart Association: Endorsed by the Infectious Diseases Society of America. Circulation 111:e394, 2005.

Bonow RO, Carabello BA, Chatterjee K, et al: 2008 focused update incorporated into the ACC/AHA 2006 guidelines for the management of patients with valvular heart disease. A report of the American College of Cardiology/American Heart Association Task Force on Practice Guidelines (writing committee to revise the 1998 guidelines for the management of patients with valvular heart disease): endorsed by the Society of Cardiovascular Anesthesiologists, Society for Cardiovascular Angiography and Interventions, and Society of Thoracic Surgeons. Circulation 118:e523, 2008.

ANSWER TO QUESTION 56

D (Braunwald, pp. 110-114; Fig. 12-5)

The volume and contour of the arterial pulse depend in part on the left ventricular stroke volume, the ejection velocity, and the compliance and capacity of the arterial system. Pulsus parvus et tardus—a small pulse with a delayed systolic peak—is characteristically seen in severe aortic stenosis and is best appreciated by palpating the carotid artery rather than a peripheral vessel such as the brachial artery. In patients with severe aortic stenosis and congestive heart failure, the delayed upstroke is not usually evident, leaving only pulsus parvus.

Pulsus bisferiens, characterized by two systolic peaks, occurs when a large stroke volume is ejected rapidly from the ventricle. It is typical of pure aortic regurgitation and of aortic regurgitation combined with aortic stenosis. It is also seen in hypertrophic cardiomyopathy with dynamic outflow obstruction.

The *peripheral* pulse rate of rise, contour, and volume is best appreciated by palpation of the brachial artery. The carotid pulse provides the most accurate representation of the *central* aortic pulse.

In coarctation of the aorta, the carotid and brachial pulses are usually bounding and rapidly rising and have large volumes. Conversely, the lower extremity pulses, such as at the femoral artery, have reduced systolic and pulse pressures with a slow rate of rise and a late peak. The femoral artery delay can be appreciated by palpating the brachial and femoral arteries simultaneously.

The normal aorta is often palpable only above the umbilicus. If the aorta is palpable below the umbilicus, an abdominal aortic aneurysm should be suspected.

REFERENCE

Vlachopoulos C, O'Rourke M: Genesis of the normal and abnormal pulse. Curr Prob Cardiol 25:297, 2000.

ANSWER TO QUESTION 57

C (Braunwald, pp. 387-390, 404)

Coronary arteriography was first performed in 1959 by Sones. It has subsequently become the most commonly used invasive procedure in cardiovascular medicine, and more than 2 million cardiac catheterization procedures are performed annually in the United States. A variety of vascular entry sites are used, including the femoral, brachial, and radial artery approaches. To decrease the risk of retroperitoneal hemorrhage when using the femoral artery approach, the puncture of the common femoral artery should be made below the inguinal ligament but proximal to the bifurcation of the superficial femoral and profunda arterial branches. If the puncture site is proximal to the inguinal ligament, it may be difficult to establish hemostasis with manual compression. If the puncture site is distal to the bifurcation, there is an increased risk for the formation of a pseudoaneurysm after sheath removal. Protamine is used to reverse the anticoagulation effects of unfractionated heparin. This drug can elicit an immune humoral response causing anaphylaxis or marked hypotension in about 2% of patients; prior exposure to protamine or NPH insulin (because of its protamine content) increases the risk of an anaphylactic reaction. Patients with a history of contrast allergy should be pretreated with glucocorticoid therapy (e.g., prednisone 60 mg the night before and again immediately before the procedure). Diphenhydramine and a histamine-2 blocker are also commonly administered before the procedure. Contrary to common belief, a history of shellfish allergy does not predispose to contrast media reactions. The allergen in shellfish appears to be the protein tropomyosin, not iodine.[1]

REFERENCE

1. Beaty AD, Lieberman PL, Slavin RG: Seafood allergy and radiocontrast media: Are physicians propagating a myth? Am J Med 121:158.e1, 2008.

ANSWER TO QUESTION 58

A (Braunwald, pp. 168-169, 511)

Exercise testing and exercise training play a critical role in the care of patients with advanced congestive heart failure. It has been demonstrated that peak oxygen consumption and anaerobic threshold, measured during cardiopulmonary exercise testing, provide independent prognostic information in this population and are superior to measures such as ejection fraction or functional class in predicting outcome. Patients with severely depressed ejection fractions exhibit a wide range of exercise capacities, with some being near normal, and exercise testing can be critical to quantifying the true functional limitation. A peak oxygen consumption of <14 mL/kg/min has been shown to predict poor survival and to identify a population in whom mortality is improved by cardiac transplantation. Patients at this level of impairment demonstrate a profound exercise limitation, with maximal exercise capacity being required for activities such as walking, golf, or raking leaves. Such a patient would be unable to complete stage I on a standard Bruce protocol. Conversely, patients who achieve a peak oxygen consumption of >14 mL/kg/min have a mortality rate similar to patients who have undergone transplantation and would be less likely to benefit from that intervention. The exercise limitation in patients with congestive heart failure is correlated most strongly with alterations in skeletal muscle metabolism. Abnormalities in autonomic and ventilatory responsiveness, increased lactate production, and inability to augment cardiac output are also contributing factors. All of these limitations improve with exercise training, and long-term moderate exercise has been shown to benefit functional capacity, reduce symptoms, and enhance quality of life.

REFERENCE

Hunt SA, Abraham WT, Chin MN, et al: ACC/AHA 2005 Guideline update for the diagnosis and management of chronic heart failure in the adult: A report of the American College/ American Heart Association Task Force on practice guidelines. Circulation 112:154, 2005.

ANSWER TO QUESTION 59

D (Braunwald, pp. 343-354, 1574-1575, 1578-1580)

Cardiac magnetic resonance (CMR) imaging is a powerful noninvasive tool for the diagnosis of several heart and vascular disorders. In recent years, there has been significant growth in the use of CMR for clinical and research applications due to a number of factors, including outstanding image quality, reproducibility, and attractive safety features (i.e., no need for ionizing radiation exposure or iodinated contrast). CMR is well suited for identification of congenital heart lesions and cardiac tumors, assessment of myocardial infarction and viability, and characterization of cardiomyopathies. CMR has been used to identify the presence of iron overload in patients with beta-thalassemia and to guide chelation therapy. CMR can define the structure and function of the right ventricle and is useful in the diagnosis of arrhythmogenic right ventricular cardiomyopathy. CMR can also be useful in the evaluation of stenotic and regurgitant valves when echocardiographic windows are inadequate. The use of CMR for pharmacologic myocardial perfusion imaging and dobutamine stress testing is a promising clinical application. Although CMR can accurately measure global left ventricular function with excellent reproducibility, echocardiography or radionuclide ventriculography remain the superior options for the patient described in answer D, in light of cost and patient comfort issues (e.g., breath holding, confined space, and relatively lengthy scan times for CMR).

Magnetic resonance angiography (MRA) is an excellent imaging technique for assessment of the aorta and peripheral arteries, and coarctation of the aorta can be readily characterized by this technique. MRA has also been validated for the noninvasive diagnosis of renal artery stenosis and is the screening test of choice for this condition at many medical centers.

REFERENCE

Hundley WG, Bluemke DA, Finn JP, et al: ACCF/ACR/AHA/NASCI/SCMR 2010 Expert consensus document on cardiovascular magnetic resonance: A report of the American College of Cardiology Foundation Task Force on Expert Consensus Documents. J Am Coll Cardiol 55:2614, 2010.

ANSWER TO QUESTION 60

D (Braunwald, pp. 261, 1640-1641)

The cardiac magnetic resonance (CMR) study shows diffuse and nodular thickening of the right atrial wall and interatrial septum, suggestive of lipomatous hypertrophy. A subsequent fat suppression technique was employed that confirmed this diagnosis. Lipomatous hypertrophy is a benign hamartoma consisting of excessive deposition of adipose tissue, most commonly in the interatrial septum, which may protrude into the right atrium. Involvement of the interatrial septum typically spares the region of the fossa ovalis, giving rise to a "dumbbell" appearance. This diagnosis is most often an incidental finding during echocardiography or other cardiac imaging studies including CMR. It has been associated with atrial arrhythmias.

Amyloidosis causes diffuse thickening of cardiac structures, including the interatrial septum, but does not display the adipose characteristics of lipomatous hypertrophy. Atrial myxoma may occur in either atrium but most commonly appears as a pedunculated mass attached to the mid-interatrial septum.

REFERENCES

Heyer CM, Kagel T, Lemburg SP, et al: Lipomatous hypertrophy of the interatrial septum: A prospective study of incidence, imaging findings, and clinical symptoms. Chest 124:2068, 2003.
Tatli S, O'Gara PT, Lambert J, et al: MRI of atypical lipomatous hypertrophy of the interatrial septum. AJR Am J Roentgenol 182:598, 2004.

ANSWER TO QUESTION 61

C (Braunwald, pp. 247-249, 1582-1586)

In hypertrophic cardiomyopathy (HCM) with outflow tract obstruction, the anterior leaflet of the mitral valve is abnormally drawn toward the hypertrophied interventricular septum during systole. This systolic anterior motion (SAM) of the valve can be readily identified by echocardiography (see Braunwald, Fig. 15-65) and plays an integral role in the development of outflow tract obstruction in this condition. In addition, characteristic systolic notching of the aortic valve is often evident, particularly by M-mode recordings, owing to the dynamic nature of the obstruction. Asymmetric hypertrophy of the interventricular septum is common in HCM and is readily identifiable by echocardiography. However, pathologic localized hypertrophy in this condition can instead be confined to the apex, lateral, or inferior segments, typically without dynamic outflow obstruction (see Braunwald, Figs. 69-1 and 69-2). Cardiac magnetic resonance imaging is complementary to echocardiography by visualizing regions that are difficult to assess by echocardiography (e.g., the anterolateral free wall).

The Doppler spectral mitral inflow pattern in HCM can be variable but usually reflects the abnormal diastolic filling of the hypertrophied ventricle. Usually there is evidence of a diminished E wave and prominent A wave. Abnormalities of diastolic function can also be identified by Doppler tissue imaging, which typically demonstrates reduced early diastolic mitral annular velocities (E') as a measure of impaired myocardial relaxation (see Braunwald, Fig. 15-65).

REFERENCE

Mohiddin SA, McKenna WJ: Hypertrophic cardiomyopathy. In Smiseth OA, Tendera M (eds): Diastolic Heart Failure. New York, Springer, 2008, pp 285-310.

ANSWER TO QUESTION 62

E (Braunwald, p. 393-396; Table 20-4; Fig. 20-10)

As summarized in the Answer to Question 23, the right atrial pressure waveform contains three positive deflections termed the *a, c,* and *v* waves. The *a* wave represents atrial systole and occurs after the P wave on the ECG. The *x* descent represents the relaxation of the atrium and downward pulling of the tricuspid annulus by right ventricular (RV) contraction. The *c* wave interrupts the *x* descent and represents the protrusion of the closed tricuspid valve into the right atrium. The *v* wave represents the passive venous filling of the atrium, which occurs during ventricular systole. The height of the *v* wave reflects atrial compliance. In the left atrium, as opposed to the right atrium, the *v* wave is generally more prominent than the *a* wave. The *y* descent follows the *v* wave, and it represents right atrial emptying after the tricuspid valve opens.

Conditions that blunt the right atrial *y* descent include cardiac tamponade, ventricular ischemia, and tricuspid stenosis. Conversely, constrictive pericarditis is associated with prominence of the *y* descent, because the very earliest phase of diastolic ventricular filling is unimpeded in this condition.

Blunting of the *x* descent can be observed in the presence of atrial fibrillation or atrial ischemia.

ANSWER TO QUESTION 63

E (Braunwald, pp. 114-118; Table 12-6)

Dynamic auscultation is the technique of altering circulatory dynamics with physiologic and pharmacologic maneuvers and then determining the effect on cardiac murmurs. Typical maneuvers include changes in respiration, the Valsalva maneuver, squatting or standing, and isometric exercise.

Patent ductus arteriosus causes a continuous murmur that is loudest at the second left intercostal space. The diastolic phase of this murmur is increased by isometric handgrip as a result of augmented systemic vascular resistance.

Hypertrophic obstructive cardiomyopathy is associated with a harsh, crescendo-decrescendo systolic murmur best heard between the apex and left sternal border. Actions that reduce left ventricular (LV) size, such as standing or the strain phase of a Valsalva maneuver, bring the anterior mitral leaflet and the interventricular septum into closer proximity, thus *intensifying* the murmur. These maneuvers are useful in differentiating hypertrophic obstructive cardiomyopathy from a fixed

orifice obstruction (i.e., aortic stenosis), in which the murmur softens with standing or the Valsalva maneuver.

The murmur of an uncomplicated ventricular septal defect is holosystolic because LV systolic pressure and systemic resistance exceed right ventricular systolic pressure and pulmonary resistance from the beginning to the end of systole. Isometric handgrip increases systemic vascular resistance and may further intensify the murmur.

Aortic regurgitation is a diastolic murmur best heard with the patient sitting forward and holding a deep expiration. The murmur may be accentuated by maneuvers that increase the arterial pressure, such as isometric handgrip.

The diastolic murmur of mitral stenosis is a low-pitched, rumbling murmur best heard at the apex. Maneuvers that increase the rate of transmitral flow, including exercise, accentuate the murmur.

ANSWER TO QUESTION 64

D (Braunwald, p. 159; Fig. 13-46)

Although the ST-segment and T wave abnormalities on this ECG may lead to concern for myocardial ischemia, the deeply inverted T waves are typical of acute cerebrovascular diseases, including subarachnoid hemorrhage. Given the presenting symptoms of headache, nausea, and dizziness, a cranial imaging study such as computed tomography should be obtained rapidly. In this scenario, antiplatelet agents and antithrombotic therapy should be withheld until intracranial bleeding has been excluded. In the absence of findings to suggest unstable myocardial ischemia, anti-ischemic therapies and cardiac catheterization are not initially appropriate. Electrocardiographic abnormalities are present in a large percentage of patients with acute cerebral events. These abnormalities may include tachyarrhythmias or bradyarrhythmias, conduction disturbances, repolarization abnormalities that resemble myocardial ischemia, prolongation of the QT interval, and prominent U waves. The mechanisms responsible for such electrocardiographic changes are unknown but appear to be related to abnormal autonomic nervous system function. Myocardial damage with release of serum markers (cardiac-specific troponins, CK-MB) and subendocardial hemorrhage can actually occur in the setting of acute severe cerebrovascular disease, believed to be related to the release of excessive local myocardial catecholamines.

In the appropriate clinical situation, diffuse deep T wave inversions are also found in some patients with hypertrophic cardiomyopathy. Giant inverted T waves in the midprecordial leads are particularly characteristic of the apical form of hypertrophic cardiomyopathy.

ANSWER TO QUESTION 65

D (Braunwald, p. 117; Table 12-5; Fig. 12-8)

Diastolic murmurs are classified according to their time of onset as early diastolic, mid-diastolic, or late diastolic (also termed *presystolic*). Early diastolic murmurs begin with the aortic component of the second heart sound (S_2) when originating on the left side of the heart. Likewise, murmurs originating from the right side begin with the pulmonic component of the S_2. Mid-diastolic murmurs begin at a clear interval after S_2, whereas late diastolic murmurs begin immediately before the first heart sound (S_1). When the murmur of aortic regurgitation (AR) radiates selectively to the right sternal border, it implies that aortic root dilatation, as occurs in Marfan syndrome, is the cause. The murmur of acute severe AR differs importantly from the murmur of chronic severe AR. The high-pitched murmur of chronic AR begins with the aortic component of S_2 and has an early peak and a dominant decrescendo pattern throughout diastole. In contrast, in acute severe AR (e.g., caused by infective endocarditis or aortic dissection), the diastolic murmur is of short duration and tends to be soft, because the aortic diastolic pressure rapidly equilibrates with the steep rise in diastolic left ventricular pressure.

Late diastolic murmurs occur immediately before S_1. The presystolic timing coincides with the ventricular filling phase that follows atrial contraction, thus implying the presence of sinus rhythm and coordinated atrial contraction. Presystolic accentuation of diastolic murmurs is typical of patients with mitral or tricuspid stenosis who are in sinus rhythm.

When pulmonic regurgitation develops in the setting of pulmonary hypertension, the murmur begins with a loud P_2 and may last throughout diastole (the Graham Steell murmur).

ANSWER TO QUESTION 66

C (Braunwald, pp. 412-417, 419-422)

The left main coronary artery arises from the superior portion of the left aortic sinus. It ranges from 3 to 6 mm in diameter and is 0 to 10 mm in length. This vessel is best visualized in the anteroposterior projection with slight caudal angulation. The left main coronary artery bifurcates into the left anterior descending artery (LAD) and the left circumflex artery (LCx). In up to 37% of patients, however, the left main trifurcates into a third vessel known as the ramus intermedius, which lies between the LAD and the LCx. The right coronary artery is the dominant vessel in 85% of patients, supplying the posterior descending artery. The LCx artery is the dominant vessel 15% of the time. The interventricular septum is the most densely vascularized area of the heart. It is supplied by septal branches of the LAD that interconnect with septal branches from the posterior descending artery, producing a network of potential collateral channels. There are a number of congenital anomalies that can cause myocardial ischemia. Coronary artery fistulas (abnormal communications between a coronary artery and a cardiac chamber or major vessel) comprise the most common congenital coronary abnormality that is of hemodynamic significance. About half of the patients with such an anomaly are asymptomatic, but the remainder develop complications including heart failure, infective endocarditis, ischemia, or rupture of an aneurysm. The figure demonstrates a congenital coronary fistula arising from branches of the LAD and circumflex coronary arteries that drains into the left ventricle (see right anterior oblique view in **A** and left anterior oblique view in **B**). Other congenital anomalies that may result in myocardial ischemia include anomalous origin of the left coronary artery from the pulmonary artery, congenital coronary stenosis, and anomalous origin of either coronary artery from the contralateral sinus of Valsalva.

REFERENCE

Angelini P: Coronary artery anomalies: an entity in search of an identity. Circulation 115:1296, 2007.

ANSWER TO QUESTION 67

A (Braunwald, pp. 114-118; see also Answer to Question 4)

Continuous murmurs and holosystolic murmurs are not synonymous. A continuous murmur begins in systole and continues uninterrupted through S_2 into all or part of diastole. The murmur does not necessarily envelop S_1, nor need it be present throughout diastole. The etiology of continuous murmurs includes aortopulmonary connections, arteriovenous connections, and disturbances of normal flow patterns in arteries and veins. The best known continuous murmur is that of patent ductus arteriosus (PDA), an aortopulmonary connection. The murmur of a PDA peaks just before and after S_2, decreases in late diastole, and may be soft or absent prior to S_1 (see Braunwald, Fig. 12-8). It is best heard at the second left intercostal space.

A continuous cervical venous hum is found commonly in healthy children and young adults. It is also detected in conditions associated with augmented cervical venous flow, such as anemia and thyrotoxicosis. The venous hum is truly continuous, although usually louder in diastole.

Arterial continuous murmurs occur in both constricted and nonconstricted arteries. An artery narrowed by atherosclerosis may display a continuous murmur that is loudest in systole or may be purely systolic. An example of a normal nonconstricted artery that displays a continuous arterial murmur is the "mammary souffle." This innocent murmur is found in late pregnancy and the puerperium, is maximal over the lactating breasts, and is typically loudest in systole.

ANSWER TO QUESTION 68

A (Braunwald, pp. 237-238, 1481-1483)

Assessment of the severity of regurgitant valvular lesions by Doppler echocardiography is less straightforward than assessment of stenotic conditions. Often a combination of findings must be visually integrated, because no one criterion has sufficient accuracy for quantification. In aortic regurgitation (AR), findings that suggest marked elevation of left ventricular (LV) end-diastolic pressure are among the more predictive indicators of lesion severity. Unlike mitral regurgitation, in which the overall jet size correlates with the degree of regurgitation, the size and depth of penetration of the AR color Doppler signal are less strongly correlated with the magnitude of the lesion. This is in part due to merging of the color jet signals of AR with normal mitral inflow into the left ventricle. Measurements of the jet width may also be misleading, because it may rapidly widen after passing through the more restricted valvular orifice, giving a falsely severe appearance. Careful imaging of the regurgitant signal in the parasternal short-axis view often gives the best sense of true jet width.

In the presence of severe AR there is rapid elevation of LV diastolic pressure such that the velocity of retrograde flow into the left ventricle quickly decays, resulting in a shortened pressure half-time. In general, a pressure half-time <250 milliseconds correlates with severe AR. In addition, the rapid rise in diastolic LV pressure can force the *mitral* valve to close prematurely. Such premature closure is often best visualized by M-mode imaging, in which the mitral leaflets coapt together before the subsequent QRS complex appears.

Although the depth of the Doppler signal in the left ventricle correlates poorly with the severity of AR, in advanced AR such flow typically extends past the tips of the papillary muscles and into the apex. Finally, detection of diastolic flow reversal in the descending thoracic aorta, imaged from the suprasternal notch, is a sign of moderate-to-severe regurgitation.

Elevated LV outflow tract systolic gradients are a sign of systolic obstruction and do not provide direct information about the severity of AR.

REFERENCE

Lancellotti P, Tribouilloy C, Hagendorff A, et al: European Association of Echocardiography recommendations for the assessment of valvular regurgitation: I. Aortic and pulmonary regurgitation (native valve disease). Eur J Echocardiogr 11:223, 2010.

ANSWER TO QUESTION 69

C (Braunwald, pp. 310-316)

Several pharmacologic stress-testing agents are available for patients who cannot exercise because of orthopedic limitations, neurologic conditions, or peripheral arterial disease.

Dipyridamole acts by inhibiting the cellular uptake and intracellular breakdown of adenosine, increasing the concentration of the latter in the circulation. The subsequent increased activation of adenosine A_{2a} receptors results in vasodilatation and increased coronary blood flow in healthy coronary arteries. However, atherosclerotic vessels tend to be maximally dilated distal to the site of significant stenosis at baseline, such that adenosine does not cause further dilatation in those territories. Therefore, perfusion imaging with either adenosine or dipyridamole in a patient with clinically significant CAD reveals regions of relatively hypoperfused myocardium adjacent to normal zones of increased myocardial blood flow, with little change in myocardial oxygen demand. As a result, in a "positive" test, the infusion of dipyridamole or adenosine results in heterogeneity of myocardial perfusion but does not actually provoke myocardial ischemia in the majority of patients with CAD, unlike standard exercise stress testing. Ischemic ST-segment depression may occur in 10% to 15% of patients receiving these vasodilators and tends to correlate with the presence of multiple perfusion defects and extensive coronary artery disease. In contrast, chest pain without electrocardiographic changes is a common symptom after infusion of these agents, is likely due to stimulation of adenosine A_1 receptors, and is of no prognostic significance. Of note, xanthine derivatives (e.g., theophylline and caffeine) compete for adenosine receptors and consumption of substances that contain these agents (e.g., coffee) before the test can result in a false-negative study.

Dobutamine is an alternative pharmacologic agent when adenosine or dipyridamole should not be used, as in patients with bronchospastic pulmonary disease (because stimulation of the adenosine A_{2b} receptor can produce bronchospasm). Dobutamine increases myocardial oxygen demand by augmenting myocardial contractility, heart rate, and blood pressure. The increase in coronary blood flow is similar to that in physical exercise but less than that caused by dipyridamole or adenosine.

In myocardial perfusion imaging, radiotracer agents such as technetium-99m sestamibi or thallium-201 should be injected 1 to 2 minutes before the end of exercise. It is important to maintain the elevated heart rate and blood pressure to allow accumulation of the radiotracer at a "steady" ischemic state.

REFERENCE

Miller DD: Pharmacologic stressors in coronary artery disease. *In* Dilsizian V, Narula J (eds): Atlas of Nuclear Cardiology. 3rd ed. New York, Springer, 2009, pp 61-78.

ANSWER TO QUESTION 70

B (Braunwald, pp. 114-118, 122)

In mitral stenosis, the opening snap is an early diastolic sound generated when superior systolic bowing of the anterior mitral valve leaflet is rapidly reversed toward the left ventricle in early diastole, as a result of the high left atrial pressure. The presence of an opening snap implies a mobile body of the anterior mitral leaflet. The first heart sound tends to be quite loud in mitral stenosis for a similar reason: it relates to the abrupt systolic movement of the body of the anterior mitral leaflet, which was recessed into the left ventricle throughout diastole because of the elevated left trial pressure.

The timing of the A_2-OS interval relates to the severity of mitral stenosis. When mitral stenosis is advanced and left atrial pressure is therefore high, left atrial and left ventricular pressures equilibrate earlier in diastole, resulting in a *shorter* A_2-OS interval. This interval varies in atrial fibrillation according to the previous cycle length. During relatively short cycles, left atrial pressure is higher (because less atrial emptying can occur) and the A_2-OS interval lessens.

REFERENCE

Perloff JK: Physical Examination of the Heart and Circulation. 4th ed. Shelton, Conn, People's Medical Publishing House, 2009.

ANSWER TO QUESTION 71

C (Braunwald, pp. 159-161, 673, 778-780, 814-815, 822-823)

Many arrhythmias may result from digitalis excess. These include bradyarrhythmias related to the markedly enhanced vagal tone (e.g., sinus bradycardia or arrest, or atrioventricular [AV] nodal blocks) and tachyarrhythmias attributed to delayed afterdepolarization-triggered activity (e.g., atrial, junctional, and ventricular tachycardias). One of the most common manifestations of excess digitalis is the appearance of ventricular premature beats (VPBs). However, because these are morphologically similar to VPBs of other causes, they are not highly specific for digitalis toxicity. When ventricular bigeminy occurs, varying morphology of the VPBs is suggestive of digitalis excess. Some forms of ventricular tachycardia are also more indicative of digitalis toxicity as the cause, including ventricular tachycardia with exit block and bidirectional ventricular tachycardia. Atrial tachycardia with block may be caused by excess digitalis but can also occur in the setting of structural heart disease without digitalis toxicity. The rhythm must be distinguished from atrial flutter; and because the amplitude of the atrial depolarization may be low, this rhythm is sometimes difficult to recognize. Nonparoxysmal junctional tachycardia (see Braunwald, Figs. 13-47 and 39-8) is highly suggestive of digitalis excess, although other causes of this rhythm must be excluded, including myocardial ischemia, recent cardiac surgery, and myocarditis. The term *nonparoxysmal* refers to the gradual appearance and disappearance of the rhythm. The majority of patients with this arrhythmia demonstrate AV dissociation due to acceleration of the AV junctional pacemaker. AV dissociation that appears in the course of digitalis therapy must be considered a sign of digitalis intoxication until proven otherwise.

ANSWER TO QUESTION 72

D (Braunwald, pp. 294-296, 308-309, 316-319, 331-332)

Myocardial perfusion and integrity of cell membranes can be assessed using thallium-201 or technetium-99m radiotracers. However, flow and metabolism can be simultaneously assessed with positron emission tomography using rubidium-82– or nitrogen-13–labeled ammonia as a flow tracer, and fluorine-18 fluorodeoxyglucose as a metabolic tracer. A mismatch pattern (preserved metabolic activity despite reduced flow), as in this case, is indicative of the presence of viable myocardium. Conversely, a true myocardial scar would demonstrate reduced flow and a matched reduction in metabolism (a perfusion-metabolism match). Additional modalities used to assess for viability include dobutamine echocardiography (which is more specific but less sensitive than radionuclide techniques) and delayed hyperenhancement assessed by gadolinium-enhanced magnetic resonance imaging, which has excellent resolution and can accurately estimate the transmural extent of myocardial scar.[1]

Observational studies have suggested that patients with ischemic cardiomyopathy and large areas of viable myocardium identified by noninvasive cardiac imaging have superior rates of survival, more substantial improvements in left ventricular function, a greater reduction in symptoms of heart failure, and better exercise tolerance after revascularization than patients with large areas of nonviable myocardium. However, the recent prospective, randomized STICH trial failed to show a difference in outcome with revascularization in patients with or without viable myocardium.[2]

REFERENCES

1. Partington SL, Kwong RY, Dorbala S: Multimodality imaging in the assessment of myocardial viability. Heart Fail Rev 16:381, 2011.
2. Bonow RO, Maurer G, Lee KL et al: Myocardial viability and survival in ischemic left ventricular dysfunction. N Engl J Med 364:1617, 2011.

ANSWER TO QUESTION 73

B (Braunwald, pp. 113-114, 121-123, 1468-1472, 1473-1474, 1588; Table 12-6)

Both aortic stenosis (AS) and hypertrophic cardiomyopathy (HCM) cause harsh systolic murmurs, but these conditions frequently can be differentiated by careful physical examination. For example, the carotid upstroke quality is different (see Braunwald, Fig. 12-5). In AS there is fixed outflow obstruction and the carotid upstrokes are diminished in amplitude and delayed (pulses parvus et tardus). In contrast, the carotid upstroke in HCM is initially brisk, then diminishes in midsystole as the left ventricular (LV) outflow gradient becomes more pronounced. Another differentiating feature is the pattern of radiation of the murmur. In AS, the systolic murmur radiates to the carotid arteries, which is not the rule in HCM. If a systolic thrill is present, it is usually located in the second right intercostal space in AS, whereas it is more likely to be felt at the fourth left intercostal space in HCM. Dynamic bedside maneuvers are helpful to distinguish AS from HCM. Physiologic maneuvers that enhance contractility increase the intensity of both murmurs. Maneuvers that reduce LV filling (e.g., strain phase of Valsalva maneuver or standing from a squatting position) decrease the intensity of the AS murmur, but in HCM the decreased intraventricular volume causes LV dynamic outflow obstruction to intensify and the murmur of HCM becomes louder. The murmur of HCM diminishes in intensity with maneuvers that augment LV filling, such as sudden squatting from the standing position.

ANSWER TO QUESTION 74

D (Braunwald, pp. 107-108, 111-112, 1076-1078; Table 53-1)

There are many causes of chest pain or discomfort unrelated to coronary artery disease. Other life-threatening disorders that may cause similar discomfort include aortic dissection, expanding thoracic aortic aneurysm, pulmonary embolism, and spontaneous pneumothorax. The chest discomfort of aortic dissection typically is persistent, is very severe, and radiates to the back and lumbar region. A blood pressure differential in the two arms of >15 mm Hg may provide a clue to that diagnosis. In the presence of an expanding thoracic aortic aneurysm, there may be erosion of thoracic vertebrae and localized, boring pain that typically is worse at night. The chest discomfort associated with pulmonary embolism is usually of sudden onset, pleuritic, and often a focal pain. A spontaneous pneumothorax produces the sudden onset of chest pain, typically in the lateral chest, with coincident acute shortness of breath. Less serious causes of noncardiac chest discomfort include esophageal disorders such as esophageal spasm. Although esophageal disorders are often accompanied by symptoms of acid reflux and worsen after eating or in the supine position, the discomfort of esophageal spasm is sometimes indistinguishable from that of myocardial ischemia and is also characteristically relieved by nitroglycerin. Esophageal spasm may interfere with swallowing, whereas coronary ischemia does not. Costochondritis is associated with both local costochondral and muscular tenderness and may be aggravated by moving, by coughing, or by direct pressure over the affected joint. In Tietze syndrome, the discomfort is localized to swollen costochondral and costosternal joints.

Herpes zoster ("shingles") can cause great discomfort before the appearance of characteristic vesicles. This affliction can be distinguished from the pain of myocardial infarction by its dermatomal localization, extreme hyperesthesia of the affected skin, and persistence.

Patients with bronchiectasis typically present with persistent cough and purulent sputum, not acute chest pain.

ANSWER TO QUESTION 75

D (Braunwald, pp. 300-302, 310-315, 326; see also Answer to Question 51)

These single-photon emission computed tomographic images demonstrate transient ischemic dilatation of the left ventricle during stress. The size of the left ventricular (LV) cavity appears larger in the exercise images than in the rest images. This phenomenon is typically due to extensive exercise-induced ischemia with transient LV dysfunction and dilatation. In some patients, the appearance of LV chamber dilatation is actually due to the development of global subendocardial ischemia with reduced tracer uptake along the internal border of the left ventricle. As a result, there is the appearance of a larger chamber without true chamber dilatation. Regardless of the precise underlying mechanism, transient LV dilatation is a high-risk marker of severe ischemia and correlates with extensive coronary artery disease (i.e., multivessel or left main coronary artery) on angiography.[1] Similarly, increased lung uptake of thallium-201 is another marker of extensive coronary artery disease and indicates increased risk for an adverse cardiac event.[1]

LV dilatation that is present both at rest and with exertion would be typical for dilated cardiomyopathy. Nuclear images of a patient with chest pain due to single-vessel disease of the left circumflex artery would likely demonstrate a reversible isolated perfusion defect at the lateral or posterior wall. For the patient with prior inferior myocardial infarction, a fixed inferior wall defect, with or without partial reversibility, would be expected. Breast attenuation artifact typically appears as a fixed defect of the anterior or anterolateral wall. A number of techniques have been developed to reduce the likelihood of a false-positive test due to breast attenuation artifact, including the use of technetium-99m–based agents and electrocardiographic gating.

REFERENCE

1. Holly TA, Abbott BG, Al-Mallah M, et al: ASNC Imaging Guidelines for Nuclear Cardiology Procedures: Single photon-emission computed tomography. J Nucl Cardiol 17:941, 2010.

ANSWER TO QUESTION 76

A (Braunwald, pp. 113-114; Fig. 12-6)

Pulsus alternans (Fig. 1-69) is a sign of marked left ventricular dysfunction characterized by alternating strong and weak ventricular contractions, which results in alternating intensity of the peripheral pulses. It is thought to reflect cyclic changes in intracellular calcium levels and action potential duration. It is more easily detectable in the femoral than in the brachial, radial, or carotid arteries and can be observed with sphygmomanometry by slowly deflating the blood pressure cuff below the systolic level. It can be elicited with maneuvers that decrease venous return, such as assumption of erect posture. Because patients with pulsus alternans generally have markedly reduced ventricular contractile function, an S_3 gallop sound is usually present.

Pulsus alternans would only rarely be accompanied by electrical alternans of the QRS complex on the ECG. The latter is more likely to be found in patients with large pericardial effusions.

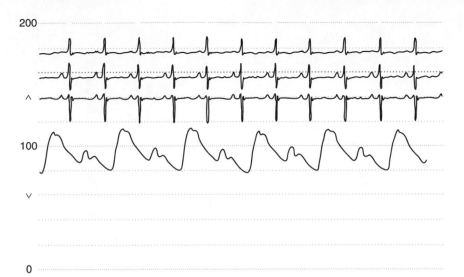

FIGURE 1-69 Pulsus alternans in a patient with severe left ventricular systolic dysfunction. The systolic pressure varies from beat to beat independently of the respiratory cycle. The rhythm is sinus throughout.

ANSWER TO QUESTION 77

A (Braunwald, pp. 184-186)

Exercise testing is often helpful in the assessment of patients with known or suspected arrhythmias. In select patients, particularly those with exercise-induced palpitations, exercise testing is a crucial component of the evaluation. In others, exercise testing can be an important adjunct to ambulatory monitoring and invasive electrophysiologic testing. In association with exercise testing, ventricular arrhythmias may occur during the recovery period, in part because circulating catecholamines continue to increase for several minutes after exertion. In fact, frequent ventricular ectopy in the early postexercise phase predicts a worse long-term cardiac prognosis than ectopy that occurs only during exercise. Supraventricular tachycardia during exercise testing occurs in 4% to 10% of normal individuals and in up to 40% of patients with underlying heart disease. Sustained supraventricular tachycardia develops in only 1% to 2% of patients and is not diagnostic for underlying ischemic heart disease. Patients with known preexcitation, such as Wolff-Parkinson-White (WPW) syndrome, only rarely experience tachyarrhythmias during exercise testing, because antegrade conduction through the atrioventricular node is favored by the catecholamine response to exercise. As such, the delta wave disappears during exercise in 20% to 50% of patients with WPW syndrome. Exercise testing is also useful to assess the response and risks of antiarrhythmic drug therapy. This is particularly important for patients on class IC antiarrhythmic agents, such as propafenone and flecainide, because QRS widening during exercise on such drugs is predictive of a proarrhythmic effect and reentrant ventricular tachycardia. In addition, prolongation of the QT interval of >10 milliseconds during exercise identifies patients at particularly high risk of a proarrhythmic effect on class IA antiarrhythmic agents.

The development of left bundle branch block (LBBB) during exercise is predictive of subsequent progression to permanent LBBB. Patients with exercise-induced LBBB also have a threefold increase in the risk of death or major cardiac events compared with patients without this abnormality.

REFERENCE

Gibbons RJ, Balady GJ, Bricker JT, et al: ACC/AHA 2002 guideline update for exercise testing: Summary article. A report of the American College of Cardiology/American Heart Association Task Force on Practice Guidelines (Committee to Update the 1997 Exercise Testing Guidelines). J Am Coll Cardiol 40:1531, 2002.

ANSWER TO QUESTION 78

D (Braunwald, pp. 114-115, 1511-1512, 1520; Figs. 12-7 and 66-36; Table 12-6)

Ejection sounds are high-frequency "clicks" that occur in early systole. They may be either aortic or pulmonic in origin, require a mobile valve for their generation, and begin at the exact time of maximal opening of the semilunar valve in question. If the valve is structurally abnormal, the ejection sound is believed to be caused by the abrupt halting of valve opening at its maximum level of ascent in early systole. If the sound is associated with a structurally normal valve, it is called a "vascular" ejection sound (e.g., associated with a dilated aortic root), in which case the origin of the sound is not clearly defined. In either case, the ejection sound starts at the moment of full opening of the valve. In valvular pulmonic stenosis, the ejection sound is loudest during expiration. With inspiration, increased venous return augments atrial systole and results in partial opening of the pulmonic

Supine

Standing

Squatting

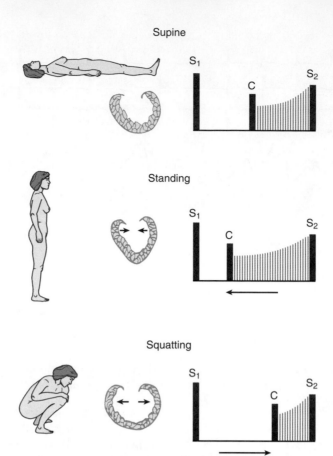

FIGURE 1-70 From Shaver JA, Leonard JJ, Leon DF: Examination of the heart: IV auscultation of the heart. Dallas, American Heart Association, 1990, p 13.

valve before ventricular systole commences. In contrast, with expiration, the pulmonic valve is forced to open from a fully closed position, thus generating a louder ejection sound as the valve's systolic movement is suddenly halted. Aortic ejection sounds do not vary with respiration.

The click of mitral valve prolapse occurs in mid or late systole and coincides with maximal systolic excursion of the prolapsed leaflet(s) into the left atrium. The generation of the click has been attributed to sudden tensing of the redundant leaflets and elongated chordae tendineae. Maneuvers that decrease left ventricular volume, such as the strain phase of the Valsalva maneuver or standing from a squatting position, move the click earlier in systole (Fig. 1-70).

ANSWER TO QUESTION 79

D (Braunwald, pp. 141-142, 157, 1713; Table 13-5; Fig. 13-20)

Chronic obstructive pulmonary disease (COPD) causes several electrocardiographic abnormalities related to changes of the position of the heart in the chest and hyperinflation of the lungs. These include reduced amplitude of the QRS complex, right-axis deviation, and *delayed* transition in the precordial leads, which may be sufficiently prominent to simulate anterior myocardial infarction (see Braunwald, Fig. 13-20).

For right ventricular hypertrophy (RVH) to be evident on the ECG, it must be severe enough to overcome the opposing effects of the larger left ventricular forces. In patients with COPD, additional electrocardiographic abnormalities that support the presence of true RVH include (1) marked right-axis deviation (>110 degrees); (2) deep S waves in the lateral precordial leads; and (3) an $S_1Q_3T_3$ pattern (S wave in lead I, prominent Q in lead III, inverted T waves in the inferior leads).

ANSWER TO QUESTION 80

C (Braunwald, pp. 121, 262-266, 352, 400-401)

Detection and quantification of shunts within the cardiac chambers or great vessels can be accomplished by cardiac catheterization, echocardiography, radionuclide scintigraphy, and magnetic resonance imaging. Shunt evaluation by cardiac catheterization involves utilizing oximetry in multiple locations and calculation of pulmonary and systemic blood flow. Comparison of pulmonary and systemic blood flows helps to establish the presence and magnitude of the shunt, whereas oximetry in multiple locations helps to localize the site of abnormal flow. "Physiologic" shunting, such as occurs in hypoventilation, pulmonary edema, and cardiogenic shock, should be correctable with the administration of 100% oxygen.

Failure to correct with 100% oxygen suggests an anatomic shunt.

A shortcoming of oximetric shunt detection is its lack of sensitivity, although most clinically relevant shunts can be detected using this method. When performing an oximetry run, multiple sites in the inferior vena cava (IVC), superior vena cava (SVC), and right atrium must be sampled because the oxygen saturation from these sites may vary widely. The IVC, because of the relatively low renal oxygen consumption, usually has the *highest* oxygen saturation. Conversely, the coronary sinus delivers venous blood with a very low oxygen saturation. The Flamm formula, the most common equation for estimating mixed venous oxygen content in the setting of an intracardiac shunt, indicates that mixed venous oxygen content is equal to [3(SVC O_2 content) + 1(IVC O_2 content)] ÷ 4.

ANSWER TO QUESTION 81

D (Braunwald, pp. 141-142, 144-145, 162-163, 1917; Table 13-8)

The normal QRS complex in lead V_1 consists of a small R wave, representing initial septal depolarization, followed by an S wave, which is inscribed as the bulk of electrical forces swing in the direction of the left ventricle.

In right ventricular hypertrophy, the increased right-sided forces cause abnormally tall R waves in leads V_1 and V_2, deep S waves in the lateral precordial leads, and right-axis deviation. The Wolff-Parkinson-White (WPW) syndrome, a form of preexcitation, is characterized by a short PR interval and an initial slur (delta wave) with prolongation of the QRS complex. When WPW is caused by a posterior or lateral left ventricular (LV) accessory pathway, the delta wave is positive in lead V_1, associated with prominence of the R wave. A tall R wave in the right precordial leads is also typical of Duchenne muscular dystrophy. In that disorder, myocardial dystrophy of the posterobasal and contiguous lateral LV wall results in deep Q waves in leads I, aVL, and V_5 and V_6, with reciprocal changes (tall R waves) in leads V_1 and V_2. Accidental placement of the right precordial leads too low on the chest wall is a common technical error that results in prominent R waves in leads V_1 and V_2.

In left anterior fascicular block, the amplitude of the R waves in the right precordial leads is often *diminished* and deep S waves are present in leads V_5 and V_6 because of the anterosuperiorly directed late QRS forces.

ANSWER TO QUESTION 82

D (Braunwald, pp. 113-114, 247-248, 393-396, 1585-1586, 1592-1593; Fig. 12-5)

The hemodynamic pressure tracing is consistent with hypertrophic obstructive cardiomyopathy (HCM). In the tracing, a large gradient exists between the midcavity of the left ventricle and the aorta as shown during the first three full beats. As the catheter is withdrawn into the subaortic left ventricular (LV) outflow tract, the gradient is no longer observed (last three beats). In patients with valvular aortic stenosis, the pressure gradient would persist in the latter location.

A bifid aortic pulse contour is demonstrated in the tracing, with a notch on the upstroke ("spike-and-dome" configuration) characteristic of HCM. This is in contrast to the slow and delayed rise of the aortic pressure tracing expected in patients with valvular aortic stenosis. In addition, LV diastolic dysfunction is common in HCM, owing to impaired LV compliance, which leads to a prominent LV *a* wave and elevation of end-diastolic pressure, as shown on the tracing.

There is no role for aortic valve replacement in the treatment of HCM. In selected patients with HCM and severe symptomatic obstruction due to septal hypertrophy, surgical myomectomy or alcohol septal ablation may be beneficial.

ANSWER TO QUESTION 83

D (Braunwald, pp. 130-131)

The normal mean QRS complex in the frontal plane ranges from −30 to +90 degrees. A mean axis more positive than +90 is referred to as *right-axis deviation*, whereas an axis more negative than −30 degrees is *left-axis deviation*. The axis is *indeterminate* (i.e., cannot be calculated in the frontal plane) if all six limb leads record isoelectric QRS complexes (i.e., equal positive and negative deflections).

The designation "vertical" heart is applied when the mean QRS complex is near +90 degrees, in which case the QRS recording in lead I would be isoelectric. A "horizontal" heart refers to a mean axis near 0 degrees, in which case there is a tall R wave in leads I and aVL and an isoelectric QRS complex in aVF.

The normal QRS complex in precordial leads V_1 and V_2 shows small R waves with more prominent S waves, reflecting early septal depolarization followed by activation of the posteriorly located left ventricle. Proceeding from V_1 to V_6, the R wave becomes gradually taller and the S wave less deep. The transition zone represents the lead in which the R wave height surpasses the depth of the S wave and is usually localized to lead V_3 or V_4. An early transition (termed *counterclockwise rotation* as viewed from under the diaphragm) is present when the height of the R wave is greater than the depth of the S wave prior to lead V_3. Conversely, a delayed transition (*clockwise rotation*) is present when the S wave depth exceeds the height of the R wave beyond lead V_4.

ANSWER TO QUESTION 84

C (Braunwald, pp. 398-400)

The pioneering work of Gorlin and Gorlin provided equations to calculate cardiac valve areas based on the measured transvalvular pressure gradient and blood flow. The valve area is proportional to:

$$\frac{F}{K \times \sqrt{\Delta P}}$$

in which F represents flow across the valve, ΔP is the mean pressure gradient across the orifice, and K is an empirical constant for the valve in question.

There are assumptions and potential pitfalls in the determination of valve area by catheterization techniques. Because flow in the Gorlin equation is assumed to be systemic (forward) cardiac output, the presence of regurgitation across the valve in question results in a falsely *low* value for F in the Gorlin equation, and therefore the calculated valve area may be underestimated. In such cases, the calculated valve area actually represents the lower limit of the true valve area.

Accurate and simultaneous determinations of cardiac output and mean pressure gradient are essential in the determination of a stenotic orifice area. Both of these measurements are subject to error. Because it is the square root of the mean pressure gradient that is used in the Gorlin formula, errors in measurement of the cardiac output have a proportionately greater influence on the calculated valve area.

ANSWER TO QUESTION 85

C (Braunwald, pp. 311-315; see also Answer to Question 69)

Exercise testing is the preferred stress modality to evaluate for coronary artery disease because it allows a correlation between exertional symptoms and objective findings of ischemia and provides substantial prognostic information. However, many patients are not capable of attaining a sufficient level of exercise (because of physical limitations or poor conditioning) and undergo phamacologic stress testing instead. The most widely used agents for pharmacologic stress testing are (1) coronary arteriolar vasodilators (adenosine, dipyridamole, and regadenoson) and (2) adrenergic agents such as dobutamine. During pharmacologic perfusion positron emission tomographic scintigraphy of a normal individual there is homogeneous uptake of the radiotracer (e.g., rubidium-82) throughout the myocardium in both the exercise and resting states. The images in the case of this patient demonstrate severe vasodilator-induced ischemia (hypoperfusion) of the anterior and anteroseptal walls. That is, there is a large region of hypoperfusion on the stress images that is predominantly *reversible:* it almost completely fills in on the resting images. A *fixed* defect is one that is present and unchanged on both exercise and rest images and corresponds to a region of prior myocardial infarction or scar. This patient subsequently underwent cardiac catheterization. A 90% stenosis at the anastomosis of the left internal mammary artery to the left anterior descending artery was found, and successful percutaneous intervention was performed.

ANSWER TO QUESTION 86

B (Braunwald, pp. 1574-1575)

This patient has an advanced form of hemochromatosis, a disease that leads to abnormal deposition of iron in tissues. The most common form of hemochromatosis is *inherited* as an autosomal recessive disorder due to a mutation in the *HFE* gene that codes for a transmembrane protein responsible for regulating iron uptake in the intestine and liver. *Acquired* hemochromatosis is the result of excess iron load due to an underlying disease process (e.g., thalassemia) or increased ingestion of iron. Normal body content of iron is maintained by the proper absorption of iron in the intestines. In hemochromatosis, mucosal absorption is inappropriately high, which leads to elevated plasma iron levels and increased transferrin saturation. The extra iron load is deposited in multiple organs, including the heart, pancreas, and liver. The classic presentation therefore is that of "bronze diabetes" due to excess iron deposition in the dermis and pancreas. Other findings include hypogonadism (impaired hypothalamic-pituitary function), arthropathy (often the small joints of the hands), and cirrhosis. The severity of cardiac involvement in hemochromatosis varies widely and may culminate in heart failure due to a mixed dilated and restrictive cardiomyopathy. Electrocardiographic findings may include supraventricular arrhythmias, varying degrees of atrioventricular block, and *low* QRS voltage. Diagnosis is based on the history, an elevated plasma iron level, normal or low total iron-binding capacity (TIBC), and markedly increased transferrin saturation (iron:TIBC ratio) and serum ferritin levels. Treatment options include phlebotomy and chelating agents (e.g., desferrioxamine).

REFERENCE

Van Bokhoven MA, Van Deirsem CT, Swinkels DW: Diagnosis and management of hereditary haemochromatosis. BMJ 342:c7251, 2011.

ANSWER TO QUESTION 87

D (Braunwald, pp. 115-118, 1511-1512; Table 12-6; Figs. 12-7 and 66-36)

Physiologic maneuvers that alter left ventricular (LV) filling can aid in the bedside diagnosis of mitral valve prolapse (MVP). Any maneuver that reduces LV volume, such as the Valsalva maneuver or standing from a supine position, causes the valve to prolapse into the left atrium sooner, such that the click and onset of the murmur occur earlier in systole and the murmur may become louder. Conversely, actions that augment impedance to LV emptying, such as isometric handgrip, increase the LV volume and thus delay the click and murmur. Squatting from a standing position will also delay the click and murmur due to the increased venous return and augmented LV volume.

Carotid sinus massage is not generally helpful in differentiating the murmur of MVP from other entities. This maneuver can be useful to slow the heart rate in a tachycardic patient to help characterize extra heart sounds.

ANSWER TO QUESTION 88

E (Braunwald, pp. 160-161; Fig. 13-49; see also Answer to Question 19)

Hyperkalemia is associated with a distinctive sequence of electrocardiographic abnormalities, beginning with narrowing and peaking (tenting) of the T wave, with a shortened QT interval. Progressive hyperkalemia reduces atrial and ventricular resting membrane potentials, which inactivates sodium channels and decreases conduction velocity. At that stage, the QRS complex begins to widen and the P wave amplitude decreases. Complete loss of observed P waves may occur. In that situation, sinus rhythm typically persists but the P wave amplitude is so small that it is not recorded on the surface ECG. Very marked hyperkalemia leads to asystole, sometimes preceded by a slow undulatory (sinusoidal wave) pattern on the ECG caused by marked QRS widening.

Hypokalemia, in contrast, is associated with hyperpolarization of the resting membrane potential and increased action potential duration. This results in resting ST-segment depression and QT interval prolongation. The T waves often become flat, whereas U waves become prominent. The QT prolongation predisposes to torsades de pointes. Hypokalemia, not hyperkalemia, predisposes to digitalis-associated tachyarrhythmias.

ANSWER TO QUESTION 89

D (Braunwald, pp. 156-157; Table 13-9)

Noninfarction Q waves can be produced by any condition that results in (1) abnormal heart position, (2) altered ventricular conduction, (3) ventricular enlargement, or (4) myocardial damage or replacement. Wolff-Parkinson-White syndrome is an example of altered ventricular conduction in which early activation of the inferoposterior wall by a bypass tract results in inferior Q waves and a pseudoinfarction pattern. Similarly, left bundle branch block is frequently associated with noninfarction Q waves due to altered ventricular activation. Any condition that displaces the mass of the left ventricle posteriorly, such as cardiomyopathy with ventricular dilatation, or chronic obstructive pulmonary disease, is associated with Q waves in the right-sided chest leads and poor R wave progression across the precordium. Incorrect superior placement of the right precordial chest leads can also result in the appearance of Q waves in those leads.

Acidosis leads to hyperkalemia with the characteristic changes of that condition (see Answer to Question 88) but not to the development of Q waves.

ANSWER TO QUESTION 90

B (Braunwald, pp. 172-175, 179-180, 185-186; Table 14-4)

Several abnormalities on the baseline ECG greatly limit the utility of standard exercise electrocardiography. These patterns include preexcitation syndromes, paced ventricular rhythms, left ventricular hypertrophy, and left bundle branch block. Digoxin can accentuate ischemic exercise-induced ST-segment changes, even if the resting ECG is without evidence of ST-segment depression.

Right bundle branch block (RBBB) is typically associated with T wave and ST-segment changes in the anterior precordial leads. Exercise-induced ST-segment depression in these leads (V_1 to V_4) is a common finding in patients with RBBB and is nondiagnostic for ischemia. Thus, RBBB decreases the sensitivity of the test; however, the ST segments in leads V_5 and V_6, and in leads II and aVF, remain interpretable in patients with this conduction disorder.

ST-segment depressions typically are not predictive of the anatomic site of ischemia. In contrast, ST-segment *elevations* in leads that do not contain pathologic Q waves are very specific for exercise-induced ischemia and are predictive of the anatomic location of ischemia.

Certain findings on exercise electrocardiography are indicative of severe (left main or multivessel) coronary artery disease and should be considered "high risk" markers. These include ≥2 mm ST-segment depressions (particularly at low levels of exercise), ST-segment depressions in more than five leads, ST-segment depressions that persist more than 5 minutes during the recovery phase, ST-segment elevations, and hypotension during exercise (see also Answer to Question 48).

REFERENCE

Gibbons RJ, Balady GJ, Bricker JT, et al: ACC/AHA 2002 guideline update for exercise testing: Summary article. A report of the American College of Cardiology/American Heart Association Task Force on Practice Guidelines (Committee to Update the 1997 Exercise Testing Guidelines). J Am Coll Cardiol 40:1531, 2002.

ANSWER TO QUESTION 91

A (Braunwald, pp. 236-240, 1493, 1504-1505)

The continuous-wave Doppler profile demonstrates combined mitral stenosis (MS) and mitral regurgitation (MR). In the figure, diastolic flow toward the transducer (into the left ventricle) is represented by velocities above the baseline while flow away from the transducer (into the left atrium) is indicated by velocities below the baseline. In a normal individual there would be no flow across the valve during systole and the peak diastolic velocity would be <1.3 m/sec. The presence of MS results in a high diastolic velocity (usually >1.5 m/sec). In addition, the persistent diastolic pressure gradient between the left atrium and left ventricle in patients with MS results in an abnormally delayed decline of the transmitral velocity signal, as shown in this case. The severity of mitral stenosis can be determined from Doppler measurements by calculating the pressure decline half-time (see Answer to Question 26).

Two-dimensional echocardiography and Doppler interrogation are also very useful techniques for assessing mitral regurgitation and determining its cause. The continuous-wave Doppler examination shown here demonstrates abnormal systolic flow directed retrograde into the left atrium. Doppler color flow imaging (not shown in this example) is one of the best echocardiographic methods to determine the magnitude of MR, which can be estimated by the area of the visualized regurgitant jet. When mitral regurgitation is severe, Doppler interrogation demonstrates reversal of systolic flow in the pulmonary veins. MR jets that are peripherally directed along the left atrial wall, rather than centrally located, may underestimate the severity of MR as determined by Doppler techniques.

ANSWER TO QUESTION 92

E (Braunwald, pp. 109, 116, 1312)

The clinical diagnosis of Marfan syndrome has historically depended on characteristic abnormalities of the skeletal, cardiovascular, and ocular systems. Genetic testing for mutations in the *FBN1* gene has not been required for routine assessment. Since 1996, the Ghent criteria have been the standard for diagnosis and rely on "major" and "minor" manifestations.[1] Major criteria include:

Skeletal findings: at least four of the following: pectus carinatum, pectus excavatum requiring surgery, arm span/height ratio >1.05, positive thumb sign (distal phalanx protrudes beyond clenched fist) and wrist sign (thumb and fifth finger overlap while encircling the wrist), scoliosis >20 degrees or spondylolisthesis, reduced elbow extension <170 degrees, pes planus (flat feet), and protrusio acetabulae

Cardiovascular findings: Dilation of sinuses of Valsalva and ascending aorta, or ascending aortic dissection

Ocular finding: Ectopia lentis (lens dislocation identified by slit lamp examination)

Central nervous system finding: Lumbosacral dural ectasia (identified by computed tomography or magnetic resonance imaging)

Family or genetic history: First-degree relative who meets diagnostic criteria or who has known Marfan mutation

Minor criteria include lesser skeletal abnormalities (joint hypermobility, nonsurgical pectus excavatum, high arched palate, and facial features such as malar hypoplasia), mitral valve prolapse, and dilation/dissection of the descending thoracic/abdominal aorta before age 50.

In the absence of a family history, the diagnosis of Marfan syndrome requires one major manifestation in two of the above organ systems, with involvement (major or minor criterion) in a third organ system, or if a mutation known to cause Marfan syndrome is found, the diagnosis is based on one major criterion plus involvement (major or minor criterion) in a second organ system.

In this patient's case, ectopia lentis is a major criterion, the other choices are minor criteria.

In 2010, an international expert committee proposed revised diagnostic nosology for Marfan syndrome that emphasizes the importance of the cardiovascular manifestations of this condition. By the new criteria, in the absence of a family history of Marfan syndrome, the combination of aortic root dilatation and ectopic lentis is sufficient to establish the diagnosis. In the absence of either of these findings, the identification of a known

FBN1 mutation or a combination of systemic findings is required for confirmation.[2]

REFERENCES

1. Judge DP, Dietz HC: Marfan's syndrome. Lancet 366:1965, 2005.
2. Loeys BL, Dietz HC, Braverman AC, et al: The revised Ghent nosology for the Marfan syndrome. J Med Genet 47:476, 2010.

ANSWER TO QUESTION 93

B (Braunwald, pp. 70-72, 1582-1591)

The microscopic specimen demonstrates marked myocyte disarray typical of hypertrophic cardiomyopathy (HCM). HCM is a genetic disorder caused by more than 900 mutations in genes that encode sarcomeric proteins. It is transmitted in an autosomal dominant fashion, and specific mutations are often unique to affected families. More than 50% of all HCM mutations occur in genes that encode β-myosin heavy chain or cardiac myosin binding protein C.

The risk of most concern for patients with HCM is sudden cardiac death. It results from ventricular tachycardia/fibrillation and may occur at any age but is most often a complication in adolescents and young adults with HCM. The risk is greatest in those with specific clinical markers, for whom primary prevention with an implantable cardioverter-defibrillator is often appropriate, particularly in younger patients: (1) a family history of HCM-related death, especially if sudden; (2) unexplained syncope; (3) hypotensive or attenuated blood pressure response on exercise testing; (4) multiple, prolonged nonsustained bursts of ventricular tachycardia on ambulatory electrocardiographic monitoring; and (5) marked left ventricular hypertrophy (wall thickness ≥30 mm).

Additional questions and answers regarding HCM and sudden cardiac death appear in Sections IV and V of this book.

REFERENCES

Watkins H, Ashrafian H, Redwood C: Inherited cardiomyopathies. N Engl J Med 364:1643, 2011.
Landstrom AP, Ackerman MJ: Mutation type is not clinically useful in predicting prognosis in hypertrophic cardiomyopathy. Circulation 122:2441, 2010.
Ho CY: Genetics and clinical destiny: Improving care in hypertrophic cardiomyopathy. Circulation 122:2430, 2010.
Maron BJ: Sudden death in hypertrophic cardiomyopathy. J Cardiovasc Trans Res 2:368, 2009.

ANSWER TO QUESTION 94

C (Braunwald, pp. 75-76, 663-664, 682, 1578-1580)

This patient has a form of arrhythmogenic right ventricular cardiomyopathy (ARVC), a condition in which fibrofatty replacement of myocardium, most commonly of the right ventricle, leads to ventricular arrhythmias and sudden cardiac death. ARVC results from mutations in genes that encode components of cardiac desmosomes, cell membrane structures that maintain structural and functional contacts between neighboring myocytes. ARVC can occur as an isolated cardiomyopathy or as a syndromic disorder. In *Naxos syndrome*, ARVC is accompanied by woolly, kinky hair and palmar-plantar keratosis. It arises from autosomal *recessive* mutations (in distinction to isolated ARVC, which is transmitted in an autosomal dominant fashion) in the gene that encodes plakoglobin, a cytoplasmic desmosomal protein. Patients with *Carvajal syndrome* display similar hair and skin findings, but the cardiomyopathic findings predominantly affect the left ventricle. The patient in this question has predominantly right ventricular involvement and therefore has Naxos syndrome.

Major diagnostic criteria for ARVC include (1) RV enlargement and dysfunction visualized by echocardiography, cardiac magnetic resonance, or angiography; (2) fibrofatty replacement of myocardium on endomyocardial biopsy (however, there is a high false-negative rate of diagnosis because of sampling error and because the RV septum [the region sampled by the bioptome] may not display characteristic changes); (3) electrocardiographic abnormalities including inverted T waves in V_1 to V_3, an epsilon wave between the QRS complex and the T wave in leads V_1 to V_3, late potentials on signal averaged electrocardiography, nonsustained or sustained ventricular tachycardia with a left bundle branch morphology, and superior axis; and (4) a confirmed family history of ARVC in a first-degree relative.

REFERENCES

Cox MGPJ, van der Zwaag PA, van der Werf C, et al: Arrhythmogenic right ventricular dysplasia/cardiomyopathy. Circulation 123:2690, 2011.

Marcus FI, McKenna WJ, Sherril D, et al: Diagnosis of arrhythmogenic right ventricular cardiomyopathy/dysplasia (ARVC/D). Circulation 121:1533, 2010.

ANSWER TO QUESTION 95

B (Braunwald, p. 75)

Mitochondria generate the energy necessary for cellular function and are present in abundance in the cytoplasm of most cells. Each mitochondrion possesses a single chromosome, which encodes for many, but not all, of the proteins involved in oxidative phosphorylation. The remainder of such genes resides in the nucleus of the cell. Thus, disorders of energy metabolism can be inherited either as mendelian traits or as nonmendelian traits owing to their location on the mitochondrial chromosome. During conception, spermatocytes contribute very little mitochondria to the zygote. Rather, the mitochondria within the fetus are essentially derived solely from the cytoplasm of the oocyte. As a result, mutations of mitochondrial chromosomes demonstrate maternal inheritance: transmission of the condition occurs through affected women but not to the offspring of affected men. Furthermore, male and female children of an affected mother are equally likely to acquire the chromosomal abnormality. All offspring of affected women may inherit the disease, although there is often substantial variability of expression within families, including apparent nonpenetrance.

MELAS is the most common inherited disorder of the mitochondrial chromosome. It is characterized by mitochondrial myopathy, encephalopathy, lactic acidosis, and stroke-like episodes along with extremity weakness and migraine-like headaches. In approximately 80% of cases it is caused by a specific mutation in the mitochondrial $tRNA^{Leu(UUR)}$ gene *(MTTL1)*. The cardiovascular manifestations include hypertrophic or dilated cardiomyopathy, which can lead to heart failure and death.

REFERENCE

Testai FD, Gorelick PB: Inherited metabolic disorders and stroke: I. Fabry disease and mitochondrial myopathy, encephalopathy, lactic acidosis, and stroke-like episodes. Arch Neurol 67:19, 2010.

ANSWERS TO QUESTIONS 96 TO 100

96-A, 97-D, 98-B, 99-C, 100-D (Braunwald, pp. 108, 885-889; Table 42-4)

Cardiac syncope is usually of rapid onset and not preceded by an aura. Patients typically regain consciousness promptly with a clear sensorium. In any patient with a history of coronary artery disease (CAD), cardiac causes of syncope should be carefully investigated, even when the presenting history is somewhat atypical. Neurologic syncope is sometimes preceded by an aura, is more characteristically associated with incontinence and tongue biting, and is notable for a clouded sensorium with slow clearing after return of consciousness. Seizure-like activity may occur at any time cerebral perfusion is impaired and is not particularly helpful in distinguishing different types of syncope.

Distinguishing cardiac syncope due to tachyarrhythmias (usually ventricular tachycardia) from that due to bradyarrhythmias can be difficult on clinical grounds alone. Patients with a history of CAD are at increased risk for ventricular tachyarrhythmias. Bradyarrhythmias are more common in patients with a history of conduction abnormalities.

A neurocardiogenic (or vasovagal) cause accounts for approximately 50% of syncopal episodes. It may be precipitated by emotional distress, fear, pain, or extreme fatigue or may occur in the setting of diminished venous return with a reduced stroke volume. Each of these situations results in high catecholamine activity with sympathetic stimulation of the heart. In susceptible individuals, the resultant hypercontractility excessively stimulates cardiac mechanoreceptors (vagal afferent C fibers), which then leads to sympathetic withdrawal, vasodilatation, and bradycardia. When extreme, this activation leads to frank syncope.

Hysterical fainting is typically not accompanied by a change in pulse, blood pressure, or skin color. It is often associated with paresthesias of the hands or face, hyperventilation, dyspnea, and other manifestations of acute anxiety.

REFERENCE

Kuriachan V, Sheldon RS: Current concepts in the evaluation and management of syncope. Curr Cardiol Rep 10:384, 2008.

ANSWERS TO QUESTIONS 101 TO 104

101–B, 102–A, 103–D, 104–C (Braunwald, pp. 114-118, 124, 139-142, 158, 160-161, 1588, 1653)

The ECG of the young man with exertional chest discomfort and a systolic murmur demonstrates marked left ventricular hypertrophy with a "strain" pattern. In this case, the systolic murmur is due to dynamic left ventricular outflow obstruction because of hypertrophic cardiomyopathy. Such a murmur becomes louder with maneuvers that decrease left ventricular preload, such as standing from a squatting position or during the strain phase of the Valsalva maneuver. The 56-year-old woman with pleuritic chest discomfort and dyspnea has a hemodynamically significant pulmonary embolism. Her ECG demonstrates borderline sinus tachycardia, an incomplete right bundle branch block, and an $S_1Q_3T_3$ pattern in the limb leads. The latter reflects a deep S wave in lead I, and a prominent Q wave with T wave inversion in lead III, a pattern that can be observed in individuals with hemodynamically significant pulmonary embolism. However, the sensitivity of this finding is low and it is observed in only a minority of such patients. The most common electrocardiographic findings of hemodynamically important pulmonary embolism are sinus tachycardia and T wave inversions in the anteroseptal leads that may mimic anterior myocardial ischemia. The 36-year-old man with sharp inspiratory chest discomfort has acute pericarditis. His ECG demonstrates diffuse ST-segment elevations. There is also subtle PR segment depression in the limb leads (especially lead II) and slight PR-segment elevation in lead aVR. All are common findings in patients with acute pericarditis. The elderly alcoholic man with vomiting and epigastric discomfort has developed hypokalemia and hypomagnesemia. His ECG is consistent with these electrolyte derangements, including a prolonged QT (actually QU) interval and low-voltage T waves.

ANSWERS TO QUESTIONS 105 TO 109

105–A, 106–C, 107–B, 108–E, 109–D (Braunwald, pp. 412-417, 419-423)

Coronary arteriography remains the benchmark to assess coronary anatomy. Coronary artery spasm (in the figure see E, Injections 1 & 2) may be due to organic vascular disease or may be induced by the mechanical stimulation of the artery by the catheter tip. In 1% to 3% of patients who do not receive vasodilators (e.g., nitroglycerin) before arteriography, spasm may be observed. Whereas the major coronary arteries usually pass along the epicardial surface of the heart, occasional short segments pass down into the myocardium, leading to myocardial bridging, as demonstrated in the figure in A (diastole and systole). Such bridging has been identified in about 5% of human hearts at autopsy. Angiographic identification of a myocardial bridge usually is most common in the left anterior descending (LAD) artery.

Intercoronary collateral vessels in the interventricular septum are normally <1 mm in diameter, are characterized by moderate tortuosity, and tend to serve as connections between numerous septal branches of the LAD and smaller posterior septal branches that arise from the posterior descending artery. Recruitment and development of such collateral vessels due to occlusion of the LAD artery are shown in part B of the figure. The most prevalent hemodynamically significant congenital coronary artery anomaly is the coronary arteriovenous fistula (see D). When the fistula drains into any of several areas—the coronary sinus, superior vena cava, pulmonary artery, or a right-sided cardiac chamber—a left-to-right shunt is created. When seen in infancy and childhood, approximately half of such patients develop symptoms of congestive heart failure, but the majority of these patients undergo evaluation because of the presence of a loud continuous murmur.

Coronary anomalies are present in 1% to 5% of patients undergoing coronary angiography. Ectopic origin of the right coronary artery (RCA) is present in approximately 2% of patients. Ectopic origin of the left circumflex from the right coronary cusp (see C) occurs in <1% of patients. Other abnormal coronary origins occur even less frequently.

ANSWERS TO QUESTIONS 110 TO 113

110–D, 111–B, 112–C, 113–A (Braunwald, pp. 226, 241, 260-261, 348-349, 351-352, 354, 1578-1580, 1640-1641)

Computed tomography (CT) provides high-resolution morphologic imaging of the heart and is very useful in the diagnosis of a number of cardiovascular disorders. The 53-year-old woman with dyspnea, embolic events, positional lightheadedness, and weight loss has a left atrial myxoma, the most common primary cardiac tumor. In this case, the myxoma is identified as a large left atrial mass attached to the interatrial septum (arrows in D of the figure). CT and magnetic resonance imaging (MRI) can supplement echocardiography in the assessment of cardiac tumors because of excellent spatial resolution.[1] The young man with recurrent syncope has arrhythmogenic right ventricular (RV) dysplasia. The computed tomogram in B demonstrates a dilated right ventricle and aneurysmal bulging of the RV free wall with a scalloped appearance (arrows). Fatty infiltration, fibrosis, and wall motion abnormalities may also be visualized on imaging studies.[2] The 69-year-old woman with prior myocardial infarction has suffered a cerebral thromboembolism due to the left ventricular apical thrombus demonstrated in C. The x-ray attenuation of the thrombus is clearly different from that of the surrounding myocardium.

The computed tomogram in A demonstrates a thickened pericardium with prominent calcification, which is consistent with constrictive pericarditis in the clinical scenario presented. A pericardial thickness >2 mm on helical CT is considered abnormal. Either CT or MRI may be used to image thickened pericardium in suspected constrictive disease; however, pericardial calcification cannot be directly visualized by MRI.[3]

REFERENCES

1. Hoey ET, Mankad K, Puppala S, et al: MRI and CT appearances of cardiac tumors in adults. Clin Radiol 64:1214, 2009.
2. Murphy DT, Shine SC, Cradock A, et al: Cardiac MRI in arrhythmogenic right ventricular cardiomyopathy. AJR Am J Roentgenol 194:W299, 2010.
3. Yared K, Baggish AL, Picard MH, et al: Multimodality imaging of pericardial diseases. J Am Coll Cardiol Cardiovasc Imaging 3:650, 2010.

ANSWERS TO QUESTIONS 114 TO 117

114–D, 115–A, 116–B, 117–C (Braunwald, pp. 220-223; Figs. 15-26 and 15-27)

Normal left ventricular (LV) filling, as recorded by Doppler imaging of diastolic mitral flow velocities, is characterized by a rapid early diastolic phase (the E wave), followed by late additional filling during atrial contraction (the A wave). The relative contribution of early versus late filling is expressed as the E/A ratio. Normally this ratio is >1 and the time required for LV deceleration in early diastole is >190 milliseconds. These relationships are altered in states of abnormal LV filling.

When impaired LV diastolic relaxation is present there is a reduced diastolic gradient between the left atrium and left ventricle, resulting in a decreased early LV filling (E wave) with a reversed E/A ratio of <1, and the early deceleration time may be prolonged.

The pseudonormalized pattern is observed in patients with more severe diastolic impairment. In this situation there is restoration of the normal early diastolic LV pressure gradient due to elevated left atrial pressure. Thus, the E wave remains taller than the A wave but the LV deceleration time is more rapid compared with normal.

The restrictive pattern of LV filling is seen in patients with infiltrative disease and other forms of restrictive cardiomyopathy. Because of the markedly elevated left atrial pressure, there is enhanced early filling of the left ventricle such that early mitral inflow (E wave) is much greater than the atrial (A wave) contribution to filling and the LV deceleration time is shortened. In this situation, atrial contraction often contributes little to LV filling and the A wave may be barely detected.

REFERENCE

Nageuh SF, Appleton CP, Gillebert TC, et al: Guidelines and standards: Recommendations for the evaluation of left ventricular diastolic function by echocardiography. J Am Soc Echocardiogr 22:107, 2009.

ANSWERS TO QUESTIONS 118 TO 121

118–A, 119–C, 120–D, 121–B (Braunwald, pp. 279-289, 1421-1422, 1426-1428, 1483, 1493, 1657-1658)

The chest radiograph in patients with abnormalities of the mitral valve commonly displays left atrial enlargement, whether the lesion is mitral stenosis or mitral regurgitation. The characteristic chest film in mitral stenosis (see A) displays a heart that is often normal in size, except for the enlargement of the left atrium, which is even more prominent in patients with atrial fibrillation. Calcification of the mitral valve may also be visible on chest films. Severe mitral stenosis is commonly accompanied by pulmonary hypertension, which may be associated with right ventricular dilatation on the chest radiograph. With advanced mitral stenosis there may be pulmonary vascular redistribution or frank interstitial edema.

A number of findings may be present on the chest radiograph in patients with aortic regurgitation (see C). Enlargement of the left ventricle results in displacement of the cardiac apex downward, to the left, and posteriorly. In addition, the ascending aorta may be dilated. In contrast, aortic stenosis tends to be more difficult to recognize on plain chest films. Abnormalities in the shape of the heart, although sometimes present, tend to be subtle. Significant left ventricular dilatation occurs only with myocardial failure in end-stage aortic stenosis. Although calcification of the aortic valve is common in aortic stenosis, it may not be appreciated on routine chest films. Similarly, routine views may not visualize the poststenotic dilatation of the ascending aorta that often occurs in this condition. The ostium secundum type of atrial septal defect (ASD; see D) is a congenital cardiac lesion that may be first identified in adults. Findings on the chest radiograph include dilatation of the main pulmonary artery, enlargement of the right ventricle, and a generalized increase in the pulmonary vascularity. Right atrial enlargement may be present. Although the chest film in a patient with a secundum ASD may be similar to that of the patient with mitral stenosis, in the latter condition there is usually left atrial enlargement and redistribution of pulmonary blood flow with dilatation of upper lobe vessels and constriction of the vessels at the lung bases. In contrast, when significant left-to-right shunting is present in an ASD, all the pulmonary vessels—including those at the bases—are dilated.

The presence of pericardial effusion (see B) leads to a characteristic set of changes in the chest roentgenogram. With increasing volumes of pericardial fluid, enlargement of the cardiac silhouette with smoothing out and loss of the normal cardiac contours occurs, leading to a symmetrically distended, flask-shaped cardiac shadow. Although such a pattern may be seen with the generalized dilatation that occurs in heart failure, the appearance of the pulmonary hila distinguishes between these two conditions. In pericardial effusion, the pericardial sac tends to cover the shadows of the hilar vessels as it is further distended. In contrast, the failing heart is usually associated with abnormally prominent hilar vessels and pulmonary vascular congestion.

ANSWERS TO QUESTIONS 122 TO 125

122–C, 123–A, 124–B, 125–D (Braunwald, pp. 133, 653-656, 771, 777-785, Fig. 39-4)

Sinus rhythm is initiated by impulses from the sinus node at rates between 60 and 100 beats/min. Because the wave of depolarization spreads downward from the right atrium toward the left atrium and ventricles, the P wave is upright in leads I, II, and aVF and is negative in lead aVR. The rate of atrial tachycardia is generally 150 to 200 beats/min, with a P wave contour that is different from that of the normal sinus P wave. This rhythm occurs most commonly in patients with structural heart disease (coronary artery disease, cor pulmonale, digitalis intoxication) but can also occur in normal hearts. Potential mechanisms of atrial tachycardia include automaticity, triggered activity, and reentry. Focal atrial tachycardia due to automaticity generally accelerates after its initiation, but the initiating P wave has the same contour as subsequent ones. In contrast, in reentrant rhythms such as atrioventricular nodal reentrant tachycardia, the first P wave is usually different in shape compared with subsequent P waves because the tachycardia is initiated by a premature atrial complex, whereas subsequent P waves derive from retrograde atrial activation.

Atrial flutter is a macroreentrant atrial rhythm. In the typical form (type I flutter) the reentrant pathway circulates in a counterclockwise direction in the right atrium, constrained anteriorly by the tricuspid annulus and posteriorly by the crista terminalis and eustachian ridge. The atrial rate during typical atrial flutter is 250 to 350 beats/min. The ECG shows recurring regular sawtooth flutter waves often best visualized in leads II, III, and aVF. In typical counterclockwise flutter, the flutter waves are inverted (negative) in these leads.

ANSWERS TO QUESTIONS 126 TO 129

126–B, 127–C, 128–A, 129–F (Braunwald, pp. 35-36, 178-179, 297-300; Table 14-2; Fig. 17-9)

Test selection depends in part on the goal of the test (i.e., is the test intended to select a subpopulation with increased probability of disease for further testing [a screening test], or is the purpose to definitively rule out the presence of disease [a confirmatory test])? Sensitivity quantifies a test's ability to detect disease when present, whereas specificity quantifies a test's ability to rule out disease. As demonstrated in the receiver operating curve, sensitivity and specificity are inversely related—as sensitivity increases, the specificity of the test decreases, and vice versa. Sensitivity and specificity can be derived from the graph: the dashed vertical line denotes 98% specificity, at which point Test A has a sensitivity of ~59%, but Test B has a sensitivity of only ~47%. Test A is thus a better test to confirm the presence of disease (i.e., better sensitivity at the high level of specificity required for a confirmatory test). In contrast, an ideal screening test has high sensitivity while minimizing false positives (i.e., maximizing specificity). In the high sensitivity range, Test B has a higher specificity (specificity ~70% at a sensitivity of 98%, denoted by the dashed line) than does Test A (specificity ~60% at the same sensitivity of 98%), making Test B the better screening test.

$$\text{Sensitivity} = \frac{\text{True Positives}}{\text{True Positives} + \text{False Negatives}}$$

$$\text{Specificity} = \frac{\text{True Negatives}}{\text{True Negatives} + \text{False Positives}}$$

Sensitivity and specificity are specific to a test, whereas positive predictive value and negative predictive value reflect the characteristics not only of the test but also of the population in which the test is being used.

Positive Predictive Value

$$= \frac{\text{True Positives}}{\text{True Positives} + \text{False Positives}} \times 100$$

Negative Predictive Value

$$= \frac{\text{True Negatives}}{\text{True Negatives} + \text{False Negatives}} \times 100$$

For the population in question with a disease prevalence of 50/1000:

True Positives = Number of people affected × Sensitivity = $50 \times 0.98 = 49$

False Negatives = Number affected − True Positives = $50 - 49 = 1$

True Negatives = Number unaffected × Specificity = $950 \times 0.6 = 570$

False Positives = Number unaffected − True Negatives = $950 - 570 = 380$

Positive Predictive Value

$$= \frac{\text{True Positives}}{\text{True Positives} + \text{False Positives}} \times 100$$

$$= \frac{49}{49 + 380} \times 100 = 11\%$$

REFERENCE

McPherson RA, Pincus MR: Henry's Clinical Diagnosis and Management by Laboratory Methods. 21st ed. Philadelphia, WB Saunders, 2006.

ANSWERS TO QUESTIONS 130 TO 133

130–D, 131–A, 132–C, 133–B (Braunwald, pp. 141-142, 147-149, 158, 160-161, 1653, 1704)

The patient with renal failure has developed hyperkalemia. The ECG was obtained when the serum potassium level was 7.2 and shows the characteristic narrow, peaked T waves of hyperkalemia (see D in the figure). The QT interval is shortened relative to baseline, and there is mild QRS widening. The P wave amplitude is normal at this time but would decrease with progressive, untreated hyperkalemia. The patient with positional, sharp chest discomfort has acute viral pericarditis, manifest on the ECG by diffuse ST-segment elevation, PR-segment depression, and a resting tachycardia (see A). The ECG of the man with lightheadedness demonstrates complete heart block. Although the initial portion of the rhythm may suggest 2:1 second-degree atrioventricular block (see C), there is actually no relationship between the P waves and QRS complexes (note that the PR interval varies). The 38-year-old woman has congenital heart disease with partially corrective surgery as a child and has subsequently developed pulmonary hypertension with a right-to-left shunt through an atrial septal defect, resulting in systemic oxygen desaturation. The ECG shows findings of right ventricular (RV) hypertrophy, including right-axis deviation in the frontal plane, deep S waves, and abnormally small R waves in the left-sided leads, with reversal of normal R wave progression across the precordium (see B). The rSR′ pattern in lead V_1 is consistent with RV conduction delay.

ANSWERS TO QUESTIONS 134 TO 142

(Braunwald, pp. 200-276)

134. Transthoracic echocardiogram, apical four-chamber view in systole. There is left ventricular enlargement with a thinned region of the distal septum and apex, which bulges outward and contains a large thrombus. There is a pericardial effusion external to the left ventricle. *Diagnosis:* Left ventricular aneurysm with thrombus and pericardial effusion.
135. Transthoracic echocardiogram, parasternal short-axis view at the aortic valve level. A bicuspid aortic valve is present (10-o'clock to 4-o'clock orientation). *Diagnosis:* Congenital bicuspid aortic valve.
136. Transthoracic echocardiogram, parasternal long-axis view. Turbulent color flow across the interventricular septum is consistent with a left-to-right shunt through a perimembranous ventricular septal defect. *Diagnosis:* Congenital ventricular septal defect.
137. Transthoracic echocardiogram, parasternal long-axis view. There is dilatation of the aortic root. *Diagnosis:* Marfan syndrome.

138. Transthoracic echocardiogram, apical four-chamber view, with color Doppler interrogation (A). The blue (retrograde flow) color Doppler signal extends to the level of the pulmonary veins, consistent with severe mitral regurgitation. In B, pulsed Doppler interrogation of a pulmonary vein confirms reversed systolic flow at that level (the systolic Doppler signal below the baseline indicates flow from the left atrium into the pulmonary vein). *Diagnosis:* Severe mitral regurgitation.
139. Doppler tissue imaging (DTI) at the lateral mitral annulus. The early diastolic relaxation velocity (the deflection below the baseline after the electrocardiographic T wave) is recorded at 7.3 cm/sec. Values <8 cm/sec are consistent with impaired diastolic relaxation. An example of a normal DTI is shown in Figure 1-71. *Diagnosis:* Diastolic dysfunction, due in this case to cardiac amyloidosis.
140. Transthoracic echocardiogram, apical four-chamber view. Images are before (left) and after (right) injection of agitated saline into an antecubital vein (a "bubble study"). A redundant and mobile interatrial septum bulges into the left atrium. Passage of "bubbles" into the left side of the heart is consistent with a right-to-left shunt. *Diagnosis:* Atrial septal aneurysm with likely patent foramen ovale and right-to-left shunt (possible paradoxical embolism as the cause of the stroke).
141. Transthoracic echocardiogram, subcostal view. There is a thickened interatrial septum that spares the fossa ovalis, creating a "dumbbell" appearance. *Diagnosis:* Lipomatous hypertrophy of the atrial septum.
142. Transthoracic echocardiogram, parasternal long-axis view. There is a large left-sided pleural effusion posterior to the left ventricle (note that the effusion extends posterior to the descending aorta; pericardial effusions accumulate *anterior* to the descending aorta). *Diagnosis:* Dyspnea due to large pleural effusion.

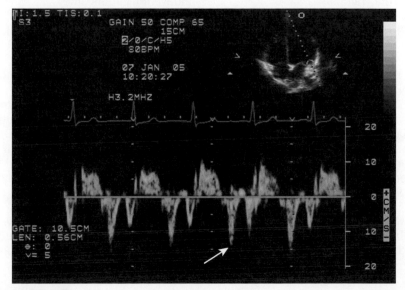

FIGURE 1-71

ANSWERS TO QUESTIONS 143 TO 167

The numbers in brackets refer to features on the electrocardiographic response form on page 46.

143. [7] Normal sinus rhythm (rate 65)
   [38] Right-axis deviation
   [52] Extensive old anterolateral myocardial infarction
   [63] Inferior nonspecific ST-segment depression and T wave abnormality
   [65] Anterolateral ST-segment elevation/T wave inversion consistent with aneurysm or recent myocardial infarction
(Patient had a prior anterior myocardial infarction with subsequent large anterior wall aneurysm)

144. [7] Normal sinus rhythm (rate 96)
   [29] Borderline first-degree atrioventricular block
   [43] Right bundle branch block
   [37] Right superior axis deviation (which is actually extreme left- or right-axis deviation, so [38] is also correct)
   [42] Left ventricular hypertrophy and right ventricular hypertrophy (R' >15 mm in lead V_1)
   [54] Possible anterior myocardial infarction, age indeterminate (Q waves in V_2 to V_3)
   [67] ST-segment/T wave abnormality secondary to hypertrophy and bundle branch block
(The ECG suggests patient has coronary artery disease and cor pulmonale)

145. [7] Normal sinus rhythm (rate 65)
   [37] Borderline left-axis deviation
   [42] Biventricular hypertrophy
      Nondiagnostic lateral Q waves
   [64, 67] Anterolateral ST-segment/T wave abnormality consistent with hypertrophy or ischemia
(The patient has asymmetric hypertrophic cardiomyopathy [85])

146. [9] Sinus bradycardia (rate 55)
   [94] Inappropriate ventricular paced beats (failure to sense and pseudofusion beat [complex 11])
   [63] Nonspecific inferior T wave abnormality
   [69] Prominent U waves
(Pacemaker malfunction)

147. [7] Normal sinus rhythm (rate 88)
   [37] Left-axis deviation
   [34] Preexcitation pattern resulting in a pseudoinfarction pattern in inferior leads and anterolateral ST-segment/T wave abnormality
(Wolff-Parkinson-White syndrome)

148. [18] Atrial flutter with 2:1 atrioventricular conduction, ventricular rate 160 (the flutter waves are seen best in the inferior leads)

149. [7] Normal sinus rhythm (rate 85)
   [5, 6] Biatrial enlargement

   [38] Right-axis deviation (+110)
   [41] Right ventricular hypertrophy (R > S and qR pattern in V1, with right-axis deviation)
   [67] ST-segment/T wave abnormality in anterior precordial leads
   [68] Prolonged QTc
(The patient has advanced mitral stenosis)

150. [19] Rapid atrial fibrillation (ventricular rate ~220)
   [37] Left-axis deviation
   [34] Preexcitation pattern
(Patient has Wolff-Parkinson-White syndrome with atrial fibrillation and rapid conduction through the accessory pathway, which is probably located in the left posteroseptal region)

151. [8] Sinus arrhythmia
   [30] Type I second-degree atrioventricular block (Wenckebach)
   [43] Right bundle branch block
(Patient was experiencing a vagal reaction during an uncomfortable medical procedure)

152. [7, 23] Normal sinus rhythm with premature ventricular depolarizations and fusion beat
   [6] Left atrial enlargement
   [37] Left-axis deviation
   [45] Left anterior fascicular block (LAFB)
   [40] Probable left ventricular hypertrophy
   [54] Possible old anteroseptal myocardial infarction (vs. small q waves in V_2 to V_3 owing to LAFB)
(This man has aortic stenosis and coronary artery disease)

153. [17] Supraventricular tachycardia (rate 160)
   [40] Left ventricular hypertrophy
   [63] Diffuse nonspecific ST-segment/T wave abnormalities
(Patient is a 43-year-old woman with a history of paroxysmal tachycardias who was successfully treated with intravenous adenosine)

154. [19] Atrial fibrillation (ventricular rate ~60)
   [43] Right bundle branch block
   [38] Right-axis deviation
   [46] Left posterior fascicular block

155. [9] Sinus bradycardia (rate 58)
      Counterclockwise rotation
   [61] Early repolarization
(Diffuse ST-segment elevation is <25% height of the T wave and there is no PR-segment depression, which helps distinguish early repolarization from pericarditis)

156. [10] Borderline sinus tachycardia (rate 100)
   [49] Intraventricular conduction delay
   [66, 74] Peaked T waves consistent with hyperkalemia
(This patient with chronic renal failure presented with a serum potassium level of 7.5 mmol/L.)

157. [9] Sinus bradycardia (rate 56)
[56, 58, 60] Old inferoposterolateral myocardial infarction
[63] Nonspecific T wave abnormality in lateral leads

158. [10] Sinus tachycardia (atrial rate 106)
[33, 27] Third-degree atrioventricular block with ventricular escape rhythm

159. [7] Normal sinus rhythm (rate 84)
[44] Incomplete right bundle branch block
[57] Acute inferior myocardial infarction

160. [7] Normal sinus rhythm (rate 66)
[29] First-degree atrioventricular block
[43] Right bundle branch block
[45] Left anterior fascicular block
[40] Left ventricular hypertrophy

161. [7] Normal sinus rhythm (atrial rate ~84)
[33, 22] Third-degree atrioventricular block with junctional escape rhythm
(Patient has congenital complete heart block related to maternal systemic lupus erythematosus)

162. [7] Normal sinus rhythm (rate 90)
[38] Borderline right-axis deviation
[6] Left atrial abnormality
[49] Right ventricular conduction delay (rsR′ in V$_1$ without prolonged QRS duration or voltage criteria for right ventricular hypertrophy)

[63] Nonspecific ST-segment/T wave abnormality in anterior leads
(A 23-year-old woman with a secundum atrial septal defect [78])

163. [7] Normal sinus rhythm (rate 82)
[68] Prolonged QT interval
(Patient with congenital prolongation of the QT interval whose subsequent ambulatory monitor showed periods of polymorphic ventricular tachycardia as the cause of her presyncopal episodes)

164. [19] Atrial fibrillation with rapid ventricular response (ventricular rate ~140)
[37] Borderline left-axis deviation
[47] Left bundle branch block

165. [22] Junctional rhythm (rate 50)
[57, 59] Acute inferior and right ventricular myocardial infarction (with possible posterior wall involvement)

166. [25] Ventricular tachycardia originating from right ventricular outflow tract (left bundle branch block morphology and inferior axis)

167. [4] Baseline artifact due to resting tremor
[9] Sinus bradycardia
[13] Atrial premature complexes
[63] Nonspecific ST-segment and T wave abnormalities
(Patient has Parkinson disease)

FUNDAMENTALS OF CARDIOVASCULAR DISEASE; MOLECULAR BIOLOGY AND GENETICS; EVALUATION OF THE PATIENT

HEART FAILURE; ARRHYTHMIAS, SUDDEN DEATH, AND SYNCOPE

DIRECTIONS: For each question below, select the ONE BEST response.

QUESTION 168

All of the following statements about natriuretic peptides are true EXCEPT:
A. Circulating levels of both atrial natriuretic peptide and brain natriuretic peptide (BNP) are elevated in patients with heart failure
B. Plasma BNP level is useful in distinguishing cardiac from noncardiac causes of dyspnea in the emergency department setting
C. Elevated plasma BNP levels predict adverse outcomes in patients with acute coronary syndromes
D. Prohormone BNP is cleaved into the biologically inactive N-terminal (NT) proBNP and biologically active BNP
E. Circulating levels of BNP and NT-proBNP levels decrease with age and worsening renal function

QUESTION 169

All of the following statements about diuretics in heart failure are true EXCEPT:
A. Mannitol is an effective diuretic in cardiac surgical patients with decompensated heart failure
B. Carbonic anhydrase inhibitors improve the alkalemia caused by other diuretic agents
C. Aldosterone receptor antagonists may cause clinically significant hyperkalemia
D. Loop diuretics often result in hypokalemia and metabolic alkalosis
E. The effectiveness of loop diuretic agents is reduced by nonsteroidal anti-inflammatory drugs

QUESTION 170

Which of the following conditions is likely to precipitate symptomatic heart failure in patients with previously compensated left ventricular contractile dysfunction?
A. Atrial fibrillation
B. Marked sinus bradycardia
C. Atrioventricular dissociation
D. Right ventricular apical pacing
E. All of the above

QUESTION 171

An 80-year-old women with a history of hypertension and type 2 diabetes is hospitalized because of progressive exertional dyspnea and orthopnea. Her examination is notable for an elevated jugular venous pressure (JVP) to the angle of the jaw, pitting peripheral edema with warm extremities, normal blood pressure, and clear mental status. After 4 days of treatment with a loop diuretic she appears clinically euvolemic with a JVP of 7 cm H_2O. However, the serum creatinine value has risen from 1.6 mg/dL at the time of admission to 2.3 mg/dL. Each of the following statements about this patient's condition is correct EXCEPT:
A. Diabetes and hypertension predispose to the development of cardiorenal syndrome
B. Worsening renal function during hospitalization for acute heart failure is an important predictor of early hospital readmission and mortality
C. Decreased renal venous pressure contributes to the cardiorenal syndrome
D. High-dose loop diuretic therapy activates neurohormones that contribute to the cardiorenal syndrome
E. A disproportionate rise in blood urea nitrogen compared with serum creatinine is a sign of renal hypoperfusion

QUESTION 172

Each of the following statements regarding therapy for systolic heart failure is correct EXCEPT:
A. Digoxin therapy decreases hospitalizations and mortality in patients with chronic heart failure
B. Angiotensin-converting enzyme (ACE) inhibitors improve survival in heart failure more than the combination of hydralazine plus isosorbide dinitrate
C. Angiotensin II receptor blockers provide morbidity and mortality benefits comparable with ACE inhibitors in patients with heart failure
D. Spironolactone reduces mortality in patients with Class III to IV heart failure symptoms

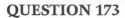

E. The aldosterone antagonist eplerenone reduces mortality in patients with Class II to III heart failure.

QUESTION 173

Each of the following statements about cardiac transplantation is true EXCEPT:
A. Use of the immunosuppressant agent cyclosporine has led to improved long-term outcomes after cardiac transplantation
B. Younger patients have better survival rates than older patients after cardiac transplantation
C. Patients with heart transplants lack the chronotropic response necessary to support the hemodynamic demands of exercise
D. Endomyocardial biopsy is the most reliable current technique to assess allograft rejection
E. Risk of death from malignancy rises with time after transplantation whereas mortality from infection declines

QUESTION 174

A 78-year-old nursing home resident is admitted via the emergency department because of fever and disorientation. His physical examination demonstrates minimal bibasilar rales and no jugular venous distention, abnormal heart sounds, or peripheral edema. The ECG shows sinus tachycardia. Notable laboratory results include an elevated white blood cell count, low platelet count, and prolonged prothrombin time. The urine sediment contains numerous polymorphonuclear leukocytes. A cardiology consultation is obtained for evaluation of the chest radiograph shown in Figure 2-1. The most likely explanation for the accompanying chest radiographic findings is:
A. Left ventricular failure
B. Pneumococcal pneumonia
C. Acute respiratory distress syndrome
D. Gram-negative pneumonia
E. Posterior wall myocardial infarction

QUESTION 175

Each of the following statements about laboratory findings in heart failure is true EXCEPT:
A. Serum electrolyte values are usually normal in patients with untreated heart failure of short duration
B. Contributors to hyponatremia in heart failure include dietary sodium restriction, diuretic therapy, and an elevated circulating vasopressin level
C. Elevated serum aspartate aminotransferase levels may accompany congestive hepatomegaly due to heart failure
D. Acute hepatic venous congestion due to heart failure may produce a syndrome that closely resembles viral hepatitis
E. Pulmonary capillary wedge pressures of 13 to 17 mm Hg are commonly responsible for pulmonary

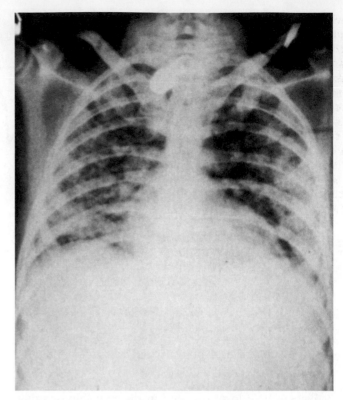

FIGURE 2-1 From Kumar V, Abbas AK, Fausto N (eds): Robbins and Cotran Pathologic Basis of Disease. 7th ed. Philadelphia, Elsevier, 2005, p 615.

vascular redistribution and interstitial edema on the chest radiograph

QUESTION 176

Each of the following statements about myocardial contraction is true EXCEPT:
A. Beta$_1$-adrenergic stimulation increases the concentration of intracellular calcium
B. Beta$_1$-adrenergic stimulation promotes production of intracellular cyclic guanosine monophosphate
C. Interaction of calcium with troponin C is essential for myocyte contraction
D. Myosin molecules are tethered to the Z line by the protein titin
E. The sarcoplasmic reticulum plays a key role in the release and uptake of calcium

QUESTION 177

A 45-year-old woman who underwent orthotopic cardiac transplantation for a familial dilated cardiomyopathy presents 2 months later for routine post-transplant surveillance. An endomyocardial biopsy is obtained (Figure 2-2). Each of the following statements is true EXCEPT:
A. Endomyocardial biopsy is the most reliable technique to assess for this complication
B. This disorder is caused by preexisting recipient antibodies to allogeneic antigens on the vascular endothelium of the donor organ

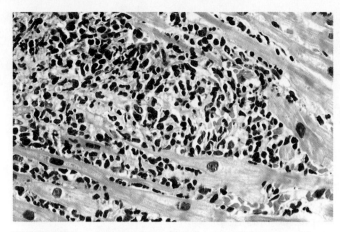

FIGURE 2-2 From Kumar V, Abbas AK, Fausto N (eds): Robbins and Cotran Pathologic Basis of Disease. 7th ed. Philadelphia, Elsevier, 2005, p 615.

C. Lymphocyte infiltration and myocyte necrosis are the most important biopsy features in the diagnosis of this disorder
D. Most episodes of this complication arise less than 6 months after transplantation
E. Pulsed corticosteroids are the therapy of choice for this finding

QUESTION 178

All of the following statements are true EXCEPT:
A. Major determinants of cardiac output are heart rate and ventricular stroke volume
B. The myocardium extracts oxygen from blood nearly maximally at rest such that the coronary sinus oxygen saturation is < 40%
C. During strenuous exercise, O_2 consumption can increase up to 18-fold
D. The peak O_2 consumption and the anaerobic threshold as measured by cardiopulmonary exercise testing are highly reproducible when measured days or weeks apart
E. A measured peak O_2 consumption of 20 mL/min/kg at exercise testing indicates severe functional impairment

QUESTION 179

Correct statements regarding structural and hemodynamic left ventricular (LV) parameters in chronic pressure- and volume-overload states include all of the following EXCEPT:
A. LV systolic stress is proportional to intracavitary pressure and chamber radius
B. Eccentric hypertrophy is characteristic of volume overload
C. Concentric hypertrophy is characteristic of pressure overload
D. LV wall thickness is greater in pressure-overload states than in volume-overload states
E. The ratio of wall thickness to chamber dimension is greater in volume-overload states

QUESTION 180

Each of the following statements concerning therapy of patients with left ventricular (LV) dysfunction is true EXCEPT:
A. Amiodarone consistently reduces mortality in patients with Class II or III heart failure
B. Implantation of a cardioverter-defibrillator is indicated in patients with the combination of LV dysfunction and unexplained syncope or resuscitated cardiac arrest
C. Patients with LV dysfunction and a transient or correctable cause of ventricular tachycardia remain at high risk for sudden death
D. Prophylactic implantation of a cardioverter-defibrillator is effective in reducing mortality in patients with coronary artery disease and severe LV dysfunction
E. Use of dronedarone in patients with moderate or severe heart failure is associated with increased mortality

QUESTION 181

A 56-year-old man with ischemic cardiomyopathy and an ejection fraction (EF) of 25% comes for an outpatient clinic visit complaining of dyspnea and fatigue with minimal exertion (Class III). His medical regimen includes lisinopril, carvedilol, eplerenone, and furosemide. Resting electrocardiography reveals sinus rhythm with a QRS complex duration of 160 milliseconds and a left bundle branch morphology. He is being considered for placement of a biventricular pacemaker. All of the following statements about cardiac resynchronization therapy (CRT) are true EXCEPT:
A. CRT reduces mortality in patients with Class III or IV heart failure only when combined with an implantable cardioverter-defibrillator (ICD)
B. Ventricular dyssynchrony is defined as a QRS complex >120 milliseconds on the surface ECG regardless of QRS morphology
C. The nonresponder rate for CRT is approximately 25%
D. CRT improves myocardial performance without increasing myocardial oxygen consumption
E. Echocardiographic measures of dyssynchrony are not part of the standard selection criteria for CRT

QUESTION 182

True statements about the syndrome of circulatory shock include all of the following EXCEPT:
A. The clinical signs of shock reflect a decrease in blood flow to multiple organs
B. Electrocardiographic signs of myocardial ischemia may appear in patients with apparently normal hearts owing to a reduction in regional coronary blood flow
C. Vasodilatory shock is characterized by an excess of circulating vasopressin
D. Vasodilatory shock is the final common pathway for long-lasting and severe shock of any cause

E. During circulatory shock, cerebral blood flow is often protected at the expense of splanchnic and renal perfusion

QUESTION 183

Each of the following statements about edema in heart failure is correct EXCEPT:
A. Edema in heart failure does not correlate well with the level of systemic venous pressure
B. Peripheral edema may be detected when extracellular fluid volume has increased by as little as 1 to 2 liters
C. Severe edema may cause rupture of the skin and extravasation of fluid
D. In patients with acute heart failure, edema may not be present
E. In patients with hemiplegia due to a cerebrovascular accident, edema is usually more apparent on the paralyzed side

QUESTION 184

A 68-year-old woman with long-standing hypertension presents to the emergency department because of progressive exertional dyspnea and fatigue over the past several months. She notes that it is increasingly difficult to put on her shoes because of ankle edema and is uncomfortable sleeping on one pillow due to a cough while recumbent. She denies chest discomfort or palpitations. Her medications include atenolol and hydrochlorothiazide.

On examination, she is an overweight woman with heart rate of 70 beats/min, respirations of 20 breaths/min, and blood pressure of 170/90 mm Hg. The jugular venous pressure is 14 cm H_2O. Examination of the chest is notable for bibasilar rales. The cardiovascular examination reveals a normal S_1, physiologically split S_2, and S_4 gallop. There is no audible murmur. The extremities demonstrate pitting edema to the midcalf bilaterally.

The ECG reveals sinus rhythm with voltage criteria for left ventricular hypertrophy. The chest radiograph shows a normal cardiac silhouette with bilateral pleural effusions with mild interstitial pulmonary edema. Echocardiography demonstrates concentric left ventricular hypertrophy. The estimated ejection fraction is 70%.

Which of the following pharmacologic agents has been shown to improve survival in this condition?
A. Digoxin
B. Perindopril
C. Verapamil
D. Candesartan
E. None of the above

QUESTION 185

Each of the following statements about physical findings in heart failure is true EXCEPT:

A. Chronic, marked elevation of systemic venous pressure may produce exophthalmos or visible systolic pulsation of the eyes
B. Pallor and coldness of the extremities are primarily due to increased adrenergic nervous system activity
C. An abdominojugular reflex reflects the combination of hepatic congestion and the inability of the right side of the heart to accept increased venous return
D. Hepatic tenderness results from long-standing right-sided heart failure with chronic stretching of the liver capsule
E. Protein-losing enteropathy may occur in patients with visceral congestion and may result in a reduced plasma oncotic pressure

QUESTION 186

A 72-year-old diabetic man with long-standing dilated cardiomyopathy presents for evaluation of dyspnea at rest. He has been hospitalized three times within the past year for decompensated heart failure and recently underwent a cardiopulmonary exercise test showing a peak oxygen consumption of 10 mL/kg/min during maximal effort. His past medical history is notable for prior placement of an implantable cardioverter-defibrillator (ICD) for primary prevention of sudden cardiac death and a prostatectomy 1 year earlier for adenocarcinoma. For the last 6 months he has been intolerant of beta-adrenergic blockers because of hypotension. He has a supportive family, adheres to therapeutic recommendations, and does not use tobacco.

Physical examination reveals a blood pressure of 92/78 mm Hg, resting heart rate of 106 beats/min, body mass index of 26 kg/m^2, jugular venous pressure of 10 cm H_2O, clear lungs, an S_3 apical gallop, and cool extremities but no evidence of hepatomegaly or ascites. Laboratory studies are notable for the following: sodium, 126 mEq/L; potassium, 4.6 mEq/L; blood urea nitrogen, 34 mg/dL; and creatinine 2.5 mg/dL. Liver function tests and the complete blood cell count are normal. Electrocardiography shows sinus tachycardia and a QRS complex duration of 96 milliseconds. Echocardiography demonstrates a dilated left ventricle with an ejection fraction of 20%, mild mitral regurgitation, and normal right ventricular size and function.

Which of the following is the most appropriate consideration for this patient?
A. Cardiac resynchronization therapy
B. Urgent listing for cardiac transplantation
C. Listing for combined heart-kidney transplantation
D. Implantation of a left ventricular assist device
E. Implantation of a biventricular assist device

QUESTION 187

All of the following statements regarding the cardiac cycle are true EXCEPT:
A. The third heart sound (S_3) corresponds to rapid early diastolic filling of the ventricles

B. The absence of an *a* wave on the right atrial pressure tracing is typical of atrial fibrillation
C. The QRS complex on the ECG corresponds to the initiation of isovolumic ventricular contraction
D. The *v* wave on the right or left atrial pressure tracing occurs before the T wave on the ECG
E. The mitral valve opens in diastole when the left ventricular pressure falls below the left atrial pressure

QUESTION 188

Each of the following statements about physical findings in heart failure is true EXCEPT:
A. Hydrothorax in heart failure is most often bilateral, but when unilateral it is usually confined to the right side of the chest
B. The absence of pulmonary rales on examination excludes the presence of an elevated pulmonary capillary pressure
C. Hepatomegaly frequently precedes the development of overt peripheral edema
D. Peripheral edema may be absent in patients with significant volume overload and systemic venous congestion
E. In left ventricular failure, P_2 is often accentuated

QUESTION 189

A 66-year-old man with a history of diabetes and hypertension presents for evaluation of exertional dyspnea. He denies associated chest discomfort but frequently awakens from sleep with shortness of breath. On examination, he has prominent jugular venous distention, a regular heart rhythm with an apical S_4 gallop, bibasilar rales, hepatomegaly, and mild bilateral pedal edema. Electrocardiography reveals sinus rhythm at a rate of 94 beats/min without ST-segment deviations or pathologic Q waves. Echocardiography is notable for a left ventricular ejection fraction of 25% and akinesis of the anterior wall. Subsequent coronary angiography reveals severe three-vessel coronary artery disease with distal targets suitable for surgical revascularization. Which of the following statements about this patient's ischemic cardiomyopathy is correct?
A. Coronary artery bypass grafting (CABG) is superior to medical therapy only if angina is present
B. In this patient's case, dobutamine echocardiography or positron emission tomography could differentiate anterior wall infarction from hibernating myocardium
C. CABG improves quality of life and survival more than medical therapy only if >50% of the myocardium is shown to be viable
D. Stunned myocardium refers to persistent contractile dysfunction caused by chronically reduced coronary blood flow
E. Surgical ventricular reconstruction should be performed along with CABG because the anterior wall is akinetic

QUESTION 190

All of the following statements about digitalis toxicity are true EXCEPT:
A. Lidocaine and phenytoin are useful agents in treating arrhythmias due to digitalis excess
B. Second- and third-degree atrioventricular blocks in this setting often respond to atropine
C. Recurrence of digitalis toxicity may occur 24 to 48 hours after the administration of antidigoxin immunotherapy
D. Direct-current cardioversion may precipitate ventricular arrhythmias in patients with digitalis intoxication and should be avoided
E. Dialysis is effective in cases of massive overdose

QUESTION 191

All of the following statements about heart failure are true EXCEPT:
A. Over the past decade, the incidence and prevalence of heart failure have increased
B. Heart failure occurs in 10% of patients older than age 75 years but only in 1% to 2% of patients ages 45 to 54 years
C. Orthopnea is a symptom that is specific for the diagnosis of heart failure
D. Pulsus alternans occurs more commonly in systolic than diastolic heart failure
E. Heart failure with preserved ejection fraction is more common in women than in men

QUESTION 192

The circulatory support device seen in the radiograph in Figure 2-3 has been shown to significantly improve

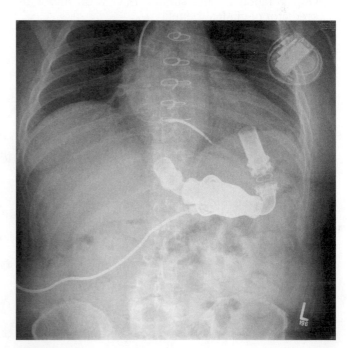

FIGURE 2-3

survival and quality of life in select patients with advanced heart failure. Common adverse events associated with this therapy include all of the following EXCEPT:
A. Stroke
B. Driveline infection
C. Pump rotor failure
D. Gastrointestinal bleeding
E. Right ventricular failure

QUESTION 193

Which of the following conditions is associated with increased left ventricular preload?
A. Sepsis
B. Right ventricular infarction
C. Mitral regurgitation
D. Dehydration
E. Pulmonary embolism

QUESTION 194

Figure 2-4 displays posteroanterior and lateral chest radiographs of a patient with an idiopathic cardiomyopathy, symptomatic heart failure, a left ventricular ejection fraction < 0.35, and left bundle branch block on the ECG. All of the following statements about the pictured device are true EXCEPT:
A. Implantation of this device reduces left ventricular dimensions and mitral regurgitation
B. Placement of this type of device is associated with improved survival
C. A complication of device implantation is phrenic nerve stimulation with diaphragmatic pacing
D. Minimization of this form of ventricular pacing is important to prevent progressive heart failure
E. QRS duration on the surface ECG is an important predictor of clinical benefit

QUESTION 195

Each of the following conditions is associated with the development of pulmonary edema EXCEPT:
A. Increased pulmonary venous pressure
B. High altitude
C. Increased plasma oncotic pressure
D. Eclampsia
E. Heroin overdose

QUESTION 196

True statements about cardiac physical findings in patients with heart failure include all of the following EXCEPT:
A. Cardiomegaly is usually absent in primary restrictive cardiomyopathy
B. Elevated jugular venous pressure and an S_4 gallop in patients with heart failure are each associated with a poor prognosis
C. Pulsus alternans results from variation of the stroke volume, likely owing to incomplete recovery of contracting myocardial cells
D. Low-grade fever may occur in advanced heart failure in the absence of underlying infection
E. Sleep-disordered breathing is common in patients with heart failure

QUESTION 197

True statements regarding the relationship between perfusion pressure and airway pressure in the upright lung include all of the following EXCEPT:
A. Pulmonary artery pressure is greater than alveolar pressure at the lung apices
B. Pulmonary venous pressure exceeds alveolar pressure at the lung bases

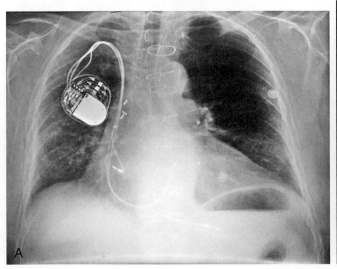
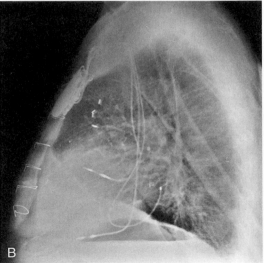

FIGURE 2-4

C. Measurement of pulmonary capillary wedge pressure is most meaningful in lung zones in which pulmonary venous and arterial pressures exceed alveolar pressure

D. Pulmonary vascular redistribution on the chest radiograph occurs when there is a relative reduction in perfusion of the bases with a relative increase in apical perfusion

QUESTION 198

Which of the following is NOT likely to be a complication of cyclosporine therapy in the cardiac transplant recipient?

A. Gingival hyperplasia
B. Myelosuppression
C. Hypertension
D. Tremor
E. Hirsutism

QUESTION 199

All of the following statements about acute heart failure are correct EXCEPT:

A. Most patients with acute heart failure present with normal or elevated blood pressure
B. Milrinone does not improve in-hospital mortality
C. Serum vasopressin levels are elevated in acute heart failure and contribute to hyponatremia, a marker of poor prognosis
D. Tolvaptan, an arginine vasopressin antagonist, reduces the risk of death and heart failure rehospitalization
E. Noninvasive ventilation in patients with acute pulmonary edema does not reduce short-term mortality compared with oxygen alone

QUESTION 200

All of the following statements about patients with symptomatic heart failure are true EXCEPT:

A. Plasma norepinephrine level is usually elevated
B. Serum B-type natriuretic peptide is elevated
C. Cardiac beta-adrenergic receptor density is increased
D. Serum aldosterone level is elevated
E. The circulating level of tumor necrosis factor-alpha is increased

QUESTION 201

All of the following statements regarding post–cardiac transplantation complications are true EXCEPT:

A. Infectious complications are responsible for approximately 20% of deaths during the year after transplantation
B. Allograft coronary artery disease is the most significant factor limiting long-term survival
C. The propensity for allograft rejection decreases with time

D. Cytomegalovirus infection is associated with development of post-transplantation lymphoproliferative disorder
E. Transplant recipients have an increased incidence of cancer compared with age-matched controls

QUESTION 202

All of the following statements regarding intra-aortic balloon (IAB) counterpulsation are true EXCEPT:

A. Patients with cardiogenic shock or mechanical complications of an acute myocardial infarction often benefit from the placement of an IAB
B. Aortic valve stenosis is a strict contraindication to the use of an IAB
C. The IAB should be timed to deflate during the isovolumetric phase of left ventricular contraction
D. The tip of the IAB should be positioned just distal to the left subclavian artery
E. Inflation of the IAB should be timed with aortic valve closure on the arterial pressure waveform

QUESTION 203

All of the following statements regarding therapy for patients with heart failure are true EXCEPT:

A. Angiotensin receptor blocking drugs are less effective than angiotensin-converting enzyme (ACE) inhibitors in the reduction of mortality in patients with heart failure
B. ACE inhibitors are indicated in patients with heart failure and left ventricular dysfunction irrespective of the functional New York Heart Association classification
C. Digoxin has been shown to decrease heart failure hospitalizations but has no effect on mortality
D. Spironolactone has been shown to decrease mortality in patients with Class III to IV symptoms
E. Regular physical exercise does not reduce mortality in patients with chronic heart failure

QUESTION 204

A 52-year-old businessman presents to the office complaining of increasing fatigue and shortness of breath. He has also recently noticed that he is more comfortable sleeping on three pillows. He denies any change in his usual habits nor has he experienced chest discomfort or pleuritic pain. His only medications are hydrochlorothiazide, 25 mg daily, and atenolol, 50 mg daily, for hypertension of 10 years' duration, with good control. His past medical history includes an appendectomy. He smokes ½ pack of cigarettes per day. He drinks whiskey socially and admits to two martinis at lunchtime each day. There is no family history of heart disease.

On examination, his heart rate is 104 beats/min, respirations are 20 breaths/min, and blood pressure is 134/84 mm Hg. There are no hypertensive changes

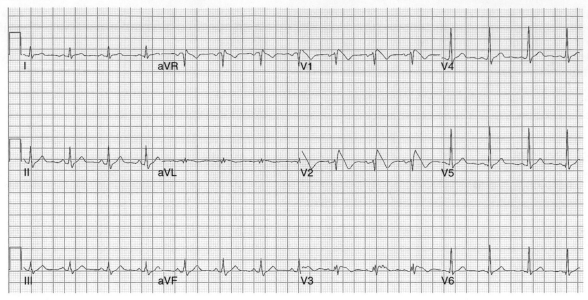

FIGURE 2-5

in the fundi. There are bibasilar rales over the lower third of the lung fields; the carotid upstrokes are normal. The apical impulse is laterally displaced and sustained. S_1 and S_2 are normal. There is a loud S_4 and a moderately loud S_3. There is a grade 2/6 holosystolic murmur that radiates to the axilla. The remainder of the examination findings are normal except for a trace of pedal edema. The chest radiograph shows left ventricular (LV) enlargement. The ECG is consistent with LV hypertrophy. The most likely cause for this man's heart failure is:

A. Hypertension
B. Alcoholic cardiomyopathy
C. Coronary atherosclerosis
D. Hypertrophic cardiomyopathy
E. Excessive beta-blocker dosage

QUESTION 205

Each of the following statements regarding dysrhythmias is true EXCEPT:

A. The prevalence of premature ventricular complexes increases with age
B. In the absence of structural heart disease, detection of premature ventricular complexes has no impact on survival
C. Class IC antiarrhythmic agents are the drugs of choice for suppression of premature ventricular complexes after myocardial infarction
D. Most concealed accessory pathways are located between the left ventricle and the left atrium
E. A concealed accessory pathway should be suspected in narrow-complex tachycardias when the retrograde P wave occurs after completion of the QRS complex

QUESTION 206

A 56-year-old man with a history of hypercholesterolemia and smoking is referred to the cardiology clinic for preoperative risk assessment before an orthopedic procedure. He denies any cardiovascular symptoms and exercises regularly. His ECG is shown in Figure 2-5. All of the following statements are true EXCEPT:

A. This syndrome is thought to account for 40% to 60% of all cases of idiopathic ventricular fibrillation
B. Genetic mutations in the sodium channel have been identified in some families with this syndrome
C. Implantable cardioverter-defibrillators are appropriate therapy for preventing sudden death
D. Antiarrhythmic therapy with procainamide reliably prevents ventricular arrhythmias in this syndrome
E. Screening of family members for this condition is recommended

QUESTION 207

True statements regarding the prevention of sudden cardiac death include all of the following EXCEPT:

A. The therapy of choice for survivors of sudden cardiac death is implantation of a cardioverter-defibrillator
B. Defibrillators reduce the risk of sudden death from arrhythmia in patients with nonischemic cardiomyopathy and left ventricular (LV) ejection fraction (EF) ≤ 35%
C. For survivors of out-of-hospital cardiac arrest not associated with a myocardial infarction, the risk of recurrent cardiac arrest at 1 year is about 30%
D. Prophylactic defibrillator implantation is appropriate for prevention of sudden death in patients with left ventricular dysfunction (LV EF ≤ 30%) and prior myocardial infarction

E. Amiodarone is the most appropriate long-term therapy for patients with hypertrophic cardiomyopathy and a prior history of syncope

QUESTION 208

True statements regarding atrioventricular (AV) block include all of the following EXCEPT:
A. In first-degree AV block, the intensity of the first heart sound is increased
B. The conduction abnormality in Mobitz type I second-degree heart block with normal QRS complex duration is almost always at the level of the AV node, proximal to the His bundle
C. In typical Mobitz type I second-degree heart block, the RR interval progressively shortens over consecutive beats, until a beat is dropped
D. In Mobitz type II second-degree heart block, the PR intervals are constant prior to the nonconducted P wave
E. The ventricular escape rate in acquired complete heart block is usually <40 beats/min

QUESTION 209

True statements about the use of ambulatory electrocardiographic monitoring in the detection of cardiac arrhythmias include all of the following EXCEPT:
A. Wenckebach-type second-degree atrioventricular block may be present in normal subjects
B. The frequency of ventricular premature beats after myocardial infarction increases over the first several weeks
C. On ambulatory electrocardiographic monitoring, sinus bradycardia with rates as low as 35 beats/min and sinoatrial exit block may be seen in normal persons
D. A long-term loop recorder is often useful for patients with frequent symptoms and an unrevealing Holter recording
E. Long-term monitoring of patients with a history of atrial fibrillation indicates that symptomatic atrial fibrillation episodes occur more commonly than asymptomatic episodes

QUESTION 210

All of the following statements regarding syncope are true EXCEPT:
A. Cardiac causes account for 10% to 20% of syncopal episodes
B. Syncope of cardiac origin is associated with a 30% 1-year mortality
C. The most common causes of syncope are vascular in origin, including reflex-mediated syncope and orthostatic hypotension
D. Supraventricular tachycardia has been identified as a common cause of syncope

E. The cause of syncope can be identified in a large percentage of patients based on history and physical examination alone

QUESTION 211

True statements about permanent pacemakers include all of the following EXCEPT:
A. AAIR pacing is appropriate for patients with sinus node dysfunction and intact atrioventricular (AV) conduction
B. Symptomatic Wenckebach AV block is an indication for permanent pacing
C. Pacemaker syndrome can be manifest in any pacing mode in which there is AV dissociation
D. Medically refractory hypertrophic cardiomyopathy is a Class I indication for the placement of a permanent dual-chamber pacemaker
E. A pacemaker mode-switching option is beneficial for patients with paroxysmal supraventricular rhythm disturbances

QUESTION 212

All of the following statements regarding pacemaker-mediated tachycardia (PMT) are true EXCEPT:
A. A dual-chamber system must be present to cause PMT
B. Intact atrial sensing is required for PMT
C. Premature ventricular contractions frequently initiate PMT
D. Shortening the postventricular atrial refractory period will prevent PMT
E. Retrograde P waves are typically present

QUESTION 213

A 76-year-old man with diabetes mellitus and exertional angina is found to have three-vessel coronary artery disease and a left ventricular ejection fraction of 40% on diagnostic angiography. He is electively admitted and undergoes successful coronary artery bypass grafting surgery. The ECG taken on the second postoperative day is shown in Figure 2-6. Preoperative administration of each of the following therapies has been shown to prevent this dysrhythmia after cardiac surgery EXCEPT:
A. Amiodarone
B. Atorvastatin
C. Atrial pacing
D. Digoxin
E. Metoprolol

QUESTION 214

Each of the following statements about procainamide is true EXCEPT:
A. At therapeutic concentrations, procainamide prolongs the QRS complex duration on the surface ECG

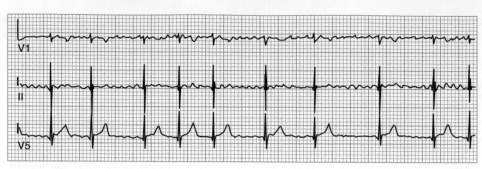

FIGURE 2-6

B. Procainamide may accelerate the ventricular rate in patients with atrial flutter

C. Procainamide suppresses conduction in the accessory pathway of patients with Wolff-Parkinson-White syndrome

D. A positive antinuclear antibody in procainamide-treated patients signals a drug-induced lupus syndrome

E. Rapid intravenous administration of procainamide may precipitate hypotension

QUESTION 215

Each of the following statements about invasive cardiac electrophysiologic study is true EXCEPT:

A. Of the common arrhythmic causes of syncope, tachyarrhythmias are most reliably initiated in the electrophysiology laboratory, followed by sinus node abnormalities and His-Purkinje block

B. Supraventricular tachycardias are characterized by a His-ventricular interval that is shorter than that recorded during normal sinus rhythm

C. Patients with sinus node dysfunction often have atrioventricular nodal conduction abnormalities

D. Sinus node recovery time is defined as the difference between the spontaneous sinus node cycle length prior to pacing and the duration to the first spontaneous sinus response after termination of pacing

E. Accessory pathways are most commonly located in the left ventricle free wall

QUESTION 216

True statements about the use of adenosine in the management of cardiac arrhythmia include all of the following EXCEPT:

A. Adenosine administration may aid in the diagnosis of wide QRS complex tachycardias

B. Slow, peripheral intravenous administration of 6 to 12 mg of adenosine is useful in terminating supraventricular tachycardias involving the atrioventricular node

C. Patients with heart transplants may have an exaggerated response to adenosine

D. Adenosine may be ineffective in patients who have consumed caffeine

E. Flushing, dyspnea, and chest pressure are all common side effects of adenosine therapy

QUESTION 217

All of the following statements regarding radiofrequency catheter ablation of atrial fibrillation are true EXCEPT:

A. Success rates vary from 70% to 90% when redo procedures are included

B. The risk of stroke is approximately 2%

C. A successful procedure requires focal ablation of premature atrial beats originating deep within the pulmonary veins

D. Ablation in the posterior left atrium is associated with a risk of atrial-esophageal fistula

E. Anomalous pulmonary venous anatomy may render the procedure less successful

QUESTION 218

Each of the following statements regarding antiarrhythmic therapy with quinidine is true EXCEPT:

A. Quinidine commonly causes gastrointestinal side effects

B. Torsades de pointes occurs in up to 3% of patients treated with quinidine

C. Periodic blood cell counts are advisable during long-term therapy with quinidine

D. Quinidine elevates the serum digoxin level

E. Quinidine is effective in the pharmacologic conversion of atrial fibrillation owing to its potentiation of vagal output

QUESTION 219

Each of the following statements concerning atrial fibrillation (AF) is true EXCEPT:

A. AF develops in up to 40% of patients after cardiac surgery

B. Patients who have been in AF for less than 48 hours can usually be safely cardioverted without the need for prolonged anticoagulation

C. Restoration of sinus rhythm is superior to chronic rate control and anticoagulation in patients with AF

D. A chronically rapid ventricular response rate in AF can result in impaired left ventricular systolic function

E. The incidence of AF approximately doubles with each decade of adult life

QUESTION 220

Each of the following statements regarding the cardiac conduction system is true EXCEPT:

A. The sinus node is innervated with postganglionic adrenergic and cholinergic nerve terminals

B. In 60% of people, the arterial supply to the atrioventricular node is derived from a branch of the left circumflex artery

C. The conduction system in the upper muscular interventricular septum receives its blood supply from branches of the anterior and posterior descending arteries

D. Inhibition of the delayed rectifier K^+ current (I_{kr}) has been implicated in the acquired form of the long QT syndrome

E. The resting transmembrane potential of the cardiac myocyte is close to the equilibrium potential of potassium

QUESTION 221

Each of the following statements regarding amiodarone is true EXCEPT:

A. The mean terminal half-life of amiodarone is about 2 months

B. Among patients with heart failure, amiodarone is of comparable efficacy with an implantable cardioverter-defibrillator in the prevention of sudden cardiac death

C. Corneal deposits develop in nearly all patients who are treated with amiodarone for more than 6 months

D. Amiodarone can cause either hypothyroidism or hyperthyroidism

E. Amiodarone-induced pulmonary toxicity may develop within the first week of therapy

QUESTION 222

Each of the following statements regarding cardiac arrhythmias is true EXCEPT:

A. In the common form of atrioventricular (AV) nodal reentry tachycardia, anterograde conduction occurs down the "slow" pathway

B. In antidromic AV reciprocating tachycardia, the activation wave travels via the accessory pathway to the ventricles and retrogradely via the AV node to the atria

C. In most patients with Wolff-Parkinson-White syndrome, the accessory pathway conducts more rapidly than the normal AV node but takes longer to recover excitability

D. Abnormal automaticity is the most common mechanism of atrial flutter

E. Mechanisms of ventricular tachycardia include reentry, triggered activity, and abnormal automaticity

QUESTION 223

A 14-year-old boy suffers two episodes of sudden syncope during gym class while jogging and is referred for further evaluation. His paternal uncle had died suddenly during physical exercise at age 20. Laboratory evaluation includes an ECG that shows normal sinus rhythm with a normal QTc interval. Cardiac magnetic resonance imaging reveals a structurally normal heart. CT angiography demonstrates normal coronary anatomy. He undergoes treadmill exercise testing, and the rhythm displayed in Figure 2-7 is noted after 3 minutes of exercise. What is the first-line treatment for this condition?

A. Magnesium

B. Dual-chamber pacemaker

C. Beta blocker and an implantable cardioverter-defibrillator

D. Exercise training with adequate hydration

E. Cardiac sympathectomy

QUESTION 224

Each of the following statements regarding Class III antiarrhythmic drugs is true EXCEPT:

A. Torsades de pointes is a potential complication of sotalol therapy

B. Sotalol can precipitate heart failure in patients with reduced baseline systolic function

C. After ibutilide administration, patients can be safely discharged 1 hour after conversion from atrial flutter to normal sinus rhythm

D. Ibutilide results in conversion to sinus rhythm in up to 60% of patients with atrial fibrillation and 70% with atrial flutter

E. The dose of dofetilide must be adjusted based on the patient's creatinine clearance

QUESTION 225

A sample tracing from an electrophysiologic study in a patient with a narrow-complex tachycardia is displayed in Figure 2-8. What is the diagnosis?

A. Sinus tachycardia

B. Atrial flutter

C. Typical (slow-fast) atrioventricular (AV) nodal reentrant tachycardia

D. Orthodromic AV reentrant tachycardia using an accessory pathway

E. Atrial tachycardia

QUESTION 226

A 75-year-old woman presents following an episode of syncope. She was watching television with her husband

3 minutes of exercise

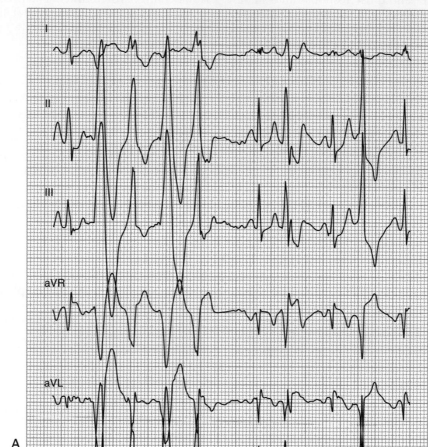

A

5 minutes of exercise

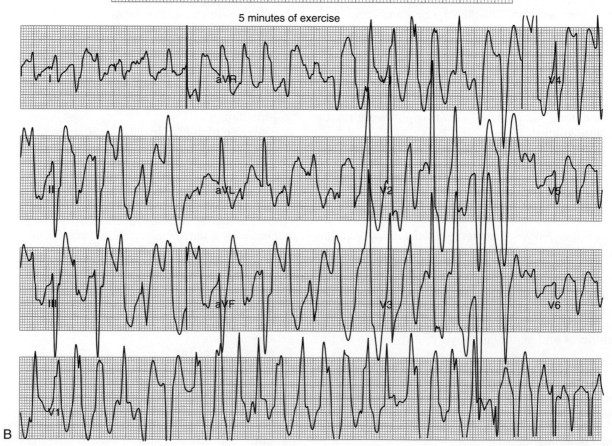

B

FIGURE 2-7

when she suddenly lost consciousness and was unresponsive for approximately 20 seconds. She awoke slightly confused but otherwise felt well. Her past medical history is unremarkable. The baseline ECG demonstrates right bundle branch block and left anterior fascicular block. An electrophysiologic study was performed, and a panel from that procedure is shown in Figure 2-9. Which of the following is the most appropriate recommendation?

A. Catheter ablation for atrioventricular nodal reentrant tachycardia
B. Beta-blocker therapy
C. Neurologic consultation
D. Permanent pacemaker implantation
E. Coronary angiography with anticipated percutaneous revascularization

QUESTION 227

All of the following statements about distinguishing ventricular tachycardia (VT) from a supraventricular tachycardia (SVT) with aberrant conduction in a patient with a wide-complex rapid rhythm are true EXCEPT:

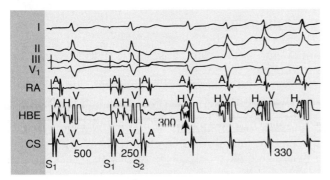

FIGURE 2-8

A. The presence of fusion beats supports the diagnosis of VT
B. Termination of the tachycardia by vagal maneuvers is consistent with an SVT
C. The presence of atrioventricular dissociation implies VT
D. Hemodynamic instability is proof of VT
E. A past history of myocardial infarction makes the diagnosis of VT more likely

QUESTION 228

All of the following statements regarding electrical cardioversion are true EXCEPT:

A. Administration of intravenous ibutilide facilitates successful cardioversion of atrial fibrillation to normal sinus rhythm
B. A synchronized shock should be delivered when electrically cardioverting supraventricular tachycardias
C. The incidence of systemic embolism after successful cardioversion of atrial fibrillation is 1% to 3%
D. Repeated shocks at the same energy level decrease chest wall impedance
E. Anticoagulation therapy can be safely discontinued 5 days after successful cardioversion of chronic atrial fibrillation to normal sinus rhythm

QUESTION 229

Each of the following may contribute to the development of the arrhythmia seen in Figure 2-10 EXCEPT:

A. Congenital severe bradycardia
B. Hypokalemia
C. Loss of function mutation in the *SCN5A* gene
D. Tricyclic antidepressant overdose
E. Disopyramide

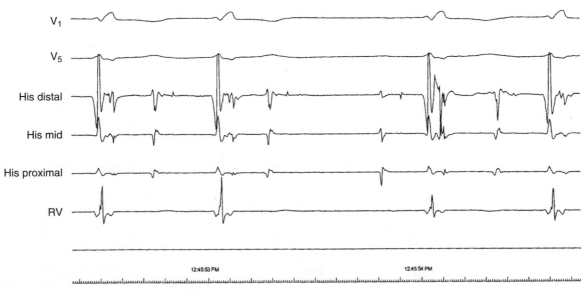

FIGURE 2-9

QUESTION 230

A 60-year-old man presents with presyncope and is found to be in a wide-complex tachycardia at 140 beats/min. An electrophysiologic study is performed and tachycardia is induced, as shown in Figure 2-11. The mechanism of this tachycardia is:

A. Atrioventricular reciprocating tachycardia utilizing an accessory pathway
B. Atrioventricular nodal reentrant tachycardia with aberrant ventricular conduction
C. Ventricular tachycardia
D. Atrial flutter with aberrant ventricular conduction
E. Sinus tachycardia

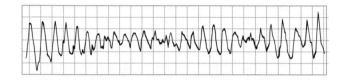

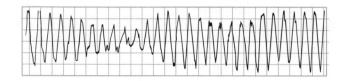

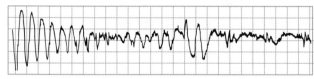

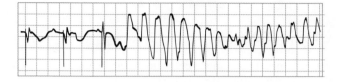

FIGURE 2-10

QUESTION 231

All of the following statements about the electrophysiologic abnormality depicted in Figure 2-12 are true EXCEPT:

A. It is associated with a benign clinical course
B. When associated with an inferior myocardial infarction, it is an indication for temporary pacing
C. It is nearly always associated with block at the level of the atrioventricular node proximal to the His bundle
D. Carotid sinus massage typically exacerbates the abnormality
E. There is typically "grouped beating" on the surface ECG

QUESTION 232

Permanent cardiac pacing is appropriate for all of the following patients EXCEPT:
A. A 35-year-old man with asymptomatic type II second-degree atrioventricular (AV) block and sinus bradycardia at 38 beats/min
B. A 70-year-old man with left ventricular hypertrophy, persistent fatigue, and lightheadedness, with marked first-degree AV block (PR interval = 0.36 second)

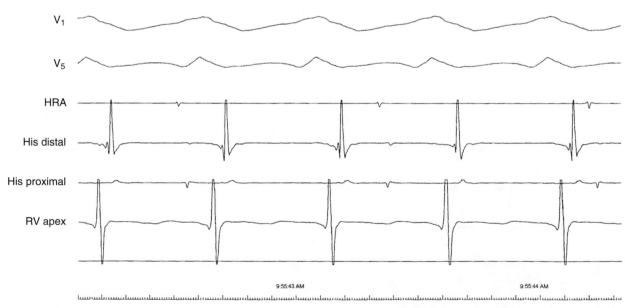

FIGURE 2-11

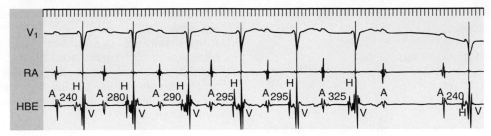

FIGURE 2-12

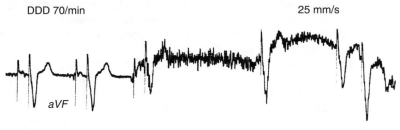

DDD 70/min   25 mm/s

aVF

FIGURE 2-13

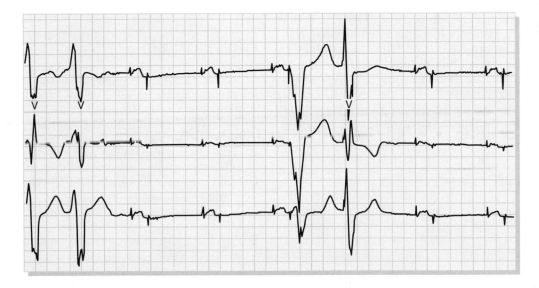

FIGURE 2-14

C. A 57-year-old man with acquired asymptomatic third-degree AV block
D. A 40-year-old woman with symptomatic congenital complete AV block
E. A 56-year-old marathon runner with 3.4-second pauses during sleep

QUESTION 233

A 62-year-old man underwent pacemaker insertion 4 years ago because of marked bradycardia. As part of his exercise program he has been using a rowing machine. Recently, he has had several episodes of near-syncope that occurred only during such exercise. An ambulatory

ECG (Holter monitor) demonstrated the rhythm strip shown in Figure 2-13 during a near-syncopal episode while rowing. Which of the following is correct?
A. There is evidence of a single-chamber pacing system
B. There is inappropriate inhibition of ventricular pacing
C. There is undersensing of atrial activity
D. There is lack of capture of the ventricles
E. There is lack of capture of the atria

QUESTION 234

The ECG in Figure 2-14 is compatible with all of the following diagnoses EXCEPT:
A. Lead insulation breach

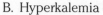
B. Hyperkalemia
C. Lead dislodgment
D. Loose set screw
E. Impending battery depletion

QUESTION 235

All of the following statements regarding sinus node function are true EXCEPT:
A. Sinus bradycardia is a common rhythm in well-trained athletes
B. During sleep, the heart rate of normal individuals can fall to 35 beats/min
C. Sinus arrest is defined as a pause that is an exact multiple of the PP interval of the underlying rhythm
D. Sinus arrest and atrioventricular block are common in patients with sleep apnea
E. In the respiratory form of sinus arrhythmia, the PP interval cyclically shortens during inspiration

QUESTION 236

Which of the following statements regarding arrhythmogenic right ventricular cardiomyopathy (ARVC) is TRUE?
A. Ventricular tachycardia in patients with ARVC typically has a right bundle branch block morphology
B. ARVC is more common in women
C. Fatty or fibrofatty infiltration of the right ventricle is the pathologic hallmark
D. Pathologic changes do not occur in the left ventricle
E. Radiofrequency ablation is successful at preventing ventricular tachycardia

QUESTION 237

Of the following patients with atrial fibrillation, which is the best candidate for aspirin rather than warfarin for stroke prophylaxis?
A. A 78-year-old diabetic man with no structural heart disease
B. A 50-year-old woman with dilated cardiomyopathy and controlled symptoms of heart failure
C. A 52-year-old man with hypertension and lower-extremity claudication
D. A 45-year-old man with a history of obesity and smoking but no structural heart disease
E. A 68-year-old woman with hypertension and left atrial enlargement by echocardiography

QUESTION 238

All of the following statements regarding the syndrome of carotid sinus hypersensitivity are true EXCEPT:
A. Atropine abolishes the cardioinhibitory form of this syndrome
B. During carotid sinus stimulation, a decrease in systolic blood pressure > 30 mm Hg and reproduction of the patient's symptoms is consistent with the vasodepressor form of this syndrome
C. A hypersensitive carotid sinus reflex is frequently found in asymptomatic individuals
D. Clonidine may exacerbate carotid sinus hypersensitivity
E. Single-chamber atrial pacing is appropriate therapy for most patients with vasodepressor carotid sinus hypersensitivity

QUESTION 239

A 30-year-old woman presents because of recurrent episodes of paroxysmal tachycardia with dyspnea and presyncope. A maternal uncle died suddenly at age 27. An electrophysiologic study is performed. The intracardiac electrograms at baseline (A) and during tachycardia (B) are shown in Figure 2-15. Of the following choices, the most appropriate therapy is:
A. Ablation of the atrioventricular nodal slow pathway
B. Ablation of an accessory pathway
C. Implantation of an automatic cardioverter-defibrillator
D. Direct-current cardioversion followed by long-term anticoagulation with warfarin
E. No further therapy is required

QUESTION 240

All of the following statements about congenital long QT syndrome (LQTS) are true EXCEPT:
A. Most forms of LQTS result from mutations in genes that code for proteins in cardiac potassium and sodium channels
B. Clinical symptomatology and risk of sudden death in LQTS syndromes vary across different genotypes
C. LQT1 patients experience a high frequency of cardiac events during swimming
D. Acoustic events are a common trigger of syncope in LQT2 patients
E. Physical exertion is the most common precipitant of sudden death in LQT3 patients

QUESTION 241

All of the following statements regarding sudden cardiac death (SCD) are true EXCEPT:
A. There are over 300,000 SCDs annually in the United States
B. The peak incidence of SCD among adults is between the ages of 45 and 75 years
C. Hereditary causes of SCD include hypertrophic cardiomyopathy, long QT syndrome, arrhythmogenic right ventricular cardiomyopathy, and the Brugada syndrome
D. SCD is more common in women than in men
E. An intraventricular conduction abnormality on the ECG is a stronger predictor of SCD than findings of left ventricular hypertrophy

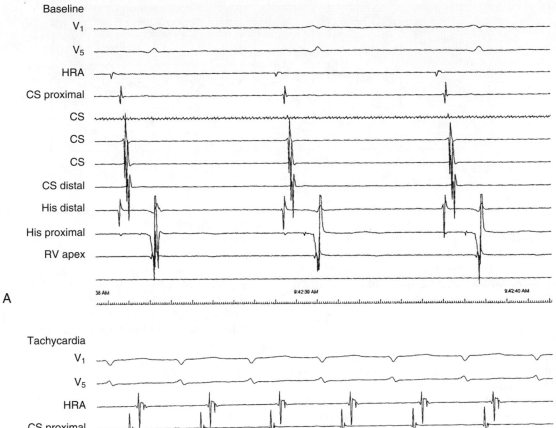

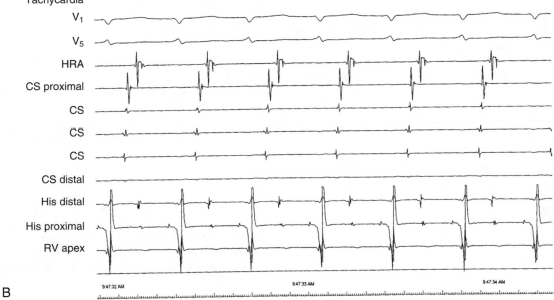

FIGURE 2-15

QUESTION 242

All of the following are likely in a patient with the ECG shown in Figure 2-16 EXCEPT:

A. A gradual increase in atrial rate with the administration of digoxin
B. An irregular atrial rate
C. Precipitation of the arrhythmia by hypokalemia
D. An absence of underlying cardiac disease in 50% of cases
E. Frequent ventricular premature beats

QUESTION 243

All of the following statements regarding sudden cardiac death (SCD) in patients with coronary artery disease are true EXCEPT:

A. SCD is the first clinical manifestation of coronary artery disease in approximately 25% of patients
B. Left ventricular dysfunction and ventricular ectopic activity after a myocardial infarction increase the risk of SCD

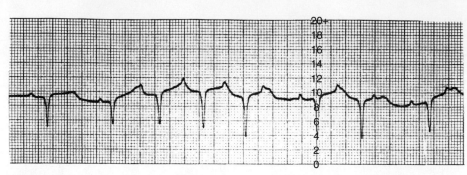

FIGURE 2-16

C. The most common mechanism of cardiac arrest is asystole

D. Onset of brain death occurs within 4 to 6 minutes of unattended ventricular fibrillation

E. The outcome of patients with bradycardic/asystolic out-of-hospital cardiac arrest is worse than if ventricular tachycardia is the initial arrhythmia

QUESTION 244

All of the following statements regarding electrophysiologic testing are true EXCEPT:

A. A long His-ventricular (HV) interval (>80 msec) identifies patients at increased risk of developing atrioventricular (AV) block

B. The HV interval has a low sensitivity but high specificity for predicting the development of complete AV block

C. A prolonged sinus node recovery time (SNRT) is very specific for identifying patients with sinus node dysfunction

D. The sensitivity of the SNRT in identifying sinus node dysfunction is 95%

E. The complication rate of electrophysiologic testing with radiofrequency ablation is 1% to 3%

QUESTION 245

Each of the following statements regarding the antiarrhythmic drug dronedarone is true, EXCEPT:

A. Its electrophysiologic properties are similar to amiodarone

B. It is safe for use in patients with heart failure symptoms

C. The prevalence of thyroid toxicity is low

D. QT prolongation is typical during use but only rarely results in proarrhythmia

E. Acute hepatic failure is a potential complication

QUESTION 246

Which of the following statements regarding cardiac pacing modes is TRUE?

A. Ventricular inhibited pacing (VVI) restores and maintains atrioventricular (AV) synchrony

B. VVI pacing provides rate responsiveness in the chronotropically incompetent patient

C. Single-chamber triggered pacing (AAT or VVT) increases the drain on the pacemaker battery

D. Atrial inhibited pacing (AAI) is an appropriate mode of pacing for patients with AV nodal dysfunction

E. Dual-chamber pacing and sensing with inhibition and tracking (DDD) is the preferred mode of pacing for patients in atrial fibrillation

QUESTION 247

All of the following statements regarding cardiac pacemakers are true EXCEPT:

A. Hyperkalemia can result in pacing and sensing threshold abnormalities

B. Lead dislodgment or inadequate initial lead placement should be suspected if true undersensing is present

C. Digital cellular telephones are unlikely to cause clinically important pacemaker interference during normal use

D. Right bundle branch block is the expected electrocardiographic pattern during right ventricular pacing

E. Pseudofusion on the surface ECG is identified by an appropriately timed pacing stimulus that does not alter the morphology of a superimposed intrinsic QRS

QUESTION 248

The finding on the chest radiograph shown in Figure 2-17 would be associated with which of the following measurements on device interrogation?

A. High-voltage threshold, high lead impedance

B. Low-voltage threshold, high lead impedance

C. High-voltage threshold, low lead impedance

D. Low-voltage threshold, low lead impedance

E. High-voltage threshold, normal lead impedance

QUESTION 249

The electrocardiographic abnormality displayed in Figure 2-18 is associated with all of the following EXCEPT:

A. An absence of underlying structural heart disease in most adults

B. Beneficial response to treatment with verapamil

C. An association with Ebstein's anomaly

D. A higher prevalence in men

E. A right posteroseptal pathway

QUESTION 250

A 65-year-old diabetic man with a history of an anterior myocardial infarction presents to your office for evaluation. He is known to have a left ventricular ejection fraction of 30% with an anterior wall motion abnormality. He is comfortable at rest but reports dyspnea with simple household activities and cannot ascend a flight of stairs without stopping to catch his breath. He does not describe chest discomfort and there is no evidence of reversible ischemia by exercise scintigraphy. His current medical regimen includes carvedilol, 25 mg twice daily, lisinopril, 20 mg daily, furosemide, 40 mg daily, spironolactone, 25 mg daily, and digoxin, 0.125 mg daily. His physical examination reveals blood pressure of 90/50 mm Hg, heart rate of 70 beats/min, normal jugular venous pressure, and clear lungs to auscultation. The apical cardiac impulse is laterally displaced toward the anterior axillary line. On auscultation there is a normal S_1, paradoxically split S_2, a soft apical S_3 gallop, and a grade 3/6 holosystolic murmur at the apex that radiates to the axilla. There is no peripheral edema. His ECG is shown in Figure 2-19. Which of the following is the most appropriate approach to device therapy in this patient?

A. No device implantation is indicated

B. Implantation of a cardioverter-defibrillator is warranted

C. Implantation of a combined cardiac resynchronization-defibrillator system is most appropriate

D. Refer the patient for echocardiography to assess dyssynchrony and, if positive, implant a cardiac resynchronization-defibrillator

E. Implantation of a cardiac-resynchronization pacemaker without defibrillation capability is most appropriate

QUESTION 251

The electrophysiologic study tracing in Figure 2-20 is obtained from a 28-year-old man with palpitations,

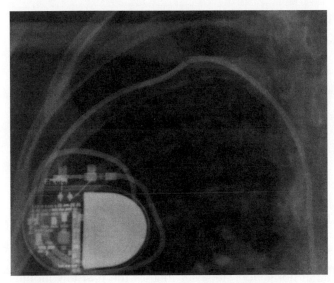

FIGURE 2-17

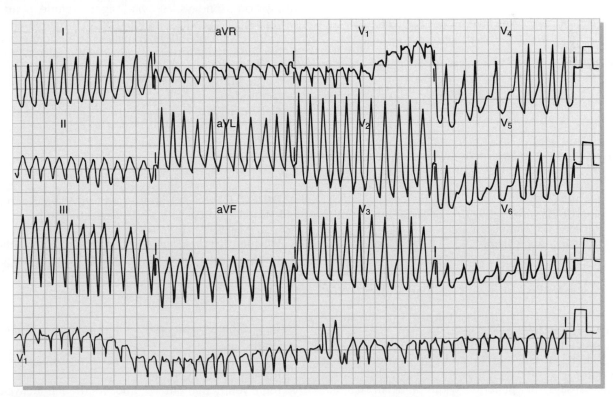

FIGURE 2-18

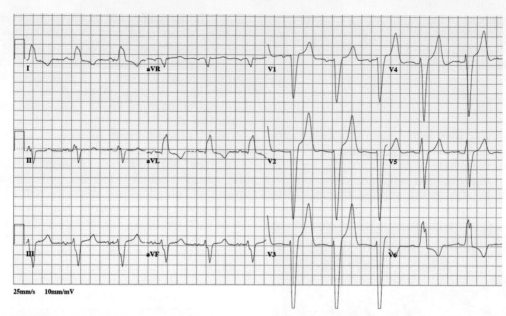

FIGURE 2-19

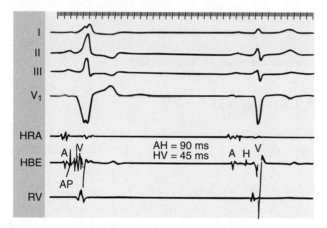

FIGURE 2-20 From Prystowsky EN, Browne KF, Zipes DP. J Am Coll Cardiol 1:468, 1983.

recurrent syncope, and a structurally normal heart. Which of the following is the most appropriate therapy?
A. Atenolol
B. Verapamil
C. Pacemaker implantation
D. Radiofrequency catheter ablation
E. Defibrillator implantation

QUESTION 252

All of the following statements are true about the antiarrhythmic drug dofetilide EXCEPT:
A. It has significant renal excretion
B. It prolongs the QT interval in a dose-dependent fashion
C. It is unsafe in patients with prior myocardial infarction
D. Patients must be admitted to the hospital for drug initiation
E. It should not be used in patients taking verapamil

QUESTION 253

A 26-year-old construction worker comes to the emergency department on the morning of January 2 in atrial fibrillation. He states that for the past few months he has had occasional episodes of palpitation, almost always on Mondays. His vital signs include heart rate of 140 beats/min, respirations of 16 breaths/min, and blood pressure of 160/95 mm Hg. His physical examination is unremarkable except for a soft systolic murmur. While being observed in the hospital, he spontaneously reverts to normal sinus rhythm. The most likely precipitating cause is:
A. Caffeine
B. Cocaine
C. Alcohol
D. Hypertension
E. Mitral valve prolapse

DIRECTIONS: Each group of questions below consists of lettered headings followed by a set of numbered questions. For each question, select the ONE lettered heading with which it is most closely associated. Each lettered heading may be used once, more than once, or not at all.

QUESTIONS 254 TO 257

For each of the following descriptions, match the appropriate disorders:
A. Jervell and Lange-Nielsen syndrome
B. Romano-Ward syndrome
C. Right ventricular outflow tract ventricular tachycardia
D. Brugada syndrome

254. Autosomal recessive disorder associated with sensorineural deafness
255. Typically, the ECG reveals a right bundle branch block morphology with ST-segment elevation in the anterior precordial leads
256. Autosomal dominant long QT syndrome with normal hearing
257. Left bundle branch block with an inferior axis

QUESTIONS 258 TO 261

Match the following antiarrhythmic drug actions with the appropriate Vaughan-Williams drug classification:
A. Predominantly block potassium channels and prolong repolarization
B. Predominantly block beta-adrenergic receptors
C. Predominantly block slow calcium channels (I Ca.L)
D. Reduce the rate of rise of the action potential upstroke (Vmax) and prolong the action potential duration
E. Block sodium channels but shorten the action potential duration and do not reduce Vmax

258. Class IA drugs
259. Class II drugs
260. Class III drugs
261. Class IV drugs

QUESTIONS 262 TO 265

Assume that you have decided to prescribe antiarrhythmic drug therapy to prevent recurrent episodes of atrial fibrillation for each of the patients described below. Match each patient with the most appropriate antiarrhythmic from the provided list:
A. Flecainide
B. Sotalol
C. Amiodarone
D. Mexiletine

262. A 64-year-old man with remote history of anterior myocardial infarction and left ventricular ejection fraction of 50%
263. A 74-year-old woman with long-standing hypertension and left ventricular hypertrophy (wall thickness = 16 mm)
264. A 58-year-old with nonischemic cardiomyopathy and Class III congestive heart failure
265. A 46-year-old otherwise healthy man with no structural heart disease

QUESTIONS 266 TO 269

For each of the following diuretic agents, match the appropriate adverse effect:
A. Ototoxicity
B. Gynecomastia
C. Metabolic acidosis
D. Hypercalcemia
E. Hyperkalemia

266. Acetazolamide
267. Metolazone
268. Torsemide
269. Eplerenone

QUESTIONS 270 TO 273

For each clinical condition, match the most appropriate pacemaker modality:
A. VAT
B. VVIR
C. DDD
D. DDDR
E. AAIR

270. A 58-year-old man with tachycardia-bradycardia syndrome who develops symptomatic sinus bradycardia with beta-blocker therapy
271. A 70-year-old woman with long-standing atrial fibrillation who complains of dizziness and is found on examination to have a ventricular rate of 30 beats/min
272. A 62-year-old man with complete heart block after aortic valve surgery
273. A 45-year-old man with symptomatic sinoatrial exit block and an appropriate junctional escape rhythm

QUESTIONS 274 TO 277

Several conditions can cause dilated cardiomyopathy (DCM) with electric instability, defined as conduction disease or arrhythmia out of proportion to the degree of left ventricular dysfunction. For each clinical description, match the corresponding etiology of DCM with electric instability:
A. Cardiac sarcoidosis
B. Giant cell myocarditis
C. Chagas disease
D. Arrhythmogenic right ventricular cardiomyopathy
E. Cardiolaminopathy

274. A 30-year-old man with a history of syncope who is found to have low-amplitude deflections on the ST segment in the right precordial leads and abnormal desmosomes on cardiac immunohistochemistry
275. A 38-year-old man with gastrointestinal dysmotility, complete heart block, and an apical aneurysm
276. A 50-year-old woman with a history of restrictive lung disease who presents with syncope in the setting of first-degree atrioventricular block and right bundle branch block
277. A 42-year-old woman with rapidly deteriorating cardiac function, frequent bursts of ventricular tachycardia, and widespread myocyte necrosis on endomyocardial biopsy

QUESTIONS 278 TO 282

For each of the following conditions, match the corresponding clinical presentations of syncope:
A. A 20-year-old woman "blacked out" during phlebotomy for a routine blood test
B. A 65-year-old woman lost consciousness after arm exercises
C. A 35-year-old man sustained syncope during exercise and has a systolic murmur that intensifies on standing upright
D. A 74-year-old man experiences sudden syncope while shaving
E. A 28-year-old woman with recurrent episodes of breathlessness, lightheadedness, and syncope after changes in body position

278. Hypertrophic cardiomyopathy
279. Subclavian steal syndrome
280. Vasovagal syncope
281. Carotid sinus hypersensitivity
282. Left atrial myxoma

QUESTIONS 283 TO 286

For each condition capable of precipitating high-output cardiac failure, match the appropriate physical findings:
A. Hyperthyroidism
B. Beriberi
C. Arteriovenous fistula
D. Carcinoid syndrome
E. Osler-Weber-Rendu syndrome

283. Nicoladoni-Branham sign
284. Hepatomegaly and abdominal bruits
285. Means-Lerman scratch
286. Paresthesias and painful glossitis

QUESTIONS 287 TO 290

For each of the following descriptions, match the appropriate medication:

A. One of the least lipid-soluble beta blockers
B. Cardioselective beta blocker with intrinsic sympathomimetic activity
C. Beta blocker with alpha-blocking activity
D. Noncardioselective beta blocker with intrinsic sympathomimetic activity

287. Atenolol
288. Carvedilol
289. Acebutolol
290. Pindolol

QUESTIONS 291 TO 294

For each disease state, match the appropriate left ventricular (LV) volume and mass data:

	END-DIASTOLIC VOLUME (mL/m²)	STROKE VOLUME (mL/m²)	LV MASS (g/m²)
Normal =	70	45	92
A.	84	44	172
B.	193	92	200
C.	199	37	145
D.	70	40	80

291. Aortic valve stenosis with peak systolic gradient >30 mm Hg
292. Myocardial disease (primary dilated cardiomyopathy)
293. Aortic regurgitation with regurgitant flow >30 mL per beat
294. Mitral valve regurgitation with regurgitant flow >20 mL per beat

HEART FAILURE; ARRHYTHMIAS, SUDDEN DEATH, AND SYNCOPE

ANSWER TO QUESTION 168

E (Braunwald, pp. 491-492, 509-510, 527; Fig. 25-7)

Natriuretic peptides are of importance in the diagnosis, and assessment of prognosis, in patients with congestive heart failure. The natriuretic peptide system consists of five structurally similar peptide hormones: atrial natriuretic peptide (ANP), urodilantin (an isoform of ANP), brain-type natriuretic peptide (BNP), C-type natriuretic peptide, and dendroaspis natriuretic peptide (DNP).[1] ANP is released by atrial myocytes in response to acute increases in atrial pressure. Prohormone BNP is released in response to hemodynamic stress from ventricular dilatation, hypertrophy, or increased wall tension. Prohormone BNP is cleaved by a circulating endoprotease into two polypeptides: the inactive N-terminal proBNP (NT-proBNP), 76 amino acids in length, and the biologically active peptide BNP, 32 amino acids in length.[2]

Circulating levels of ANP and BNP are elevated in patients with heart failure. Both ANP and BNP promote vasodilatation and natriuresis, thereby counteracting the salt- and water-retaining effects of the adrenergic, renin-angiotensin-aldosterone, and vasopressin systems. BNP and NT-proBNP levels *rise* with increasing age and worsening renal function. In contrast, BNP levels have an inverse relationship with body mass index.

CNP is derived predominantly from endothelial cells in the peripheral vasculature. The precise roles of CNP, urodilantin, and DNP in cardiovascular physiology remain unclear.

A large, multicenter study of patients in the emergency department undergoing evaluation for acute dyspnea showed that a BNP level of > 100 pg/mL is 90% sensitive and 76% specific in identifying a cardiac etiology.[3] A BNP level > 400 pg/mL rendered the diagnosis of heart failure likely. Analogous results were found for NT-proBNP—patients in acute heart failure had mean levels > 4000 pg/mL compared with 130 pg/mL in those without heart failure.[4]

A substudy of the TACTICS-TIMI 18 trial demonstrated that an elevated BNP level in patients presenting with acute coronary syndromes is associated with a higher risk of subsequent congestive heart failure and death.[5]

REFERENCES

1. Daniels LB, Maisel AS: Natriuretic peptides. J Am Coll Cardiol 50:2357, 2007.
2. Braunwald E: Biomarkers in heart failure. N Engl J Med 358:2148, 2008.
3. Maisel AS, Krishnaswamy P, Nowak RM, et al: Rapid measurement of B-type natriuretic peptide in the emergency diagnosis of heart failure. N Engl J Med 347:161, 2002.
4. Januzzi JL Jr, Camargo CA, Anwaruddin S, et al: The N-terminal pro-BNP investigation of dyspnea in the emergency department (PRIDE) study. Am J Cardiol 95:948, 2005.
5. Morrow DA, deLemos JA, Sabatine MS, et al: Evaluation of B-type natriuretic peptide for risk assessment in unstable angina/non-ST-elevation myocardial infarction: B-type natriuretic peptide and prognosis in TACTICS-TIMI 18. J Am Coll Cardiol 41:1264, 2003.

ANSWER TO QUESTION 169

A (Braunwald, pp. 551-556, Figs. 28-10 and 28-11; Table 28-7)

Mannitol is an inert osmotic agent that expands the extracellular fluid volume; its use is *contraindicated* in patients with decompensated heart failure.

Carbonic anhydrase inhibitors induce a metabolic acidosis by increasing the urinary excretion of bicarbonate. As a result, they can be used temporarily in edematous patients with hypochloremic metabolic alkalosis resulting from long-term use of loop diuretics.

Mineralocorticoid receptor antagonists (spironolactone and eplerenone) act at the renal distal convoluted tubule and cortical collecting tubule to reduce sodium reabsorption and inhibit K^+ and H^+ excretion. Although only weak diuretics, they have been shown to reduce morbidity and mortality in systolic heart failure.[1] However, aldosterone receptor antagonists may contribute to clinically significant hyperkalemia, particularly when used in combination with angiotensin-converting enzyme (ACE) inhibitors and/or angiotensin II receptor blockers (ARBs).[2]

Loop diuretics, such as furosemide, torsemide, and bumetanide, are inhibitors of the $Na^+/K^+/2Cl^-$ cotransporter in the thick ascending limb of the loop of Henle. Inhibition of this cotransporter markedly increases the fractional excretion of sodium and chloride. However, the delivery of large amounts of sodium and fluid to the distal nephron increases K^+ and H^+ secretion, leading to hypokalemia and metabolic alkalosis.

Nonsteroidal anti-inflammatory agents (NSAIDs) may impair renal function and diminish the action of diuretics by inhibiting the production of vasodilator prostaglandins. All NSAIDs, including aspirin, have this potential effect, which can contribute to diuretic resistance in individuals with an initially favorable diuretic response.[3]

REFERENCES

1. Zannad F, McMurray JJV, Krum H, et al: Eplerenone in patients with systolic heart failure and mild symptoms. N Engl J Med 364:11, 2011.
2. Juurlink DN, Mamdani MM, Lee DS, et al: Rates of hyperkalemia after publication of the Randomized Aldactone Evaluation Study. N Engl J Med 351:543, 2004.
3. Jessup ML, Abraham WT, Casey DE, et al: 2009 focused update: ACCF/AHA Guidelines for the Diagnosis and Management of Heart Failure in Adults. A report of the American College of Cardiology Foundation/American Heart Association Task Force on Practice Guidelines: Developed in collaboration with the International Society for Heart and Lung Transplantation. Circulation 119:1977, 2009.

ANSWER TO QUESTION 170

E (Braunwald, pp. 523, 527; Table 26-6)

Cardiac arrhythmias are common in patients with structural heart disease, can contribute to worsening intracardiac hemodynamics, and may precipitate acute decompensated heart failure.[1] Cardiac output is dependent on maintenance of adequate stroke volume and heart rate. Tachyarrhythmias (most commonly atrial fibrillation with rapid ventricular response) increase myocardial oxygen demand and reduce the time available for ventricular filling in diastole, compromising ventricular stroke volume and cardiac output. Because stroke volume is compromised in patients with left ventricular dysfunction, maintenance of cardiac output is largely dependent on an adequate heart rate. Thus, excessive heart rate slowing (i.e., bradyarrhythmias) may also depress cardiac output.

Dissociation between atrial and ventricular contraction (as in high-grade atrioventricular block) reduces the atrial contribution to ventricular filling, impairing subsequent stroke volume and cardiac output in patients with systolic or diastolic dysfunction. Abnormal intraventricular conduction, as in ventricular tachycardia or right ventricular apical pacing, may impair myocardial performance because of the loss of synchronized ventricular contraction.[2] Optimization of atrioventricular and ventriculoventricular synchrony is the primary mechanism of benefit from cardiac resynchronization therapy (biventricular pacing) in patients with left ventricular dysfunction and heart failure.

REFERENCES

1. Benza RL, Tallaj JA, Felker GM, et al: The impact of arrhythmias in acute heart failure. J Card Fail 10:279, 2004.
2. Wang NC, Maggioni AP, Konstam MA, et al: Clinical implications of QRS duration in patients hospitalized with worsening heart failure and reduced left ventricular ejection fraction. JAMA 299:2656, 2008.

ANSWER TO QUESTION 171

C (Braunwald, pp. 508-509, 522-524, 547; Figs. 27-3 and 28-5)

The cardiorenal syndrome is characterized by worsening renal function during a heart failure hospitalization, or soon after discharge, despite symptomatic improvement with diuretic therapy and maintenance of adequate intravascular volume.[1,2] Underlying chronic kidney disease (e.g., associated with diabetes or hypertension) increases the risk of cardiorenal syndrome, as does neurohormonal activation resulting from impaired cardiac output and excessive loop diuretic therapy.

Renal function is an important prognostic indicator in patients with acute heart failure syndromes. Impaired baseline renal function, and worsening renal function during hospitalization or early after discharge, are potent predictors of adverse outcomes, including early readmission rates and mortality.[3] *Elevated*, not reduced, systemic venous pressure appears to be an important contributing factor to the development of cardiorenal syndrome, because venous congestion contributes to elevated intra-abdominal pressure that can impair glomerular filtration.[4]

An increase in blood urea nitrogen (BUN) out of proportion to serum creatinine is a sign of renal hypoperfusion, resulting from low forward cardiac output or intravascular volume depletion because of high doses of intravenous diuretics. The neurohormonal activation accompanying renal hypoperfusion increases proximal sodium and urea reabsorption, while creatinine handling is unaffected, leading to an elevated BUN/creatinine ratio.

REFERENCES

1. Gheorghiade M, Pang PS: Acute heart failure syndromes. J Am Coll Cardiol 53:557, 2009.
2. Bock JS, Gottlieb SS: Cardiorenal syndrome: New perspectives. Circulation 121:2592, 2010.
3. Damman K, Navis G, Voors AA, et al: Worsening renal function and prognosis in heart failure: Systematic review and meta-analysis. J Card Fail 13:599, 2007.
4. Mullens W, Abraham Z, Francis GS, et al: Importance of venous congestion for worsening of renal function in advanced decompensated heart failure. J Am Coll Cardiol 53:589, 2009.

ANSWER TO QUESTION 172

A (Braunwald, pp. 558-565)

The effectiveness of digoxin was studied in the DIG trial, which enrolled 6800 patients with Class I to III heart failure, with a mean left ventricular (LV) ejection fraction of 28%.[1] Over 37 months of follow-up there was a significant decrease in heart failure hospitalizations but no significant improvement in total mortality with digoxin therapy compared with placebo.

Angiotensin-converting enzyme (ACE) inhibitors are the cornerstone of therapy for patients with chronic heart failure or asymptomatic LV dysfunction because of their favorable hemodynamic effects and unsurpassed benefit on long-term mortality. The Vasodilator Heart Failure Trial II (V-HEFT II) compared the ACE inhibitor enalapril with the combination of hydralazine plus isosorbide dinitrate in the treatment of chronic moderate congestive heart failure. Survival in the enalapril-treated group proved superior.[2]

There is also significant benefit of angiotensin II receptor blockers (ARBs) in patients with heart failure. The

VALIANT[3] trial randomized patients with LV dysfunction after myocardial infarction to valsartan, captopril, or both and found similar benefit with the ACE inhibitor or ARB in reducing mortality. The incremental benefit of ARBs in patients already treated with ACE inhibitors is less clear. ARBs are currently accepted as appropriate substitutes for patients with LV dysfunction who are intolerant of ACE inhibitors.

In the RALES trial, the aldosterone antagonist spironolactone was shown to reduce mortality when added to standard heart failure therapy in patients with Class III to IV heart failure with an ejection fraction < 35%.[4] In the more recent EMPHASIS trial, eplerenone, a selective aldosterone antagonist, significantly reduced mortality compared with placebo when added to standard heart failure therapy in patients with Class II or III systolic heart failure.[5]

REFERENCES

1. The Digitalis Investigation Group: The effect of digoxin on mortality and morbidity in patients with heart failure. N Engl J Med 336:525, 1997.
2. Cohn JN, Johnson G, Zeische S, et al: A comparison of enalapril with hydralazine-isosorbide dinitrate in the treatment of chronic congestive heart failure. N Engl J Med 325:303, 1991.
3. Pfeffer MA, McMurray JJV, Velazquez EJ, et al: Valsartan, captopril, or both in patients with myocardial infarction complicated by heart failure, left ventricular dysfunction, or both. N Engl J Med 349:1893, 2003.
4. Pitt B, Zannad F, Remme WJ, et al: The effect of spironolactone on morbidity and mortality in patients with severe heart failure. Randomized Aldactone Evaluation Study Investigators. N Engl J Med 341:709, 1999.
5. Zannad F, McMurray JJ, Krum H, et al: Eplerenone in patients with systolic heart failure and mild symptoms. N Engl J Med 364:11, 2011.

ANSWER TO QUESTION 173

C (Braunwald, pp. 608-615; Fig. 31-13; Table 31-4)

Cardiac transplantation has been performed since 1967. Long-term outcomes after transplantation improved dramatically with the introduction of the calcineurin inhibitor cyclosporine as the cornerstone of immunosuppression. The median survival of all cardiac transplant patients is now 10 years, with a median survival of 13 years among those patients who are alive 1 year after transplant.[1] By the first year after transplantation, 90% of surviving patients report no functional limitations.[2]

The selection of candidates for transplantation is a complex process that integrates assessment of hemodynamics, comorbidities that might limit post-transplantation survival, and psychosocial factors that may impair compliance. Optimal candidates for heart transplantation are younger patients with advanced heart failure, minimal comorbid illness or end-organ damage, a history of adherence to prescribed medical therapy, and a strong family and social network.

The transplanted heart is denervated and relies on atypical adaptive mechanisms to meet varying demands for cardiac output. As a result of increased venous return at the onset of exercise, the transplanted heart responds with the intrinsic Frank-Starling mechanism to increase cardiac output. Circulating catecholamine levels rise as exercise ensues, providing a delayed chronotropic response. This mechanism allows near-normal hemodynamic function at rest, and the capacity to support at least moderate exercise in a large majority of long-term survivors. Of note, beta blockers may impair the heart rate response and should be used cautiously after heart transplantation.

Allograft rejection is monitored most reliably by surveillance right ventricular endomyocardial biopsy, which is carried out on a routine schedule during the post-transplantation period and over the life of the transplant. High-grade rejection may be signaled by the development of clinical heart failure, atrial arrhythmias, low QRS voltage on the ECG, or echocardiographic evidence of left ventricular dysfunction; however, definitive diagnosis or identification of early or subtle lower-grade rejection requires histologic examination of the myocardium.

Allograft rejection and infection are the most common causes of death early after transplant. By contrast, the risk of fatal malignancy increases progressively in the years thereafter. The most common fatal early malignancies are post-transplant lymphoproliferative disorder and lung cancer. The risk of infection diminishes with time as the intensity of immunosuppression therapy is reduced.

REFERENCES

1. Stehlik J, Edwards LB, Kucheryavaya AY et al: The Registry of the International Society of Heart and Lung Transplantation: Twenty-seventh official adult heart transplant report—2010. J Heart Lung Transplant 29:1089, 2009.
2. Grady KL, Naftel DC, Young JB, et al: Patterns and predictors of physical functional disability at 5 to 10 years after heart transplantation. J Heart Lung Transplant 26:1182, 2007.

ANSWER TO QUESTION 174

C (Braunwald, pp. 507-508)

Many medical and surgical conditions are associated with a chest radiographic pattern consistent with pulmonary edema, as in the accompanying radiograph. The physical examination of this patient was nearly normal, without dramatic chest examination findings, jugular venous distention, or a third heart sound. This suggests that, in this patient, the edema was primarily caused not by an alteration in the Starling forces across pulmonary capillaries but rather by abnormal permeability of the alveolar-capillary membrane. This situation is consistent with acute respiratory distress syndrome (ARDS). Among the conditions that have been associated with ARDS are pneumonia, inhaled toxins, circulating foreign substances (including bacterial endotoxins), aspiration of gastric contents, acute radiation pneumonitis, release of endogenous vasoactive substances, disseminated intravascular coagulation, shock lung in association with nonthoracic trauma, and acute hemorrhagic pancreatitis.

Whereas the pathophysiology of ARDS is incompletely understood, it is likely that epithelial injury leading to increased permeability of the alveolar-capillary barrier is a critical initiating event. An imbalance between proinflammatory cytokines and anti-inflammatory mediators likely contributes to recruitment of neutrophils, release of toxic inflammatory substances, loss of endothelial integrity, reduced surfactant production, and impaired removal of edema fluid from the alveolar space.

REFERENCE

Ware LB, Matthay MA: Clinical practice: Acute pulmonary edema. N Engl J Med 353:2788, 2005.

ANSWER TO QUESTION 175

E (Braunwald, pp. 286-287, 507-509; Fig. 16-16)

A variety of laboratory abnormalities may be noted in patients with congestive heart failure. Alterations in serum electrolyte values usually occur only after patients have begun treatment or in more long-standing, severe cases of heart failure. Hyponatremia may be present for a variety of reasons, including sodium restriction, intensive diuretic therapy, a decrease in the ability to excrete water related to reductions in renal blood flow and glomerular filtration rate (GFR), and elevations in the concentration of circulating vasopressin.[1] Hypokalemia may result from aggressive diuretic therapy. Conversely, hyperkalemia may occasionally occur in patients with severe heart failure who have marked reductions in GFR or who are receiving aldosterone receptor antagonists (spironolactone or eplerenone).

Congestive hepatomegaly due to "backward" failure and cardiac cirrhosis from long-standing heart failure is often accompanied by impaired hepatic function, reflected by abnormal circulating liver enzymes. In acute hepatic venous congestion, severe jaundice may result, with bilirubin levels as high as 15 to 20 mg/dL, dramatic elevations of serum aspartate aminotransferase levels, and prolongation of the prothrombin time. Although the clinical and laboratory profiles of such an event may resemble viral hepatitis, the diagnosis of hepatic congestion due to heart failure is confirmed by rapid normalization of these values with successful treatment of heart failure. In patients with long-standing heart failure and secondary severe hepatic damage, albumin synthesis may become impaired. Rarely, more severe sequelae may occur, including hepatic hypoglycemia, fulminant hepatic failure, and hepatic coma.

Elevations in pulmonary capillary pressure are reflected by the appearance of the vasculature on the chest radiograph. With minimal elevations (i.e., ~13 to 17 mm Hg), early equalization in the size of the vessels in the apices and bases is first discernible. It is not until greater pressure elevations occur (~18 to 20 mm Hg) that actual pulmonary vascular redistribution occurs. When pressure exceeds 20 to 25 mm Hg, frank interstitial pulmonary edema is usually observed. Importantly, however, in patients with *chronic* left ventricular failure, higher pulmonary pressures can be accommodated with few clinical and radiologic signs of congestion due to enhanced lymphatic drainage.

REFERENCE

1. De Luca L, Klein L, Udelson JE, et al: Hyponatremia in patients with heart failure. Am J Cardiol 96:19L-23L, 2005.

ANSWER TO QUESTION 176

B (Braunwald, pp. 460-468; Figs. 24-1 and 24-6)

The binding of a beta-adrenergic agonist to its myocyte receptor initiates a complex system of messengers within the sarcolemma and cytosol of the cell. The beta$_1$ receptor is coupled, via G-proteins, to activation of adenylate cyclase and formation of cyclic *adenosine* monophosphate (cAMP). This molecule acts via protein kinases to phosphorylate proteins and enzymes within the cell. Such action stimulates enhanced entry of calcium ions through voltage-dependent L-type calcium channels, followed by additional calcium-induced calcium release from the sarcoplasmic reticulum. The rise in cytosolic calcium increases calcium–troponin C interaction, a necessary step for subsequent contraction. The activated troponin C binds tightly to the inhibitory molecule troponin I, thus removing inhibition of actin-myosin cross-bridge formation, and contraction ensues.

Whereas cAMP is a second messenger for the beta-adrenergic system, another cyclic nucleotide, cyclic guanosine monophosphate (cGMP), acts as a second messenger during *cholinergic* stimulation. In vascular smooth muscle, cGMP acts as an intracellular messenger after nitric oxide stimulation.

Titin is a large protein that provides elasticity and supports the myosin molecule by tethering it to the myocyte Z line.

REFERENCE

Opie LH: Heart Physiology: From Cell to Circulation. 4th ed. Philadelphia, Lippincott Williams & Wilkins, 2004.

ANSWER TO QUESTION 177

B (Braunwald, pp. 611-12; Table 31-1)

Rejection is a ubiquitous concern after solid organ transplantation. It results from cell- or antibody-mediated allograft injury owing to recognition of the allograft as non-self tissue. Three major types of rejection have been identified: hyperacute, acute, and chronic. *Hyperacute* rejection occurs within minutes to hours after heart transplantation and is mediated by preexisting antibodies to allogeneic antigens on the vascular endothelium that fix complement. This results in occlusion of graft vasculature and overwhelming graft failure. In contrast, the biopsy specimen in this question shows a dense lymphocytic infiltrate and myocyte damage typical of *acute* cellular allograft rejection. Acute cellular rejection is a T-cell–mediated process that develops in the first weeks to 6 months after transplantation. *Chronic* rejection, or late graft failure, is an irreversible deterioration of graft function years after transplant mediated by antibodies or progressive graft loss from ischemia.

Risk factors for rejection include female gender, black recipient race, recipient-positive cytomegalovirus serology, prior infections, and the number of HLA mismatches.[1] Patients who do not experience acute rejection within the first 6 months after transplantation have a lower incidence of late rejection.

There are no reliable serologic markers for rejection, so endomyocardial biopsy remains the gold standard for routine post-transplant surveillance. The procedure is performed under fluoroscopic or echocardiographic guidance using a bioptome inserted percutaneously via the right internal jugular vein. Potential complications include pneumothorax, transient rhythm disturbances, myocardial perforation, and tricuspid regurgitation.

The most important feature of the post-transplant biopsy specimen is the detection of lymphocyte infiltration and the presence of myocyte necrosis. A revised continuum scale has been established for grading cardiac biopsies from no rejection (grade OR) to diffuse damaging inflammatory cell infiltrates with encroachment of myocytes and disruption of normal cell architecture (grade 3R).[2] Appropriate therapy for acute cellular rejection depends on the timing and severity of the rejection episode. Episodes that occur within the first 3 months, or episodes that are moderate to severe, are initially treated with pulsed-dose methylprednisolone. If steroid therapy is ineffective, then more aggressive therapy with OKT3 monoclonal antibody or ATGAM (horse antithymocyte globulin) may be necessary.[3]

REFERENCES

1. Kobashigawa JA, Starling RC, Mehra MR, et al: Multicenter retrospective analysis of cardiovascular risk factors affecting long-term outcome of de novo cardiac transplant recipients. J Heart Lung Transplant 25:1063, 2006.
2. Stewart S, Winters GL, Fishbein MC, et al: Revision of the 1990 working formulation for the standardization of nomenclature in the diagnosis of heart rejection. J Heart Lung Transplant 24:1710, 2005.
3. Jessup M, Brozena S: State-of-the-art strategies for immunosuppression. Curr Opin Organ Transplant 12:536, 2007.

ANSWER TO QUESTION 178

E (Braunwald, pp. 477-478, 511, 608)

The four primary determinants of cardiac output (CO) are (1) heart rate; (2) preload, which is closely related to left ventricular (LV) end-diastolic volume; (3) afterload, which is closely related to aortic impedance (i.e., the sum of the external factors that oppose ventricular ejection); and (4) contractility, a fundamental property of cardiac muscle that reflects the level of activation of crossbridge formation. Preload, afterload, and contractility determine the ventricular stroke volume (SV), and cardiac output = Heart rate × SV.

Unlike other organs, the myocardium extracts oxygen from blood nearly maximally. Thus, even at rest, the oxygen saturation in coronary venous blood (measured at the coronary sinus) is quite low, usually <40%.

The body's oxygen consumption at peak exercise is an indirect measure of the CO.[1] The peak oxygen uptake ($\dot{V}_{O_2}$ max) is defined as the value achieved when $\dot{V}_{O_2}$ plateaus despite a continued increase in the intensity of exercise. The anaerobic threshold is indicated by the $\dot{V}_{O_2}$ at which carbon dioxide production starts to rise, resulting in an increase in the $\dot{V}_{CO_2}/\dot{V}_{O_2}$ ratio. Both the peak oxygen consumption and the anaerobic threshold are reproducible when measured days or weeks apart. During exercise, the CO of a normal heart increases up to 6-fold and the body's oxygen consumption can increase up to 18-fold.

In patients with left ventricular dysfunction, cardiopulmonary exercise tests are often performed to determine functional capacity. A peak oxygen consumption of >20 mL/min/kg reflects mild or no functional impairment. Conversely, a peak oxygen consumption of <12 mL/kg/min indicates severe impairment and a poor prognosis. Serial tests can be performed over time to assess the response to pharmacologic therapies in patients with heart failure and can help guide the need for aggressive interventions such as cardiac transplantation or placement of a ventricular assist device.

REFERENCE

1. Balady GJ, Arena R, Sietsema K, et al: Clinician's guide to cardiopulmonary exercise testing in adults: A scientific statement from the American Heart Association. Circulation 122:191, 2010.

ANSWER TO QUESTION 179

E (Braunwald, pp. 478-479, 483-484; Fig. 24-21)

By the law of Laplace, LV wall stress (σ) is directly proportional to intracavitary pressure and chamber radius and inversely proportional to wall thickness (σ = [Pressure × radius]/wall thickness). Ventricular hypertrophy is therefore an adaptive mechanism that serves to reduce ventricular wall stress. Myocardial hypertrophy and remodeling proceed in different patterns based on the timing and nature of the provocative stimulus. When the primary stimulus is pressure overload (as in aortic stenosis or hypertension), an increase in wall stress during ventricular systole triggers the addition of new myofibrils in parallel, leading to wall thickening at the expense of chamber size, in a pattern of *concentric* hypertrophy. When the primary stimulus is volume overload (as in chronic mitral regurgitation), increased wall stress during ventricular diastole triggers the replication of sarcomeres in series, elongation of myocytes, and ventricular cavity dilatation, in a pattern of *eccentric* hypertrophy. Therefore, although both chronic pressure and volume overload are associated with a compensatory increase in LV mass, the pattern of hypertrophy is distinct in each case.

With the use of echocardiography, concentric hypertrophy can be distinguished from eccentric hypertrophy visually, or on the basis of the ratio between wall thickness and the LV internal diameter during diastole (i.e., the relative wall thickness = [2 × posterior wall thickness]/LV internal dimension). A relative wall thickness <0.45 suggests eccentric hypertrophy, whereas a higher ratio is more consistent with concentric hypertrophy.

ANSWER TO QUESTION 180

A (Braunwald, pp. 582-584, 722-724, Fig. 29-5; Fig. 29-6)

Amiodarone has been studied extensively in patients with left ventricular (LV) dysfunction. It effectively suppresses ventricular and supraventricular arrhythmias and appears to be safe for use in this subset of patients. However, convincing evidence of mortality reduction has not been shown. In the SCD-HeFT study of patients with Class II to III heart failure and a left ventricular ejection fraction of 35% or less, amiodarone did not improve survival compared with placebo.[1]

Dronedarone is a derivative of amiodarone that shares its electrophysiologic properties but does not contain iodine and is associated with lower rates of lung and thyroid toxicity. Dronedarone is approved to facilitate maintenance of sinus rhythm in patients with atrial fibrillation or atrial flutter. It should not be prescribed in Class III to IV heart failure because its use was associated with increased mortality in such patients in the ANDROMEDA trial.[2]

The results of several randomized, controlled clinical trials support the benefit of implantable cardioverter-defibrillator therapy in reducing mortality among patients with LV dysfunction. The Antiarrhythmics Versus Implantable Defibrillators (AVID) study randomized patients with reduced LV ejection fraction and prior resuscitated cardiac arrest, or symptomatic sustained ventricular tachycardia (VT), to therapy with amiodarone or an implantable cardioverter-defibrillator (ICD). ICD therapy was associated with a 29% reduction in all-cause mortality compared with amiodarone. A concurrent registry of patients with transient or correctable causes of VT or ventricular fibrillation not enrolled in the primary trial revealed that the risk of mortality in these patients remains comparable with those with primary VT or ventricular fibrillation.[3] ICD therapy is therefore recommended as the standard of care for secondary prevention of sudden cardiac death or symptomatic ventricular tachyarrhythmias in patients with LV dysfunction.

The data for ICD efficacy in primary prevention of sudden cardiac death are also compelling. The results of the Multicenter Automatic Defibrillator Implantation II Trial (MADIT II) confirm that, in patients with coronary artery disease, prior myocardial infarction, and LV ejection fraction ≤30%, prophylactic implantation of a defibrillator reduces mortality by 31% relative to conventional medical therapy.[4] The results of the Sudden Cardiac Death in Heart Failure Trial (SCD-HeFT) have extended the benefits of ICD therapy to patients with nonischemic cardiomyopathy.[1] Thus, current ACC/AHA guidelines indicate that patients with mild to moderate heart failure and an LV ejection function ≤35% on optimal medical therapy are potential candidates for ICD implantation.

REFERENCES

1. Bardy GH, Lee KL, Mark DB, et al: Amiodarone or an implantable defibrillator in advanced chronic heart failure. N Engl J Med 352:225, 2005.
2. Kober L, Torp-Pederson C, McMurray JJ, et al: Increased mortality after dronedarone therapy for severe heart failure. N Engl J Med 358:2678, 2008.
3. Wyse DG, Friedman PL, Brodsky MA, et al: Life-threatening ventricular arrhythmias due to transient or correctable causes: High risk for death in follow up. J Am Coll Cardiol 38:1718, 2001.
4. Moss AJ, Zareba W, Hall WJ, et al: Prophylactic implantation of a defibrillator in patients with myocardial infarction and reduced ejection fraction. N Engl J Med 346:877, 2002.

ANSWER TO QUESTION 181

A (Braunwald, pp. 578-582; Figs. 29-3 and Fig. 29-4)

Ventricular dyssynchrony is defined as a QRS duration >120 milliseconds on the surface ECG regardless of the QRS morphology. Ventricular conduction delay alters the timing of ventricular activation and places an already failing ventricle under further mechanical disadvantage by reducing contractility and ventricular filling and prolonging the duration of mitral regurgitation.[1] Cardiac resynchronization therapy (CRT), also known as biventricular pacing, helps to optimize atrioventricular delay and resynchronize left ventricular (LV) contraction, leading to improved ventricular performance and reduced LV filling pressures.

CRT improves ventricular function without increasing myocardial energy consumption, in contrast to the effects of inotropic agents such as dobutamine. CRT may also reverse LV remodeling over time, reducing LV mass and end-diastolic dimension while increasing the ejection fraction.

The CARE-HF trial demonstrated that CRT alone, without a defibrillator, reduces mortality in patients with Classes III and IV heart failure, left ventricular ejection fraction ≤35%, and ventricular dysynchrony.[2] CRT combined with an implantable cardioverter-defibrillator (CRT-D) has been shown to reduce death and hospitalization rates in patients with Classes II and III heart failure and LV systolic dysfunction.[3] The mortality benefit of CRT alone (without a defibrillator) remains uncertain for patients with Class I or II heart failure with a reduced ejection fraction and dyssynchrony on electrocardiography.

Approximately 25% of patients receiving CRT under current indications are nonresponders. Contributing factors to nonresponse include coronary venous anatomy that precludes optimal LV lead placement, the presence of ventricular scar, or suboptimal atrioventricular or ventriculoventricular activation timing.

Echocardiography is a promising means to identifying mechanical dyssynchrony, but it is not part of the current selection criteria for CRT.

REFERENCES

1. Jarcho JA: Biventricular pacing. N Engl J Med 355:288, 2006.
2. Cleland JG, Daubert JC, Erdmann E, et al: The effect of cardiac resynchronization on morbidity and mortality in heart failure. N Engl J Med 352:1539, 2005.

3. Tang AS, George GA, Talajic M, et al: Cardiac-resynchronization therapy for mild-to-moderate heart failure. N Engl J Med 363:2385, 2010.

ANSWER TO QUESTION 182

C (Braunwald, pp. 520-522)

The hallmark of circulatory shock is a marked reduction of blood flow to vital organs. This occurs either because of a dramatic fall in cardiac output (as a result of cardiac pump failure or massive volume loss) or as a result of an acute loss of systemic vascular tone (due to sepsis, anaphylaxis, or spinal cord injury). Regulatory mechanisms permit maintenance of cerebral and coronary blood flow, at the expense of splanchnic and renal perfusion, until the most advanced stages. A decrease in mental alertness or the development of electrocardiographic abnormalities (including ischemic ST-segment and T wave changes) is an ominous sign and reflects progressive cerebral or regional myocardial hypoperfusion.

Sepsis is the most frequent cause of vasodilatory shock, but loss of vascular tone is also the final common pathway for severe and long-lasting shock of any cause. In patients with marked hypotension and decreased tissue perfusion due to hemorrhagic or cardiogenic shock, for example, correction of the initial problem may not cure the hypotension because excessive vasodilatation has supervened. The common mechanisms responsible for the vasodilatation and resistance to vasopressor medications that occur in vasodilatory shock include activation of adenosine triphosphate–sensitive potassium channels in the plasma membrane of vascular smooth muscle, activation of the inducible form of nitric oxide synthase, and *deficiency* of the hormone vasopressin. Exogenous vasopressin administration in patients with vasodilatory shock may therefore be of clinical usefulness in improving arterial pressure.

REFERENCE

Landry DW, Oliver JA: The pathogenesis of vasodilatory shock. N Engl J Med 345:588, 2001.

ANSWER TO QUESTION 183

B (Braunwald, pp. 505-508)

Although peripheral edema is a common and important physical finding in congestive heart failure, its presence does not correlate well with the level of systemic venous pressure. The excess volume of extracellular fluid is a more important determinant of edema. In adults, a minimum of 4 liters of excess extracellular fluid volume usually must accumulate before peripheral edema is manifested. In patients with chronic left ventricular failure and a low cardiac output, peripheral edema may develop in the presence of normal or minimally elevated systemic venous pressure because of a gradual but persistent accumulation of extracellular fluid volume.

Edema generally accumulates in dependent portions of the body such as the ankles or feet of ambulatory patients or the sacrum of bedridden patients. As heart failure progresses, edema becomes more severe and may become massive and generalized (anasarca). In rare instances, especially when edema develops suddenly and severely, frank rupture of the skin with extravasation of fluid may result. Edema is usually more marked on the paralyzed side of patients with hemiplegia; unilateral edema may also result from unilateral venous obstruction.

ANSWER TO QUESTION 184

E (Braunwald, pp. 586-590)

This patient's presentation is most consistent with the syndrome of heart failure with normal ejection fraction (HFnlEF). She exhibits many of the typical demographic features including advanced age, a history of hypertension, and elevated body mass index as well as clinical signs and symptoms of decompensated heart failure.

In contrast to heart failure with a reduced EF, there are only limited data from prospective, randomized clinical trials to guide appropriate management of this large population of patients. Although aggressive management of hypertension in this disorder is beneficial,[1] no specific therapy has been clearly associated with a survival benefit. In the subgroup of HFnlEF patients enrolled in the Digitalis Investigators Group (DIG) trial, digoxin did not improve the composite primary end point of heart failure hospitalization or cardiovascular mortality.[2]

The PEP-CHF[3] trial randomized a population of patients with heart failure, normal or near normal EF, and age >70 years to treatment with the angiotensin-converting enzyme inhibitor perindopril or placebo and failed to demonstrate a benefit in the primary endpoint of all-cause mortality or unplanned heart failure hospitalizations.

The CHARM-Preserved trial randomized patients with chronic heart failure and EF > 40% to treatment with the angiotensin receptor blocker candesartan or placebo.[4] Fewer hospitalizations for heart failure occurred in the candesartan group, but cardiovascular survival was not improved. The I-PRESERVE trial studied patients >60 years old with symptomatic heart failure and EF ≥ 45%. After randomization to irbesartan or placebo there was no significant effect on mortality or hospitalizations from a cardiovascular cause.[5]

No multicenter clinical trial has examined the use of verapamil in HFnlEF.

REFERENCES

1. Jessup ML, Abraham WT, Casey DE, et al: 2009 focused update: ACCF/AHA Guidelines for the Diagnosis and Management of Heart Failure in Adults. A report of the American College of Cardiology Foundation/American Heart Association Task Force on Practice Guidelines: Developed in collaboration with the International Society for Heart and Lung Transplantation. Circulation 119:1977, 2009.
2. Ahmed A, Rich MW, Fleg JL, et al: Effects of digoxin on morbidity and mortality is diastolic heart failure: The ancillary digitalis investigation group trial. Circulation 114:397, 2006.
3. Cleland JG, Tendera M, Adamus J, et al: The perindopril in elderly people with chronic heart failure (PEP-CHF) study. Eur Heart J 27:2338, 2006.

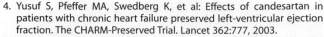

HEART FAILURE; ARRHYTHMIAS, SUDDEN DEATH, AND SYNCOPE

4. Yusuf S, Pfeffer MA, Swedberg K, et al: Effects of candesartan in patients with chronic heart failure preserved left-ventricular ejection fraction. The CHARM-Preserved Trial. Lancet 362:777, 2003.
5. Massie BM, Carson PE, McMurray JJ, et al: Irbesartan in patients with heart failure and preserved ejection fraction. N Engl J Med 359:2456, 2008.

ANSWER TO QUESTION 185

D (Braunwald, pp. 507-508, 526, Table 27-6)

A variety of physical examination findings are present in patients with heart failure. Characteristic findings include jugular venous distention, hepatomegaly, peripheral edema, accentuation of the P_2 component of S_2, gallop heart sounds (in particular, an S_3) and pulmonary rales. Chronic, marked elevation of systemic venous pressures may result in severe tricuspid regurgitation with visible systolic pulsation of the neck veins and even the eyes. Low cardiac output results in sympathetic nervous system activation and systemic arterial vasoconstriction, which helps to support blood pressure and maintain end-organ perfusion. Sustained arteriolar vasoconstriction commonly produces pallor and coldness of the extremities and, in severe cases, digital cyanosis.

In patients with mild right-sided heart failure, the jugular venous pressure may appear normal at rest but may rise with compression of the right upper quadrant. Formally, a positive abdominojugular reflux test is defined as a sustained increase in jugular venous pressure of >3 cm that persists during prolonged abdominal compression (up to 1 minute). If present, this sign indicates that intracardiac filling pressures are elevated and the right side of the heart is unable to accommodate increased venous return.

Hepatomegaly is a common finding in patients with heart failure and often occurs before lower extremity edema develops. If hepatomegaly occurs rapidly, as in cases of sudden onset of heart failure, acute stretching of the liver capsule ensues that can result in right upper quadrant tenderness. However, in long-standing heart failure this tenderness abates, even if the liver remains enlarged. Ascites may follow as a result of increased visceral capillary permeability, long-standing systemic venous hypertension, and hepatic venous congestion. Rarely, persistent visceral congestion due to severe heart failure may result in a protein-losing enteropathy. The resultant reduction in plasma oncotic pressure may exacerbate the underlying tendency to form ascites.

ANSWER TO QUESTION 186

D (Braunwald, pp. 608-610, 617-623; Table 32-1; Figs. 31-11, 32-1, 32-5, and 32-6)

The patient in this vignette has New York Heart Association (NYHA) Class IV and American College of Cardiology/American Heart Association stage D congestive heart failure. He is not a candidate for cardiac resynchronization therapy because the QRS complex duration is normal (see Answer to Question 181). Repeated hospitalizations for heart failure, hyponatremia, intolerance to beta-adrenergic blockade, and a markedly reduced peak oxygen uptake of 10 mL/kg/min are all markers of poor prognosis and, taken together, predict mortality >50% in the next year. Such a patient should be considered for advanced therapies, including heart transplantation and mechanical circulatory support. Given the limitations of donor supply, cardiac transplantation is generally reserved for younger patients with few comorbid conditions. In addition, because of renal insufficiency and the recent diagnosis of cancer, this patient is unlikely to be eligible for transplantation (either heart alone or combined heart-kidney). Furthermore, the typically long waiting time for a donor heart renders transplantation an impractical immediate solution for this patient with a very limited predicted short-term survival.

Durable mechanical circulatory devices (i.e., ventricular assist devices) can extend survival and enhance the quality of life in patients with advanced heart failure. Mechanical support can be used as a "bridge to transplantation" and also as permanent "destination therapy" in patients for whom cardiac transplantation is not feasible. Such devices may also be used as a "bridge to recovery" in rare cases of an identifiable, potentially reversible cause of cardiac decompensation, such as acute myocarditis, postcardiotomy syndrome, or peripartum cardiomyopathy. Because this patient is ineligible for transplantation, destination therapy would be the most appropriate mechanical support strategy.

The Randomized Evaluation of Mechanical Assistance for the Treatment of Congestive Heart Failure (REMATCH) trial evaluated patients with NYHA Class IV symptoms and left ventricular ejection fraction < 25%, most of whom were on continuous intravenous inotropes.[1] REMATCH demonstrated the superiority of an early-generation pulsatile left ventricular assist device (LVAD) compared with medical therapy, but by 2 years of follow-up only 23% of the patients with the assist devices were still alive.

The HeartMate II, a next-generation rotary LVAD providing continuous blood flow, has been approved by the U.S. Food and Drug Administration both as a bridge to transplantation and as destination therapy. Continuous-flow pumps are relatively low profile devices that allow implantation in smaller patients and offer mechanical durability but do expose patients to the risk of stroke, infection, and bleeding. The HeartMate II LVAD confers an actuarial survival of 68% at 1 year and 58% at 2 years, while dramatically improving the quality of life in the majority of patients.[2,3] Of note, patients being considered for destination LVAD therapy must have adequate native right ventricular (RV) function, because postoperative RV failure is associated with high mortality.

Although mechanical biventricular support is also available as a bridge to transplantation, it is not currently approved as destination therapy. Because this patient has adequate right ventricular function by echocardiography, he should be well supported by an isolated LVAD.

Finally, palliative and hospice level care are playing increasingly important roles in the care of stage D heart failure patients for whom the just-mentioned options are not practical and there are no reasonable prospects for improvement in quality or length of life.

REFERENCES

1. Rose EA, Gelijns AC, Moskowitz AJ, et al: Long-term mechanical left ventricular assistance for end-stage heart failure. N Engl J Med 345:1435, 2001.
2. Slaughter MS, Rogers JG, Milano CA, et al: Advanced heart failure treated with continuous-flow left ventricular assist device. N Engl J Med 361:2241, 2009.
3. Wilson SR, Mudge GH, Stewart GC, et al: Evaluation for a ventricular assist device: Selecting the appropriate candidate. Circulation 119:2225, 2009.

ANSWER TO QUESTION 187

D (Braunwald, pp. 475-477; Table 24-3. Fig. 24-18)

The Wiggers diagram of the cardiac cycle graphically demonstrates the important temporal relationships between the electrical and mechanical events of cardiac contraction and relaxation (Fig. 2-21). Nearly

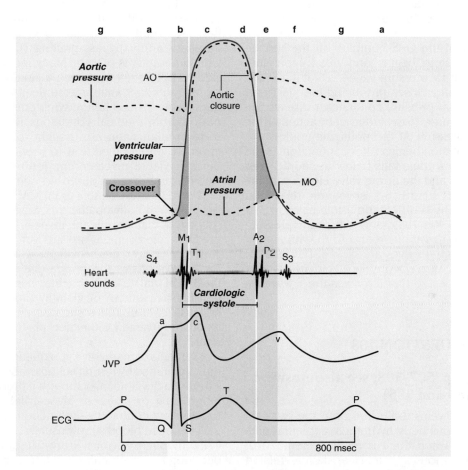

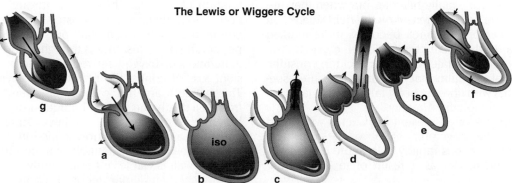

FIGURE 2-21 From Opie LH: Heart Physiology: From Cell to Circulation. Philadelphia, Lippincott Williams & Wilkins, 2004; copyright L. H. Opie, 2004.

simultaneous events occur in the right and left sides of the heart during the cardiac cycle; here we concentrate on the left-sided events. Filling of the left ventricle begins in early diastole when the left ventricular (LV) pressure falls below left atrial pressure and the mitral valve opens. The subsequent early phase of rapid ventricular filling corresponds to the timing of the third heart sound (S_3), which may be audible when filling pressures are increased (as in patients with heart failure).

As the pressures in the left atrium and ventricle equalize, ventricular filling slows. Filling is then augmented at end diastole owing to atrial contraction, which generates the *a* wave on the left atrial pressure tracing. Temporally, the *a* wave occurs just after the P wave on the surface ECG and coincides with timing of the fourth heart sound (S_4). In atrial fibrillation, organized atrial contraction is absent and a discrete *a* wave is usually not evident.

With the onset of the QRS complex on the surface ECG, ventricular systole begins and the LV pressure begins to rise. When LV pressure exceeds that in the left atrium, the mitral valve closes, producing the first heart sound (S_1). Ventricular pressure continues to rise at constant ventricular volume (isovolumic contraction) until it exceeds aortic pressure. At this point, the aortic valve opens and rapid ejection begins. After contraction, as the pressure in the left ventricle falls below the aortic pressure, ejection ceases and the aortic valve closes, generating the second heart sound (S_2). Isovolumic relaxation then occurs, beginning ventricular diastole again.

The *v* waves on the right and left atrial pressure tracings correspond to venous return to the atria when the tricuspid and mitral valves are closed. The peak of the *v* wave is usually inscribed after electrical repolarization of the ventricles, so that it *follows* the T wave on the ECG.

ANSWER TO QUESTION 188

B (Braunwald, pp. 507-508; see also Answers to Questions 183 and 185)

Because the pleural veins drain into both the systemic and pulmonary venous beds, hydrothorax (pleural effusion) may develop when there is marked elevation of pressure in either venous system. Heart failure–related pleural effusions are usually bilateral, but when they are unilateral they are usually present on the right side. When hydrothorax develops, dyspnea becomes more marked because of a further reduction in vital capacity. The absence of pulmonary rales does not exclude considerable elevation of the pulmonary capillary pressure, especially in patients with chronic heart failure who may have well-developed lymphatic drainage.

Hepatomegaly is often present in patients with heart failure before the development of overt peripheral edema. When it develops rapidly with acute congestion, the liver may be tender as a result of rapid capsular distention.

Peripheral edema often does not correlate well with the degree of systemic venous congestion. Usually, a substantial gain of extracellular fluid volume (>4 L in adults) must occur before peripheral edema develops.

With the development of left ventricular failure, pulmonary artery pressures rise and the pulmonic component of the second heart sound is accentuated. A systolic murmur of mitral regurgitation may also become audible owing to ventricular cavity dilatation.

ANSWER TO QUESTION 189

B (Braunwald, pp. 601-603, 606-607; Figs. 31-1 and 31-3)

The patient in the vignette has an ischemic cardiomyopathy due to multivessel obstructive coronary artery disease (CAD). Patients with left ventricular (LV) dysfunction and heart failure due to CAD may benefit from coronary artery bypass grafting (CABG) regardless of whether angina is present. Many factors should be considered before referring such a patient for CABG, including the coronary anatomy, the degree of LV dysfunction, the severity of heart failure symptoms, and the magnitude of comorbid medical conditions. Because the benefits of revascularization are thought to result in part from improvement in blood flow to previously underperfused but still viable myocardium, testing to assess cellular viability has been utilized to identify patients likely to derive greatest benefit from CABG.[1] In patients with ischemic cardiomyopathy, the weight of evidence has suggested that significant myocardial viability (≥25%) predicts improvement in survival and quality of life with CABG over medical therapy alone. However, preliminary results of the myocardial viability substudy of the STICH trial call this conclusion into question, suggesting that assessment of viability alone is not sufficient, because comorbidities such as diabetes, renal impairment, and overall LV function play important predictive roles.[2]

Segments of markedly hypokinetic or akinetic myocardium identified by resting echocardiography may contain substantially viable myocardium if those areas are simply hibernating or stunned. Myocardial *hibernation* refers to persistent contractile dysfunction caused by a chronically reduced blood supply, usually a result of multivessel CAD. In such regions, irreversible damage has not occurred and ventricular function can improve with restoration of adequate blood flow through revascularization.[3] Myocardial *stunning* refers to reversible postischemic contractile dysfunction that persists for a prolonged period after reperfusion. It is thought to be caused by the generation of oxygen-derived free radicals or the transient loss of contractile filament sensitivity to calcium. This patient's anterior wall akinesis may have resulted from cell death due to prior infarction, or it may represent hibernating myocardium. Viability testing with thallium perfusion imaging, positron emission tomography, or dobutamine echocardiography can confirm whether the anterior wall is viable or permanently scarred.

Surgical ventricular reconstruction (SVR) involves the resection of an aneurysmal or akinetic segment after transmural myocardial infarction and reconstruction with a patch. The exclusion of thinned, scarred myocardium restores an elliptical shape to the left ventricle with the goal of diminishing wall stress, mitral regurgitation, and residual ischemia. The results of the SVR portion of the STICH trial indicate that routine performance of SVR at the time of coronary artery bypass surgery is *not* associated with improved clinical outcomes.[4]

REFERENCES

1. Hunt SA, Abraham WT, Chin MH, et al: ACC/AHA 2005 Guideline Update for the Diagnosis and Management of Chronic Heart Failure in the Adult. A report of the American College of Cardiology/American Heart Association Task Force on Practice Guidelines (Writing Committee to Update the 2001 Guidelines for the Evaluation and Management of Heart Failure): Developed in collaboration with the American College of Chest Physicians and the International Society for Heart and Lung Transplantation: Endorsed by the Heart Rhythm Society. Circulation 112:e154, 2005.
2. Bonow RO, Maurer G, Lee KL, et al: Myocardial viability and survival in ischemic left ventricular dysfunction. N Engl J Med 364:1617-1625, 2011.
3. Carnici PG, Prasad SK, Rinoldi OE: Stunning, hibernation, and assessment of myocardial viability. Circulation 117:103, 2008.
4. Jones RH, Velazquez EJ, Michler RA, et al: STICH Hypothesis 2 Investigators: Coronary artery bypass surgery with or without surgical ventricular reconstruction. N Engl J Med 260:1705, 2009.

ANSWER TO QUESTION 190

E (Braunwald, pp. 564-565)

Disturbances of cardiac rhythm are important and potentially life-threatening complications of cardiac glycoside administration. Side effects can be minimized by maintaining therapeutic levels of digoxin between 0.5 and 1.0 ng/mL. Although overt digitalis toxicity is usually manifest at serum levels > 2.0 ng/mL, adverse drug effects may occur at lower levels, particularly if hypokalemia or hypomagnesemia is present. Digitalis toxicity may be manifest by neurologic symptoms (visual abnormalities, confusion), gastrointestinal disturbance (nausea, vomiting), or ventricular or supraventricular tachycardias and bradyarrhythmias. Common rhythm disturbances include junctional or ventricular ectopic beats, varying grades of atrioventricular (AV) block, accelerated AV junctional rhythm, paroxysmal atrial tachycardia with block, excessively slow ventricular response to atrial fibrillation, or bidirectional ventricular tachycardia. Lidocaine and phenytoin may be helpful in managing ventricular arrhythmias due to digoxin toxicity, and vagally mediated AV block in this setting often responds to therapeutic doses of atropine. Conversely, direct-current cardioversion can precipitate serious ventricular arrhythmias in patients with overt digitalis toxicity and elective cardioversion should be avoided.

Owing to its significant binding to plasma proteins and its large volume of distribution, digoxin is not efficiently removed by dialysis. However, in cases of life-threatening overdose, antidigoxin immunotherapy can prove lifesaving. Doses of purified antidigoxin Fab are administered on the basis of estimated dose of digoxin ingested, or total body burden. Although rare, recurrence of toxicity can occur, usually 24 to 48 hours after administration of antidigoxin immunotherapy.

REFERENCE

Bauman JL, Didomenico RJ, Galanter WL: Mechanisms, manifestations, and managements of digoxin toxicity in the modern era. Am J Cardiovasc Drugs 6:77, 2006.

ANSWER TO QUESTION 191

C (Braunwald, pp. 506-508, 543-544, 586-588)

Heart failure is a common disorder, and its prevalence and incidence continue to rise. Over 5.7 million people in the United States are actively being treated for heart failure, with 670,000 new cases diagnosed annually.[1] The prevalence of heart failure increases with age, occurring in up to 10% of patients older than the age of 75 years but only in 1% to 2% of those ages 45 to 54. Orthopnea refers to dyspnea that develops quickly after lying in the recumbent position, relieved by sitting upright. Although common in patients with heart failure, orthopnea is a nonspecific symptom that may occur in any condition in which pulmonary vital capacity is decreased, such as ascites, a large pleural effusion, or obstructive lung disease.

In severe heart failure, the stroke volume is reduced and is reflected by a reduced pulse pressure. Pulsus alternans is characterized by a regular heart rhythm with an alternating strong and weak peripheral pulse. This sign occurs most commonly in systolic, rather than diastolic, heart failure. It signifies advanced myocardial disease and is likely due to cyclical alteration in the left ventricular stroke volume due to incomplete myocardial recovery after contraction. It often disappears with successful treatment of heart failure.

Heart failure with preserved ejection fraction ("diastolic heart failure") occurs most commonly in patients who are elderly, female, and hypertensive.[2]

REFERENCES

1. Roger VL, Go AS, Lloyd-Jones DM, et al: Heart disease and stroke statistics—2001 update: A report from the American Heart Association. Circulation 123:e18, 2011.
2. Owan T, Hodge D, Herges D, et al: Heart failure with preserved ejection fraction: Trends in prevalence and outcomes. N Engl J Med 355:308, 2006.

ANSWER TO QUESTION 192

C (Braunwald, pp. 617-624, Fig. 32-2)

This radiograph displays a continuous-flow left ventricular assist device (LVAD) in the center of the figure. This rotary, axial flow pump is implanted below the diaphragm, with an inflow cannula inserted in the LV apex and an outflow cannula connected to the ascending aorta. Continuous-flow LVADs have a smaller profile, lower weight, and greater durability than earlier generation pulsatile LVADs and very low mechanical failure rates. The HeartMate II continuous-flow LVAD has been approved by the U.S. Food and Drug Administration for use both as a bridge to cardiac transplantation and as permanent destination therapy in patients not eligible for transplantation. In a pivotal destination therapy trial, patients with a HeartMate II had an actuarial survival of 68% at 1 year and 58% at 2 years, a significant improvement over the earlier-generation pulsatile device.[1]

Despite improved pump design and survival, disabling strokes remain a common complication of continuous-flow LVAD therapy, with rates approaching 10% per year. Device-related infections are the second leading cause of death after cardiac failure. Bacterial pathogens dominate and are found most commonly in the blood or the percutaneous driveline. Device endocarditis requires systemic antibiotics and device explantation. Gastrointestinal bleeding is more common with continuous flow LVADs compared with earlier generation pulsatile pumps and may be related to either an acquired von Willebrand factor defect (secondary to shear-related damage of high molecular weight von Willebrand factor multimers) or to enhanced development of gastrointestinal arteriovenous malformations (perhaps as a consequence of low pulse pressure). Bleeding complications may be further exacerbated by the requirement for both antiplatelet and anticoagulant therapy to prevent device-related thromboembolism.[2] LVAD therapy is associated with a high rate of right-sided heart failure, which may prolong hospitalization and reduces survival. Right-sided heart failure may be the consequence of underlying right-sided heart disease and LVAD-related hemodynamic alterations. A continuous-flow LVAD generates increased right-sided venous return and can produce interventricular septal shifts that can further impair right ventricular performance.[3] Therefore, patients with preoperative right ventricular dysfunction may not be candidates for isolated left-sided mechanical support.

The device in the upper left chest in the radiograph is an implantable cardioverter-defibrillator.

REFERENCES

1. Slaughter MS, Rogers JG, Milano CA, et al: Advanced heart failure treated with continuous-flow left ventricular assist device. N Engl J Med 361:2241, 2009.
2. Slaughter MS, Pagani FD, Rogers JG, et al: Clinical management of continuous-flow left ventricular assist devices in advanced heart failure. J Heart Lung Transplant 29:S1, 2010.
3. Kormos RL, Teuteberg JJ, Pagani FD, et al: Right ventricular failure in patients with the HeartMate II continuous-flow left ventricular assist device: Incidence, risk factors, and effect on outcomes. J Thorac Cardiovasc Surg 139:1316, 2010.

ANSWER TO QUESTION 193

C (Braunwald, pp. 477-478)

Preload represents the load on the ventricle just before contraction. It reflects the venous filling pressure, and left ventricular (LV) preload is most often approximated by the pulmonary capillary wedge pressure or the LV end-diastolic pressure. According to Starling's law, as preload increases, so does the stroke volume, and that relationship is graphically demonstrated by the Frank-Starling ventricular performance curves. Because stroke volume is a major determinant of cardiac output (cardiac output = stroke volume × heart rate), increased preload contributes to augmented cardiac output as well. Conditions that reduce filling of the left ventricle, such as sepsis (due to vasodilatation), dehydration, or right ventricular (RV) infarction (due to decreased RV output) lower the preload and therefore decrease stroke volume. Conversely, mitral regurgitation or increased intravascular volume (as may occur in renal failure) results in increased LV filling and preload.

ANSWER TO QUESTION 194

D (Braunwald, pp. 578-581)

The chest radiographs illustrate a biventricular pacing system, implanted for the purpose of cardiac resynchronization therapy (CRT). Three pacing leads are present, including standard leads in the right atrium and right ventricle and a third lead placed via the coronary sinus into a lateral marginal vein for left ventricular (LV) pacing. For patients with LV ejection fraction ≤ 0.35, prolonged QRS duration (>0.12 sec) on the surface ECG, and symptomatic heart failure (Class II to IV) despite optimal medical therapy, there is compelling evidence that CRT, either alone or with defibrillator capability, is associated with improvements in functional capacity, quality of life, and mortality. For example, the RAFT trial of CRT in patients with Class II to III heart failure, ejection fraction ≤ 0.30, and prolonged QRS complex demonstrated a 25% reduction in all-cause mortality and a 32% reduction in heart failure hospitalizations, confirming the results previously shown in MADIT-CRT.[1]

Improvements in ventricular mechanical delay with CRT are associated with reductions in the end-systolic volume index and mitral regurgitation and an augmented LV ejection fraction. These data support a potential "reverse remodeling" benefit of CRT in patients with heart failure and reduced ejection fraction.

To date, the QRS complex duration (a marker of delayed electrical activation) is the most extensively validated criterion in selection of patients for CRT. Although it is an imperfect surrogate for mechanical ventricular dyssynchrony, QRS complex duration predicts acute hemodynamic improvement after CRT, especially among patients with left bundle branch block in sinus rhythm.

Because the left ventricular lead is typically placed over the surface of the left ventricle via a coronary sinus branch, inadvertent phrenic nerve stimulation and diaphragmatic pacing may complicate device implantation.

To achieve the clinical and hemodynamic benefits of CRT, biventricular pacing must be continuous. This is in distinction to isolated right ventricular apical pacing, a mode that can *contribute* to dyssynchrony and a higher risk of heart failure symptoms.[2]

REFERENCES

1. Tang AS, Wells GA, Talajic M, et al: Cardiac-resynchronization therapy for mild-to-moderate heart failure. N Engl J Med 363:2385, 2010.

2. Yu CM, Chan JY, Zhang Q, et al: Biventricular pacing in patients with bradycardia and normal ejection fraction. N Engl J Med 361:2123, 2009.

ANSWER TO QUESTION 195

C (Braunwald, pp. 520-521, 526)

Pulmonary edema is initiated by an imbalance of Starling forces. Such an imbalance results from (1) increased pulmonary capillary pressure, (2) *decreased* plasma oncotic pressure, (3) increased negativity of interstitial pressure, or (4) increased interstitial oncotic pressure. An increased pulmonary venous pressure (e.g., due to mitral stenosis or left ventricular failure) raises the pulmonary capillary pressure and can result in pulmonary edema.

High-altitude pulmonary edema may occur in individuals who rapidly ascend to altitudes >2500 meters and then perform strenuous physical exercise before they have become acclimated.[1] The pathogenesis appears to involve hypoxic pulmonary vasoconstriction leading to increased capillary pressure. Symptoms respond quickly to descent to a lower altitude or to administration of a high inspiratory concentration of oxygen.

Acute pulmonary edema may develop in women with preeclampsia or eclampsia, most commonly in the postpartum period.[2] Multiple factors likely contribute, including the increased afterload of acute systemic hypertension, hypervolemia, hypoalbuminemia, and increased vascular permeability.

Many prescription drugs and drugs of abuse can cause lung injury or pulmonary edema. Heroin overdose is a well-recognized cause of pulmonary edema. The precise mechanism is not known but may relate to an alveolar-capillary membrane leak induced by the drug.

REFERENCES

1. Scherrer U, Rexhaj E, Jayet PY, et al: New insights in the pathogenesis of high-altitude pulmonary edema. Prog Cardiovasc Dis 52:485, 2010.
2. Bauer ST, Cleary KL: Cardiopulmonary complications of pre-eclampsia. Semin Perinatol 33:158, 2009.

ANSWER TO QUESTION 196

B (Braunwald, pp. 507-508, 566-567; Fig. 28-19)

Systolic dysfunction sets into motion a cascade of neurohormonal events that promote ventricular remodeling and progressive left ventricular cavity enlargement. As a consequence, cardiomegaly is common in patients with heart failure and reduced systolic function. However, many patients develop heart failure without apparent systolic dysfunction. This group of patients with heart failure and preserved ejection fraction comprises a diverse group of patients with primary diastolic heart failure, pericardial disease, valvular heart disease, hypertrophic heart disease, or primary restrictive cardiomyopathy. A clue to identifying these syndromes is the presence of signs and symptoms of heart failure in the absence of cardiomegaly.

Analysis of the Studies of Left Ventricular Dysfunction (SOLVD) treatment trial has demonstrated that the physical examination carries important prognostic information in patients with heart failure. In particular, elevated jugular venous pressure and a *third* heart sound are each independently associated with adverse outcomes, including progression of heart failure.[1]

Pulsus alternans is characterized by a regular rhythm with an alternating strong and weak peripheral pulse (see also Answer to Question 191). It signifies advanced myocardial disease and is likely the result of cyclic alteration in left ventricular stroke volume due to incomplete myocardial recovery after contraction. It often disappears with successful treatment of heart failure.

The presence of fever in congestive heart failure should always alert the physician to the possibility of underlying infection, pulmonary infarction, or infective endocarditis. In severe heart failure, low-grade fever may be seen as a consequence of cutaneous vasoconstriction and impairment of heat loss from sustained adrenergic nervous system activation. Sleep-disordered breathing is common in heart failure and is an independent risk factor for death and need for cardiac transplantation. *Central* sleep apnea, commonly referred to as Cheyne-Stokes breathing, is present in approximately 40% of patients with a reduced LV ejection fraction, whereas *obstructive* sleep apnea is present in another 10%. Sleep-disordered breathing causes recurrent apnea-related hypoxemia and sleep arousal, contributing to chronic neurohormonal activation, peripheral vasoconstriction, and reduced cardiac performance.[2]

REFERENCES

1. Drazner MH, Rame JE, Stevenson LW, Dries DL: Prognostic importance of elevated jugular venous pressure and a third heart sound in patients with heart failure. N Engl J Med 345:574, 2001.
2. Bradley TD, Floras JS. Obstructive sleep apnoea and its cardiovascular consequences. Lancet 373:82, 2009.

ANSWER TO QUESTION 197

A (Braunwald, pp. 286-287, 508)

The lung can be divided into three zones on the basis of the relationship between pulmonary arterial, alveolar, and pulmonary venous pressures. In zone 1 (at the apex), the alveolar pressure exceeds both pulmonary arterial and pulmonary venous pressures, so that there is ventilation without perfusion (dead space). In zone 2, alveolar pressure exceeds the venous but not the arterial pressure at some stage of the respiratory cycle. In zone 3, the alveolar pressure does not exceed either arterial or venous pressures. Zone 3 alveoli are therefore the best perfused and in the upright patient are situated in the dependent areas of the lung.

Measurement of the pulmonary capillary wedge pressure using a balloon-tipped catheter will be misleading if the catheter tip is wedged in a zone 1 or zone 2 arterial branch. In these zones, the wedge pressure measures alveolar pressure rather than the true left atrial pressure. In most spontaneously breathing patients, a flow-directed balloon-tipped catheter is naturally directed to zone 3 (because these areas are best perfused) and the pulmonary artery occlusion pressure is a truer estimate of the left atrial pressure.

Pulmonary vascular redistribution on the chest radiograph reflects a relative reduction of perfusion of the bases and a relative increase in apical perfusion. This phenomenon is likely due to compression of vessels at the lung bases owing to dependent edema in that zone.

ANSWER TO QUESTION 198

B (Braunwald, p. 611)

The calcineurin inhibitors (cyclosporine and tacrolimus) interfere with T-cell activation and have become the cornerstone of immunosuppression in solid organ transplantation. Despite reducing episodes of rejection and prolonging survival after transplantation, cyclosporine use is associated with a number of potential complications. Hypertension and nephrotoxicity are common, and cyclosporine levels must be monitored carefully to limit progressive renal failure. Adverse gastrointestinal tract side effects include hepatotoxicity and cholelithiasis, leading to dose-dependent abnormalities in liver function tests. Fine tremors, paresthesias, and occasionally seizures are potential neurologic side effects of cyclosporine therapy. Many patients who receive cyclosporine develop hypertrichosis (hirsutism) or gingival hyperplasia. The latter complication is reported to occur more frequently in those treated simultaneously with nifedipine. Myelosuppression in transplant patients is most commonly associated with azathioprine, not cyclosporine.

Tacrolimus has a different side-effect profile. Hirsutism and gingival hyperplasia do not occur with tacrolimus, and this drug is associated with a lower incidence of hypertension and dyslipidemia than cyclosporine. However, hyperglycemia and neurologic toxicity may be more common with tacrolimus.

REFERENCE

Lindenfeld J, Miller GG, Shakar SF, et al: Drug therapy in the heart transplant recipient: II. Immunosuppressive drugs. Circulation 110:3858, 2004.

ANSWER TO QUESTION 199

D (Braunwald, pp. 525, 534-535; Table 27-3; Figs. 27-7 and 27-9)

Acute heart failure syndromes (AHFS) are responsible for > 1 million hospitalizations annually in the United States. Systolic blood pressure is usually normal or high (≥180 mm Hg) in patients with AHFS regardless of ejection fraction, likely related to enhanced sympathetic tone. Fewer than 10% of patients are hypotensive (<90 mm Hg), usually in association with advanced left ventricular (LV) systolic dysfunction and reduced cardiac output with systemic vasoconstriction. Patients with low cardiac output may benefit hemodynamically from infusion of intravenous inotropes with vasodilating properties, such as the phosphodiesterase-3 inhibitor milrinone for short-term support. However, milrinone use has not been shown to improve hospital mortality rates and can be associated with hypotension, arrhythmias, and myocardial ischemia and should be used only for patients who do not respond to diuretics and noninotropic vasodilators.[1]

Arginine vasopressin, also known as antidiuretic hormone, mediates (1) vasoconstriction via binding to the V_{1a} receptor on vascular smooth muscle, and (2) free water retention via the V_2 receptor at the renal collecting duct. Vasopressin levels are elevated in both acute and chronic heart failure and are thought to be a major contributor to hyponatremia, an adverse prognostic marker. Tolvaptan, an orally available V_2 antagonist, has been shown to improve the pulmonary capillary wedge pressure and to normalize serum sodium concentrations. However, the Efficacy of Vasopressin Antagonism in Heart Failure Outcome Study with Tolvaptan (EVEREST) trial failed to demonstrate a reduction in mortality or rehospitalizations for heart failure with use of this agent.[2]

Initial management of AHFS with noninvasive ventilation reduces respiratory distress and improves LV function by lowering afterload. Noninvasive mask ventilation may be administered by continuous positive airway pressure (CPAP) or noninvasive intermittent positive-pressure ventilation (NIPPV). The Three Interventions in Cardiogenic Pulmonary Oedema (3CPO) Trial demonstrated that noninvasive ventilation improves dyspnea, hypercapnia, and acidosis compared with standard therapy but does not reduce mortality or the need for intubation in patients with pulmonary edema.[3]

REFERENCES

1. Felker GM, Benza RL, Chandler AB, et al: Heart failure etiology and response to milrinone in decompensated heart failure: results from the OPTIME-CHF study. J Am Coll Cardiol 41:997, 2003.
2. Konstam MA, Gheorghiade M, Burnett JC Jr, et al: Effects of oral tolvaptan in patients hospitalized for worsening heart failure: the EVEREST outcome trial. JAMA 297:1319, 2007.
3. Masip J, Mebazaa A, Filippatos GS: Noninvasive ventilation in acute cardiogenic pulmonary edema. N Engl J Med 359:2068, 2008.

ANSWER TO QUESTION 200

C (Braunwald, pp. 487-495)

Neurohormonal activation is an important aspect of heart failure syndromes.[1] Although initially a beneficial compensatory response to falling cardiac output, sustained neurohormonal activation ultimately contributes to ventricular remodeling and heart failure progression. Neurohormonal modulation is consequently a cornerstone of modern heart failure treatment.

Reduced cardiac output in patients with heart failure triggers adrenergic nervous system stimulation and increased norepinephrine (NE) release. The degree of elevation in the plasma NE concentration correlates with the severity of left ventricular dysfunction, and plasma NE levels are a potent predictor of mortality in heart failure patients. Low forward cardiac output also activates the renin-angiotensin system, increasing circulating levels of angiotensin II and aldosterone and promoting salt and water retention. Increased preload and afterload in the failing heart contribute to mechanical atrial and ventricular stretch, which triggers the release of natriuretic peptides. These peptides, in particular atrial natriuretic peptide and B-type natriuretic peptide (BNP), promote a compensatory vasodilatation and natriuresis. Circulating levels of inflammatory cytokines, including tumor necrosis factor-alpha, are also increased in heart failure and may contribute to the cachexia seen in patients with end-stage disease.[2]

The initial myocardial response to neurohormonal stimulation may wane with time. In many patients with heart failure, there is progressive *downregulation* of cardiac beta-adrenergic receptors, proportional to disease severity.

REFERENCES

1. Floras JS: Sympathetic nervous system activation in human heart failure: Clinical implications of an updated model. J Am Coll Cardiol 54:375, 2009.
2. Anker SD, von Haehling S: Inflammatory mediators in chronic heart failure: An overview. Heart 90:464, 2004.

ANSWER TO QUESTION 201

D (Braunwald, pp. 608-615)

Mortality from infection accounts for approximately 20% of deaths over the first year after transplantation.[1] Infections in the first postoperative month tend to involve nosocomial bacterial and fungal pathogens. Later post-transplantation infections are more diverse and involve opportunistic infections such as cytomegalovirus (CMV), herpes simplex, *Candida, Pneumocystis jiroveci* (formerly *Pneumocystis carinii*), *Nocardia,* and *Toxoplasma gondii.*

CMV infection is one of the most frequent post-transplantation infections. CMV-negative recipients who receive a CMV-positive allograft are at highest risk, but prior seropositivity does not fully protect against this complication. Prophylactic therapy with trimethoprim-sulfamethoxazole (TMP-SMZ) is prescribed to prevent infections by *Pneumocystis* and *T. gondii.* For patients allergic to TMP-SMZ, oral atovaquone prophylaxis against *Pneumocystis* pneumonia is commonly prescribed.

Allograft rejection is a very important potential complication of heart transplantation, but the likelihood is substantially reduced with effective immunosuppression. Immunologic tolerance to the donor organ develops in the recipient over time, making rejection less likely, which permits a gradual decrease in the intensity of immunosuppressive drugs.

More than 1 year from heart transplantation, the leading cause of death is the development of coronary artery disease in the allograft. It is pathologically distinct from typical atherosclerosis and is associated with intimal hyperplasia and smooth muscle cell proliferation that lead to progressive obliteration of the vessel lumen and loss of tertiary branching.[2] Patients with CMV infection appear to be at higher risk. The diagnosis of this complication is established by surveillance angiography, which is typically performed on an annual basis in patients after transplantation.

Transplant recipients have a markedly increased incidence of various cancers compared with age-matched controls. This increased risk is related to the intensity and chronicity of immunosuppression therapy. Skin cancers are the most common malignancy after transplantation, followed by lymphoproliferative disorders (which are associated with Epstein-Barr virus infection, not CMV). Other common malignancies after transplantation include adenocarcinomas of the prostate, lung, bladder, and kidney.

REFERENCES

1. Stehlik J, Edwards LB, Kucheryavaya AY, et al: The Registry of the International Society for Heart Lung Transplant: Twenty-seventh official adult heart transplant report. J Heart Lung Transplant 29:1089, 2010.
2. Schmauss D, Weis M: Cardiac allograft vasculopathy: Recent developments. Circulation 117:2131, 2008.

ANSWER TO QUESTION 202

B (Braunwald, p. 1145)

The intra-aortic balloon (IAB) is a catheter-mounted counterpulsation device first developed more than 40 years ago. IABs are now most commonly inserted percutaneously through the common femoral artery and positioned in the descending aorta just distal to the left subclavian artery. The balloon timing should be adjusted such that inflation occurs at the dicrotic notch of the arterial pressure waveform, which coincides with the timing of aortic valve closure. The resultant diastolic rise in aortic pressure increases coronary blood flow. The IAB is timed to deflate during the isovolumic phase of left ventricular (LV) contraction. That relative reduction of afterload decreases peak LV pressure and myocardial oxygen consumption.

IAB counterpulsation is valuable in the treatment of cardiogenic shock after cardiac surgery, acute myocardial infarction (MI), or during high-risk coronary interventions.[1] IAB therapy is indicated in patients compromised by mechanical complications of acute MI such as mitral regurgitation or ventricular septal defect. IAB may also be useful as a treatment of refractory angina or ventricular arrhythmias and as a means to stabilize critically ill patients awaiting cardiac transplantation before insertion of a ventricular assist device. Absolute contraindications to the use of an IAB include aortic valve *insufficiency* and aortic dissection. An IAB should not be inserted via the femoral artery in patients with an abdominal aortic aneurysm or severe calcific aortoiliac or femoral arterial disease.

The complication rate of IAB usage ranges from 5% to 47%. Major complications include limb ischemia, aortic dissection, aortoiliac laceration or perforation, and deep wound infection.

In recent years, novel temporary percutaneous cardiac assist devices that can directly augment cardiac output have begun to replace IAB counterpulsation for the treatment of cardiogenic shock.[2]

REFERENCES

1. Sjauw KD, Engstrom AE, Vis MM, et al: A systematic review and meta-analysis of intra-aortic balloon pump therapy in ST-elevation myocardial infarction: Should we change the guidelines? Eur Heart J 30:459, 2009.
2. Naidu SS: Novel percutaneous cardiac assist devices: The science of and indications for hemodynamic support. Circulation 123:533, 2011.

ANSWER TO QUESTION 203

A (Braunwald, pp. 558-565; Table 28-8)

The annual mortality rate of patients with ventricular dysfunction and heart failure ranges from 2% to 5% in asymptomatic patients (Class I) to greater than 25% in those who are severely symptomatic (Class IV).

Many clinical trials have confirmed that angiotensin-converting enzyme (ACE) inhibitors should be the mainstay of treatment for patients with left ventricular (LV) dysfunction. In patients with asymptomatic LV dysfunction (Class I), ACE inhibitors slow progression to symptomatic heart failure. In patients who have established symptomatic heart failure (Class II to IV), ACE inhibitors significantly reduce mortality. For individuals who are intolerant of ACE inhibitors, an angiotensin receptor blocker (ARB) or the combination of hydralazine plus long-acting nitrates should be considered, because both of these strategies have shown outcome benefits in patients with symptomatic heart failure. The CHARM trial demonstrated that ARB therapy results in comparable outcomes as ACE inhibition in patients with chronic heart failure.[1] In heart failure patients of African-American descent, data from the A-HeFT trial show that addition of hydralazine plus isosorbide dinitrate to standard therapy results in improved clinical endpoints.[2] Beta blockers (in particular carvedilol or long-acting metoprolol) should also be prescribed to heart failure patients in stable condition (those without substantial fluid retention or recent episodes of acute decompensation requiring inotropic therapy).

The DIG trial demonstrated that digoxin decreases hospitalizations for heart failure in patients with Class II to IV symptoms but has no effect on overall mortality. The RALES trial showed that the addition of spironolactone to standard heart failure therapy decreases mortality in patients with advanced (Class III to IV) symptoms.[3]

Historically, patients with chronic heart failure were instructed to avoid physical exercise and to rest in bed. This practice is no longer recommended because regular exercise has been shown to improve functional capacity. In addition, exercise may improve excessive neurohormonal activation and quality of life.[4] However, moderate levels of exercise have not been demonstrated to improve the natural history of heart failure.

REFERENCES

1. Pfeffer MA, Swedberg K, Granger CB, et al: Effects of candesartan on mortality and morbidity in patients with chronic heart failure. The CHARM-Overall programme. Lancet 362:759, 2003.
2. Taylor AL, Ziesche S, Yancy C, et al: Combination of isosorbide dinitrate and hydralazine in blacks with heart failure. N Engl J Med 351:2049, 2004.
3. Pitt B, Zannad F, Remme WJ, et al: The effect of spironolactone on morbidity and mortality in patients with severe heart failure. N Engl J Med 341:709, 1999.
4. Flynn KE, Pena IL, Whellan DJ, et al: Effects of exercise training on health status in patients with chronic heart failure: HF-ACTION randomized controlled trial. JAMA 301:1451, 2009.

ANSWER TO QUESTION 204

B (Braunwald, pp. 1628-1631)

This 52-year-old man has symptoms and signs of heart failure. There are several possible contributors to his left ventricular (LV) dysfunction based on the clinical history. The history of smoking and hypertension put him at high risk for coronary artery disease, but there is no evidence of angina or prior myocardial infarction by history or ECG. Long-standing, severe, uncontrolled hypertension may ultimately lead to heart failure owing to progressive LV hypertrophy and diastolic dysfunction; however, this patient's hypertension has been well controlled in recent years. The evidence by chest radiograph and physical examination for an enlarged heart with decompensated heart failure is most consistent with a dilated cardiomyopathy. His confessed alcohol use is moderate; however, patients with excessive alcohol intake may underreport their true consumption. Of the choices presented, the best unifying diagnosis is alcoholic cardiomyopathy.

Heavy alcohol consumption is the leading cause of nonischemic dilated cardiomyopathy in the United States for both men and women. In general, alcoholic cardiomyopathy is associated with heavy alcohol consumption, although the precise amount of alcohol that is "safe" for any given individual is variable. Excessive alcohol consumption causes abnormalities of both systolic and diastolic function as well as progressive LV cavity enlargement. Frequently, individuals with alcoholic cardiomyopathy develop atrial fibrillation or ventricular arrhythmias. It has been observed that the toxic effects of alcohol are more dramatic in hypertensive individuals and those with LV hypertrophy.

There is no definitive diagnostic test for alcoholic cardiomyopathy. As a result, it is often recommended that patients with dilated cardiomyopathy abstain completely from alcohol consumption. Total cessation in the early stages of the disease frequently leads to resolution of the manifestations of congestive heart failure and the return of the heart size to normal. Continued alcohol consumption leads to further myocardial damage and fibrosis, with the development of refractory heart failure. Patients with alcoholic cardiomyopathy benefit from treatment with standard medical therapies for heart failure, including angiotensin-converting enzyme inhibitors and beta blockers. Because nutritional deficiencies are common in alcoholics and may contribute to myocardial dysfunction, vitamin supplementation (in particular, thiamine) should be considered.

REFERENCE

Laonigro I, Correale M, Di Biase M, et al: Alcohol abuse and heart failure. Eur J Heart Fail 11:453, 2009.

ANSWER TO QUESTION 205

C (Braunwald, pp. 785-787, 796-798; Fig. 39-12)

Premature ventricular complexes (PVCs) are common and the prevalence increases with age. Their frequency may be exacerbated by a variety of factors, including electrolyte imbalances (especially hypokalemia and hypomagnesemia), infection, hypoxia, and excessive use of tobacco, caffeine, or alcohol. In the absence of structural heart disease, isolated PVCs have no impact on survival. Conversely, after myocardial infarction (MI), PVCs identify patients who are at increased risk for ventricular tachycardia or sudden death. In the Cardiac Arrhythmia Suppression Trial (CAST), the use of Class IC antiarrhythmic drugs (encainide and flecainide) to suppress asymptomatic ventricular arrhythmias after acute MI was associated with an *increased* rate of death, and such agents should not be used in the setting of coronary artery disease.

Approximately 30% of patients with paroxysmal supraventricular tachycardias referred for electrophysiologic study are found to have a concealed accessory pathway, most commonly between the left ventricle and the left atrium. These concealed pathways conduct unidirectionally from the ventricles to the atria but not in the opposite direction. Thus, the ventricle is not preexcited and the ECG does not demonstrate a delta wave during normal sinus rhythm. Nonetheless, concealed pathways may participate in reentrant AV tachycardias. This mechanism should be suspected during tachycardias when the QRS complex is of normal width (due to anterograde conduction down the atrioventricular node) and the retrograde P wave occurs *after* completion of the QRS complex, in the ST segment or T wave.

REFERENCE

Wellens HJ: Twenty-five years of insights into the mechanisms of supraventricular arrhythmias. J Cardiovasc Electrophysiol 14:1020, 2003.

ANSWER TO QUESTION 206

D (Braunwald, pp. 805-806)

The ECG demonstrates right bundle branch block with prominent ST-segment elevation in the anterior precordial leads, typical of Brugada syndrome. This condition can lead to sudden cardiac death due to ventricular fibrillation despite the fact that the heart is structurally normal.[1] The clinical presentation is distinguished by male predominance and appearance of arrhythmic events at an average age of 40 years. It is believed that this syndrome accounts for 40% to 60% of cases of idiopathic ventricular fibrillation. The mechanism that produces the electrocardiographic abnormalities and development of ventricular fibrillation remains unknown. In many families the syndrome segregates in an autosomal dominant fashion and is associated with mutations in the sodium channel *(SCN5A)*.[2] Screening of family members, including an ECG, is therefore important. Pharmacologic therapies are not effective in treating ventricular arrhythmias associated with Brugada syndrome. Administration of sodium channel blocking agents such as procainamide may be useful in bringing out the typical electrocardiographic phenotype in patients with a history of aborted sudden death and an equivocal ECG. Implantation of a defibrillator is the therapy of choice for prevention of sudden cardiac death.

REFERENCES

1. Morita H, Zipes DP, Wu J: Brugada syndrome: Insights on ST elevation, arrhythmogenicity, and risk stratification from experimental observations. Heart Rhythm 6:S34, 2009.
2. Ruan Y, Liu N, Priori SG: Sodium channel mutations and arrhythmias. Nat Rev Cardiol 6:337, 2009.

ANSWER TO QUESTION 207

E (Braunwald, pp. 582-583, 758-761; Fig. 29-6; see also Answer to Question 180)

The preferred therapy for survivors of cardiac arrest at risk for recurrence is an implantable cardioverter-defibrillator (ICD), rather than antiarrhythmic drug therapy.[1] Among survivors of out-of-hospital cardiac arrest not associated with an myocardial infarction, the risk of recurrent cardiac arrest after 1 year is 30% and after 2 years it is about 45%. In the AVID trial, ICD implantation resulted in a 27% relative risk reduction in total mortality over 2 years of follow-up.

A number of studies directed at the primary prevention of sudden cardiac death (SCD) in high-risk patients have been reported. In patients with left ventricular (LV) dysfunction (ejection fraction ≤30%) and prior history of myocardial infarction, prophylactic ICD implantation is associated with a reduction in all-cause mortality.[2] Defibrillator implantation also reduces death rates in patients with symptomatic systolic heart failure from nonischemic causes. In the SCD-HeFT trial of patients with Class II to III heart failure and LV ejection fraction ≤35%, ICD implantation reduced overall mortality by 23% and was superior to amiodarone therapy.[2]

ICDs are also an appropriate consideration in primary and secondary prevention of SCD in high-risk individuals with hypertrophic cardiomyopathy. High-risk features include a history of syncope, a family history of SCD, the presence of marked LV hypertrophy (wall thickness > 30 mm), and the finding of nonsustained ventricular tachycardia on noninvasive monitoring.[3]

REFERENCES

1. Epstein AE, DiMarco JP, Ellenbogen KA, et al: ACC/AHA/HRS 2008 guidelines for device-based therapy of cardiac rhythm abnormalities: A report of the ACC/AHA Task Force on Practice Guidelines. Circulation 117:e350, 2008.
2. Bardy GH, Lee KL, Mark DB, et al: Amiodarone or an implantable cardioverter-defibrillator for congestive heart failure. N Engl J Med 352:225, 2005.
3. Maron BJ, Spirito P, Shen W-K, et al: Implantable cardioverter-defibrillators and prevention of sudden cardiac death in hypertrophic cardiomyopathy. JAMA 298:405, 2007.

ANSWER TO QUESTION 208

A (Braunwald, pp. 818-821)

Atrioventricular (AV) block is present when atrial impulses are conducted to the ventricles with abnormal delay or are not conducted at all. There are three categories. *First-degree AV block* is present when the PR interval is prolonged (>0.20 second) in a constant fashion and every atrial impulse conducts to the ventricle. In *second-degree heart block*, some impulses fail to conduct from the atria to the ventricles. Second-degree block is divided into two groups: *Mobitz type I* and *Mobitz type II*. In the former type (also termed *Wenckebach block*), the PR interval progressively increases (and the RR interval usually progressively shortens) until an atrial impulse fails to conduct to the ventricles. In Mobitz type II block, the PR intervals are constant and without warning there is intermittent failure of an atrial impulse to conduct to the ventricles. *Third-degree heart block* is present when all atrial impulses fail to conduct to the ventricles such that the atrial and the ventricular rhythms are independent of one another.

In first-degree heart block, the delay between atrial and ventricular contraction allows the leaflets of the mitral and tricuspid valves to drift toward a partially closed position prior to ventricular systole. Therefore, the intensity of the first heart sound is *diminished*. First-degree heart block and Mobitz type I second-degree heart block often arise in normal healthy adults and well-trained athletes, owing to increased vagal tone.

Mobitz type I second-degree heart block with a normal QRS duration almost always occurs at the level of the AV node, proximal to the His bundle. Conversely, type II second-degree heart block, especially when accompanied by a bundle branch block QRS morphology, usually reflects a more serious abnormality in the His-Purkinje system.

In third-degree heart block there is complete AV dissociation. As a result, the ventricular rate is governed not by the atrial rate but by an independent ventricular escape pacemaker. In acquired forms of third-degree heart block, the ventricular rate is usually <40 beats/min. The ventricular rate tends to be faster in patients with congenital complete heart block, about 50 beats/min.

ANSWER TO QUESTION 209

E (Braunwald, pp. 691-693, 702-704)

Prolonged ambulatory electrocardiographic (Holter) monitoring of patients engaged in normal daily activity is useful to document the nature and frequency of underlying cardiac arrhythmias and to correlate a patient's symptoms with rhythm disturbances. Although significant rhythm disturbances are uncommon in healthy persons, a variety of arrhythmias, including sinus bradycardia (with rates as low as 35 beats/min), sinus arrhythmia, sinoatrial exit block, Wenckebach second-degree atrioventricular block (especially during sleep), and junctional escape complexes may be seen in normal persons. In addition, the prevalence of arrhythmias in normal subjects increases with older age. Persons with ischemic heart disease, especially those recovering from acute myocardial infarction, exhibit ventricular premature beats (VPBs) when long-term recordings of the heart rhythm are obtained. The frequency of VPBs increases over the first several weeks after infarction and decreases about 6 months after infarction. Frequent and complex ventricular ectopy is associated with a twofold to fivefold increased risk of sudden cardiac death after myocardial infarction.

Long-term electrocardiographic recordings have been useful for the detection of underlying rhythm disturbances in patients with hypertrophic cardiomyopathy and mitral valve prolapse, as well as in patients who have unexplained syncope or transient cerebrovascular symptoms. In normal subjects and in patients with underlying rhythm disturbances, the cardiac rhythm may vary dramatically from one long-term recording period to the next.

On many occasions, the relatively brief period of recording provided by standard Holter monitoring may be inadequate to identify an abnormal rhythm responsible for a patient's symptoms. Longer term monitoring in such patients, using an external event recorder, may help to establish a diagnosis. For patients with very infrequent symptoms, *implantable* loop recorders are available that can remain in place for several months. These devices have proven useful in establishing a diagnosis in patients with recurrent syncope and negative evaluations using standard techniques. Variants have also been used to document a high frequency of asymptomatic recurrence of atrial fibrillation in patients treated with antiarrhythmic drugs for that condition. Evidence suggests that, in patients with atrial fibrillation, the frequency of asymptomatic episodes exceeds that of symptomatic episodes, which has important implications for the risk of discontinuing anticoagulant medications.

REFERENCE

Zimetbaum P, Goldman A: Ambulatory arrhythmia monitoring: Choosing the right device. Circulation 122:1629, 2010.

ANSWER TO QUESTION 210

D (Braunwald, pp. 885-892; Table 42-2; Fig. 42-1)

Syncope may result from vascular, cardiac, neurologic, and metabolic causes. Vascular causes of syncope are by far the most common, accounting for about one third of all episodes. Vascular causes include orthostatic hypotension and reflex-mediated syncope, such as carotid sinus hypersensitivity and neurocardiogenic (vasovagal) syncope.

Cardiac abnormalities, especially tachyarrhythmias and bradyarrhythmias, represent the second most common causes of syncope, accounting for 10% to 20% of episodes. Ventricular tachycardia is the rhythm disorder that most frequently causes loss of consciousness. Bradyarrhythmias such as sick sinus syndrome and advanced atrioventricular blocks can also result in syncope, but less commonly. Supraventricular tachycardias are much more likely to present as less severe symptoms such as palpitations or lightheadedness rather than loss of consciousness. Although the prognosis of patients with noncardiac causes of syncope tends to be benign, those who have syncope of cardiac origin have a 30% mortality rate over the next year.

The history and physical examination are by far the most important part of the evaluation of patients presenting with syncope. Studies estimate that, in up to one fourth of cases, an accurate diagnosis can be made on the basis of history and physical examination alone. The ECG is the most useful initial diagnostic test; any abnormality of the baseline ECG in patients with syncope is an independent predictor of mortality and indicates the need to pursue a cardiac etiology.

REFERENCE

Moya A, Sutton R, Ammirati F, et al: Guidelines for the diagnosis and management of syncope (version 2009): The Task Force for the Diagnosis and Management of Syncope of the European Society of Cardiology (ESC). Eur Heart J 30:2631, 2009.

ANSWER TO QUESTION 211

D (Braunwald, pp. 753-755, Tables 38-1 and 38G-8)

Current nomenclature for pacemaker coding has five positions. The first position reflects the chamber that is being paced (O = none, A = atrium, V = ventricle, D – dual [both atrium and ventricle are paced]); the second position reflects the chamber being sensed (O, A, V, and D as above); the third position corresponds to the response to sensing (O = none, T = triggered, I = inhibited, D = dual); and the fourth position reflects programmability and rate modulation (e.g., O = none, R = rate modulation). The fifth position of the code is used to indicate whether multisite pacing is present in (0) none of the cardiac chambers, (A) one or both atria, (V) one or both ventricles, or (D) any combination of atria and ventricles. As an example, a patient with a dual-chamber, rate-adaptive pacemaker

with biventricular stimulation would have a DDDRV code.

Rate-adaptive pacemakers incorporate a sensor that can modulate the pacing rate independently of intrinsic cardiac activity by monitoring physiologic processes such as physical activity or minute ventilation. Mode switching is a useful feature in which the pacemaker mode automatically changes (e.g., from DDDR to DDIR) in response to inappropriate rapid atrial rhythms. This is particularly beneficial for patients with paroxysmal supraventricular tachyarrhythmias, such as atrial fibrillation or flutter, to avoid rapid ventricular pacing during those episodes.

"Pacemaker syndrome" refers to the deterioration of hemodynamics with associated patient symptoms, or a limitation of optimal functional status, despite a normally functioning pacing system. This is observed most commonly with VVI pacing but may occur in any pacing mode in which atrioventricular (AV) synchrony is lost. Patients may experience a sensation of fullness in the head and neck, syncope or presyncope, hypotension, cough, dyspnea, congestive heart failure, or weakness. Physical findings include cannon *a* waves in the jugular venous pulsations and a fall in blood pressure during pacing compared with normal sinus rhythm (Fig. 2-22). Symptomatic AV block of any kind (including Wenckebach) is an indication for permanent pacing. In patients with hypertrophic cardiomyopathy, dual-chamber pacing has been shown to reduce the left ventricular outflow tract gradient and lead to symptomatic improvement. There is, however, a significant placebo effect from pacing, and some studies have not confirmed this benefit. Thus, the American College of Cardiology/American Heart Association guidelines consider pacemaker placement a Class IIb indication in patients with medically refractory hypertrophic cardiomyopathy and outflow tract obstruction.

REFERENCE

Epstein AE, DiMarco JP, Ellenbogen KA, et al: ACC/AHA/HRS 2008 guidelines for device-based therapy of cardiac rhythm abnormalities: A report of the ACC/AHA Task Force on Practice Guidelines. Circulation 117:e350, 2008.

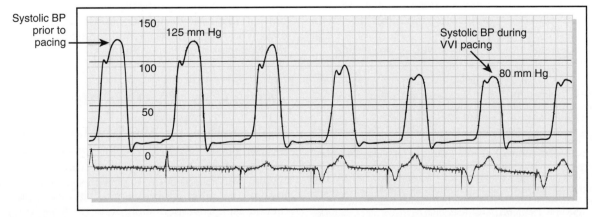

FIGURE 2-22

ANSWER TO QUESTION 212

D (Braunwald, p. 755, Fig. 38-1)

Pacemaker-mediated tachycardia (PMT), or endless loop tachycardia, is a syndrome of upper rate behavior that occurs when there is intact ventriculoatrial conduction resulting in retrograde P waves. If these retrograde P waves are sensed by the atrial sensing circuit, the pacemaker atrioventricular interval is initiated and a paced ventricular contraction follows, which generates another retrograde P, and so on, generating a perpetual "loop." The diagnosis should be suspected in patients with a dual-chamber device who present with a paced tachycardia near the maximum tracking limit of the device. It is managed by *increasing* the postventricular atrial refractory period, which prevents atrial sensing of the retrograde P wave. Because episodes of PMT are often triggered by a premature ventricular contraction (PVC), some commercially available devices offer automatic extension of the postventricular refractory period after a PVC to recognize and terminate PMT.

ANSWER TO QUESTION 213

D (Braunwald, pp. 835, 843; Fig. 40-1)

Postoperative atrial fibrillation (AF) occurs in up to 40% of patients undergoing coronary artery bypass grafting or valvular surgery. This dysrhythmia is associated with an increased stroke risk in this setting and is the most common cause of prolonged hospitalization after cardiac surgery.[1] Risk factors for postoperative AF include advanced age (>70 years), male gender, diabetes, obesity, chronic lung disease, and left ventricular dysfunction. Several antiarrhythmic drugs have been shown to reduce the risk of developing AF after cardiac surgery. Oral beta blockers such as metoprolol lower the risk by 31% and unless contraindicated have a Class IA recommendation for use in this setting.[2] Other effective prophylactic antiarrhythmic agents are the Class III agents amiodarone and sotalol. Digoxin may have a role in rate control of atrial fibrillation when it occurs but has not been shown to prevent postoperative AF. Atrial pacing using temporary electrodes attached to either the right atrium or both atria reduces the probability of postoperative AF. Atorvastatin, an HMG-CoA reductase inhibitor, has been shown to reduce postoperative AF by 62%, an effect that is likely independent of its lipid-lowering properties.[3]

REFERENCES

1. Burgess DC, Kilborn MJ, Keech AC: Interventions for prevention of post-operative atrial fibrillation and its complications after cardiac surgery: A meta-analysis. Eur Heart J 27:2846, 2006.
2. Fuster V, Ryden LE, Cannom DS, et al: ACC/AHA/ESC 2006 guidelines for the management of patients with atrial fibrillation: Executive summary. A report of the American College of Cardiology/American Heart Association Task Force on Practice Guidelines and the European Society of Cardiology Committee for Tractive Guidelines (Writing Committee to Revise the 2001 Guidelines for the Management of Patients with Atrial Fibrillation). J Am Coll Cardiol 48:854, 2006.
3. Patti G, Chello M, Candura D, et al: Randomized trial of atorvastatin for reduction of postoperative atrial fibrillation in patients undergoing cardiac surgery: Results of the ARMYDA-3 (Atorvastatin for Reduction of Myocardial Dysrhythmia After cardiac surgery) study. Circulation 114:1455, 2006.

ANSWER TO QUESTION 214

D (Braunwald, pp. 716-717)

Procainamide, a Class IA antiarrhythmic agent, is effective in the management of both supraventricular and ventricular arrhythmias. As a sodium channel–blocking agent it acts to depress phase 0 depolarization, thereby slowing conduction. In addition, it has moderate potassium channel–blocking activity (largely owing to the action of its metabolite N-acetyl-procainamide [NAPA]), which leads to slowing in the rate of repolarization and a prolongation of the action potential duration. Prolongation of the QRS complex duration is seen at therapeutic concentrations owing to slowing of conduction in the Purkinje system and ventricular muscle. QT interval prolongation occurs with rising serum concentrations and may precipitate ventricular arrhythmias.

In patients with atrial fibrillation or flutter, procainamide may lead to chemical cardioversion to normal sinus rhythm. Although procainamide slows the atrial rate, it may facilitate rapid 1:1 conduction through the atrioventricular node and actually increase the ventricular response rate in atrial flutter or fibrillation unless a nodal blocking agent (e.g., a beta blocker) is co-administered. In patients with atrial fibrillation and Wolff-Parkinson-White syndrome, procainamide is effective at prolonging the effective refractory period of the bypass tract and suppresses extranodal atrioventricular conduction.

Multiple noncardiac side effects of procainamide have been reported, including rashes, myalgias, digital vasculitis, Raynaud phenomenon, gastrointestinal side effects, and central nervous system toxicity. Higher doses of the drug may depress myocardial contractility and diminish myocardial performance; rapid intravenous administration has been associated with hypotension due to a reduction in systemic vascular resistance. Chronic administration of procainamide is associated with a positive antinuclear antibody in almost all patients, particularly slow acetylators. However, symptoms of drug-induced lupus (arthritis, arthralgias, pleuritis) occur only in 15% to 20% of patients. Many of these patients exhibit positive antihistone antibodies, and the syndrome resolves after drug discontinuation.

ANSWER TO QUESTION 215

B (Braunwald, pp. 696-701; Table 36G-6)

Invasive electrophysiologic study (EPS) is employed for the evaluation of patients with disturbances of cardiac rhythm and conduction. It provides information about the type of rhythm abnormality and its electrophysiologic mechanism. Therapeutically, it is possible during EPS to terminate tachycardias by electrical stimulation, to evaluate the effects of antiarrhythmic therapies, and to ablate myocardium responsible for tachycardias.

EPS is the gold standard for evaluation of arrhythmic causes of syncope, including the three most common: sinus node dysfunction, His-Purkinje block, and tachyarrhythmias. Of the three, tachyarrhythmias are most reliably initiated in the electrophysiology laboratory, followed by sinus node abnormalities and His-Purkinje block.

EPS allows the measurement of intracardiac conduction times and the sequence of myocardial activation using catheter electrodes capable of sensing and pacing. In patients with acquired atrioventricular (AV) block and related symptoms, EPS evaluates the length of the His-ventricular (HV) interval, in order to assess infranodal conduction abnormalities that might prompt pacemaker implantation. HV intervals > 55 milliseconds are associated with organic heart disease, a greater likelihood of developing trifascicular block, and higher mortality.

EPS is helpful in the management of patients with suspected sinus node dysfunction. The sinus node recovery time (SNRT) is used to assess the effects of overdrive suppression on sinus node automaticity. The SNRT is measured by subtracting the spontaneous sinus node cycle length before pacing from the time delay to the first spontaneous sinus response after termination of pacing. Normal values are generally < 525 milliseconds, and prolongation of the SNRT suggests abnormal sinus node function. Because many patients with impaired sinus node function also exhibit abnormal AV conduction, it is important also to evaluate AV nodal and His-Purkinje function in this population.

In patients with wide-QRS complex tachycardias, EPS may be used to differentiate supraventricular tachycardia with aberrancy from ventricular tachycardia, because the sequence of, and relation between, atrial and ventricular activation can be determined. Supraventricular tachycardias are characterized in part by the presence of an HV interval during tachycardia equal to or greater than that recorded during normal sinus rhythm. Shortening of the HV interval during tachycardia suggests either VT or the presence of an accessory pathway. EPS is also used to locate and ablate accessory pathways in preexcitation syndromes. Left free wall accessory pathways are most common, followed by posteroseptal, right free wall, and anteroseptal locations.

REFERENCE

Calkins H: Syncope. In Zipes DP, Jalife J (eds): Cardiac Electrophysiology: From Cell to Bedside. 5th ed. Philadelphia, WB Saunders, 2009, pp. 913-922.

ANSWER TO QUESTION 216

B (Braunwald, p. 727)

Intravenous administration of adenosine slows the sinus rate and conduction through the atrioventricular (AV) node, causing transient AV block. Its AV nodal effects, in combination with its extremely short half-life (1.5 seconds), make adenosine a safe and effective drug for the diagnosis and treatment of reentrant supraventricular tachycardias (SVTs) involving the AV node. AV nodal reentrant tachycardia (AVNRT) and AV reentrant tachycardia (AVRT) nearly always terminate after adenosine administration. In addition, the transient AV block induced by adenosine may help to unmask other underlying supraventricular arrhythmias such as atrial tachycardia or atrial flutter. Because of its short half-life, adenosine must be administered as a *rapid* intravenous bolus to achieve adequate blood and tissue levels. Short duration of action also implies a brief period of side effects, which differentiates adenosine from other drugs (e.g., beta blockers, calcium channel blockers) that are used to treat SVTs.

Adenosine may also be helpful in the differentiation of wide QRS complex tachycardia. Ventricular tachycardia is usually unaffected by adenosine, whereas SVT with aberrant conduction will either terminate or be exposed by transient AV block. However, a theoretical risk of adenosine use in these patients is acceleration of conduction through an accessory pathway, if one is present, as in patients with the Wolff-Parkinson-White syndrome. Transient side effects are common with adenosine, occurring in up to 40% of patients. The most common are dyspnea, chest pressure, and flushing, all of which are fleeting and generally resolve within 1 minute. Adenosine may provoke bronchospasm in patients with severe asthma or obstructive lung disease. Patients after heart transplantation appear to be particularly sensitive to the effects of adenosine, and appropriate caution should be exercised in this population. Because caffeine and theophylline antagonize the adenosine receptor, adenosine is unlikely to be effective in patients receiving these substances.

ANSWER TO QUESTION 217

C (Braunwald, pp. 833-835)

Many patients with atrial fibrillation (AF) have a focal origin of the arrhythmia within the pulmonary veins, which has led to the development of methods to localize and ablate the responsible source. Initial techniques were aimed at ablating sites of premature atrial contractions at their origin deep within the pulmonary veins. However, only a small number of patients have sufficient atrial premature beats to serve as such a target, and ablation deep within these veins can result in pulmonary vein stenosis. Subsequently, techniques shifted to electrical isolation of the pulmonary veins by creating a circumferential line of block encircling the venous ostia, so as to prevent spread of impulses from the site of initiation to the remainder of the atria.[1] At high-volume centers, the single-procedure 1-year success rates are 70% to 80% in patients with paroxysmal AF and approximately 50% in patients with persistent AF. After a redo procedure, a success rate of approximately 90% is realistic for patients with paroxysmal AF compared with approximately 75% for patients with persistent AF. Noninvasive imaging of the pulmonary veins, using high-resolution computed tomography or magnetic resonance imaging, is helpful before the procedure to exclude anomalous pulmonary venous anatomy, which can interfere with successful ablation.[2]

The risk of a major complication from radiofrequency catheter ablation of AF occurs in 5% to 6% of patients.[3] The most common are cardiac tamponade, pulmonary vein stenosis, and cerebral thromboembolism, each of which occur in approximately 1% of patients. Rarely, pulmonary vein stenosis results from the procedure, and left atrial-esophageal fistula has been reported as a complication of ablation within the posterior left atrium. Esophageal temperature monitoring or real-time esophageal imaging may be helpful in avoiding the latter complication.

REFERENCES

1. Oral H, Pappone C, Chugh A, et al: Circumferential pulmonary-vein ablation for chronic atrial fibrillation. N Engl J Med 354:934, 2006.
2. Burkhardt JD, Natale A: New technologies in atrial fibrillation ablation. Circulation 120:1533, 2009.
3. Calkins H, Reynolds MR, Spector P, et al: Treatment of atrial fibrillation with antiarrhythmic drugs or radiofrequency ablation: Two systematic literature reviews and meta-analyses. Circ Arrhythm Electrophysiol 2:349, 2009.

ANSWER TO QUESTION 218

E (Braunwald, pp. 715-717)

Quinidine is a Class IA antiarrhythmic agent that simultaneously inhibits the upstroke velocity of the action potential and prolongs the action potential duration. It has a wide spectrum of activity against a broad variety of atrial and ventricular tachyarrhythmias. Quinidine can produce early afterdepolarizations, which may be responsible for torsades de pointes, a complication that develops in 1% to 3% of patients.[1] Hypokalemia, hypomagnesemia, and severe left ventricular dysfunction increase the risk of this proarrhythmic side effect.

The most common side effects of quinidine are gastrointestinal, including nausea, vomiting, abdominal pain, and diarrhea. Quinidine can also result in cinchonism—neurologic toxicity that includes tinnitus, hearing loss, visual disturbances, confusion, and delirium. Other potential complications of quinidine include immune-mediated thrombocytopenia and hemolytic anemia.

Quinidine decreases the total-body clearance and volume of distribution of digoxin, thereby raising its serum level. The elimination half-life of oral quinidine is 6 to 8 hours, and it is metabolized by the cytochrome P-450 system. Approximately 20% is excreted unchanged in the urine. Quinidine's elimination can be reduced by, and its dosage should be lowered in, patients with congestive heart failure, liver disease, or renal dysfunction.

Quinidine is now infrequently used for the pharmacologic conversion of atrial fibrillation due to the availability of more effective and better tolerated agents. Although quinidine may slow the atrial rate, it can enhance the efficacy of atrioventricular (AV) conduction (because of its *vagolytic* effect) and paradoxically increase the ventricular response rate in atrial fibrillation. Thus, when administered for this condition, it should be combined with a negatively chronotropic drug (e.g., beta blocker, verapamil, or digoxin) to prevent enhanced AV nodal conduction.

REFERENCE

1. Heist EK, Ruskin JN: Drug induced arrhythmia. Circulation 122:1426, 2010.

ANSWER TO QUESTION 219

C (Braunwald, pp. 825-838)

Atrial fibrillation (AF) is an irregularly irregular rhythm characterized by total disorganization of atrial depolarization without effective atrial contractions. It occurs due to random reentry of multiple activation wavefronts in an abnormal atrial-tissue substrate that collide, extinguish, re-form, and follow an apparently random path to the atrioventricular node.

AF commonly occurs in patients with hypertensive heart disease, hyperthyroidism, rheumatic heart disease, cardiomyopathy, coronary artery disease, or atrial septal defect or after cardiac surgery (in up to 40% of patients). The incidence of AF approximately doubles with each decade of adult life. It is an independent risk factor for mortality, even after adjustment for other risk factors, including age, diabetes, hypertension, congestive heart failure, rheumatic and nonrheumatic valvular disease, and myocardial infarction. The presence of AF also increases the risk of stroke by threefold to fivefold.

Treatment of AF varies depending on the clinical presentation but includes three components: (1) assessment of the need for, proper timing of, and appropriate method for the restoration of sinus rhythm; (2) anticoagulation to prevent embolic stroke; and (3) medication to control the ventricular rate (to reduce symptoms and prevent the development of tachycardia-related cardiomyopathy). The results of the AFFIRM trial demonstrate that a strategy of sinus rhythm maintenance with antiarrhythmic drugs offers no survival advantage over a strategy of long-term rate control in patients with AF and that long-term anticoagulation is imperative in all high-risk patients to prevent thromboembolic complications.[1]

In patients presenting with AF of < 48 hours' duration, electrical or chemical cardioversion for restoration of sinus rhythm can be performed without the need for prolonged anticoagulation. In those presenting with AF of longer duration, anticoagulation with warfarin for at least 3 weeks is advised before cardioversion, given the potential for dislodging formed thrombus within the left atrial appendage. If intra-atrial thrombus is first excluded by transesophageal echocardiography, more expeditious cardioversion may be safely performed in these patients as well.[2]

REFERENCES

1. The Atrial Fibrillation Follow-up Investigation of Rhythm Management (AFFIRM) Investigators: A comparison of rate control and rhythm control in patients with atrial fibrillation. N Engl J Med 347:1825, 2002.
2. Klein AL, Grimm RA, Murray JA, et al: Use of transesophageal echocardiography to guide cardioversion in patients with atrial fibrillation. N Engl J Med 344:1411, 2001.

ANSWER TO QUESTION 220

B (Braunwald, pp. 653-658, 669, 675-676)

The sinus node is composed of nodal cells, transitional cells, and atrial muscle cells and is richly innervated by both postganglionic adrenergic and cholinergic nerve terminals. Vagal stimulation releases acetylcholine and slows the discharge rate of the sinus node, whereas adrenergic stimulation releases norepinephrine and speeds the discharge rate.

The arterial supply to the atrioventricular node arises from a branch of the right coronary artery in 85% to 90% of human hearts and from a branch of the circumflex in 10% to 15%. The upper muscular interventricular septum is supplied by both the anterior and posterior descending arteries.

Phase 3 (final rapid depolarization) of the cardiac cycle results from activation of repolarizing K^+ currents and the inactivation of the inward calcium current. Interference with potassium currents by genetic mutation or drugs can result in prolongation of the QT interval. For example, a number of medications, including erythromycin, terfenadine, and ketoconazole, can inhibit the delayed rectifier K^+ current (I_{Kr}), resulting in an acquired form of the long QT syndrome, thereby predisposing to the ventricular arrhythmia torsades de pointes.

Phase 4 of the cardiac cycle is the resting membrane potential period. During this phase there is an abundance of open potassium channels, which maintains the cardiac transmembrane potential close to the equilibrium potential of potassium.

ANSWER TO QUESTION 221

B (Braunwald, pp. 722-724)

Amiodarone is a Class III antiarrhythmic agent that is used to suppress a wide spectrum of supraventricular and ventricular arrhythmias. The onset of action of the intravenous form is within 1 to 2 hours. After oral administration, the onset of action is delayed by days or weeks but is shortened by large loading doses. Elimination is primarily by hepatic excretion into bile with some enterohepatic recirculation. Renal and plasma elimination of amiodarone is negligible and the dose does not need to be adjusted in renal failure. Amiodarone's elimination half-life is multiphasic, with an initial 50% reduction in plasma concentration 3 to 10 days after drug cessation, followed by a terminal half-life ranging from 26 to 107 days, with a mean of about 53 days.

Unlike many other antiarrhythmic drugs, amiodarone is tolerated by patients with left ventricular dysfunction and it is not associated with increased mortality in patients with heart failure. However, all prospective, randomized comparisons have shown that implanted defibrillators are superior for the prevention of sudden cardiac death in this population.

Amiodarone is associated with a number of significant extracardiac toxicities. Of great significance is the development of pulmonary toxicity, which may reflect a hypersensitivity reaction. This complication can occur as early as 6 days after amiodarone's initiation or may appear after long-term use.

Additional adverse effects of amiodarone include hepatic toxicity, neurologic dysfunction, photosensitivity, and bluish skin discoloration. Both hypothyroidism (2% to 4%) and hyperthyroidism (1% to 2%) have been reported with the use of this drug. Corneal deposits, visualized by slit lamp examination, occur in almost all patients who are treated with amiodarone for more than 6 months, but resultant visual impairment is unusual. Optic neuritis is a more serious potential adverse ophthalmic effect but is very rare.

REFERENCE

Bardy GH, Lee KL, Mark DB, et al: Amiodarone or an implantable cardioverter-defibrillator for congestive heart failure. N Engl J Med 352:225, 2005.

ANSWER TO QUESTION 222

D (Braunwald, pp. 777-778, 780-792, 798-799; Figs. 39-8 and 39-15)

Mechanisms of cardiac arrhythmias can be classified into those of disordered impulse formation (e.g., abnormal automaticity, triggered activity) and those of disordered impulse conduction (e.g., conduction blocks, reentry). Common examples of reentry include atrioventricular nodal reentrant tachycardia (AVNRT), AV reciprocating tachycardia (AVRT), and atrial flutter.

AVNRT is due to reentry involving dual AV nodal pathways. In the common form of AVNRT, the anterograde conduction occurs down the "slow" pathway and retrograde conduction occurs up the "fast" pathway. As a result, retrograde P waves on the ECG are typically superimposed on the terminal portion of the QRS complex.

In the *uncommon* form of AVNRT, anterograde conduction occurs down the "fast" pathway and retrograde conduction is delayed as it proceeds up the "slow" pathway. Thus, in this form, retrograde P waves occur later, after the QRS complex. In most cases of AVRT due to preexcitation, such as those seen in Wolff-Parkinson-White syndrome, the accessory pathway conducts more rapidly than the normal AV node but takes a longer time to recover excitability (i.e., the accessory pathway has a longer anterograde refractory period than the AV node). The consequence is that a premature atrial complex may be blocked in the accessory pathway, continue to the ventricle over the normal AV node and His bundle, and return to the atrium retrograde via the accessory pathway. This creates a continuous conduction loop for generation of a narrow complex, *orthodromic* AVRT. In *antidromic* AVRT, anterograde conduction to the ventricles occurs down the accessory pathway with retrograde conduction up the AV node, resulting in a wide QRS complex tachycardia.

The typical form of atrial flutter ("counterclockwise" flutter) is due to reentry within the right atrium. Radiofrequency ablation of the cavotricuspid isthmus often interrupts the reentrant pathway and eliminates recurrence of the arrhythmia.

Ventricular tachycardias can be caused by numerous mechanisms, including reentry (e.g., bundle branch reentry), triggered activity (e.g., right ventricular outflow tachycardias), or abnormal automaticity. Optimal therapy may vary depending on the underlying pathophysiologic mechanism.

ANSWER TO QUESTION 223

C (Braunwald, p. 805, Fig. 39-30)

In the absence of structural heart disease or coronary artery anomalies, a history of recurrent, exertionally related syncope in a young person is of concern for an underlying predisposition to ventricular dysrhythmias. His ECG during exercise confirms the likely cause of syncope with the onset of polymorphic ventricular tachycardia. This constellation of findings, the family history of sudden cardiac death during exertion, and the normal corrected QTc interval at rest suggests the diagnosis of *catecholaminergic polymorphic ventricular tachycardia (CPVT)*, a rare inherited form of ventricular tachycardia. CPVT is triggered by stress, which first induces sinus tachycardia, followed by ventricular premature beats, followed by polymorphic or bidirectional VT, as shown in the figure. Approximately 30% of CPVT patients have a family history of sudden death or stress-induced syncope.[1] Mutations in the ryanodine receptor gene have been linked to an autosomal dominant form of CPVT that accounts for half of all cases.[2]

The treatment of choice for CPVT is beta-blocker therapy (to blunt the impact of catecholamine surges) along with an implantable cardioverter-defibrillator for prevention of sudden death. Patients with CPVT should be counseled to avoid vigorous exercise. Cardiac sympathectomy has been reported to be effective in a few cases but is not considered first-line therapy.[3] Magnesium has not been shown to be effective in patients with CPVT.

REFERENCES

1. Liu N, Ruan Y, Prior SG: Catecholaminergic polymorphic ventricular tachycardia. Prog Cardiovasc Dis 51:23, 2008.
2. Gyorke S: Molecular basis of catecholaminergic polymorphic ventricular tachycardia. Heart Rhythm 6:123, 2009.
3. Wilde AA, Bhulyan ZA, Crotti L, et al: Left cardiac sympathetic denervation for catecholaminergic polymorphic ventricular tachycardia. N Engl J Med 258:2024, 2008.

ANSWER TO QUESTION 224

C (Braunwald, pp. 722-725)

Examples of Class III antiarrhythmic drugs include sotalol, ibutilide, dofetilide, dronedarone, and amiodarone. Sotalol is a nonspecific beta blocker that also prolongs repolarization. It is approved by the U.S. Food and Drug Administration for the treatment of life-threatening ventricular tachyarrhythmias and for atrial fibrillation. It should be used cautiously in patients with reduced contractile function because its negative inotropic effect may cause a further decline in cardiac index and precipitate heart failure. The most common and serious cardiac side effect of sotalol use is proarrhythmia; new or worsened ventricular tachyarrhythmias occur in about 4% of cases, and this complication is due to torsades de pointes in about 2.5%. The risk of torsades de pointes is dose dependent and higher in patients with a history of sustained ventricular tachycardia.

Ibutilide is available intravenously for the acute termination of atrial flutter and fibrillation. Up to 60% of patients with atrial fibrillation and 70% with atrial flutter convert to sinus rhythm after ibutilide therapy. It has also been used at the time of electrical cardioversion to enhance the successful termination of atrial fibrillation. The most significant adverse effect of ibutilide is torsades de pointes (~2% of cases), which can arise within 4 to 6 hours after administration, and all patients should be monitored for at least that long after receiving the drug.

Dofetilide is another oral Class III agent and is approved for the treatment of atrial flutter and fibrillation. It acts by blocking the rapid component of the delayed rectifier potassium current (I_{Kr}), thereby prolonging repolarization. The most important adverse effect is torsades de pointes, which occurs in 2% to 4% of patients. The risk of torsades de pointes can be minimized by calculating the drug's dose based on the patient's creatinine clearance and by carefully monitoring the QT interval.

The other Class III agents, amiodarone and dronedarone, are discussed in the Answers to Questions 180 and 221.

REFERENCE

Smith TW, Cain ME: Class III antiarrhythmic drugs: Amiodarone, ibutilide and sotalol. In Zipes DP, Jalife J (eds): Cardiac Electrophysiology: From Cell to Bedside. 5th ed. Philadelphia, WB Saunders, 2009, pp 932-941.

ANSWER TO QUESTION 225

C (Braunwald, pp. 782-785; Fig. 39-10)

The figure depicts the initiation of a narrow-complex tachycardia during electrophysiologic study by rapid atrial pacing from the coronary sinus. A train of stimuli is delivered at a cycle length of 500 milliseconds (S_1), followed by a premature stimulus (S_2) at an S_1-S_2 interval of 250 milliseconds. The effects of this premature stimulus on intracardiac conduction are seen in the His bundle recording (HBE). The AH interval, reflecting the conduction time from the atrium to the His bundle, is markedly prolonged after the premature stimulus, increasing to 300 milliseconds. This occurs because, in this patient with dual atrioventricular (AV) nodal pathways, the premature atrial stimulus encounters a refractory *fast* pathway and conducts anterograde through the *slow* pathway instead. In a patient without such dual AV nodal pathways, the premature stimulus would merely extinguish in the AV node. In this case, the slowed conduction through the AV node initiates a narrow-complex tachycardia. Such a "jump" in the AH interval during rapid atrial pacing is the electrophysiologic signature of dual AV nodal physiology. Examination of the sequence of atrial activation in the subsequent tachycardia reveals that the earliest atrial activation is in the His bundle recording (low right atrium, HBE lead), later progressing to the high right atrium (RA) and coronary sinus (CS, reflecting left atrial activation). These features identify this rhythm as an AV nodal reentrant tachycardia.

ANSWER TO QUESTION 226

D (Braunwald, pp. 819-821; Fig. 39-50)

The electrogram depicted demonstrates spontaneous infrahisian block, consistent with infrahisian conduction disease. Four QRS complexes are shown, with two surface electrocardiographic leads (V_1 and V_5), three His catheter electrograms (proximal, mid, and distal pole), and a right ventricular (RV) electrogram. The surface ECG shows right bundle branch block and sinus rhythm with a single dropped beat after the second QRS complex. After the second QRS complex, deflections are present on the three His catheter channels representing atrial depolarization. This event is followed by a small, sharp deflection evident only on the distal His channel, representing the His electrogram. That His bundle deflection fails to conduct to the ventricles because there is no QRS complex immediately following it. Together with bifascicular block evident on the surface ECG, this is a Class I indication for permanent pacing.

REFERENCE

Epstein AE, DiMarco JP, Ellenbogen KA, et al: ACC/AHA/HRS 2008 guidelines for device-based therapy of cardiac rhythm abnormalities: A report of the ACC/AHA Task Force on Practice Guidelines. Circulation 117:e350, 2008.

ANSWER TO QUESTION 227

D (Braunwald, pp. 799-801; Fig. 39-28)

The differential diagnosis of wide-QRS complex tachycardia includes ventricular tachycardia (VT) and supraventricular tachycardia (SVT) with aberrancy. Several features of the clinical history and surface ECG may assist in making this differentiation, although none is absolute. The clinical scenario is important, because a past history of myocardial infarction makes the diagnosis of VT more likely. On the ECG, the presence of fusion beats (which indicate activation of the ventricle from two different foci, one of ventricular origin), capture beats (intermittent narrow complex QRS at an interval shorter than the rate of tachycardia), or atrioventricular dissociation all support the diagnosis of VT. Concordance of the QRS complex in the precordial leads (all complexes are positively directed or all are negatively directed) favors VT over SVT. Slowing or termination of the tachycardia by vagal maneuvers is consistent with SVT. Hemodynamic stability is not a useful criterion for differentiating SVT from VT.

Specific QRS contours are also helpful. For example, a triphasic QRS complex (rSR') in lead V_1 supports the presence of SVT. Conversely, monophasic or biphasic QRS complexes in lead V_1 are more consistent with VT. VT with a left bundle branch block configuration typically demonstrates a small Q–large R (qR) or QS pattern in lead V_6 and a broad, prolonged (>40 msec) R wave in lead V_1. VT with a right bundle branch pattern demonstrates a monophasic or biphasic QRS in lead V_1 and small R–large S waves or QS complexes in lead V_6.

REFERENCE

Goldberger ZD, Rho RW, Page RL, et al: Approach to the diagnosis and initial management of the stable adult patient with a wide complex tachycardia. Am J Cardiol 101:1456, 2008.

ANSWER TO QUESTION 228

E (Braunwald, pp. 728-730)

Electrical cardioversion is very effective for termination of supraventricular and ventricular tachyarrhythmias, particularly those due to reentry. Except in patients with ventricular fibrillation or rapid ventricular flutter, a *synchronized* shock (delivered during the QRS complex) should be used to minimize the risk of firing on the ST segment or T wave, which might precipitate ventricular fibrillation. The minimal effective energy should be used initially to reduce the risk of myocardial damage, with upward titration as required. If the "maximum" energy level of the electrical cardioverter fails to terminate the abnormal rhythm, repeated shocks at the same energy level can decrease the chest wall impedance and may succeed. Ibutilide pretreatment may also enhance the success of cardioversion in patients with atrial fibrillation. Direct-current cardioversion is contraindicated in suspected digitalis-induced tachyarrhythmias because of the potential for ventricular proarrhythmia.

The risk of thromboembolism is 1% to 3% in patients successfully cardioverted from atrial fibrillation to normal sinus rhythm. Thus, for patients who have been in atrial fibrillation or flutter for longer than 48 hours, elective cardioversion should be postponed for at least 3 weeks of therapeutic anticoagulation. In emergency situations requiring more urgent cardioversion, transesophageal echocardiography can be performed to exclude the presence of left atrial thrombus. After successful cardioversion, anticoagulation should be continued for an additional 3 to 4 weeks because full recovery of atrial mechanical activity often lags behind the return of normal electrical function and persistent blood stasis could permit thrombus formation.

REFERENCE

Reiffel JA: Cardioversion for atrial fibrillation: Treatment options and advances. Pacing Clin Electrophysiol 32:1073, 2009.

ANSWER TO QUESTION 229

C (Braunwald, pp. 806-809, Fig. 39-32)

The arrhythmia in the figure is *torsades de pointes*, a form of polymorphic ventricular tachycardia that can develop in patients with delayed ventricular repolarization, manifest by a prolonged QT interval on the ECG. Torsades de pointes is thought to be triggered by early afterdepolarizations during the vulnerable period of ventricular repolarization, producing QRS complexes of changing amplitude twisting around the isoelectric line at a rate of 200 to 250 beats/min.

A prolonged corrected QT interval on the surface ECG is defined as >0.46 millisecond in men or >0.47 millisecond in women. A long QT interval, the electrocardiographic substrate for torsades de pointes, can be either congenital or acquired. Congenital forms include those associated with congenital severe bradycardia or loss of function mutations in the *KCNQ1* (LQT1) and *KCNQ2* (LQT2) potassium channel genes or a *gain* of function mutation in the *SCN5A* sodium channel gene, which is responsible for LTQ3.[1] *Loss* of function mutations in the *SNC5A* gene (which result in accelerated sodium channel recovery or inactivated sodium channels) are associated with Brugada syndrome (and ventricular fibrillation) rather than prolongation of the QT interval and torsades de pointes.

Multiple drugs, both in toxic and therapeutic doses, can result in prolongation of the QT interval and an increased risk of torsades de pointes, including commonly used agents such as tricyclic antidepressants, erythromycin, and pentamidine. Antiarrhythmic drugs that prolong the QT interval and predispose to torsades de pointes include quinidine, procainamide, disopyramide, sotalol, and dofetilide.[2] Electrolyte disturbances, including hypokalemia or hypomagnesemia, may also contribute to a long QT interval and torsades de pointes.

REFERENCES

1. Rhoden DM: The long-QT syndrome. N Engl J Med 358:169, 2008.
2. Heist EK, Ruskin JN: Drug-induced arrhythmia. Circulation 122:1426, 2010.

ANSWER TO QUESTION 230

C (Braunwald, pp. 698-699, 798-801)

Intracardiac electrograms are shown depicting electrical activity in the high right atrium (HRA), in the bundle of His (His proximal and His distal), and at the right ventricular (RV) apex. The surface electrocardiographic leads V$_1$ and V$_5$ also are shown. The surface ECG demonstrates a wide-complex tachycardia at approximately 140 beats/min with a right bundle branch block morphology. The His distal and RV apical electrograms show deflections corresponding to each QRS complex, which represent ventricular depolarization. Smaller, periodic deflections at a slower rate are evident on the HRA and His proximal electrograms that represent atrial depolarizations. The lack of relationship between the atrial and ventricular depolarizations confirms the presence of AV dissociation. Thus, this rhythm represents ventricular tachycardia.

ANSWER TO QUESTION 231

B (Braunwald, pp. 819-821)

The electrophysiologic tracing in the figure depicts type I (Wenckebach) second-degree atrioventricular (AV) block. This is evident both in the surface electrocardiographic channel, which demonstrates progressive PR interval prolongation followed by a nonconducted P wave, and in the His bundle tracing (HBE), which shows progressive AH interval prolongation followed by block within the AV node. In contradistinction, in patients with type II second-degree heart block, there is sudden block of impulse conduction (a P wave not followed by a QRS complex) without prior lengthening of the PR interval.

Type I second-degree AV block with normal QRS duration often portends a benign clinical course, and no specific intervention is indicated in the absence of symptoms. When type I AV block occurs in acute myocardial infarction (MI), it is usually in the setting of an inferior wall infarction. Such occurrences are usually transient and do not typically require therapy. The presence of higher degrees of AV block, including type II second-degree block, in acute MI indicates greater myocardial damage and predicts higher mortality.

The surface ECG allows a reasonably reliable differentiation of the site of conduction abnormality in second-degree AV block. Type I AV block with a normal-width QRS complex almost always occurs at the level of the AV node proximal to the His bundle. In contrast, type II AV block, especially when it occurs in association with bundle branch block morphology of the QRS, may be localized to the His-Purkinje system. Type I AV block in a patient with a bundle branch block may be due to block either in the AV node or more distally in the His-Purkinje system. In patients with a 2:1 pattern of AV block, it can be difficult to distinguish whether type I or type II block is present. However, if the QRS duration is normal, Mobitz type I is more likely.

Vagal maneuvers, such as carotid sinus massage, may enhance type I AV block by further prolonging AV nodal conduction and may therefore be useful in differentiating type I from type II AV block.

ANSWER TO QUESTION 232

E (Braunwald, pp. 765-766, 818-822, Table 38G-1)

Acquired atrioventricular (AV) blocks are most commonly idiopathic and related to aging. However, many defined conditions can impair AV conduction, including coronary artery disease, infections (e.g., Lyme disease, Chagas disease, endocarditis), collagen vascular diseases (e.g., rheumatoid arthritis, scleroderma, dermatomyositis), infiltrative diseases (e.g., sarcoid, amyloid), neuromuscular disorders, and drug effects.

Indications for permanent pacing in AV conduction disorders have been described in detail. Among the major indications, permanent pacing is appropriate for (1) permanent or intermittent complete (third-degree) heart block, (2) permanent or intermittent type II second-degree AV block, and (3) type I second-degree AV block if accompanied by symptoms or evidence of block at, or inferior to, the bundle of His.

Pacing is not indicated in asymptomatic first-degree AV block or type I second-degree AV block above the level of the bundle of His. Occasionally, patients with first-degree AV block with marked prolongation of the PR interval (>300 msec) are hemodynamically symptomatic because of the loss of effective AV synchrony. In that case, consideration of a pacemaker is appropriate if reversible contributors to the AV block are not identified. Because of vagal influences, many normal persons (particularly those with high resting vagal tone, such as conditioned athletes) may exhibit pauses significantly longer than 3 seconds during sleep; in and of itself, therefore, this observation is not sufficient to warrant permanent pacemaker implantation.

Controversy exists about the appropriate timing of permanent pacing in congenital complete heart block. Because of the high incidence of unpredictable syncope, the tendency now is to implant permanent pacemakers in adults with this condition, even if they are asymptomatic.

REFERENCE

Epstein AE, DiMarco JP, Ellenbogen KA, et al: ACC/AHA/HRS 2008 guidelines for device-based therapy of cardiac rhythm abnormalities: A report of the ACC/AHA Task Force on Practice Guidelines. Circulation 117:e350, 2008.

ANSWER TO QUESTION 233

B (Braunwald, p. 756)

Some dual-chamber pacemakers operate with unipolar leads, as in this case. The metal capsule of the generator serves as the indifferent electrode. This can result in oversensing, in which skeletal muscle potentials result in inappropriate inhibition or triggering of pacing.

The first two beats in the tracing show appropriate dual-chamber atrial and ventricular sensing and pacing at a rate of 70 beats/min. There is no evidence of lack of capture (all pacing stimuli cause myocardial depolarizations) or undersensing (because there are no native atrial or ventricular complexes).

After the third complex there is a long pause during which no pacemaker activity is observed. There is significant baseline artifact (due to muscle contractions) during this period. The lack of pacemaker activity during the pause indicates that the ventricular lead has sensed the electrical activity generated by the arm and chest muscles and has inappropriately inhibited pacemaker output.

In cases of suspected oversensing, placing the pacemaker in an asynchronous mode (with application of a magnet) will abolish the symptoms caused by pacemaker malfunction and aid in the diagnosis. Conversion of the lead system to a bipolar configuration frequently eliminates oversensing of myopotentials.

ANSWER TO QUESTION 234

D (Braunwald, pp. 756-757; Fig. 38-22)

The figure is an electrocardiographic tracing from a patient with a dual-chamber pacemaker. Atrial pacing artifacts with effective atrial depolarization are seen throughout the tracing. However, all but one ventricular pacing artifact (complex 5) fail to result in ventricular depolarization. Because the pacemaker generates appropriate output but not consistent, effective ventricular depolarization, this is an example of intermittent failure to capture of the ventricular lead.

Failure to capture most commonly occurs due to dislodgment of the pacemaker lead from the endocardial surface, a complication that usually occurs within the first few weeks after implantation. Newer designs for active and passive fixation of pacemaker leads are associated with a much lower frequency of lead dislodgment. Failure to capture may also occur due to a lead insulation break, which allows some of the electrode current to dissipate into the surrounding tissues. Even if the lead system is intact and in contact with the myocardium, failure to capture may occur if the pacing threshold required to depolarize the myocardium exceeds the programmed voltage amplitude and pulse duration. This can occur in the setting of exit block, in which an inflammatory reaction or fibrosis at the electrode-myocardium interface raises the depolarization threshold; the risk of this complication is greatly reduced through the use of a steroid-eluting lead. Pacing thresholds (and the likelihood of failure to capture) may also be increased in the setting of marked metabolic abnormalities (e.g., hyperkalemia) or therapy with antiarrhythmic drugs (e.g., flecainide).

Impending total battery depletion may also result in a subthreshold pacing stimulus and failure to capture. Total battery depletion usually results in complete failure to output, which is not the case here, because consistent atrial and ventricular pacing and atrial capture are seen. In patients with a unipolar pacemaker, air in the pacemaker pocket may act as an insulator and reduce the effective pacemaker output, resulting in noncapture.

A loose set screw (which helps secure the lead to the generator) is a cause of failure to output but not failure to capture. This diagnosis is inconsistent with this tracing, because consistent ventricular pacing artifacts are seen.

ANSWER TO QUESTION 235

C (Braunwald, pp. 771-774, 813-816; Fig. 39-39)

Sinus bradycardia in adults is defined as a sinus node discharge <60 beats/min. It is generally a benign arrhythmia and well tolerated in most patients. It can result from excessive vagal stimulation or decreased sympathetic discharge and is common in well-trained athletes. During sleep, the heart rate in normal individuals can decrease to 35 to 40 beats/min and pauses of 2 to 3 seconds or even longer are not uncommon. Asymptomatic sinus bradycardia does not require specific therapy. Symptomatic patients can be treated acutely with intravenous atropine or sympathetic stimulants. For chronic, symptomatic sinus bradycardia, electronic pacing may be required.

Sinus arrest (which is distinct from sinus exit block) is identified by a pause in the sinus rhythm and a PP interval surrounding the pause that is not a multiple of the underlying PP rate. Sinus arrest can be due to sinus node ischemia during an acute myocardial infarction, degenerative fibrotic changes, digitalis toxicity, or excessive vagal tone. A large proportion of patients with sleep apnea have periods of sinus arrest as well as atrioventricular (AV) block.

Sinus arrhythmia is defined as phasic variations in the sinus cycle length, and it can appear in two forms: respiratory and nonrespiratory. In the respiratory form the PP interval shortens in a cyclical fashion during inspiration owing to inhibition of vagal tone. In the nonrespiratory form, as seen in digitalis toxicity, the phasic variation is unrelated to the respiratory cycle. Symptoms are very uncommon, and therapy is generally not necessary.

Sinus tachycardia in adults is manifest by a sinus rate exceeding 100 beats/min. This arrhythmia can be caused by a number of different physiologic stresses, including fever, hypotension, anemia, hyperthyroidism, hypovolemia, ischemia, pulmonary embolism, and alcohol or caffeine exposure. Sinus tachycardia generally has a gradual onset and termination, unlike reentrant tachycardia such as AV nodal tachycardia or sinoatrial tachycardia. Management of sinus tachycardia should focus on elimination of the underlying cause.

REFERENCE

Monfredi O, Dobrzynski H, Mondal T, et al: The anatomy and physiology of the sinoatrial node—a contemporary review. Pacing Clin Electrophysiol 33:1392, 2010.

ANSWER TO QUESTION 236

C (Braunwald, pp. 804-805; Fig. 39-29)

Arrhythmogenic right ventricular cardiomyopathy (ARVC) is a cardiomyopathy, more common in males, in which there is fatty or fibrofatty infiltration of the right ventricular (RV) wall.[1] Clinically, the disease is characterized by life-threatening ventricular arrhythmias in apparently healthy young people. The prevalence is estimated at 1 in 5000 individuals, although the difficulty of diagnosis makes the true prevalence difficult to estimate. In its familial form, genetic abnormalities have been found in desmosomal proteins, the ryanodine receptor, and transforming growth factor-beta$_3$. Immunohistochemistry of desmosomal proteins, such as plakoglobin, in endomyocardial biopsy samples has been shown to be a sensitive and specific diagnostic test for ARVC.[2] Most patients with ARVC demonstrate RV abnormalities by echocardiography, computed tomography, RV angiography, or magnetic resonance imaging. In advanced forms, the left ventricle is commonly involved.

The ECG in patients with ARVC in sinus rhythm may demonstrate a complete or incomplete right bundle branch block, with a terminal notch in the QRS complex,

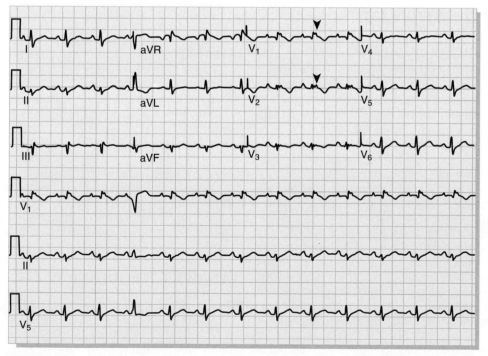

FIGURE 2-23

known as an *epsilon wave* (see arrowheads in Fig. 2-23). Ventricular tachycardia (VT) occurs commonly in patients with ARVC, usually with a *left* bundle branch block morphology due to its RV origin.

Because of the progressive nature of this disease and the multiple morphologies of the VT it produces, radiofrequency catheter ablation is not often successful. Use of an implantable cardioverter-defibrillator is usually the treatment of choice, even in asymptomatic patients.[3]

REFERENCES

1. Basso C, Corrado D, Marcus FI, et al: Arrhythmogenic right ventricular cardiomyopathy. Lancet 373:1289, 2009.
2. Asimaki A, Tandri H, Huang H, et al: A new diagnostic test for arrhythmogenic right ventricular cardiomyopathy. N Engl J Med 360:1075-1084, 2009.
3. Marcus FI, Zareba W, Calkins H, et al: Arrhythmogenic right ventricular cardiomyopathy/dysplasia clinical presentation and diagnostic evaluation: Results from the North American Multidisciplinary Study. Heart Rhythm 6:984, 2009.

ANSWER TO QUESTION 237

D (Braunwald, pp. 828-829)

A major objective of therapy in patients with atrial fibrillation (AF) is the prevention of stroke and other thromboembolic complications. Whereas warfarin is more effective than aspirin for this purpose, warfarin is also more likely to result in bleeding complications, so it should be prescribed only to patients for whom the thromboembolic risk exceeds the likelihood of hemorrhage. A widely used algorithm to facilitate decision making between warfarin and aspirin in this setting is the CHADS$_2$ score, which assigns points to stroke risk factors, including congestive heart failure (1 point), hypertension (1 point), age $\geq$75 years (1 point), diabetes mellitus (1 point), and prior stroke or transient ischemic attack (2 points). Patients with a CHADS$_2$ score of 0 have an expected stroke rate of <2%/year and may be safely treated with aspirin as the antithrombotic agent, whereas those with CHADS$_2$ scores >1 are at sufficiently high risk for stroke that warfarin is preferred. Of the selections listed, patient A has a CHADS$_2$ score of 2; patients B, C, and E have scores of 1, and patient D has a score of 0, making patient D the most appropriate candidate for aspirin therapy.

Recently, a refinement of the CHADS$_2$ score, the CHADS$_2$-VASc score, has been proposed to improve risk stratification. It encompasses additional stroke risk factors, including peripheral vascular disease (1 point), age 65-74 (1 point), and sex category (female gender = 1 point). In this modification, age $\geq$75 years receives an incremental weight of 2 points. Using this algorithm the scores for patients B, C, and E each increase to 2, reinforcing the appropriateness of warfarin, while patient D still has a score of 0, confirming aspirin as the preferred prophylactic agent.

REFERENCES

Camm AJ, Kirchhof P, Lip GY, et al: Guidelines for the management of atrial fibrillation. The Task Force for the Management of Atrial Fibrillation of the European Society of Cardiology (ESC). Eur Heart J 19:2369-2429, 2010.

Fuster V, Ryden LE, Cannom DS, et al: ACC/AHA/ESC 2006 Guidelines for the Management of Patients with Atrial Fibrillation. Circulation 114:e257-e354, 2006.

ANSWER TO QUESTION 238

E (Braunwald, pp. 816-817, 887; Fig. 39-44)

Two types of carotid sinus hypersensitivity have been described: cardioinhibitory and vasodepressor. In the *cardioinhibitory* type, a period of ventricular asystole exceeding 3 seconds is produced by carotid sinus stimulation. The *vasodepressor* type is defined as a decrease in systolic blood pressure of 50 mm Hg or more without slowing of the heart rate or as a decrease in systolic blood pressure of 30 mm Hg or more with reproduction of the patient's symptoms. The mechanism responsible for carotid sinus hypersensitivity is not known. Carotid sinus hypersensitivity is identified in nearly one third of elderly patients who present with syncope or falls but is also frequently observed in asymptomatic individuals.

Acutely, cardioinhibitory carotid sinus hypersensitivity can be prevented by atropine. Long-term therapy generally requires placement of a permanent pacemaker, usually a dual-chamber device, because AV block can occur during periods of hypersensitive carotid reflex.

Atropine and electronic pacing are not sufficient to prevent the fall in the blood pressure in patients with the vasodepressor type of carotid sinus hypersensitivity, which may result from inhibition of sympathetic vasoconstrictor activity. In such individuals, sodium-retaining drugs, elastic support hose, and avoidance of intravascular volume depletion may be beneficial. Drugs that enhance the response to carotid sinus massage, such as beta blockers, digoxin, and clonidine, should be avoided.

REFERENCE

Tan MP, Newton JL, Chadwick TJ, et al: The relationship between carotid sinus hypersensitivity, orthostatic hypotension, and vasovagal syncope: A case-control study. Europace 10:1400, 2008.

ANSWER TO QUESTION 239

B (Braunwald, pp. 785-792; Table 39-4)

The two intracardiac electrograms include surface electrocardiographic leads V$_1$ and V$_5$, a recording from a catheter in the high right atrium (HRA), a series of five recordings from a multiple-pole catheter placed in the coronary sinus (displayed from the proximal to distal CS), recordings from a bundle of His position catheter (His proximal and His distal), and a recording from a catheter at the right ventricular (RV) apex.

The baseline electrogram demonstrates preexcitation: the surface ECG shows that the QRS complex occurs nearly simultaneously with the small, sharp His potential deflection on the His distal electrogram. This implies that ventricular activation occurs well before depolarization of the His-Purkinje system.

In the electrogram recorded during tachycardia, the surface ECG leads show a narrow-complex rhythm at approximately 160 beats/min. The intracardiac electrograms demonstrate ventricular depolarizations at the His and RV apical catheters corresponding to the QRS complex on each surface ECG. Each ventricular depolarization is preceded by a His depolarization. Atrial depolarization is apparent in the His catheter positions and throughout the CS electrograms. The sequence of atrial activation begins at the distal CS electrogram and proceeds to the proximal and His catheters. These observations are consistent with orthodromic AV reciprocating tachycardia via an accessory pathway. Specifically, the location of the accessory pathway is likely to be left lateral based on the sequence of atrial activation.

ANSWER TO QUESTION 240

E (Braunwald, pp. 81-84, 807-809)

Congenital long QT syndrome (LQTS) is an inherited disorder characterized by delayed repolarization of the myocardium (QTc > 480 msec) and susceptibility to life-threatening ventricular arrhythmias (torsades de pointes).[1,2] Hundreds of causal mutations have been identified in 12 LQTS susceptibility genes.

Approximately 75% of disease-causing mutations occur in three genes, comprising the most common forms of this condition: LQT1 (mutations in the *KCNQ1* gene that encodes the alpha subunit of the I_{Ks} potassium channel, causing loss of function), LQT2 (mutations in *KCNH2*, the gene that encodes the alpha subunit of the I_{Kr} potassium channel, causing loss of function), and LQT3 (mutations in the *SCN5A* gene, which encodes the cardiac sodium channel, causing gain of function).

Clinical symptomatology in LQTS is highly variable and is related in part to the genetic locus that is affected. LQT1 patients experience the majority of cardiac events during physical (especially swimming) or emotional stress, suggesting a connection with sympathetic nervous system activation. In contrast, LQT2 patients are at highest risk for lethal events by auditory triggers or during the postpartum period. Cardiac events during sleep or at rest are most common in LQT3.

For patients who have congenital LQTS but no history of syncope, ventricular arrhythmias, or family history of sudden cardiac death, generally no therapy or treatment with a beta blocker (to reduce triggered activity) is appropriate. Permanent pacing is indicated in select patients with atrioventricular block or pause-dependent torsades de pointes. In patients deemed at high risk for sudden death (e.g., those with a history of syncope or resuscitated cardiac arrest), an implantable cardioverter-defibrillator is the therapy of choice.

REFERENCES

1. Rhoden DM: The long-QT syndrome. N Engl J Med 358:169, 2008.
2. Goldenberg I, Moss AJ. Long QT syndrome. J Am Coll Cardiol 51:2291, 2008.

ANSWER TO QUESTION 241

D (Braunwald, pp. 845-860; Fig. 41-1; Tables 41-1 and 41-3)

Sudden cardiac death (SCD) is defined as a natural death due to cardiac causes, in which abrupt loss of consciousness occurs within 1 hour of the onset of acute symptoms. An estimated 300,000 to 350,000 cases occur in the United States annually, accounting for one half of all cardiovascular deaths. There are two peak age distributions of sudden death: (1) from birth to 6 months of age (i.e., sudden infant death syndrome) and (2) between 45 and 75 years of age. Coronary artery disease is the structural basis for 75% to 80% of SCDs, and prophylactic cardioverter-defibrillator implantation in high-risk patients with coronary artery disease is now the standard of care. SCD is more common in men than woman, with a fourfold to sevenfold excess of SCD in men compared with women before age 65. At older ages, the difference decreases to 2:1 or less. A number of hereditary conditions can result in SCD, including hypertrophic cardiomyopathy, the long QT syndrome, arrhythmogenic right ventricular cardiomyopathy, and Brugada syndrome. This observation allows potential screening and preventive therapy for individuals at high risk.

Hypertension and cigarette smoking, but not hypercholesterolemia, have been established as risk factors for SCD. Interestingly, in the Framingham study, intraventricular conduction abnormalities on the ECG (but not left ventricular hypertrophy or nonspecific ST-T wave abnormalities) were associated with an increased risk of SCD. Psychosocial factors such as social isolation and a high level of life stress were also found to increase the risk of sudden death.

ANSWER TO QUESTION 242

D (Braunwald, pp. 728, 778-779)

The ECG illustrated shows atrial tachycardia with block. In this condition, an atrial rate of 130 to 200 beats/min, with a ventricular response less than or equal to the atrial rate is present. Digitalis toxicity accounts for this rhythm in 50% to 75% of cases, and in such instances the atrial rate may show a gradual increase if digoxin is continued. Other signs of digitalis excess are often present, including frequent premature ventricular complexes.

In nearly one half of all patients with atrial tachycardia with block, the atrial rate is irregular and demonstrates a characteristic isoelectric interval between each P wave, in contrast to the morphology of atrial flutter waves. Most instances of this rhythm occur in patients with significant organic heart disease. Causes other than digitalis toxicity include ischemic heart disease, myocardial infarction, and cor pulmonale. In patients taking digitalis, potassium depletion may precipitate the arrhythmia and the oral administration of potassium, and the withholding of digoxin often will allow reversal to normal sinus rhythm. Because atrial tachycardia with block is seen primarily in patients with serious underlying heart disease, its onset may lead to significant clinical deterioration.

ANSWER TO QUESTION 243

C (Braunwald, pp. 852-854, 864-871; see also Answer to Question 241)

Sudden cardiac death (SCD) is the first clinical manifestation of coronary artery disease in approximately 25% of patients. However, a previous myocardial infarction (MI) can be identified in about 75% of patients who die suddenly. The extent of left ventricular dysfunction and the presence of premature ventricular complexes after MI are both powerful predictors of SCD.

The arrhythmias that most commonly cause cardiac arrest, in decreasing order of frequency, are ventricular fibrillation (VF), bradyarrhythmias/asystole or pulseless electrical activity, and sustained ventricular tachycardia (VT). Survival after an out-of-hospital cardiac arrest is best for those patients in whom sustained VT was the initial recorded rhythm. Patients with bradycardic/asystolic cardiac arrest have the worst prognosis.

Unattended VF results in irreversible brain damage within 4 to 6 minutes. As a result, the probability of a favorable outcome deteriorates rapidly as a function of time. This has led to the proliferation of automatic external defibrillators in public places (e.g., airports, shopping malls) to improve the response time for patients with cardiac arrest.

REFERENCE

Eisenberg MS, Psaty BM: Defining and improving survival rates from cardiac arrest in US communities. JAMA 301:860, 2009.

ANSWER TO QUESTION 244

D (Braunwald, pp. 696-699)

In patients with an intraventricular conduction delay, invasive electrophysiologic study (EPS) provides useful information on the duration of the His-ventricular (HV) interval. A prolonged HV interval (>80 msec) identifies patients at increased risk of developing complete AV block, with a high specificity (approximately 80%) but low sensitivity (approximately 66%). Atrial pacing and infusion of procainamide during EPS can help expose abnormal His-Purkinje conduction.

The sinus node recovery time (SNRT), measured during EPS, is the interval between the last paced high right atrial complex and the first spontaneous sinus response after termination of pacing. Because the spontaneous sinus rate influences the SNRT, this number must be corrected by subtracting the spontaneous sinus cycle length from the SNRT. This corrected measurement, the CSNRT, is useful in the evaluation of sinus node function. Prolongation of the CSNRT (e.g., >525 msec) is found in patients suspected of having sinus node dysfunction. However, the sensitivity of the SNRT is only about 50%. The specificity for sinus node dysfunction, when combined with measurements of the sinoatrial

conduction time, is about 88%. Thus, if the SNRT is abnormal, the patient likely has sinus node dysfunction, but if it is normal, such dysfunction is not excluded.

The complication rate of EPS is low. For example, EPS with radiofrequency ablation has a risk of complications ranging from 1% to 3%, with procedure-related death occurring in about 0.2%. Because most EPS procedures do not require entry into the left side of the heart, the risk of stroke, myocardial infarction, or systemic embolism is lower than for coronary arteriography. The major risks include myocardial perforation by a catheter, provocation of arrhythmias, and complications at the groin entry sites.

ANSWER TO QUESTION 245

B (Braunwald, p. 724)

Dronedarone is an antiarrhythmic drug derived from amiodarone and the two agents share electrophysiologic properties, including blockade of the delayed rectifier potassium current (Class III effect), inhibition of the rapid sodium and l-type calcium currents, and antiadrenergic effects. However, unlike amiodarone, dronedarone does not contain iodine molecules, a property that likely accounts for its much lower rate of thyroid and pulmonary toxicity.

Dronedarone is approved by the U.S. Food and Drug Administration to facilitate the maintenance of sinus rhythm in patients with atrial fibrillation or atrial flutter.[1] It is orally absorbed, is hepatically metabolized, and has a much shorter elimination half-life than amiodarone (only 13 to 19 hours). Like amiodarone, the QT interval may become prolonged but the risk of proarrhythmia is small.

In the Antiarrhythmic Trial with Dronedarone in Moderate-to-Severe Heart Failure Evaluating Morbidity Decrease (ANDROMEDA), patients on dronedarone had *increased* mortality compared with those taking a placebo (8.1% vs. 3.8%), thus the drug should *not* be used in patients with recent or current heart failure.[2] In addition, rare cases of acute severe liver injury have been reported with dronedarone therapy.[3]

REFERENCES

1. Hohnloser SH, Crijns HJ, van Eickels M, et al: Effect of dronedarone on cardiovascular events in atrial fibrillation. N Engl J Med 260:668, 2009.
2. Kober L, Torp-Pedersen C, McMurray JJ, et al: Increased mortality after dronedarone therapy for severe heart failure. N Engl J Med 358:2678, 2008.
3. U.S. Food and Drug Administration: FDA Drug Safety Communication: Severe liver injury associated with the use of dronedarone (marketed as Multaq). Available at http://www.fda.gov/Drugs/DrugSafety/ucm240011.htm. Accessed June 30, 2011.

ANSWER TO QUESTION 246

C (Braunwald, pp. 748-755; Table 38-1; see also Answer to Question 211 for discussion of nomenclature)

Selection of the appropriate mode of cardiac pacing depends on many factors, including the underlying rhythm disturbance, the patient's exercise capacity, and the chronotropic response to exercise. Ventricular inhibited pacing (VVI) inhibits ventricular pacemaker output if a ventricular event is sensed but it does not sense or pace the atrium. This mode protects against bradycardias but does not restore or maintain atrioventricular (AV) synchrony, so that AV dissociation is common. In addition, in chronotropically incompetent patients in whom the sinus heart rate does not increase with exercise, this mode does not provide rate responsiveness. These deficiencies may result in the "pacemaker syndrome" of reduced functional capacity, shortness of breath, dizziness, and fatigue, which can occur in up to 20% of patients with normally functioning VVI pacing.

Single-chamber triggered pacing (AAT or VVT) generates an output pulse every time a native event is sensed. As a result, it accelerates the rate of battery depletion. This mode of pacing is not frequently used.

Atrial inhibited pacing (AAI) inhibits atrial pacemaker output if an atrial event is sensed. It does not sense or pace the ventricle. It is an appropriate mode for patients with sinus node dysfunction who have normal AV conduction but should not be used in individuals with AV nodal disease. Dual-chamber pacing and sensing with inhibition and tracking (DDD) is typically the preferred mode of pacing for patients with combined sinus and AV node dysfunction, because physiologic pacing reduces the frequency of the pacemaker syndrome and may reduce the incidence of atrial fibrillation. However, no randomized trial has demonstrated any effect of pacing mode choice (DDD vs. VVI) on mortality in patients with sinus node dysfunction.

In patients with atrial fibrillation, standard DDD or DDDR is not desirable because P-synchronous pacing is not possible and sensing of the chaotic atrial rhythm could trigger an accelerated ventricular pacing response. To compensate for this deficiency, modern DDD and DDDR devices have an automatic mode switching feature that, when atrial fibrillation develops, inhibits atrial-sensed ventricular pacing.

REFERENCE

Epstein AE, DiMarco JP, Ellenbogen KA, et al: ACC/AHA/HRS 2008 guidelines for device-based therapy of cardiac rhythm abnormalities: A report of the ACC/AHA Task Force on Practice Guidelines. Circulation 117:e350, 2008.

ANSWER TO QUESTION 247

D (Braunwald, pp. 753-758; Fig. 38-27)

Pacemaker malfunction may be manifested by impaired pacemaker output or failure to capture or sense the appropriate cardiac chamber. On the ECG, failure to capture is identified when a pacing "spike" is present without evidence of subsequent myocardial depolarization (a P wave or QRS complex). This condition can result from an abnormally elevated electrical threshold, lead dislodgment or perforation, impending battery depletion, or circuit failure. Threshold alterations may be due to medications (e.g., Class IC antiarrhythmic agents)

or electrolyte and metabolic abnormalities, including hyperkalemia, severe acidosis and alkalosis, hypercapnia, hypoxemia, and myxedema. Failure to sense can result from lead dislodgment or inadequate initial lead placement, lead insulation or circuit failure, electromagnetic radiation, or battery depletion.

Patients with pacemakers should be cautioned about electromagnetic interference that could potentially result in malfunction. An example is industrial-strength welding equipment (>500 Å); close contact should be avoided. Patients with pacemakers should be warned not to lean on or linger near electronic antitheft devices (situated at the exits of many stores) because pacemaker malfunction has been reported in that setting; simply walking past or through such devices is not problematic. Cellular telephones can also interfere with the function of cardiac pacemakers; however, when they are placed in the normal position over the ear, rather than over the device, this interference does not pose a significant risk.

Left bundle branch block morphology is the expected electrocardiographic pattern during standard right ventricular pacing owing to the delay in depolarization of left ventricular myocardium. The presence of right bundle branch block after right ventricular pacemaker implantation is suggestive of accidental lead placement or migration into the left ventricle.

Pseudofusion is present on the surface ECG when a pacing spike does not alter the normal morphology of a superimposed instrinsic QRS complex (Fig. 2-24). This results when a pacing impulse is delivered at the appropriate escape interval into myocardium whose action potentials are in the absolute refractory period owing to slightly earlier intrinsic activation. Pseudofusion can be distinguished from a *fusion beat*, in which the QRS complex represents the combination of intrinsic ventricular activation and *effective* pacemaker depolarization, producing a morphology intermediate between intrinsic and paced beats.

ANSWER TO QUESTION 248

A (Braunwald, pp. 756-758)

The figure depicts a close-up view of a chest radiograph in a patient with a single-chamber pacemaker. The finding of note is a fracture at the point where the lead dives below the clavicle (arrow in Fig. 2-25). The patient presented with intermittent failure to capture and intermittent failure to output on the ventricular lead. Lead impedance was greatly elevated.

The telemetric measurement of voltage and current thresholds, lead impedance, and electrograms can be very helpful in differentiating the causes of pacemaker malfunction. When a pacemaker wire has fractured, both the voltage threshold and the lead impedance are high. In the case of an insulation break, the voltage threshold and the lead impedance are low. In the setting of a dislodged lead, the voltage threshold is high but the lead impedance is normal. Exit block may occur as the result of an inflammatory reaction at the point of contact between the pacemaker lead and the myocardium. When

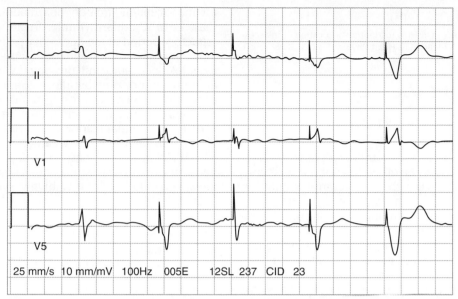

FIGURE 2-24 Three-channel tracing from an ambulatory monitor. The first QRS is intrinsic. The second and fourth beats represent fusion; the third beat is pseudofusion, that is, the underlying morphology is nearly identical to the intrinsic QRS; and the final QRS represents paced depolarization.

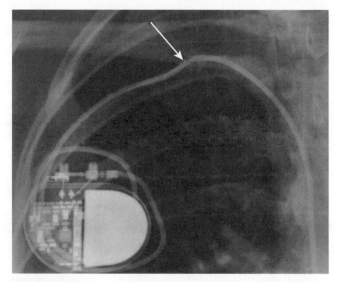

FIGURE 2-25

this occurs, the measured voltage and current thresholds are high but lead impedance is normal.

ANSWER TO QUESTION 249

B (Braunwald, pp. 785-795)

The ECG in the figure depicts atrial fibrillation with rapid ventricular rate and aberrant conduction in a patient with Wolff-Parkinson-White (WPW) syndrome and a right posteroseptal accessory pathway. The latter localization is possible because of the negative initial deflections in leads II, III, aVF, and V₁, with upright initial forces in leads I and aVL. Acute treatment of this dysrhythmia must include agents that prolong refractoriness in the accessory pathway, such as intravenous procainamide or amiodarone. In hemodynamically unstable patients, direct-current cardioversion is the treatment of choice. Intravenous verapamil prolongs conduction time in the atrioventricular node without affecting conduction through the accessory pathway. Thus the administration of verapamil to a patient with WPW in atrial fibrillation may *accelerate* conduction through the bypass tract and precipitate ventricular fibrillation, such that it should not be used in this setting.

Electrocardiographic evidence of the WPW syndrome is present in approximately 0.25% of healthy individuals. Three basic features characterize the electrocardiographic abnormalities of the syndrome: the presence of a PR interval <120 milliseconds during sinus rhythm; a QRS duration >120 milliseconds with a slurred, slowly rising onset of the QRS in some leads (the delta wave); and secondary ST-segment/T wave changes generally directed opposite to the major QRS vector. The axis of the delta waves on the surface ECG can be used to localize the position of the accessory pathway in the heart. Left free wall accessory pathways are the most common, followed by the posteroseptal, right free wall, and anteroseptal locations.

The prevalence of WPW is higher in men and decreases with age; however, the frequency of paroxysmal tachycardia associated with the syndrome apparently increases with age. Most such tachycardias are reciprocating tachycardias (80%), with 15% to 30% presenting as atrial fibrillation and 5% as atrial flutter. Although most adults with the WPW syndrome have normal hearts, a number of cardiac defects are occasionally associated with this syndrome, including Ebstein's anomaly. In patients with Ebstein anomaly, multiple accessory pathways are often present and are located on the right side of the heart, with preexcitation localized to the atrialized ventricle.

REFERENCE

Fox DJ, Klein GJ, Skanes AC, et al: How to identify the location of an accessory pathway by the 12-lead ECG. Heart Rhythm 5:1763, 2008.

ANSWER TO QUESTION 250

C (Braunwald, pp. 578-581, 767)

This patient has ischemic cardiomyopathy with a reduced left ventricular ejection fraction of 30% and left bundle branch block with a QRS complex duration of ~190 milliseconds on the surface ECG. He is on optimal medical therapy with apparently normal filling pressures by physical examination and has persistent Class III symptoms. Accordingly, he meets guideline-based criteria for cardiac resynchronization therapy (CRT).[1] In addition, based on the reduced ejection fraction and persistent symptoms, he qualifies for implantation of a cardioverter-defibrillator for primary prevention of sudden cardiac death. The results of the COMPANION trial suggest incremental mortality benefit from a device capable of combined cardiac resynchronization and defibrillation (CRT-D) over cardiac resynchronization alone in this population.[2] The PROSPECT study did not support the use of echocardiographic measures of dyssynchrony as selection criteria for CRT in patients with a QRS duration ≥ 120 milliseconds.[3]

REFERENCES

1. Epstein AE, DiMarco JP, Ellenbogen KA, et al: ACC/AHA/HRS 2008 guidelines for device-based therapy of cardiac rhythm abnormalities: A report of the ACC/AHA Task Force on Practice Guidelines. Circulation 117:e350, 2008.
2. Bristow MR, Saxon LA, Boehmer J, et al: Cardiac-resynchronization therapy with or without an implantable defibrillator in advanced chronic heart failure. N Engl J Med 350:2140, 2004.
3. Chung ES, Leon AR, Tavazzi A, et al: Results of the predictors of response to CRT (PROSPECT) trial. Circulation 117:2608, 2008.

ANSWER TO QUESTION 251

D (Braunwald, pp. 785-795)

The electrophysiologic tracing depicts a recording of ventricular depolarization over an accessory pathway. The first QRS complex is preexcited, with a short PR interval and delta wave on the surface ECG. The His bundle activation is buried within the ventricular complex (see lead HBE). During the second beat, the accessory pathway is refractory and normal conduction over the atrioventricular (AV) node ensues, generating a normal QRS complex. In this normal complex, His bundle activation clearly precedes ventricular activation, with a measurable His-ventricular (HV) interval of 45 milliseconds. Ventricular preexcitation in association with a delta wave is consistent with a diagnosis of Wolff-Parkinson-White (WPW) syndrome.

Patients with ventricular preexcitation and frequent symptomatic tachyarrhythmia require therapy. Options for management include pharmacologic therapy with Class IA or IC antiarrhythmic drugs (which prolong the refractory period in the accessory pathway) and invasive treatment with radiofrequency catheter ablation. Both atenolol and verapamil prolong AV nodal conduction time but do not directly affect conduction through the accessory pathway. As a result, in patients with WPW syndrome and atrial fibrillation, these drugs may actually *enhance* ventricular response and precipitate ventricular fibrillation. Radiofrequency catheter ablation in patients with WPW syndrome has a high success rate and low frequency of complications and is cost effective. It is the therapy of choice in this highly symptomatic young patient.

REFERENCE

Tischenki A, Fox DJ, Yee R, et al: When should we recommend catheter ablation for patients with the Wolff-Parkinson-White syndrome? Curr Opin Cardiol 23:32, 2008.

ANSWER TO QUESTION 252

C (Braunwald, p. 725)

Dofetilide is a Class III antiarrhythmic drug whose sole electrophysiologic effect appears to be blockade of the rapid component of the delayed rectifier potassium current (I_{Kr}). Its effect is most pronounced in the atria, and the drug is currently approved for the acute conversion of atrial fibrillation to sinus rhythm as well as chronic suppression of recurrent atrial fibrillation. Its role in therapy for ventricular arrhythmias is not well established. Dofetilide has a neutral effect on mortality (i.e., it does not increase it) in patients after myocardial infarction.

Dofetilide is well absorbed orally, with over 90% bioavailability. Fifty percent to 60% of the drug is excreted in the urine, whereas the remainder undergoes hepatic metabolism to inert compounds. The drug's dosage must be carefully adjusted based on the creatinine clearance (Ccr), and it should not be administered to patients with a Ccr <20 mL/min. The most important adverse effect of dofetilide is QT interval prolongation with development of torsades de pointes, occurring in 2% to 4% of patients receiving the drug. The risk is highest in patients with hypokalemia, those taking other drugs that prolong repolarization, and those with baseline QT interval prolongation. For this reason, dofetilide currently is approved only for inpatient initiation so that the QT interval can be closely monitored. Patients with a corrected baseline QT interval >440 milliseconds are not candidates for dofetilide therapy. Verapamil, ketoconazole, and trimethoprim all increase the serum dofetilide concentration and should not be used concurrently with this antiarrhythmic drug.

REFERENCE

MyKytsey A, Bauman JL, Razminia M, et al: Observations on the safety and effectiveness of dofetilide in patients with paroxysmal atrial fibrillation and normal left ventricular function. J Cardiovasc Pharmacol Ther 12:36, 2007.

ANSWER TO QUESTION 253

C (Braunwald, pp. 827-828, 1630-1631)

This 26-year-old man presents with atrial fibrillation (AF) after the New Year holiday. Furthermore, most of his episodes of AF have occurred on Mondays. These facts should prompt consideration of the "holiday heart syndrome," which is the occurrence of palpitations, chest discomfort, and syncope after a binge of alcohol consumption.

The most common arrhythmia associated with this syndrome is AF, followed by atrial flutter and frequent ventricular premature beats. Electrophysiologic testing in subjects without heart disease suggests that alcohol enhances the vulnerability of the heart to induction of atrial arrhythmias. The mechanism of this proarrhythmic effect is unclear but may be related to metabolic derangements (hypokalemia, hypomagnesemia) owing to the diuretic effects of alcohol ingestion. AF in this situation usually occurs several hours after the last drink and may also be related to the onset of early withdrawal symptoms, especially sympathetic hyperactivity. Treatment is typically conservative, with a focus on abstinence from alcohol.

Regular excess alcohol consumption is also an important cause of hypertension and left ventricular systolic dysfunction. In fact, ethanol abuse is the leading cause of nonischemic dilated cardiomyopathy in industrialized nations, accounting for approximately one half of patients with this diagnosis. The likelihood of developing cardiomyopathy appears to correlate with the amount and duration of daily alcohol consumption, but there are wide variations in the susceptibility of individual patients to myocardial toxicity. With abstinence from alcohol, left ventricular systolic and diastolic dysfunction often improve.

Cocaine is associated with multiple cardiovascular complications, most commonly myocardial ischemia and infarction due to coronary artery vasoconstriction and cocaine-enhanced platelet aggregation. Long-term cocaine use is also associated with left ventricular hypertrophy and systolic dysfunction, perhaps the sequelae of repeated, profound sympathetic stimulation. The direct arrhythmogenic potential of cocaine is not well established.

REFERENCE

Kodama S, Saito K, Tanaka S, et al: Alcohol consumption and risk of atrial fibrillation: A meta-analysis. J Am Coll Cardiol 57:427, 2011.

ANSWERS TO QUESTIONS 254 TO 257

254—A, 255—D, 256—B, 257—C (Braunwald, pp. 798-812; see also Answers to Questions 229 and 240)

Many specific syndromes associated with ventricular tachycardia (VT) have been identified. The *long QT syndromes*, either familial or acquired, can result in ventricular arrhythmias (e.g., torsades de pointes) and sudden death. The *familial* forms include (1) the autosomal recessive Jervell and Lange-Nielsen syndrome and (2) the autosomal dominant Romano-Ward syndrome. The former is associated with sensorineural deafness, whereas patients with the latter condition have normal hearing. Genetic abnormalities in potassium and sodium channels cause the familial long QT syndromes, and specific mutations carry varying degrees of risk for the development of ventricular arrhythmias. The *acquired* form of long QT syndrome can result from many medications, including quinidine, procainamide, sotalol, terfenadine, tricyclic antidepressants, erythromycin, and ketoconazole. Electrolyte abnormalities such as hypokalemia, hypomagnesemia, and hypocalcemia can also result in significant prolongation of the QT interval and predispose to ventricular arrhythmias.

Right ventricular outflow tract VT is a type of idiopathic VT with a characteristic left bundle branch block morphology and an inferior axis. The electrophysiologic mechanism of this rhythm appears to be related to early or delayed afterdepolarizations.[1] Vagal maneuvers and adenosine administration terminate the VT, whereas exercise or isoproterenol infusion can initiate it. Beta blockers and verapamil may suppress VT in this disorder, and catheter ablation can be curative in many patients. The prognosis is generally good.

Brugada syndrome is a form of idiopathic ventricular fibrillation associated with characteristic abnormalities on the surface ECG and a high risk of sudden cardiac death.[2] The ECG in sinus rhythm typically demonstrates a right bundle branch block morphology with unusual ST-segment elevation in the anterior precordial leads. Mutations in a gene responsible for the cardiac sodium channel (*SCN5A*) have been identified in some families with this syndrome. Pharmacologic therapy has not been very successful in preventing the associated ventricular arrhythmias. As a result, the general recommendation is for cardioverter-defibrillator implantation in patients with this condition.

REFERENCES

1. Bala R, Marchlinski FE: Electrocardiographic recognition and ablation of outflow tract ventricular tachycardia. Heart Rhythm 4:366, 2007.
2. Antzelevitch C, Brugada P, Borggrefe M, et al: Brugada syndrome: Report of the second consensus conference: endorsed by the Heart Rhythm Society and the European Heart Rhythm Association. Circulation 111:659, 2005.

ANSWERS TO QUESTIONS 258 TO 261

258—D, 259—B, 260—A, 261—C (Braunwald, pp. 710-713; Tables 37-1 and 37-3)

The Vaughan-Williams classification is a commonly used system for grouping similarly acting antiarrhythmic agents. Not all drugs within a class have identical effects, and drug actions are more complex than those depicted by this classification scheme.

Class I drugs predominantly block the fast sodium channels and are divided into three subgroups. Class IA drugs (e.g., quinidine, procainamide, disopyramide) reduce the rate of rise of the action potential upstroke (Vmax) and prolong the action potential duration. Class IB drugs (e.g., lidocaine, mexiletine, phenytoin) reduce Vmax to only a minimal degree and *shorten* the action potential duration. Class IC drugs (e.g., flecainide, propafenone) reduce Vmax, slow conduction, and minimally prolong refractoriness.

Class II drugs are beta-adrenergic receptor blockers (e.g., metoprolol, timolol, propranolol). Class III drugs (e.g., sotalol, amiodarone, ibutilide, dofetilide, bretylium) primarily block potassium channels and prolong repolarization. Class IV drugs are slow calcium channel ($I_{Ca.L}$) blockers (e.g., verapamil, diltiazem).

ANSWERS TO QUESTIONS 262 TO 265

262—B, 263—C, 264—C, 265—A (Braunwald, pp. 830-832)

Many antiarrhythmic drugs are available to maintain sinus rhythm in patients with a history of atrial fibrillation (AF). Standard beta blockers are sometimes usefulfor this purpose and are generally well tolerated. Conversely, when more potent antiarrhythmic agents are required, the benefit of the drug must be weighed against the risk of potentially dangerous adverse effects. Such risk can be minimized by choosing a drug that is appropriate for the patient's underlying cardiac disease. For example, Vaughn-Williams Class IC drugs (e.g., flecainide or propafenone) are well tolerated and are reasonably safe drugs for patients without ischemic or structural heart disease but are associated with increased morbidity and mortality in patients with these conditions. Similarly, Class IA agents (e.g., quinidine) and the Class III drug sotalol should not be used in patients with a prolonged QT interval or left ventricular (LV) hypertrophy (e.g., ≥1.4 cm) because of the risk of precipitating torsades de pointes. The class III drug amiodarone is the most potent agent available to prevent recurrent atrial fibrillation. It is only rarely proarrhythmic, even in patients with underlying structural heart disease. It is, however, associated with significant noncardiac toxicities (especially affecting the lungs, liver, and thyroid), and therefore therapy with this drug must be monitored carefully.

Table 2-1 summarizes general recommendations for long-term rhythm control in patients with a history of AF.

REFERENCE

Lafuente-Lafuente C, Mouly S, Longas-Tejero MA, et al: Antiarrhythmic drugs for maintaining sinus rhythm after cardioversion for atrial fibrillation: A systematic review of randomized controlled trials. Arch Intern Med 166:719, 2006.

ANSWERS TO QUESTIONS 266 TO 269

266—C, 267—D, 268—A, 269—E (Braunwald, pp. 551-558)

Diuretics are frequently used in the management of heart failure and hypertension. Collectively, they act to lower

TABLE 2-1

CARDIAC CONDITION	FIRST-LINE DRUG	SECOND-LINE DRUG
Structurally normal heart without coronary disease	Class IC agent (e.g., flecainide, propafenone), sotalol, dronedarone	Amiodarone
Hypertension with LV wall thickness >1.3 cm	Amiodarone	
Coronary artery disease with preserved LV function	Sotalol, dofetilide, dronedarone	Amiodarone
Heart failure	Amiodarone, dofetilide	

plasma volume by increasing excretion of sodium and water. Diuretics can be classified into four categories based on mechanism and site of action in the nephron: (1) carbonic anhydrase inhibitors (e.g., acetazolamide), which act at the proximal tubule; (2) loop diuretics, which inhibit the $Na^+/K^+/Cl^-$ transporter in the thick ascending limb of the loop of Henle (e.g., furosemide, torsemide, bumetanide, and ethacrynic acid); (3) thiazide-like diuretics, which inhibit the Na^+/Cl^- cotransporter in the distal convoluted tubule (e.g., chlorothiazide, hydrochlorothiazide, metolazone, indapamide, and chlorthalidone); and (4) potassium-sparing diuretics, which block sodium reabsorption in the collecting duct. Potassium-sparing diuretics are available in two classes: (1) those that directly inhibit epithelial sodium channels (e.g., triamterene, amiloride) and (2) those that antagonize the mineralocorticoid type I receptor, inhibiting the effects of aldosterone (spironolactone and eplerenone).

Each type of diuretic is associated with potential adverse effects. For example, acetazolamide, a carbonic anhydrase inhibitor, may result in increased urinary excretion of sodium, potassium, and bicarbonate, leading to metabolic acidosis. As a result of this "adverse effect," it can be useful in treating alkalemia caused by other diuretics.

Metolazone is a thiazide-like diuretic that can elevate the serum calcium and uric acid levels. It can also result in hypokalemia and hypomagnesemia, particularly when utilized in combination with loop diuretics. Hydrochlorothiazide, which is in the same family as metolazone, can cause elevations in serum low-density lipoproteins and triglyceride levels.

Torsemide, like other loop diuretics, may cause ototoxicity. High doses of loop diuretics should be used cautiously in combination with aminoglycoside antibiotics due to an additive ototoxic effect.

The aldosterone antagonists may be associated with hyperkalemia, particularly in patients with renal insufficiency, owing to their inhibition of potassium excretion in the collecting duct. This side effect can be favorably exploited to help limit potassium wasting caused by loop diuretics. Spironolactone, in contrast to eplerenone, has potent antiandrogenic side effects and may be associated with gynecomastia in male patients.

ANSWERS TO QUESTIONS 270 TO 273

270–D, 271–B, 272–C, 273–E (Braunwald, pp. 765-768; Table 38G-11)

The preceding examples are all consistent with Class I (definite) indications for pacing, as recommended by the American College of Cardiology/American Heart Association/Heart Rhythm Society guidelines. In general, dual-chamber pacemakers should be used only in patients who require sensing or pacing of both the atria and the ventricles. Similarly, rate-modulating pacemakers should be used in patients with chronotropic incompetence due to abnormal or absent sinus node function.

In the 58-year-old man with tachycardia-bradycardia syndrome who developed symptomatic sinus bradycardia with beta-blocker therapy, the most appropriate pacemaker mode would be DDDR. Ventricular pacing is necessary here because there is a risk of atrioventricular (AV) block due to beta blockers, and the rate-modulating function is important because of the abnormal sinus node function. Use of a non–rate-responsive (DDD) pacemaker in this patient would most likely result in lower rate pacing most of the time, with inappropriate response to physical activity.

In the 70-year-old woman with atrial fibrillation who complains of dizziness and is found on examination to have a ventricular rate of 30 beats/min, VVIR pacing is most appropriate. Atrial sensing or pacing is not possible because of chronic atrial fibrillation, and the rate-modulating function is necessary because of the evident chronotropic dysfunction.

In the 62-year-old man with complete heart block after aortic valve surgery, there is no indication of sinus node disease and DDD pacing should be sufficient.

In the 45-year-old man with symptomatic sinoatrial exit block and junctional escape rhythm, loss of sinus mechanism requires atrial pacing and rate modulation. There is no evidence of AV block and ventricular pacing support is therefore not necessary, so the AAIR pacing mode is appropriate.

REFERENCE

Epstein AE, DiMarco JP, Ellenbogen KA, et al: ACC/AHA/HRS 2008 guidelines for device-based therapy for cardiac rhythm abnormalities: A report of the ACC/AHA Task Force on Practice Guidelines. Circulation 117:e350, 2008.

ANSWERS TO QUESTIONS 274 TO 277

274–D, 275–C, 276–A, 277–B (Braunwald, pp. 804-805, 1602, 1611-1618)

Multiple disease processes produce a clinical phenotype of dilated cardiomyopathy (DCM) with electrical instability. Sarcoidosis is a systemic inflammatory disease of unknown etiology that often has cardiac involvement. Patients with sarcoid often have concurrent thoracic lymphadenopathy, interstitial lung disease, and cardiomyopathy of variable severity accompanied by either heart block or ventricular tachycardia (VT). Although the identification of noncaseating granulomas on endomyocardial biopsy is necessary for definitive diagnosis, suggestive findings of cardiac inflammation may be apparent on cardiac magnetic resonance imaging and fluorodeoxyglucose positron emission tomography.

Giant cell myocarditis is notable for its rapidly progressive clinical course, widespread necrosis with giant cells on histology, and association with autoimmune disease and thymoma. Prompt diagnosis via endomyocardial biopsy along with early institution of mechanical circulatory support and immunosuppression is critical, because the prognosis is generally poor, with many cases progressing to cardiac transplant or death.

Chagas disease is caused by the protozoan parasite *Trypanosoma cruzi* endemic to Central and South America. A common noncardiac manifestation of Chagas disease is gastrointestinal dysmotility. Cardiac involvement is notable for conduction disease, an infarct pattern on the ECG, apical aneurysm formation often with mural thrombus, and VT. Chagas disease is a common cause of heart failure leading to transplantation in South America.

Arrhythmogenic right ventricular cardiomyopathy (ARVC) is a heritable disorder of the cardiac desmosome characterized by fibrofatty infiltration of the right ventricular myocardium. The hallmark of ARVC on the surface ECG (apparent in ~50% of cases) is a low-amplitude "notch" in the ST segment near the terminal portion of the QRS complex in the right precordial leads V_1 to V_3 (termed an *epsilon wave*). Additional electrocardiographic findings include right-sided T wave inversions and ventricular tachycardia with a left bundle branch block morphology indicating its origin in the right ventricle. The cardinal pathologic feature of ARVC, typically apparent on immunohistochemistry, is evidence of disruption in the desmosomes connecting cardiomyocytes, leading to abnormal cell-to-cell signaling and loss of structural integrity.

Cardiolaminopathy is a common cause of autosomal dominant familial DCM resulting from a mutation in the *LMNA* gene, encoding the nuclear envelope protein lamin A/C. The clinical course is highly variable, with typically subtle initial manifestations of conduction system disease (e.g., first-degree atrioventricular block) frequently delaying recognition until adulthood when more significant heart block or subsequent ventricular dysfunction become apparent.

REFERENCE

Lakdawala NK, Givertz MM: Dilated cardiomyopathy with conduction disease and arrhythmia. Circulation 122:527, 2010.

ANSWERS TO QUESTIONS 278 TO 282

278–C, 279–B, 280–A, 281–D, 282–E (Braunwald, pp. 885-888; Table 42-2)

The approach to the patient with syncope begins with a careful clinical history and physical examination, which can often suggest a specific cause. For example, syncope in patients with hypertrophic cardiomyopathy typically occurs with exertion, and examination may demonstrate the typical murmur associated with dynamic left ventricular outflow tract obstruction. Syncope with exertion is also typical of patients with the long QT syndrome (LQT1 in particular), aortic stenosis, pulmonary hypertension, mitral stenosis, coronary artery disease, and idiopathic ventricular tachycardia.

Patients with the subclavian steal syndrome may present with syncope after arm exercises. In this condition, atherosclerotic stenosis of a subclavian artery is present proximal to the origin of the vertebral artery. Retrograde blood flow through the ipsilateral vertebral artery, enhanced by exercise involving the affected arm, can induce cerebral ischemia. Auscultation over the supraclavicular fossa may demonstrate a bruit caused by the subclavian stenosis, and the blood pressure is usually diminished in the affected arm.

Vasovagal (neurocardiogenic) syncope occurs after a sudden unexpected pain, an unpleasant sight, sound, or smell, prolonged standing, or a stressful situation. This common form of syncope is characterized by the abrupt onset of hypotension with or without bradycardia.

In some individuals, carotid sinus hypersensitivity is manifest during stimulation of the carotid sinus baroreceptors. Syncopal events in patients with this disorder may be associated with head rotation or application of pressure to the carotid sinus with shaving or wearing tight shirt collars. The physiologic response to carotid hypersensitivity syndrome can be cardioinhibitory (e.g., marked bradycardia), vasodepressor (e.g., decrease in blood pressure in the absence of bradycardia), or mixed.

Left atrial myxoma is a rare cause of syncope. Symptoms may be positional as the tumor shifts and transiently obstructs the mitral orifice.

REFERENCE

Moya A, Sutton R, Ammirati F, et al: Guidelines for the diagnosis and management of syncope. The Task Force for the Diagnosis and Management of Syncope of the European Society of Cardiology (ESC). Eur Heart J 30:2631, 2009.

ANSWERS TO QUESTIONS 283 TO 286

283–C, 284–E, 285–A, 286–B (Braunwald, pp. 1836-1838)

Each of the conditions listed is associated with sustained increases in cardiac output that may precipitate heart failure in the appropriate clinical setting. Clinical findings in hyperthyroidism include constitutional changes such as nervousness, diaphoresis, heat intolerance, and fatigue, as well as cardiovascular manifestations such as palpitations, atrial fibrillation, and sinus tachycardia with a hyperkinetic heart action. Cardiovascular examination may reveal tachycardia, widened pulse pressure, brisk arterial pulsations, and a variety of findings associated with the hyperkinetic state. These may include a prominent S_1, the presence of an S_3 or S_4 or both, and a midsystolic murmur along the left sternal border secondary to increased flow. When a particularly hyperdynamic cardiac effect is seen, this murmur may have an unusual scratching component known as the *Means-Lerman*

scratch. This is thought to be caused by the rubbing together of normal pleural and pericardial surfaces.

Systemic arteriovenous (AV) fistulas may be acquired as a result of trauma, or they may be congenital. The increase in cardiac output that such lesions create is related to the size of the communication and the resultant reduction in the systemic vascular resistance that it promotes. In general, systemic AV fistulas lead to a widened pulse pressure, brisk arterial pulsations, and mild tachycardia. The *Nicoladoni-Branham sign,* defined as the slowing of heart rate after manual compression of the fistula, is commonly present. The maneuver may also raise arterial and lower venous pressure.

Osler-Weber-Rendu disease, or hereditary hemorrhagic telangiectasia, is an inherited condition that may be associated with AV fistulas, especially in the liver and the lungs. The disease may produce a hyperkinetic circulation with abdominal bruits and hepatomegaly due to intrahepatic AV connections.

Beriberi heart disease is a rare condition caused by severe thiamine deficiency that leads to impaired oxidative metabolism. It occurs most frequently in the Far East; in Western society, alcoholic cardiomyopathy may contribute to, or overlap with, this syndrome because of the tendency for alcoholics to become vitamin deficient. Patients with beriberi may present with a high-output state and severe generalized malnutrition. Typical findings include peripheral neuropathy with paresthesias of the extremities, decreased or absent knee and ankle jerks, hyperkeratinized skin lesions, and painful glossitis. The presence of edema characterizes "wet beriberi" and differentiates this condition from the "dry" form.

The carcinoid syndrome is an uncommon disease that results from the release of serotonin and other vasoactive substances by carcinoid tumors. Physical findings may include cutaneous flushing, telangiectasia, diarrhea, and bronchial constriction due to release of humoral mediators.

REFERENCE

Mehta PA, Dubrey SW: High output heart failure. QJM 102:235, 2009.

ANSWERS TO QUESTIONS 287 TO 290

287–A, 288–C, 289–B, 290–D (Braunwald, pp. 720-722)

Beta blockers are classified by their degree of cardioselectivity, that is, their ability to block the beta$_1$-adrenergic receptors in the heart compared with the beta$_2$-adrenergic receptors in the bronchi, peripheral blood vessels, and other sites. Beta blockers can be further classified into those that possess intrinsic sympathomimetic activity (ISA) versus those that do not. Beta blockers with ISA induce an agonist response but at the same time block the greater agonist effects of endogenous catecholamines. The result is to lower blood pressure similar to other beta blockers but to cause less bradycardia.

Acebutolol is a selective beta blocker with ISA. Atenolol, metoprolol, and esmolol are examples of selective beta blockers without ISA. Atenolol and nadolol are less lipid soluble than other beta blockers; as a result, they cause fewer central nervous system side effects.

Pindolol, carteolol, and penbutolol are nonselective beta blockers with ISA. Nadolol, propranolol, timolol, and sotalol are examples of nonselective beta blockers without ISA.

Carvedilol is a minimally beta$_1$-receptor selective agent that also expresses high affinity for alpha$_1$-adrenergic receptors and is used primarily in patients with heart failure. Because of its potent vasodilating property, orthostatic symptoms can occur and upward dose titration must be undertaken carefully.

ANSWERS TO QUESTIONS 291 TO 294

291–A, 292–C, 293–B, 294–B (Braunwald, pp. 495-496; Fig. 25-9)

Left ventricular mass increases in response to chronic pressure or volume overload or secondary to primary myocardial disease. With predominant pressure overload, as in aortic stenosis, there is an increase in mass with little change in chamber volume (concentric hypertrophy, as exemplified by patient A). In contrast, chronic volume overload (as in aortic or mitral regurgitation), or primary dilated cardiomyopathy, results in ventricular dilatation with only a small increase in wall thickness (eccentric hypertrophy). In chronic regurgitant disease (patient B), there is usually an increased stroke volume in the compensated state, whereas in cardiomyopathy there is impaired systolic function and a reduced stroke volume (patient C).

HEART FAILURE; ARRHYTHMIAS, SUDDEN DEATH, AND SYNCOPE

PREVENTIVE CARDIOLOGY; ATHEROSCLEROTIC CARDIOVASCULAR DISEASE

DIRECTIONS: For each below, select the ONE BEST response.

QUESTION 295

Each of the following statements regarding high-sensitivity C-reactive protein (hsCRP) is true EXCEPT:
A. Statins reduce hsCRP in a manner directly related to their low-density lipoprotein–lowering effect
B. An hsCRP level > 3 mg/L in a patient with unstable angina is associated with an increased risk of recurrent coronary events
C. An elevated level of hsCRP is predictive of the onset of type 2 diabetes mellitus
D. Statin therapy has been shown to reduce cardiovascular events in apparently healthy individuals with elevated hsCRP even if the baseline LDL-C is <130 mg/dL
E. The cardiovascular benefit of aspirin therapy appears to be greatest in patients with elevated hsCRP levels

QUESTION 296

All of the following interventions have a blood pressure–lowering effect EXCEPT:
A. A diet that reduces caloric intake by 1000 calories per day
B. Reduction of dietary sodium
C. Daily magnesium supplements
D. Tobacco cessation
E. Reduction of ethanol consumption to less than 1 oz (30 mL)/d

QUESTION 297

With respect to renovascular disease, all of the following statements are true EXCEPT:
A. Worsening renal function with angiotensin-converting enzyme inhibitor therapy suggests bilateral renovascular disease
B. Atherosclerotic disease most commonly involves the proximal third of the main renal artery

C. The most common form of fibroplastic renovascular disease in adults involves the media
D. The incidence of renovascular hypertension declines with increased age
E. Patients with severe, accelerated hypertension have the highest prevalence of renovascular disease

QUESTION 298

Each of the following statements regarding hypertension is true EXCEPT:
A. Pure "white coat" hypertension is found in 20% to 30% of patients
B. Renal parenchymal disease is the second most common cause of hypertension after essential hypertension
C. Pseudohypertension may occur in patients with sclerotic brachial arteries
D. When measuring the blood pressure, an inappropriately small cuff size results in a spuriously low systolic measurement
E. Coarctation of the aorta, Cushing disease, and pheochromocytoma together account for < 1% of all hypertensive patients

QUESTION 299

An asymptomatic 68-year-old man presents with newly diagnosed hypertension. The electrocardiogram (ECG) demonstrates left ventricular hypertrophy (LVH) with "strain" pattern. Which of the following statements is TRUE?
A. Electrocardiography is more sensitive than echocardiography for the detection of LVH
B. Hypertensive patients with LVH are more likely to develop heart failure than those without LVH
C. The presence of LVH is expected in hypertension and has no bearing on mortality rates
D. A beta-blocker such as atenolol reduces cardiovascular morbidity and mortality more than other pharmacologic agents in hypertensive patients with LVH
E. LVH is a compensatory protective mechanism that prevents further hypertensive damage to the heart

QUESTION 300

Each of the following statements regarding the association of oral contraceptive pills and hypertension is correct EXCEPT:
A. Among oral contraceptive users, the likelihood of developing hypertension is increased by alcohol consumption
B. The incidence of hypertension is about twice as great in pill users as in nonusers
C. The likelihood of developing hypertension is dependent on the age of the user
D. Hypertension resolves in the vast majority of patients after discontinuation of oral contraceptives
E. The mechanism for contraceptive-induced hypertension likely involves renin-aldosterone–mediated volume expansion

QUESTION 301

Each of the following statements regarding pheochromocytoma is true EXCEPT:
A. Approximately 15% of pheochromocytomas are extra-adrenal
B. Ten percent of pheochromocytomas are malignant
C. Ten percent of adrenal pheochromocytomas are bilateral
D. Hypertension related to pheochromocytoma only rarely causes chronic persistent hypertension
E. Multiple adrenal tumors are common in familial forms of pheochromocytoma

QUESTION 302

Each of the following statements regarding antihypertensive agents is true EXCEPT:
A. Pericardial effusions have been reported with the use of minoxidil
B. Flushing and tachycardia may result from hydralazine
C. More than 5% of patients taking an angiotensin-converting enzyme (ACE) inhibitor develop a cough
D. ACE inhibitor–induced cough reliably resolves within 3 days after discontinuation of the drug
E. Calcium channel blockers commonly result in ankle edema

QUESTION 303

Thiazide diuretics can contribute to each of the following metabolic effects EXCEPT:
A. Hypomagnesemia
B. Hypouricemia
C. Hypercalcemia
D. Hypercholesterolemia
E. Hyponatremia

QUESTION 304

Each of the following statements regarding the effects of HMG-CoA reductase inhibitors ("statins") is true EXCEPT:
A. The rate of cholesterol formation is decreased
B. Expression of hepatic low-density lipoprotein receptors is increased
C. Hepatic production of very low-density lipoprotein is decreased
D. Reversible elevation of serum hepatic transaminases develops in 10% of patients
E. Concurrent administration of erythromycin increases the risk of myositis

QUESTION 305

True statements regarding the effect of medications on the serum lipid profile include all of the following EXCEPT:
A. Nonselective beta-blockers increase high-density lipoprotein (HDL) levels
B. Thiazide diuretics increase triglyceride levels
C. Estrogen replacement therapy raises HDL and triglyceride levels
D. Immunosuppressive agents increase triglyceride levels
E. Protease inhibitors raise total cholesterol and triglyceride levels

QUESTION 306

True statements regarding genetic lipoprotein disorders include all of the following EXCEPT:
A. Patients with familial combined hyperlipidemia are at increased risk for coronary artery disease
B. Patients with familial hypertriglyceridemia typically develop xanthomas or xanthelasmas
C. Familial hypercholesterolemia results from mutations in the low-density lipoprotein receptor gene
D. Dysbetalipoproteinemia develops in patients who are homozygous for the apo E2 allele
E. Familial defective apo B100 is often clinically indistinguishable from familial hypercholesterolemia

QUESTION 307

All of the following statements regarding nicotinic acid are correct EXCEPT:
A. It acts primarily by reducing hepatic synthesis of very low-density lipoprotein and by reduction of free fatty acid release from tissues
B. It reduces low-density lipoprotein by 10% to 25% and triglycerides by 20% to 50%
C. It reduces serum levels of lipoprotein (a)
D. Hepatic toxicity is reduced by the use of sustained-release forms
E. Preadministration of aspirin reduces flushing

QUESTION 308

True statements about apolipoproteins include all of the following EXCEPT:
A. Apo AI is a major component of high-density lipoprotein
B. Combined AI/CIII deficiency is a genetic disorder associated with premature atherosclerosis
C. Apo B48, synthesized by the small intestine, and apo B100, secreted by the liver, are synthesized by two distinct genes
D. Apo B100 is the major apoprotein in low-density lipoproteins
E. Type III hyperlipoproteinemia is a disorder of apoprotein E

QUESTION 309

Each of the following statements regarding hypertriglyceridemia is true EXCEPT:
A. Hypertriglyceridemia is associated with diabetes mellitus, chronic renal failure, and obesity
B. Cigarette smoking and excessive alcohol consumption are associated with secondary hypertriglyceridemia
C. In epidemiologic studies, adjustment for high-density lipoprotein levels and other factors diminishes the role of hypertriglyceridemia as an independent predictor of coronary artery disease
D. There is a stronger relationship between hypertriglyceridemia and cardiovascular risk in women than in men
E. The addition of fenofibrate to simvastatin lowers triglyceride levels and has been shown to reduce major coronary events in type 2 diabetic patients, compared with simvastatin alone

QUESTION 310

Each of the following statements regarding lipoprotein (a) [Lp(a)] is true EXCEPT:
A. One component of Lp(a) is structurally identical to low-density lipoprotein and another is similar to plasminogen
B. Lp(a) levels do not vary significantly between racial groups
C. Lp(a) levels vary little with changes in dietary fat intake
D. Observational studies have associated elevated Lp(a) levels with cardiovascular events
E. Nicotinic acid lowers serum levels of Lp(a)

QUESTION 311

True statements regarding lipid-lowering medications include each of the following EXCEPT:
A. Fibric acid derivatives lower triglycerides, raise high-density lipoprotein (HDL) levels, and may increase LDL cholesterol levels
B. Fish oil therapy raises triglyceride levels
C. Niacin, administered in doses 200 times the recommended daily allowance, raises HDL levels
D. Other medications should not be taken within 1 hour before or within 3 hours after taking a bile acid–binding resin
E. Ezetimibe selectively inhibits cholesterol uptake by intestinal epithelial cells and significantly lowers the circulating low-density lipoprotein cholesterol level

QUESTION 312

Each of the following statements regarding hypertension is true EXCEPT:
A. The prevalence of hypertension in the United States rises progressively with age in both men and women
B. Systolic and diastolic hypertension are each associated with an increased risk of coronary heart disease
C. Drug therapy for hypertension benefits patients older than 80 years of age
D. Patients with prehypertension (systolic 120 to 139 mm Hg or diastolic 80 to 89 mm Hg) benefit from lifestyle modifications, including weight reduction, regular exercise, and smoking cessation
E. The target blood pressure for hypertensive patients with cardiovascular disease or diabetes is <140/90 mm Hg

QUESTION 313

Which of the following statements regarding the secondary prevention of stroke is correct?
A. Clopidogrel monotherapy is superior to aspirin plus dipyridamole for secondary prevention of noncardioembolic stroke
B. Hypertension should not be a target of secondary prevention after an ischemic stroke because elevated blood pressure is necessary to maintain adequate cerebral perfusion
C. Treatment with HMG-CoA reductase inhibitors reduces the risk of recurrent stroke
D. The combination of aspirin plus clopidogrel is superior to aspirin alone for prevention of recurrent stroke
E. Compared with aspirin alone, chronic warfarin therapy reduces the risk of recurrent stroke

QUESTION 314

All of the following statements are true regarding the relationship between alcohol and coronary artery disease EXCEPT:
A. Moderate alcohol intake (1 or 2 drinks daily) is associated with a lower incidence of coronary heart disease than is no alcohol intake
B. Alcohol consumption reduces platelet aggregation
C. Heavy alcohol intake is associated with increased cardiovascular mortality
D. Alcohol lowers low-density lipoprotein levels
E. Alcohol raises high-density lipoprotein levels

QUESTION 315

Each of the following statements regarding smoking cessation is correct EXCEPT:
A. Smoking cessation reduces coronary heart disease mortality by more than 35% compared with patients who continue to smoke
B. Patients who continue to smoke after a myocardial infarction have twice the mortality rate of those who stop smoking
C. Patients who successfully quit usually do so after five or more unsuccessful attempts
D. Physician counseling alone is as effective as pharmacologic aids in achieving smoking cessation
E. Varenicline is more efficacious than placebo or bupropion at achieving continuous abstinence

QUESTION 316

All of the following statements regarding exercise training and rehabilitation of patients with coronary artery disease are true EXCEPT:
A. Home programs should emphasize exercise to the onset of mild dyspnea, because many patients cannot adequately monitor their heart rates during activity
B. Augmented cardiac output during exercise is due more to an increase in heart rate than in stroke volume
C. During exercise, increased myocardial oxygen supply is provided more by a rise in coronary blood flow than by augmented oxygen extraction
D. Despite achieving improvements in physical capacity there is no evidence that exercise-based cardiac rehabilitation improves mortality rates
E. Approximately half of the improvement in exercise performance with physical training is due to increased cardiac output and half to peripheral adaptations that improve tissue oxygen extraction

QUESTION 317

All of the following statements regarding homocysteine are true EXCEPT:
A. Inherited defects of methionine metabolism may cause extremely high serum levels of homocysteine and premature atherothrombosis
B. Polymorphisms in the methylene tetrahydrofolate reductase gene are associated with elevated homocysteine levels
C. Epidemiologic studies have linked mild hyperhomocystinemia with an increased risk of coronary events
D. Folic acid and other vitamin B supplements reduce serum homocysteine levels
E. Dietary supplementation with a combination of B vitamins (folic acid, B_6 and B_{12}) reduces the risk of atherothrombotic events

QUESTION 318

Each of the following is a component of the atherogenic "metabolic syndrome" EXCEPT:
A. Hyperglycemia
B. Elevated serum triglycerides
C. Abdominal obesity
D. Serum low-density lipoprotein > 140 mg/dL
E. Hypertension

QUESTION 319

A 52-year-old woman presents for routine outpatient management. She is interested in nonpharmacologic approaches to tobacco cessation and blood pressure reduction. Which of the following statements is TRUE?
A. Acupuncture is an effective modality to achieve smoking cessation
B. Hypnotherapy has established long-term effectiveness in smoking cessation
C. Hypnotherapy provides no benefit in lowering blood pressure
D. Regular adherence to qigong (Chinese meditative practice using slow graceful movements and controlled breathing) reduces blood pressure
E. The practice of yoga substantially reduces blood pressure, equivalent to the effect of dual antihypertensive drug therapy

QUESTION 320

Clinical trials of each of the following dietary interventions have shown significant improvements in coronary artery disease endpoints EXCEPT:
A. Cholesterol-lowering diet rich in polyunsaturated fats
B. Mediterranean-style diet supplemented with alpha-linolenic acid
C. Very low-fat diet
D. Low-carbohydrate, high-protein, high-fat diet (e.g., Atkins-style diet)
E. Increased omega-3 fatty acid diet

QUESTION 321

Each of the following statements about pharmacologic therapy for secondary prevention of coronary artery disease is correct EXCEPT:
A. Long-term aspirin use after myocardial infarction (MI) reduces cardiovascular mortality, re-infarction, and stroke rates
B. After MI, beta-blocker use reduces mortality by 30% to 40% over the next 2 to 3 years
C. Angiotensin-converting enzyme inhibitors administered after MI confer a mortality reduction only in patients with left ventricular dysfunction
D. Administration of HMG-CoA reductase inhibitors reduces cardiovascular deaths after MI in patients with average cholesterol levels

E. After an acute MI, intensive lipid-lowering with a high-dose statin confers improved clinical outcomes compared with only moderate lipid lowering

QUESTION 322

Each of the following statements regarding heterozygous familial hypercholesterolemia is correct EXCEPT:
A. It is a relatively common disorder with a gene frequency of 1 in 500 persons in the population
B. Tendon xanthomas and arcus corneae are common but nonspecific findings
C. It is inherited as a recessive trait
D. Cutaneous planar xanthomas occur only in homozygotes
E. The fundamental defect is the presence of only half of the normal number of low-density lipoprotein surface receptors

QUESTION 323

All of the following are characteristics of familial hypertriglyceridemia EXCEPT:
A. Plasma low-density lipoprotein is usually low
B. Plasma triglyceride levels can exceed 1000 mg/dL after a meal
C. Plasma high-density lipoprotein cholesterol is usually reduced
D. It is accompanied by a fivefold increased incidence of atherosclerosis
E. Hypertriglyceridemia is usually not manifest until puberty or early adulthood

QUESTION 324

Each of the following statements about coronary stent thrombosis is correct EXCEPT:
A. The strongest predictor of late stent thrombosis is premature discontinuation of dual antiplatelet therapy
B. Stent thrombosis has been reported to occur more than a year after the placement of drug-eluting stents
C. Implantation of a drug-eluting stent should be avoided in a patient for whom noncardiac surgery is planned within 12 months
D. Stent thrombosis is associated with a mortality rate of 5% to 10%
E. Late stent thrombosis is more likely to occur in individuals with diabetes or renal failure than in patients without these conditions

QUESTION 325

A 60-year-old man was admitted to the hospital with an acute anterior myocardial infarction (MI). He underwent urgent catheterization and successful reperfusion was achieved after a complex coronary angioplasty with stent placement. The patient's hospital course was complicated by rising serum creatinine and urea nitrogen

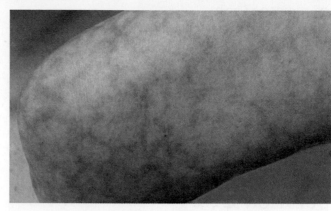

FIGURE 3-1 From Firestein: Kelley's Textbook of Rheumatology. 8th ed. Philadelphia, Elsevier Saunders, 2008.

levels. In addition, a purple, net-like discoloration developed on his lower extremities (Fig. 3-1). Each of the following statements is correct EXCEPT:
A. These findings likely resulted from the catheterization procedure rather than from the presenting MI
B. The urinalysis likely reveals an active sediment with cells and casts
C. A low serum complement level is common
D. Transient eosinophilia may be part of this syndrome
E. Progression to end-stage renal failure may follow

QUESTION 326

Correct statements with respect to low-density lipoprotein (LDL) include all the following EXCEPT:
A. LDL is the major cholesterol-carrying components of plasma
B. Apo AI is the dominant protein present in LDL
C. LDL is formed mainly from metabolism of very low-density lipoprotein (VLDL)
D. The major lipid components of LDL are triglyceride and esterified cholesterol
E. The minority of patients with elevated LDL levels have familial hypercholesterolemia

QUESTION 327

All the following statements about the Heart Protection Study (HPS) are true EXCEPT:
A. The HPS enrolled patients with, or at increased risk of, coronary artery disease
B. Simvastatin treatment was associated with a 24% relative risk reduction in cardiovascular events
C. The mortality benefit of simvastatin was only seen in patients with low-density lipoprotein cholesterol levels > 125 mg/dL
D. Patients enrolled in the HPS would not have met existing criteria for lipid-lowering therapy
E. The HPS found no benefit of antioxidant vitamins in preventing cardiovascular events

QUESTION 328

All of the following are features of renovascular hypertension due to fibromuscular hyperplasia, as opposed to atherosclerosis EXCEPT:
A. Age typically < 50 years
B. Female gender
C. No family history of hypertension
D. Progression more likely to complete renal artery occlusion
E. Absence of carotid bruits

QUESTION 329

A newly diagnosed diabetic patient presents with multiple blood pressure (BP) readings that are 155/95 mm Hg or higher. All of the following statements about treatment of this patient's hypertension are correct EXCEPT:
A. Current guidelines recommend BP <130/80 in diabetics
B. Control of BP reduces cardiovascular event rates more in diabetics than in nondiabetics
C. Pharmacologic blockade of the renin-angiotensin system reduces the risk of both microvascular and macrovascular events
D. Antihypertensive therapy with dihydropyridine calcium channel blockers reduces cardiovascular event rates
E. Aggressive BP control (target systolic BP < 120 mm Hg) in diabetics has been shown to reduce cardiovascular event rates compared with a target systolic BP <140 mm Hg

QUESTION 330

True statements regarding the clinical history of patients with acute myocardial infarction (MI) include all of the following EXCEPT:
A. A clear precipitating factor or prodromal symptoms can be identified in 90% of patients with acute MI
B. Between 20% and 60% of nonfatal MIs are unrecognized by the patient and are identified only by a subsequent routine ECG
C. One third of patients with an MI prodrome have had symptoms for 1 to 4 weeks before hospitalization
D. Patients who report a high level of stress after an acute coronary syndrome have an increased risk of subsequent MI
E. The peak frequency of MI onset is between 6 AM and noon

QUESTION 331

Each of the following statements regarding the use of percutaneous coronary intervention (PCI) as a primary therapy in acute myocardial infarction (MI) is true EXCEPT:
A. PCI is associated with lower rates of intracranial hemorrhage than thrombolysis
B. The primary success rate for PCI during acute MI is approximately 90%
C. In trials comparing primary PCI with thrombolysis, patients randomized to primary PCI had a lower incidence of death or re-infarction by hospital discharge and at 6-month follow-up
D. Primary PCI is associated with a worse outcome compared with thrombolysis for acute MI patients presenting with cardiogenic shock
E. When performed in experienced centers, hospital length of stay and follow-up costs are significantly less than for patients treated with thrombolysis

QUESTION 332

True statements about atrial infarction include all of the following EXCEPT:
A. Atrial infarction is found in < 20% of autopsy-proven cases of myocardial infarction
B. Atrial infarction typically occurs in conjunction with left ventricular infarction
C. Rupture of the atrial wall is a recognized complication
D. Atrial infarction commonly leads to supraventricular arrhythmias
E. Infarction of the left atrium occurs more commonly than infarction of the right atrium

QUESTION 333

True statements regarding ventricular free wall rupture complicating myocardial infarction (MI) include all of the following EXCEPT:
A. It is more likely to occur in patients with a history of prior MI
B. It typically occurs within the first 4 days after infarction
C. It occurs in approximately 2% of patients with MI
D. It is more common in elderly patients and in women
E. A history of hypertension is a risk factor for free wall rupture

QUESTION 334

True statements about right ventricular infarction (RVI) include all of the following EXCEPT:
A. RVI may result in Kussmaul's sign
B. ST-segment elevation in lead V_4 is commonly present
C. Echocardiography typically demonstrates right ventricular enlargement and hypokinesis
D. A marked hypotensive response to nitroglycerin administration is consistent with this diagnosis
E. Atrioventricular sequential pacing offers greater hemodynamic benefit than single-chamber ventricular pacing in patients with RVI

QUESTION 335

A 60-year-old man is admitted to the coronary care unit after 14 hours of chest pain that had resolved by the time of hospital presentation. The initial ECG reveals 0.5 mm ST-segment elevations with T wave inversions and pathologic Q waves in leads II, III, and aVF. The initial cardiac examination is unremarkable. On the second day, a faint late systolic murmur is heard at the apex, and by the third day this murmur has increased to grade 3/6. The patient has mild dyspnea, and a chest radiogram shows pulmonary vascular redistribution. The most likely explanation for the murmur is:
A. Ruptured posterior papillary muscle
B. Ruptured anterior papillary muscle
C. Infarcted posterior papillary muscle
D. Infarcted anterior papillary muscle
E. Ruptured chordae tendineae

QUESTION 336

True statements about pericarditis and pericardial effusion in the setting of acute myocardial infarction (MI) include all of the following EXCEPT:
A. Post-MI pericardial effusions are found most often in patients with larger infarcts, in those with congestive heart failure, and in the setting of an anterior wall MI
B. When it arises, early post-MI pericarditis typically manifests between the first and second weeks after an acute MI
C. When present, Dressler syndrome manifests 2 to 10 weeks after infarction
D. Modern therapy of MI has been associated with a decreased incidence of Dressler syndrome
E. Tamponade due to pericarditis in the setting of acute MI is uncommon

QUESTION 337

True statements about conduction disturbances in acute myocardial infarction (MI) include all of the following EXCEPT:
A. Most patients with acute MI and first-degree atrioventricular (AV) block have an intranodal conduction disturbance
B. Sinus bradycardia in acute MI often results from increased vagal tone
C. Of patients with acute MI and second-degree AV block, the majority have Mobitz type I (Wenckebach) block
D. Mobitz type II second-degree AV block occurs more commonly in anterior infarction than in inferior infarction
E. In patients with anterior infarction who develop third-degree AV block, the conduction disturbance almost always appears without prior intraventricular conduction abnormalities

QUESTION 338

True statements regarding the use of fibrinolytic therapy in acute myocardial infarction (MI) include all of the following EXCEPT:
A. Fibrinolytic therapy reduces the mortality of ST-segment elevation MI by 15% to 20% at 1 month
B. Compared with patients with anterior ST-segment elevation, those who present with a bundle branch block have a similar risk reduction with fibrinolytic therapy
C. Compared with patients with anterior ST-segment elevation, patients with inferior ST-segment elevation demonstrate a greater risk reduction with fibrinolytic therapy
D. Clinical trial data demonstrate no mortality benefit of fibrinolysis administered more than 12 hours after the onset of symptoms
E. Patients older than age 75 years experience an absolute reduction in mortality similar to that of patients younger than 55 years

QUESTION 339

True statements regarding acute coronary syndromes that are not treated with acute reperfusion strategies include all of the following EXCEPT:
A. Occlusive coronary thrombosis is typically responsible for ST-segment elevations
B. Q waves develop in approximately 75% of patients with ST-segment elevation myocardial infarction
C. The presence of pathologic Q waves reliably indicates the transmural involvement of myocardial infarction
D. Nonocclusive coronary thrombosis typically results in ST-segment depressions and/or T wave inversions

QUESTION 340

True statements regarding catheter-based reperfusion therapy in acute myocardial infarction, performed by experienced operators, include all of the following EXCEPT:
A. Primary angioplasty results in higher coronary artery patency rates than fibrinolysis
B. Primary angioplasty results in lower mortality than fibrinolysis
C. Primary angioplasty results in lower stroke rates than fibrinolysis
D. Primary stenting compared with angioplasty reduces mortality and recurrent infarction
E. Stenting in acute myocardial infarction decreases the need for subsequent target vessel revascularization

QUESTION 341

Each of the following statements about left ventricular (LV) aneurysm after myocardial infarction (MI) is correct EXCEPT:
A. LV aneurysm complicating acute MI is usually due to total occlusion of the left anterior descending artery

B. Aneurysms typically range from 1 to 8 cm in diameter
C. Inferoposterior aneurysms are more common than apical aneurysms
D. The presence of an aneurysm increases the mortality rate compared with patients with similar ejection fractions without an aneurysm
E. Persistent ST-segment elevation on the ECG does not necessarily indicate aneurysm formation

A. This rhythm confers a significant increase in mortality
B. This rhythm is observed in up to 20% of patients with acute MI
C. It often occurs as a result of slowing of the sinus rhythm
D. Approximately 50% of such episodes are initiated by a premature beat
E. This is the most common arrhythmia after reperfusion by fibrinolytic therapy

QUESTION 342

The rhythm shown in Figure 3-2 developed in a 72-year-old man on the second day of hospitalization for an acute ST-segment elevation myocardial infarction (STEMI). Each of the following statements is correct EXCEPT:
A. The presence of this rhythm in STEMI is associated with increased mortality
B. This rhythm may result from left ventricular failure, pericarditis, or left atrial ischemia in the setting of STEMI
C. If associated with hemodynamic compromise, it should be treated by immediate electrical conversion
D. This rhythm tends to be persistent, rather than transient, in the setting of acute STEMI
E. Treatment with an angiotensin-converting enzyme inhibitor reduces the incidence of this rhythm in acute STEMI

QUESTION 344

Each of the following statements concerning the utility of cardiac biomarkers in patients with acute coronary syndromes is correct EXCEPT:
A. Levels of C-reactive protein (CRP) are greatly elevated in patients with an acute coronary syndrome (ACS) compared with patients with stable coronary disease
B. CRP and cardiac-specific troponin levels offer complementary information in the prognosis of patients with ACS
C. In patients with unstable angina, an elevated myeloperoxidase level is associated with increased risk of death
D. Patients with elevated levels of B-type natriuretic peptide have a twofold to threefold increased risk of adverse events
E. Patients with non–ST-elevation MI and elevated white blood cell (WBC) counts have similar mortality rates as those with normal WBC counts

QUESTION 343

Each of the following statements about the arrhythmia illustrated in Figure 3-3, observed in the setting of an acute myocardial infarction (MI), is correct EXCEPT:

QUESTION 345

A 45-year-old man with elevated low-density lipoprotein cholesterol (LDL), hypertension, and a family history of premature coronary disease presents to his physician's

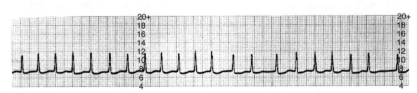

FIGURE 3-2

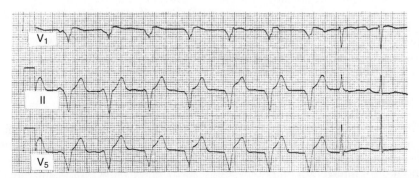

FIGURE 3-3

office for routine evaluation. He does not have diabetes. He smokes 1 pack of cigarettes per day and is exploring means to quit. He also has a history of supraventricular tachycardia that has been successfully suppressed by verapamil, after not tolerating a beta blocker. He is currently taking simvastatin, 20 mg daily, verapamil, sustained-release 180 mg daily, and aspirin, 81 mg daily. His blood pressure is 128/70 mm Hg. Laboratory studies include total cholesterol, 240 mg/dL; HDL cholesterol, 40 mg/dL; LDL cholesterol, 166 mg dL; and triglycerides, 170 mg/dL. The hepatic transaminase levels are normal. Which of the following is the appropriate recommendation regarding lipid-altering therapy?

A. He does not have active coronary artery disease—no further adjustment in medication is required
B. Simvastatin should be increased to 40 mg daily
C. Simvastatin should be increased to 80 mg daily
D. Simvastatin should be transitioned to a higher-potency statin
E. Gemfibrozil should be added

QUESTION 346

True statements about the progression of atherosclerosis after coronary artery bypass graft (CABG) surgery include all of the following EXCEPT:

A. Between 12% and 20% of vein grafts are occluded by the end of the first year after CABG
B. The annual rate of saphenous vein graft occlusion between years 2 through 5 after CABG is about 2%
C. At 10 years, the overall occlusion rate for a saphenous vein graft approaches 50%
D. The atherosclerotic process that occurs in venous grafts is histologically different from that which occurs in native arterial vessels
E. Progression of disease in native coronary arteries occurs at a rate of 18% to 38% over the first decade after operation

QUESTION 347

All of the following statements regarding myocardial stunning are true EXCEPT:

A. Stunning is a state of depressed myocardial function due to chronic hypoperfusion
B. Stunning can be global or regional
C. Stunning can follow cardiac surgery with cardiopulmonary bypass
D. Oxygen free radicals and excess intracellular calcium likely contribute to stunning
E. Stunning affects both systolic and diastolic function

QUESTION 348

Each of the following statements regarding antithrombotic therapies in the treatment of unstable angina is correct EXCEPT:

A. Aspirin reduces the incidence of cardiovascular death and nonfatal myocardial infarction (MI)

B. The combination of aspirin and unfractionated heparin is superior to aspirin alone in prevention of death and nonfatal MI
C. The early beneficial cardiac outcome effects of clopidogrel in acute coronary syndromes persist for 12 months after hospital discharge
D. Acute treatment with the low-molecular-weight heparin enoxaparin has been shown to be superior to unfractionated heparin in reducing the rate of death, nonfatal MI, and recurrent ischemia
E. Compared with enoxaparin, treatment of acute coronary syndromes with the factor Xa inhibitor fondaparinux results in excess major bleeding

QUESTION 349

True statements regarding coronary collateral circulation include all of the following EXCEPT:

A. Preexisting collateral vessels open immediately after coronary occlusion
B. Increased flow through preexisting collateral vessels triggers a maturation process that produces a vessel nearly indistinguishable structurally from a normal coronary artery
C. Exercise does not increase collateral circulation formation
D. Collateral vessels can provide nearly as much blood flow as the native coronary circulation
E. In the setting of an acute myocardial infarction (MI), the presence of preexisting collateral vessels decreases infarct size and improves survival

QUESTION 350

All of the following statements regarding medical therapy versus percutaneous coronary intervention (PCI) for chronic stable angina are correct EXCEPT:

A. PCI results in greater symptomatic relief than does medical therapy
B. In patients with severe proximal left anterior descending artery stenoses, PCI is superior to medical therapy for reduction of exercise-induced ischemia
C. PCI is superior to medical therapy alone in reducing cardiovascular mortality in patients with chronic stable angina
D. In patients with stable angina and one- to two-vessel coronary artery disease, aggressive lipid lowering (atorvastatin, 80 mg daily) without PCI leads to fewer ischemic events than a strategy of PCI plus less intense lipid lowering

QUESTION 351

True statements regarding the surgical management of abdominal aortic aneurysms include all of the following EXCEPT:

A. Large aneurysms enlarge faster than smaller ones
B. Aortic aneurysms grow and rupture at similar rates in men and women

C. Aneurysms > 5.5 cm in diameter should undergo surgical repair

D. In men, surgical repair of aneurysms with diameters of 4.0 to 5.5 cm offers no mortality benefit over continued surveillance

E. With aneurysmal rupture, 60% of patients die before reaching the hospital

QUESTION 352

All of the following statements regarding the abnormality in Figure 3-4 are correct EXCEPT:

A. Without treatment, mortality exceeds 25% in the first 24 hours

B. Outcomes with surgical repair is superior to pharmacologic therapy in the management of this condition when it occurs proximally

C. Initial pharmacologic therapy without surgery is recommended when this condition is distal in location and uncomplicated

D. Aortic valve replacement is universally required when there is accompanying aortic regurgitation

E. Labetalol is an appropriate initial agent to lower arterial pressure in patients with this condition

QUESTION 353

A 65-year-old man with cirrhosis and chronic stable angina presents to the cardiovascular clinic for evaluation. He describes typical angina climbing one flight of stairs, despite beta-blocker and long-acting nitrate therapies. Stress testing with nuclear perfusion imaging confirms exercise-induced reversible ischemia of the anterior left ventricular wall; the left ventricular (LV) ejection fraction is 50%. Coronary angiography reveals a long occlusion of the left anterior descending artery in its mid

segment with collateral perfusion to the distal vessel from the right coronary artery. The lesion is not amenable to percutaneous intervention. You are hesitant to increase the beta-blocker and nitrate dosages because his resting heart rate is 50 beats/min and the blood pressure is 102/78 mm Hg. Which of the following statements is correct?

A. Ranolazine would decrease the blood pressure and heart rate further and should be avoided

B. Ranolazine does not offer incremental antianginal benefit to patients already taking beta-blocker, long-acting nitrate, or calcium channel blocker therapies

C. Compared with placebo, ranolazine increases the risk of torsades de pointes

D. Ranolazine is metabolized in the liver and it should be avoided in this patient

E. The most common side effect of ranolazine is diarrhea

QUESTION 354

True statements regarding the abnormality labeled "A" in Figure 3-5 include all of the following EXCEPT:

A. The majority are asymptomatic

B. Physical examination tends to overestimate the size

C. Ultrasonography and computed tomography are highly accurate means to quantitate the size

D. Although magnetic resonance angiography can define the size, it cannot accurately determine the proximal extent of disease

E. The mean rate of expansion is approximately 0.4 cm per year

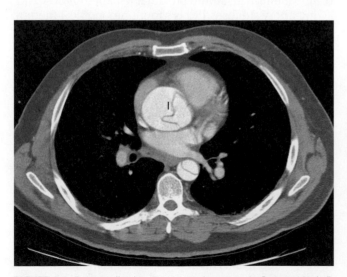

FIGURE 3-4 From Isselbacher EM: Aortic dissection. *In* Creager MA (ed): Atlas of Vascular Disease. 2nd ed. Philadelphia, Current Medicine, 2003.

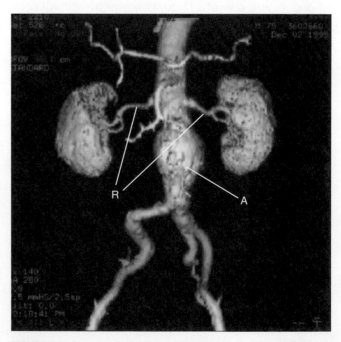

FIGURE 3-5 Courtesy of John A. Kaufman, MD, Division of Vascular Radiology, Massachusetts General Hospital, Boston.

QUESTION 355

All of the following statements regarding the use of platelet glycoprotein (GP) IIb/IIIa inhibitors in percutaneous coronary intervention procedures are correct EXCEPT:
A. They decrease the need for urgent revascularization over the next 30 days
B. They decrease the rate of subsequent myocardial infarction
C. The major reduction of clinical events with GP IIb/IIIa inhibitors occurs within the first 48 hours
D. Reductions in cardiac ischemic events observed with GP IIb/IIIa inhibition continue to accrue over the month after the acute intervention
E. For patients with acute ST-segment elevation myocardial infarction who have received aspirin plus clopidogrel there is no significant benefit of routine GP IIb/IIIa inhibitor administration before transport to the catheterization laboratory

QUESTION 356

All of the following statements regarding Prinzmetal (variant) angina are true EXCEPT:
A. The majority of coronary sites that manifest focal vasospasm have evidence of underlying atherosclerosis
B. Nitrates are useful in treating and preventing attacks of Prinzmetal angina
C. Calcium channel blockers are useful in treating and preventing attacks of Prinzmetal angina
D. Provocative testing is indicated in patients with nonobstructive lesions on coronary angiography, a clinical picture consistent with vasospasm, and documented transient ST-segment elevations on electrocardiography
E. Patients with Prinzmetal angina have a rate of sudden cardiac death of < 5% at 5 years

QUESTION 357

True statements about the condition shown in Figure 3-6 include all of the following EXCEPT:
A. The most common cause is surgical manipulation of an atherosclerotic aorta
B. Cardiac catheterization may lead to this condition
C. Hepatitis is an important complication of this disorder
D. Stigmata of this disorder may be visible on direct inspection of the retinal arteries
E. Livedo reticularis is a recognized manifestation

QUESTION 358

True statements regarding nitric oxide (NO) include all of the following EXCEPT:
A. NO production by endothelial cells is augmented by hypoxia, thrombin, and adenosine diphosphate
B. In atherosclerotic vessels, acetylcholine causes unopposed smooth muscle constriction

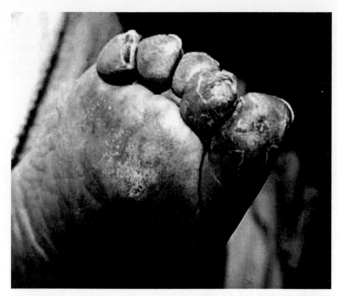

FIGURE 3-6 Modified from Beckman JA, Creager MA: *In* Creager MA, Dzau VJ, Loscalzo J (eds): Vascular Medicine: A Companion to Braunwald's Heart Disease. Philadelphia, Elsevier, 2006, p 259.

C. NO is formed in endothelial cells by the actions of NO synthase on the substrate L-arginine
D. NO stimulates increased cyclic adenosine monophosphate formation in vascular smooth muscle cells
E. The vasodilatory effects of nitroglycerin and prostacyclin are independent of endothelial NO production

QUESTION 359

All of the following statements regarding aortic intramural hematoma are true EXCEPT:
A. This condition results from an intimal tear in the aorta
B. A history of hypertension and aortic atherosclerosis is typical
C. Computed tomography is more sensitive than aortography for diagnosis
D. Intramural hematomas of the descending aorta have a more favorable prognosis than those in the ascending aorta
E. Symptoms are indistinguishable from those of classic aortic dissection

QUESTION 360

The following statements regarding low-molecular-weight heparins are correct EXCEPT:
A. They possess greater anti–factor Xa activity than anti–factor IIa activity
B. They cause significant elevations in the activated partial thromboplastin time, which is useful for monitoring the anticoagulant effect
C. Their clearance is affected by renal impairment
D. They are not neutralized by platelet factor 4
E. They are contraindicated in patients with type II heparin-induced thrombocytopenia

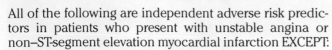

QUESTION 361

All of the following are independent adverse risk predictors in patients who present with unstable angina or non–ST-segment elevation myocardial infarction EXCEPT:
A. Increased cardiac troponin level
B. ST-segment deviation ≥ 0.05 mV
C. Diabetes mellitus
D. Lack of prior aspirin use
E. Increased C-reactive protein level

QUESTION 362

Each of the following statements regarding the epidemiology and pathophysiology of peripheral arterial disease (PAD) is correct EXCEPT:
A. The prevalence of PAD is more than 20% in patients older than 75 years
B. Dyslipidemia is a more powerful risk factor than cigarette smoking
C. Claudication symptoms are present in only 10% to 30% of patients with PAD
D. PAD tends to develop at arterial branch points
E. The earliest site of fatty streak and atheroma development is in the abdominal aorta

QUESTION 363

Each of the following statements about the clinical manifestations of aortic dissection is correct EXCEPT:
A. Men are more frequently affected than women
B. Severe pain is the most common presenting symptom
C. Patients with aortic dissection usually present with hypotension
D. Aortic regurgitation is more common in proximal aortic dissection than in distal dissection
E. Pulse deficits are more common in proximal than in distal aortic dissection

QUESTION 364

Each of the following statements about patients with peripheral arterial disease (PAD) is correct EXCEPT:
A. Intermittent claudication is characterized by pain precipitated by walking as well as by standing upright for several minutes
B. On examination, arterial bruits, diminished distal pulses, and hair loss of the affected extremity are common
C. Segmental pressure measurements demonstrate gradients of >20 mm Hg in the lower extremities or >10 mm Hg in the upper extremities
D. The ankle/brachial index is frequently < 1.0
E. Magnetic resonance angiography is >90% sensitive and specific for the diagnosis of PAD in the aorta, iliac, femoral-popliteal, and tibial-peroneal arteries

QUESTION 365

Each of the following statements regarding anticoagulation therapy in percutaneous coronary intervention (PCI) procedures is true EXCEPT:
A. Routine administration of intravenous unfractionated heparin (UFH) after PCI procedures results in a reduced number of ischemic complications
B. In patients pretreated with clopidogrel, bivalirudin is associated with a lower rate of major bleeding complications than UFH but no difference in ischemic complications
C. Clinical outcomes are similar for patients treated with fixed-dose UFH or weight-adjusted UFH during PCI
D. In conjunction with platelet glycoprotein IIb/IIIa inhibitor therapy, standard-dose UFH results in a similar rate of ischemic complications but a higher rate of hemorrhagic complications when compared with low-dose UFH
E. No additional anticoagulation is required during PCI if a patient has received a dose of the low-molecular-weight heparin enoxaparin within the previous 8 hours

QUESTION 366

Each of the following statements regarding nitrates in ischemic heart disease is correct EXCEPT:
A. Nitrates directly relax vascular smooth muscle
B. The vasodilator effects of nitrates predominate in the venous circulation
C. Coronary arteries containing significant atherosclerotic plaque often dilate in response to nitrates
D. N-acetylcysteine may counteract tolerance to long-term nitroglycerin therapy
E. An intact endothelium is required for nitrate-induced vasodilatation

QUESTION 367

All of the following statements regarding glycoprotein (GP) IIb/IIIa inhibitors are true EXCEPT:
A. Abciximab administration before transport to the cardiac catheterization laboratory reduces ischemic complications in patients with ST-segment elevation myocardial infarction pretreated with clopidogrel who undergo percutaneous intervention
B. Eptifibatide is a cyclic heptapeptide related to pygmy rattlesnake venom
C. Tirofiban has a half-life of approximately 2 hours
D. GP IIb/IIIa inhibitors should be administered with heparin
E. Human antichimeric antibodies develop in approximately 5% of patients treated with abciximab

QUESTION 368

All of the following statements about atherosclerotic renal artery stenosis and percutaneous renal artery intervention are correct EXCEPT:

A. Renal percutaneous transluminal angioplasty has a technical success rate of > 90% for nonostial lesions
B. Compared with surgical revascularization, percutaneous renal artery interventions result in similar blood pressure control and stabilization of renal function
C. Stenting of hemodynamically significant renal artery stenosis allows discontinuation of antihypertensive medications in the majority of patients
D. Stenting of renal artery stenosis significantly reduces restenosis compared with balloon angioplasty alone
E. Potential procedural complications of percutaneous revascularization include peripheral gangrene leading to toe or limb amputation

QUESTION 369

Each of the following statements regarding patients with chest pain and normal coronary angiograms ("syndrome X") is correct EXCEPT:
A. During stress testing, many patients with this syndrome develop chest pain and scintigraphic evidence of ischemia
B. During periods of increased myocardial oxygen demand, patients with this syndrome consistently produce elevated myocardial lactate
C. Estrogen therapy for postmenopausal women with this syndrome often improves symptoms
D. Microvascular dysfunction, enhanced pain sensitivity, and psychiatric disorders have all been associated with this syndrome
E. The incidence of coronary calcification by multislice computed tomography is greater than in control subjects

QUESTION 370

All of the following statements regarding endovascular repair of abdominal aortic aneurysms are true EXCEPT:
A. Anatomic constraints limit the use of endografts
B. Primary success rates for aneurysm exclusion are >75%
C. Endoleaks are a serious complication after implantation
D. Thirty-day mortality rates are lower with endovascular repair compared with open surgical repair
E. Long-term outcomes are better with endografts than with open surgical repair

QUESTION 371

All of the following statements regarding treatment of peripheral arterial disease are correct EXCEPT:
A. Pentoxifylline's actions are mediated through its hemorheologic properties
B. Cilostazol's benefits arise via calcium channel blockade
C. Supervised exercise training programs improve maximum walking distances by 50% to 200%

D. Percutaneous transluminal angioplasty of the iliac artery results in 4-year patency rates of 60% to 80%
E. Aortobifemoral bypass results in 10-year patency rates of nearly 90%

QUESTION 372

Each of the following steps is appropriate in the management of patients with acute aortic dissection EXCEPT:
A. Intravenous sodium nitroprusside
B. Intravenous beta-blocker therapy
C. Urgent surgical repair for proximal dissection
D. Urgent surgical repair for distal dissection
E. Use of narcotics for pain relief

QUESTION 373

Which of the following statements regarding diabetes mellitus as a cardiovascular risk factor is correct?
A. The prevalence of diabetes is decreasing in the developed world
B. A glycosylated hemoglobin (hemoglobin A1c) level >7.0% is required to make a diagnosis of diabetes
C. Statin therapy reduces coronary events only in diabetics with abnormal cholesterol levels
D. Fibric acid derivatives are the lipid-lowering agents of choice for the prevention of coronary events in diabetics
E. Lifestyle modifications significantly reduce the rate of diabetes development in at-risk individuals

QUESTION 374

All of the following statements regarding blood flow in the subendocardium as compared with the subepicardium are true EXCEPT:
A. Systolic flow is less in the subendocardium
B. Under normal conditions, total subendocardial flow is equal to or greater than subepicardial flow
C. An elevation of ventricular end-diastolic pressure will reduce subendocardial flow to a greater extent than subepicardial flow
D. The reserve for vasodilatation in the subendocardium is greater than in the subepicardium

QUESTION 375

Each of the following statements regarding myocardial stunning and hibernation is correct EXCEPT:
A. Stunning refers to myocardial dysfunction that persists after periods of severe ischemia
B. Molecular contributors to stunning include oxygen-derived free radicals, calcium overload, and reduced sensitivity of myofilaments to calcium
C. Stunned myocardium does not respond to inotropic agents

D. Hibernating myocardium reflects decreased myocardial function due to chronically decreased coronary blood flow that can be reversed with revascularization

E. Histopathologic studies of hibernating myocardium reveal dedifferentiation and apoptosis

QUESTION 376

All of the following statements regarding atherosclerotic plaque in unstable angina are true EXCEPT:

A. Approximately 15% of patients presenting with unstable angina have no significant coronary artery disease on angiography

B. The culprit lesion in unstable angina typically exhibits an eccentric stenosis

C. Coronary microvascular dysfunction can be demonstrated in fewer than 5% of patients who present with unstable angina in the absence of critical coronary obstructions

D. On angioscopy, "white" thrombi are typically observed in patients with unstable angina

E. Intravascular ultrasonography often reveals vulnerable plaques in unstable angina to be echolucent, consistent with a lipid-rich core with a thin fibrous cap

QUESTION 377

In patients with stable coronary artery disease, each of the following statements about the role of percutaneous coronary intervention (PCI) versus coronary artery bypass graft (CABG) surgery is correct EXCEPT:

A. In the majority of patients there is no mortality advantage of one treatment strategy compared with the other

B. CABG is associated with a lower rate of subsequent myocardial infarction

C. PCI is associated with a higher rate of recurrent angina

D. Patients with diabetes and severe multivessel disease demonstrate a greater reduction in mortality with CABG

E. In patients with single-vessel disease (>70% stenosis) of the left anterior descending coronary artery, there is no difference between PCI and CABG in the rates of subsequent myocardial infarction or cardiovascular death

QUESTION 378

Each of the following statements regarding high-dose statin therapy (80 mg/d) is correct EXCEPT:

A. High-dose simvastatin results in a greater degree of skeletal myopathy compared with low-dose (20 mg/d) therapy

B. High-dose atorvastatin results in measurable regression of atherosclerotic coronary stenosis

C. High-dose simvastatin has been shown to reduce coronary events after an acute coronary syndrome compared with less intensive therapy

D. Compared with less intensive statin therapy, high-dose atorvastatin reduces subsequent mortality in patients after an acute coronary syndrome

QUESTION 379

Each of the following statements regarding oral antiplatelet agents is correct EXCEPT:

A. Aspirin's principal antiplatelet action is via inhibition of cyclooxygenase

B. Clopidogrel and prasugrel are reversible inhibitors of the platelet P2Y12 adenosine diphosphate receptor

C. Prasugrel displays a more rapid onset of action than clopidogrel

D. Nonsteroidal anti-inflammatory drugs such as ibuprofen may inhibit the effect of aspirin

E. Cilostazol's mechanism of action is via inhibition of platelet phosphodiesterase-3

QUESTION 380

Each of the following statements regarding pharmacologic inhibition of the renin-angiotensin system in patients with ST-segment elevation myocardial infarction (STEMI) is true EXCEPT:

A. Oral angiotensin-converting enzyme (ACE) inhibitors reduce mortality in patients with STEMI

B. In patients with STEMI and left ventricular dysfunction, an angiotensin receptor blocker in combination with an ACE inhibitor results in better cardiovascular outcomes than an ACE inhibitor alone

C. In short-term trials, one third of the mortality benefit of ACE inhibitors in STEMI occurs within the first 2 days of therapy

D. Oral administration of the selective aldosterone inhibitor eplerenone is associated with reduced mortality in patients with STEMI and left ventricular dysfunction

QUESTION 381

A 42-year-old man with an extensive smoking history presents with claudication and rest pain of his right calf and foot. An angiogram of his posterior tibial artery is shown in Figure 3-7. Each of the following statements about this condition is true EXCEPT:

A. It affects primarily the small and medium vessels of the arms and legs

B. High-dose statin therapy improves symptoms

C. Smoking cessation improves outcomes

D. Vascular surgery is usually not beneficial

E. More than 75% of patients with this condition are men

QUESTION 382

All the following characteristics are typical of hypertensive crises EXCEPT:

A. Diastolic blood pressure >120 mm Hg

B. Retinal hemorrhages

C. Constriction of cerebral arterioles with decreased vascular permeability
D. Proteinuria
E. Microangiopathic hemolytic anemia

QUESTION 383

Each of the following conditions has been associated with the abnormality demonstrated in the transesophageal echocardiogram shown in Figure 3-8 EXCEPT:

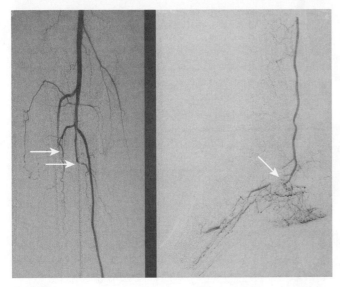

FIGURE 3-7

A. Heroin use
B. Hypertension
C. Marfan syndrome
D. Bicuspid aortic valve
E. Pregnancy

QUESTION 384

Each of the following is an appropriate therapy for a patient with acute ST-segment elevation myocardial infarction and cardiogenic shock EXCEPT:
A. Percutaneous left ventricular assist device
B. Fibrinolytic therapy
C. Urgent percutaneous intervention
D. Vasopressor drugs
E. Coronary artery bypass surgery

QUESTION 385

True statements about the diagnosis and treatment of right ventricular infarction (RVI) include all of the following EXCEPT:
A. Hypotension in response to small doses of nitroglycerin in patients with inferior infarction suggests RVI
B. Unexplained systemic hypoxemia in RVI raises the possibility of a patent foramen ovale
C. Hemodynamic parameters in RVI often resemble those of patients with pericardial disease

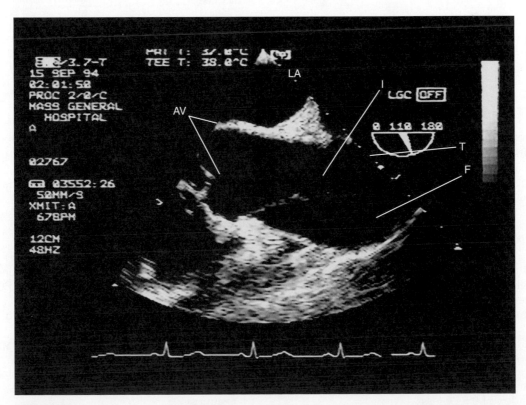

FIGURE 3-8

PULSE VOLUME RECORDING

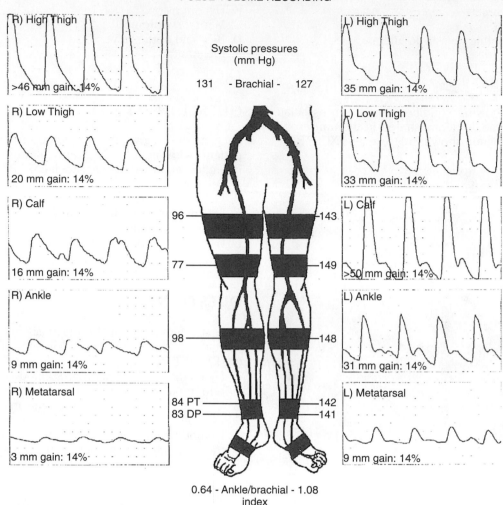

R) High Thigh
>46 mm gain: 14%

R) Low Thigh
20 mm gain: 14%

R) Calf
16 mm gain: 14%

R) Ankle
9 mm gain: 14%

R) Metatarsal
3 mm gain: 14%

L) High Thigh
35 mm gain: 14%

L) Low Thigh
33 mm gain: 14%

L) Calf
>50 mm gain: 14%

L) Ankle
31 mm gain: 14%

L) Metatarsal
9 mm gain: 14%

Systolic pressures
(mm Hg)

131 - Brachial - 127

96 —— ——143
77 —— ——149
98 —— ——148
84 PT —— ——142
83 DP —— ——141

0.64 - Ankle/brachial - 1.08
index

FIGURE 3-9

D. Loop diuretics are usually the preferred initial therapy for patients with RVI and intact left ventricular contractile function

E. ST-segment elevation in lead V_4R is a sensitive and specific sign of RVI

QUESTION 386

A 65-year-old man presents with several months of right lower extremity discomfort and fatigue while walking. Segmental pressure measurements were obtained as shown in Figure 3-9. Each of the following statements is true EXCEPT:

A. An ankle/brachial index >0.85 is considered normal

B. A pressure difference >20 mm Hg between successive cuffs is evidence of significant arterial stenosis

C. Critical limb ischemia is associated with an ankle/brachial index of 0.5 or less

D. The sensitivity of the ankle/brachial index for the diagnosis of peripheral arterial disease is decreased in severely calcified arteries

E. This patient has evidence of right iliac and right common femoral artery stenoses

QUESTION 387

Each of the following statements regarding restenosis after percutaneous coronary intervention (PCI) is correct EXCEPT:

A. Bare metal stents are associated with a 20% to 25% rate of angiographic in-stent restenosis

B. Plain balloon angioplasty is associated with a 30% to 40% rate of restenosis

C. Direct coronary atherectomy and rotational atherectomy are the preferred therapies for in-stent restenosis

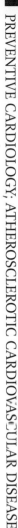

D. Brachytherapy impairs neointimal proliferation and reduces the rate of recurrent in-stent restenosis

QUESTION 388

Each of the following statements regarding clinically approved drug-eluting stents (DES) is correct EXCEPT:
A. DES have been shown to suppress local neointimal proliferation
B. The rate of angiographic restenosis after DES implantation is <10%
C. Paclitaxel stabilizes microtubules and prevents cell division
D. DES systems that incorporate everolimus prevent restenosis less effectively than those that incorporate paclitaxel
E. DES implantation results in superior outcomes compared with brachytherapy in treatment of in-stent stenosis within bare metal stents

QUESTION 389

Each of the following is a beneficial effect of regular exercise EXCEPT:
A. Favorable changes in the fibrinolytic system
B. Decreased heart rate variability
C. Increased expression of nitric oxide synthase
D. Decreased triglyceride levels
E. Improved systolic and diastolic blood pressures

QUESTION 390

Each of the following is a major contributor to myocardial oxygen demand (MVO_2) EXCEPT:
A. Ventricular wall tension
B. Plasma hemoglobin level
C. Myocardial contractile state
D. Heart rate
E. Left ventricular volume

QUESTION 391

A 63-year-old man with long-standing insulin-requiring diabetes presented to the physician's office for management of hypertension (160/94 mm Hg). Urine and serum chemistries at that time were normal except for serum creatinine = 1.6 mg/dL and blood urea nitrogen (BUN) = 30 mg/dL. A potassium-sparing diuretic (triamterene hydrochlorothiazide) was prescribed. When he returns 2 weeks later, the serum potassium level is 6.8 mmol/L with no significant change in BUN or creatinine level. The most likely contributing mechanism is:
A. Excessive consumption of tomatoes and bananas
B. A recent urinary tract infection
C. Primary hyperaldosteronism
D. Hyporeninemic hypoaldosteronism
E. Cushing syndrome

QUESTION 392

Each of the following statements about the use of prasugrel is correct EXCEPT:
A. Compared with clopidogrel, platelet aggregation is more effectively inhibited by prasugrel
B. Compared with clopidogrel, prasugrel reduces the risk of stent thrombosis
C. Compared with clopidogrel, bleeding complications associated with prasugrel are lower
D. Prasugrel is contraindicated in patients with a history of stroke
E. The risk of bleeding with prasugrel is higher in patients >75 years of age.

DIRECTIONS: The group of questions below consists of lettered headings followed by a set of numbered items. For each numbered item, select the ONE lettered heading with which it is MOST closely associated. Each lettered heading may be used once, more than once, or not at all.

QUESTIONS 393 TO 396

Match the following cell types potentially involved in atherogenesis with the appropriate descriptive phrase:
A. Endothelial cell
B. Smooth muscle cells
C. Macrophage
D. Platelet

393. Demonstrate(s) proliferation in the intima in atherosclerosis
394. Is (are) the principal cell(s) of the fatty streak
395. Secrete(s) prostacyclin
396. Is (are) capable of little or no protein synthesis

QUESTIONS 397 TO 400

For each statement, match the corresponding beta blocker:
A. Atenolol
B. Carvedilol
C. Propranolol
D. Pindolol

397. Has alpha- and beta-receptor blocking activity
398. Is most hydrophilic
399. Has inherent sympathomimetic activity
400. Has shortest half-life

QUESTIONS 401 TO 405

For each statement, match the most appropriate complication following myocardial infarction:
A. Aneurysm
B. Pseudoaneurysm
C. Both
D. Neither

401. Low risk of rupture
402. Narrow base
403. Due to true myocardial rupture
404. Associated thrombus is common
405. Surgical repair is usually required

QUESTIONS 406 TO 409

For each statement, match the corresponding anticoagulant(s):
A. Unfractionated heparin (UFH)
B. Low-molecular-weight heparin (LMWH)
C. Bivalirudin
D. UFH and bivalirudin
E. LMWH and bivalirudin

406. Binds directly to thrombin, independent of antithrombin
407. Dose(s) should be adjusted if creatinine clearance is < 30 mL/min
408. Degree of anticoagulation can be monitored using the activated partial thromboplastin time
409. Least likely to trigger type II heparin-induced thrombocytopenia

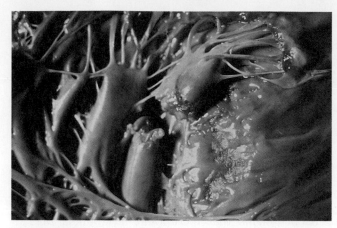

FIGURE 3-10 From Schoen FJ: The heart. *In* Kumar V, Abbas AK, Fausto N (eds): Robbins & Cotran Pathologic Basis of Disease. 8th ed. Philadelphia, Saunders, 2010, pp 529-587.

QUESTIONS 410 TO 414

Match the descriptions with the appropriate cell type:
A. Monocytes
B. Smooth muscle cells
C. Both
D. Neither

410. Migrate into the arterial intima from the media in response to chemoattractants
411. Primary constituent(s) of fibrous plaques
412. Require low-density lipoprotein receptor to become foam cells
413. Rely on chemoattractants to enter into developing atherosclerotic intimal lesions
414. Adhesion molecules such as VCAM-1 and ICAM-1 regulate adherence to endothelial cells

QUESTIONS 415 TO 419

For each statement, match the most appropriate fibrinolytic agent:
A. Streptokinase
B. Alteplase
C. Reteplase
D. Tenecteplase

415. Shortest half-life
416. Most fibrin-specific
417. Administered as a single bolus
418. Lowest intracranial hemorrhagic risk
419. Antigenic

QUESTIONS 420 TO 423

For each statement, match the most likely complication following acute myocardial infarction:
A. Acute ventricular septal rupture
B. Acute mitral regurgitation
C. Both
D. Neither

420. The murmur may decrease in intensity as arterial pressure falls
421. Pulmonary artery wedge pressure tracing demonstrates large v waves
422. Associated with the pathologic process shown in Figure 3-10
423. Occurs primarily with large infarctions

QUESTIONS 424 TO 427

For each of the following prospective lipid-lowering trials, match the most appropriate statement.
A. Statistically significant reduction in nonfatal myocardial infarction
B. Statistically significant reduction in overall mortality
C. Both
D. Neither

424. Scandinavian Simvastatin Survival Study (4S)
425. The Heart Protection Study (HPS)
426. Anglo-Scandinavian Cardiac Outcomes Trial (ASCOT-LLA)
427. Rosuvastatin to Prevent Vascular Events in Men and Women with Elevated C-Reactive Protein (JUPITER)

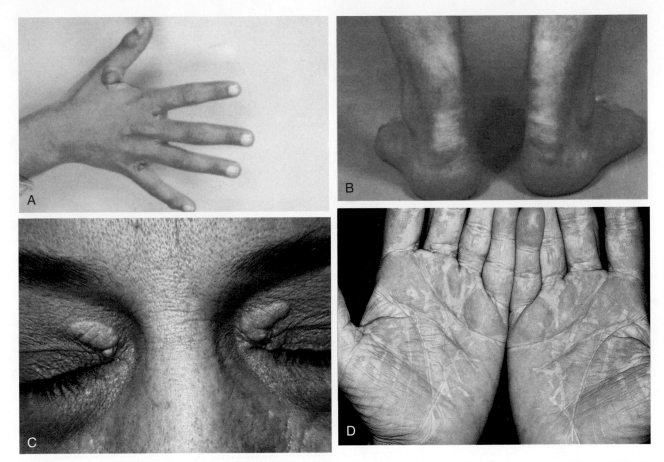

FIGURE 3-11 A AND B from Gotto A: Cholesterol Education Program: Clinician's Manual. Dallas, American Heart Association, 1991, pp. 34-36. By permission of the American Heart Association, Inc; C and D from Habif: Clinical Dermatology. 5th ed, St. Louis, Mosby Elsevier, 2009.

QUESTIONS 428 TO 431

For each pharmacologic agent, match the associated lipoprotein effect:
A. Elevate(s) high-density lipoprotein cholesterol
B. Elevate(s) low-density lipoprotein (LDL) cholesterol
C. Have (has) no significant effect on lipoproteins
D. Lower(s) HDL cholesterol
E. Lower(s) very low-density lipoprotein cholesterol

428. Corticosteroids
429. Propranolol
430. Second-generation antipsychotic medications (e.g., olanzapine)
431. Calcium channel antagonists

QUESTIONS 432 TO 435

For each clinical feature in Figure 3-11, match the appropriate condition:
A. Familial hypercholesterolemia
B. Type III hyperlipoproteinemia (familial dysbetalipoproteinemia)
C. Both
D. Neither

432. See part A
433. See part B
434. See part C
435. See part D

PREVENTIVE CARDIOLOGY; ATHEROSCLEROTIC CARDIOVASCULAR DISEASE

ANSWER TO QUESTION 295

A (Braunwald, pp. 922-926)

C-reactive protein (CRP), a circulating member of the pentraxin family, plays an important role in innate immunity. It is formed primarily in the liver but is also elaborated from coronary arteries, especially atherosclerotic intima. Levels of CRP are elevated in inflammatory states and may directly affect vascular vulnerability, thereby promoting atherosclerosis. Multiple epidemiologic studies have demonstrated that CRP levels measured by high-sensitivity assays (hsCRP) are strongly and independently associated with myocardial infarction, stroke, peripheral arterial disease, and sudden death.[1] hsCRP levels can be classified as low (<1 mg/L), intermediate (1 to 3 mg/L), or high (>3 mg/L). In patients with acute coronary events, high hsCRP levels are associated with worse outcomes, including increased mortality.[2]

An elevated level of hsCRP also predicts the onset of type 2 diabetes, perhaps because it correlates with insulin sensitivity, endothelial dysfunction, and hypofibrinolysis. Many medications lower hsCRP levels, in particular statins, fibrates, and niacin. Statin therapy reduces hsCRP levels largely unrelated to the low-density lipoprotein–lowering effect.[3] Furthermore, statin therapy has been shown to benefit patients with relatively normal LDL, if the hsCRP is elevated. In the JUPITER trial, rosuvastatin resulted in a 44% reduction in vascular events in apparently healthy individuals with baseline LDL < 130 mg/dL and hsCRP > 2 mg/L.[4]

Aspirin does not directly lower hsCRP levels but appears to have the greatest cardiovascular benefit in patients with elevated baseline hsCRP levels.

REFERENCES

1. Ridker PM: C-reactive protein and the prediction of cardiovascular events among those at intermediate risk: moving an inflammatory hypothesis toward consensus. J Am Coll Cardiol 49:2129, 2007.
2. Morrow DA, de Lemos JA, Sabatine MS, et al: Clinical relevance of C-reactive protein during follow-up of patients with acute coronary syndromes in Aggrastat-to-Zocor Trial. Circulation 114:281, 2006.
3. Albert MA, Danielson E, Rifai N, Ridker PM, PRINCE Investigators: Effect of statin therapy on C-reactive protein levels. The pravastatin Inflammation/CRP Evaluation (PRINCE): A randomized trial and cohort study. JAMA 286:64, 2001.
4. Ridker PM, Danielson E, Fonseca FA, et al: Rosuvastatin to prevent vascular events in men and women with elevated C-reactive protein. N Engl J Med 359:2195, 2008.

ANSWER TO QUESTION 296

C (Braunwald, pp. 956-959)

Lifestyle modifications benefit most individuals with hypertension.[1] Obesity contributes to elevated blood pressure (BP) and even small degrees of weight loss can lower it, no matter what type of diet is employed.[2]

Modest sodium restriction can also improve hypertension. Reduction of dietary sodium intake to < 100 mmol/d (2.4 g of sodium or 6 g sodium chloride) decreases systolic BP approximately 2 to 8 mm Hg. Not all hypertensive individuals respond to lower salt intake, and some patients (African Americans and the elderly) may be particularly sensitive to sodium reduction.[3] Adoption of the DASH (Dietary Approaches to Stop Hypertension) eating plan—rich in fruits, vegetables, and low-fat dairy products and low in total and saturated fat—has been shown to reduce BP by 11.4/5.5 mm Hg. Even greater reductions are manifest by combining the DASH diet with reduced sodium intake.[3] Magnesium supplements have not been demonstrated to significantly reduce blood pressure.

Ethanol consumption of no more than 1 oz/d (24 oz beer, 10 oz wine, 3 oz 80-proof liquor for a normal-size man and less for a woman) is associated with decreased cardiac mortality, but excessive alcohol intake exerts a pressor effect, so that alcohol abuse is actually a cause of reversible hypertension.

REFERENCES

1. Joint National Committee: The seventh report of the Joint National Committee on Prevention, Detection, Evaluation, and Treatment of High Blood Pressure (JNC-7 Express). JAMA 289:2560, 2003.
2. Sacks FM, Bray GA, Carey VJ, et al: Comparison of weight-loss diets with different compositions of fat, protein, and carbohydrates. N Engl J Med 360:859, 2009.

3. Sacks FM, Svetky LP, Vollmer WM, et al: Effects on blood pressure of reduced dietary sodium and the Dietary Approaches to Stop Hypertension (DASH) diet. DASH-Sodium Collaborative Research Group. N Engl J Med 344:3, 2001.

ANSWER TO QUESTION 297

D (Braunwald, pp. 946-948)

Renovascular disease is one of the most common causes of secondary hypertension and has two main etiologies. The most common cause (80% to 90% of cases) is atherosclerotic disease affecting the proximal third of the main renal artery, typically seen in older men. The prevalence of atherosclerotic renovascular disease is higher with advanced age, diabetes, and evidence of atherosclerosis in other arterial beds.

The second, and less common, form of renal artery stenosis is fibrodysplasia, which primarily afflicts young women. It involves mainly the distal two thirds of the main renal artery, and, although all layers of the vessel may be involved, fibrodysplasia of the media is most common.

A renovascular etiology of hypertension should be suspected in patients who develop high blood pressure before age 30, or after age 50 with the abrupt onset of severe and resistant hypertension and signs of atherosclerosis elsewhere, or in patients with recurrent sudden unexplained pulmonary edema. *Bilateral* renal artery stenosis should be suspected if renal insufficiency is present, especially if renal function worsens following initiation of angiotensin-converting enzyme inhibitor or angiotensin receptor blocker therapy.

REFERENCE

Dworkin LD, Cooper CJ: Renal-artery stenosis. N Engl J Med 361:1972-1978, 2009.

ANSWER TO QUESTION 298

D (Braunwald, pp. 943-946, 950)

Essential hypertension accounts for approximately 90% of patients with elevated blood pressure.[1] Renal parenchymal disease is the second most common cause, responsible for approximately 5%. Grouped together, coarctation of the aorta, Cushing disease, and pheochromocytoma contribute to < 1%. Primary aldosteronism accounts for ~1% of hypertension in the general population but a higher percentage (~11%) in patients with resistant hypertension.[2]

Pure "white coat" hypertension, in which blood pressures taken in the office are persistently elevated but out-of-office readings are not, is found in 20% to 30% of patients. Most patients with white coat hypertension are found to be free of target organ damage and have an excellent 10-year prognosis with respect to cardiovascular disease.

When measuring the blood pressure, the correct cuff size should be used. The cuff bladder should encircle and cover two thirds of the length of the arm. If the cuff bladder is too small, blood pressure readings may be spuriously *high*.[3]

In elderly patients, the brachial arteries are often sclerotic and may not become occluded until the blood pressure cuff is inflated to a very high pressure. As a result, the recorded cuff pressure may be much higher than that measured intra-arterially, resulting in "pseudohypertension."

REFERENCES

1. Chobanian AV, Bakris GL, Black HR, et al: The Seventh Report of the Joint National Committee on Prevention, Detection, Evaluation, and Treatment of High Blood Pressure: The JNC 7 report. JAMA 289:2560, 2003.
2. Douma S, Petidis K, Doumas M, et al. Prevalence of primary hyperaldosteronism in resistant hypertension: A retrospective observational study. Lancet 371:1921-1926, 2008.
3. Ogedegbe G, Pickering T: Principles and techniques of blood pressure measurement. Cardiol Clin 28:571-586, 2010.

ANSWER TO QUESTION 299

B (Braunwald, pp. 941, 944-945, 959-961)

Target organ damage in hypertension results from the increased workload on the heart and vascular damage from the combined effects of elevated pressure and accelerated atherosclerosis. Hypertensive heart disease, cerebrovascular disease, large-vessel disease (leading to peripheral arterial disease, aortic aneurysm and dissection), and chronic kidney disease can develop simultaneously, contributing to the long-term complications of hypertension.

In hypertensive individuals, the presence of left ventricular hypertrophy (LVH) powerfully predicts morbidity and mortality. Electrocardiographic LVH is present in 5% to 10% of hypertensive patients, and patients with LVH and strain pattern are at increased risk of further hypertensive cardiac disease and subsequent heart failure.[1] Echocardiography is even more sensitive and detects LVH in approximately 30% of unselected hypertensive adults.

The treatment of hypertension with LVH should be similar to that for other hypertensive patients, and first-line agents include diuretics, calcium channel blockers, angiotensin-converting enzyme inhibitors, angiotensin receptor blockers (ARBs), and beta blockers. However, in the LIFE trial, the ARB losartan was compared with the beta-blocker, atenolol in high-risk hypertensive patients with electrocardiographic LVH, the majority of whom were also treated with a diuretic. Despite a similar reduction in blood pressure, the individuals who received losartan demonstrated reduced cardiovascular morbidity and mortality compared with those who received the beta blocker.[2]

REFERENCES

1. Okin PM, Devereux RB, Nieminen MS, et al: Electrocardiographic strain pattern and prediction of new-onset congestive heart failure in hypertensive patients: The Losartan Intervention for Endpoint Reduction in Hypertension (LIFE) study. Circulation 113:67, 2006.

2. Dahlof B, Devereux RB, Kjeldsen SE, et al: Cardiovascular morbidity and mortality in the Losartan Intervention For Endpoint reduction in hypertension study (LIFE): A randomised trial against atenolol. Lancet 359:995, 2002.

ANSWER TO QUESTION 300

D (Braunwald, pp. 950-951)

The use of oral contraceptive pills may be the most common cause of secondary hypertension in young women, resulting in a relative risk of developing elevated blood pressure of 1.8 compared with those not using these pills. The likelihood is increased by alcohol consumption, age > 35 years, and obesity and is probably related to the estrogen content of the agent. Because estrogen increases the hepatic production of angiotensinogen, a probable mechanism for hypertension induced by oral contraceptives is activation of the renin-angiotensin system with subsequent sodium retention and volume expansion. Nonetheless, angiotensin-converting enzyme inhibitors do not influence blood pressure to a greater degree in women with contraceptive-induced hypertension than in those with primary essential hypertension.

Blood pressure returns to normal in only about 50% of women within 3 to 6 months after discontinuation of oral contraceptives, but it is not known if the pill is the cause of permanent hypertension or simply unmasks women who are prone to essential hypertension.

REFERENCE

Shufelt CL, Barey Merz CN: Contraceptive hormone use and cardiovascular disease. J Am Coll Cardiol 53:221-231, 2009.

ANSWER TO QUESTION 301

D (Braunwald, pp. 950, 1841)

Pheochromocytomas account for only 0.1% of all cases of hypertension. Most pheochromocytomas arise in the adrenal medulla, where 10% are bilateral and 10% are malignant. Approximately 15% of pheochromocytomas are extra-adrenal (paragangliomas).

Pheochromocytomas should be suspected in patients with paroxysmal hypertension who have symptoms of catecholamine excess (sweating, tachycardia, weight loss) and/or marked variability of the blood pressure. However, more than 50% of patients with pheochromocytoma actually have chronic persistent hypertension. Laboratory confirmation of pheochromocytoma can be made by measuring a 24-hour urine assay for total metanephrine, the catecholamine metabolite least affected by interfering substances. However, urinary metanephrine excretion can be increased in patients taking sympathomimetic or dopaminergic drugs or the alpha/beta-blocker labetalol. A single plasma free metanephrine assay is as, or more, sensitive for the diagnosis than urinary catecholamine assays but is less specific and may produce false-positive results. Pheochromocytomas may be inherited alone, or in combination with other abnormalities, most commonly multiple endocrine neoplasia (MEN) type 2A or 2B. Multiple adrenal tumors are particularly common in the familial forms.

REFERENCE

Yu R, Nissen NN, Chopra P, et al: Diagnosis and treatment of pheochromocytoma in an academic hospital from 1997 to 2007. Am J Med 122:85, 2009.

ANSWER TO QUESTION 302

D (Braunwald, pp. 965-968)

All antihypertensive medications have potential side effects that may limit their use. Minoxidil is a direct vasodilator that is effective and occasionally used in patients with renal failure and severe hypertension. Its side effects include a reflex increase in cardiac output, fluid retention, and hirsutism. Approximately 3% of patients who take minoxidil develop a pericardial effusion, even in the absence of renal or cardiac dysfunction.

Hydralazine is a direct vasodilator with potential adverse effects that include tachycardia, flushing, and headaches. These side effects can be prevented, and the antihypertensive effect increased, by co-administration of a beta blocker.

Angiotensin-converting enzyme (ACE) inhibitors lower blood pressure by blocking the formation of angiotensin II and by increasing the circulating concentration of the vasodilator bradykinin. Rare side effects include angioedema, rash, loss of taste, and leukopenia. The most common side effect is an annoying dry, hacking cough that occurs in more than 10% of women and 5% of men taking ACE inhibitors.[1] That side effect may persist for more than 3 weeks after discontinuation of the medication. Substitution with an angiotensin receptor blocker results in a similar antihypertensive effect, without producing cough in the majority of affected patients.

Calcium channel blockers vasodilate and lower blood pressure by interacting with plasma membrane L-type calcium channels. Common side effects of such vasodilatation include headache, flushing, and ankle edema.

REFERENCE

1. Dicpinigaitis PV: Angiotensin-converting enzyme inhibitor-induced cough: ACCP evidence-based clinical practice guidelines. Chest 129:169s, 2006.

ANSWER TO QUESTION 303

B (Braunwald, pp. 961-963)

Thiazide diuretics are the most frequently prescribed first-line agents for the treatment of hypertension. They have a number of important side effects. The most common metabolic disturbance is hypokalemia; the serum potassium level falls an average 0.7 mmol/L after institution of 50 mg/d of hydrochlorothiazide, and 0.4 mmol/L with 25 mg/d, but there is almost no decline with 12.5 mg/d.[1] Hypomagnesemia is usually mild but may prevent the restoration of an intracellular deficit of potassium; therefore, it should be corrected.

*Hyper*uricemia is present in one third of untreated hypertensive persons, and it develops in another third during therapy with thiazides. This is likely a result of increased proximal tubular reabsorption of urate.[1] Thiazides may increase the total blood cholesterol in a dose-related fashion. Low-density lipoproteins and triglycerides also increase. There may also be a rise in serum calcium (usually < 0.5 mg/dL) on thiazide therapy, which is probably secondary to increased proximal tubular reabsorption. Hyponatremia may occur with thiazide therapy, especially in the elderly.

REFERENCE

1. Hunter DJ, York M, Chaisson CE, et al: Recent diuretic use and the risk of recurrent gout attacks: The online case-crossover gout study. J Rheumatol 33:1341, 2006.

ANSWER TO QUESTION 304

D (Braunwald, p. 987)

The HMG-CoA reductase inhibitors (statins) are competitive inhibitors of the rate-limiting enzyme in cholesterol synthesis, primarily in the liver. By reducing the intracellular cholesterol concentration, the expression of cell-surface low-density lipoprotein (LDL) receptors is increased, resulting in enhanced removal of LDL particles from the circulation. These agents also inhibit hepatic synthesis of very low-density lipoprotein (VLDL), the precursor of LDL cholesterol. As a result of these actions, total and LDL cholesterol levels fall, as do triglycerides, the major component of VLDL particles. Statins are very well tolerated. Approximately 1% of patients show elevations of hepatic transaminases (ALT, AST) to levels more than three times normal, a side effect that is usually asymptomatic and reversible on stopping the drug. Myopathy, consisting of muscle aching or weakness in association with serum creatine kinase levels more than 10 times normal, occurs in <0.1% of patients. This adverse effect should prompt immediate discontinuation of the drug. The risk of myopathy is increased when there is concurrent therapy with other drugs that interfere with cytochrome P-450 metabolism of many of the statins. Examples of such drugs include erythromycin, cyclosporine, and antifungal agents.

REFERENCES

Beltowski J, Wojcicka G, Jamroz-Wisniewska A: Adverse effects of statins: Mechanisms and consequences. Curr Drug Saf 4:209:2009.

ANSWER TO QUESTION 305

A (Braunwald, pp. 986, 1624; Tables 47-5 and 72-6)

Many medications have the potential to alter a patient's lipid profile. Beta blockers, particularly non–beta$_1$-selective agents, increase triglyceride levels and lower high-density lipoprotein (HDL) levels. Thiazides tend to increase triglyceride levels. Nonetheless, both beta blockers and diuretics are effective antihypertensive agents that reduce the frequency of vascular events.

Hormonal replacement therapy with estrogen increases both HDL and triglyceride levels. Despite the augmented HDL effect, the use of estrogen to improve the lipid profile is not recommended because of the associated increase in cardiovascular events.[1] Immunosuppressive drugs and corticosteroids tend to raise triglyceride levels.

Protease inhibitors, for patients with human immunodeficiency virus infection, can induce a dyslipidemic syndrome characterized by elevated triglyceride and total cholesterol levels with decreased HDL levels. Chronic use of protease inhibitors has been associated with an increased risk of myocardial infarction compared with antiretroviral regimens that do not include a protease inhibitor.[2,3]

REFERENCES

1. Mosca L, Banka CL, Benjamin EJ, et al: American Heart Association evidence-based guidelines for cardiovascular disease prevention in women: 2007 update. J Am Coll Cardiol 49:1230, 2007.
2. The DAD Study Group: Class of antiretroviral drugs and the risk of myocardial infarction. N Engl J Med 356:1723-1735, 2007.
3. Ho JE, Hsue PY: Cardiovascular manifestations of HIV infection. Heart 95:1193-1202, 2009.

ANSWER TO QUESTION 306

B (Braunwald, pp. 982-985; Tables 47-3 and 47-4)

Most clinically encountered lipoprotein disorders arise from an interaction between diet, lack of exercise, excessive weight, and an individual's genetic composition. Genetic lipoprotein disorders may affect low-density lipoprotein (LDL), high-density lipoprotein (HDL), triglycerides, lipoprotein (a), and remnant lipoprotein molecules.

Familial combined hyperlipidemia (FCH) is a common polygenic disorder with abnormalities that include elevations of LDL and/or triglycerides, a reduction in HDL, and elevated apo B levels. Patients with FCH have an increased risk of coronary artery disease (CAD), and there can be considerable clinical overlap between FCH and the insulin-resistance metabolic syndrome. Physical findings such as corneal arcus or xanthomas are rare.

Familial hypertriglyceridemia (type IV hyperlipoproteinemia) is also a polygenic disorder and is characterized by elevated triglycerides with normal or low LDL levels and reduced HDL. Patients do not develop xanthomas or xanthelasmas, and the relationship with CAD is not as strong or consistent as with FCH.

Familial hypercholesterolemia (FH) is an autosomal co-dominant disorder that results from defects in the LDL receptor. More than 1000 different mutations of the LDL receptor gene have been described.[1] Patients with FH have LDL levels > the 95th percentile for age and gender. Corneal arcus, tendinous xanthomas, and xanthelasmas are common. Men with heterozygous FH usually develop CAD by the third or fourth decade. Affected women present 8 to 10 years later. Familial defective apo B100, which results from mutations in the apo B gene, can be clinically indistinguishable from FH. It results in a reduced affinity of affected LDL particles for the LDL receptor.

Dysbetalipoproteinemia (type III hyperlipoproteinemia) is a rare genetic disorder that arises in patients who are homozygous for the apo E2 allele. This condition results in an accumulation of remnant lipoprotein particles, and serum levels of both total cholesterol and triglycerides are elevated. Affected individuals are at increased risk for CAD. Pathognomonic clinical manifestations include tuberous xanthomas and striated palmar xanthomas.[2]

REFERENCES

1. Souter AK, Naoumova RP: Mechanisms of disease: Genetic causes of familial hypercholesterolemia. Nat Clin Pract Cardiovasc Med 4:214, 2007.
2. Schaefer JR: Unraveling hyperlipidemia type III (dysbetalipoproteinemia) slowly. Eur J Hum Genet 17:541-542, 2009.

ANSWER TO QUESTION 307

D (Braunwald, p. 988)

Nicotinic acid (niacin) is a B vitamin with lipid-lowering effects that occur when taken at pharmacologic doses. Its primary action is to reduce very low-density lipoprotein secretion from the liver, which causes a subsequent reduction in intermediate-density lipoprotein and low-density lipoprotein (LDL) levels. In addition, nicotinic acid decreases the release of free fatty acids from adipocytes (which are used by the liver for triglyceride synthesis), thus reducing triglyceride levels. In therapeutic doses, nicotinic acid reduces LDL cholesterol by 10% to 25% and triglycerides by 20% to 50%. It also increases high-density lipoprotein (HDL) cholesterol by 15% to 35%. The increase in HDL cholesterol is caused by decreased catabolism of HDL and apo AI.[1] Nicotinic acid also reduces circulating levels of lipoprotein (a). Despite these important effects on the lipid profile and proven clinical benefits,[2,3] its widespread use has been limited because of side effects. The most common adverse effect is flushing, which can be reduced by preadministration of aspirin or other prostaglandin inhibitors. Hepatotoxicity is a serious and potentially life-threatening complication that has been reported more often with sustained-release, compared with the immediate-release, preparations.

REFERENCES

1. Ruparelia N, Digby JE, Choudhury RP: Effects of niacin on atherosclerosis and vascular function. Curr Opin Cardiol 26:66-70, 2011.
2. Brown BG, Zhao XQ, Chait A, et al: Simvastatin and niacin, antioxidant vitamins, or the combination for the prevention of coronary disease. N Engl J Med 345:1583, 2001.
3. Taylor AJ, Villines TC, Stanek EJ, et al: Extended-release niacin or ezetimibe and carotid intima–media thickness. N Engl J Med 361:2113-2122, 2009.

ANSWER TO QUESTION 308

C (Braunwald, pp. 975-978)

The apoprotein components of lipoproteins have several functions, including structural support, receptor recognition, and, in some cases, enzymatic activity. Apo AI is the major protein in high-density lipoprotein (HDL) that has been inversely correlated with arteriographic evidence of coronary disease.[1] The apo AI protein also activates the enzyme lecithin-cholesterol acyltransferase (LCAT). LCAT allows the HDL particle to convert cholesterol obtained from peripheral tissues to cholesteryl ester, an important step in the "reverse" cholesterol transport pathway.

The two forms of apoprotein B (apo B48 and apo B100) arise from a *single* gene that displays a unique editing mechanism that allows for synthesis of both proteins.[2] Apo B100 is the primary apoprotein of low-density lipoprotein (LDL), allowing recognition of the particle by the LDL receptor on cell surfaces.

Apoprotein E may be found in very low-density lipoproteins (VLDL) particles as well as in chylomicrons, in intermediate-density lipoprotein (IDL) particles, and, to a small extent, in HDL. Most patients with type III hyperlipoproteinemia are homozygous for the apoprotein E2/2 genotype. This disorder is characterized by premature atherosclerosis and is notable for both hypercholesterolemia and hypertriglyceridemia owing to an increase in IDL and/or VLDL particle populations.

REFERENCES

1. Di Angelantonio E, Sarwar N, Perry P, et al: Major lipids, apolipoproteins, and risk of vascular disease. JAMA 302:1993-2000, 2009.
2. Bransteitter R, Prochnow C, Chen XS: The current structural and functional understanding of APOBEC deaminases. Cell Mol Life Sci 66:3137, 2009.

ANSWER TO QUESTION 309

E (Braunwald, pp. 983-984, 993)

The relation between triglyceride levels and coronary artery disease (CAD) remains controversial.[1] Although hypertriglyceridemia has been shown to be a risk factor for CAD in univariate analyses, its significance has typically been weakened in multivariable analyses. This is likely due to the association of elevated triglyceride levels with other degenerative conditions, such as diabetes mellitus, chronic renal failure, obesity, cigarette smoking, and excessive alcohol consumption. In addition, it would be difficult to design a trial to isolate the benefits of triglyceride reduction because most antilipidemic agents have multiple effects on the lipid profile. The association between hypertriglyceridemia and cardiovascular risk appears to be stronger in women than in men.[2]

In the recent ACCORD trial, type 2 diabetic patients already treated with simvastatin achieved a marked reduction in triglycerides with the addition of fenofibrate. However, compared with placebo, clinical outcomes (fatal cardiovascular events, nonfatal myocardial infarction, or stroke) were not reduced by the addition of fenofibrate.[3]

REFERENCES

1. Jialal I, Amess W, Kaur M: Management of hypertriglyceridemia in the diabetic patient. Curr Diabetes Rep 10:316, 2010.
2. Nordestgaard BG, Benn M, Schnohr P, et al: Nonfasting triglycerides and risk of myocardial infarction, ischemic heart disease, and death in men and women. JAMA 298:299, 2007.
3. The ACCORD Study Group. Effect of combination lipid therapy in type 2 diabetes mellitus. N Engl J Med 362:1563-1574, 2010.

ANSWER TO QUESTION 310

B (Braunwald, pp. 927, 983)

Lp(a) consists of a low-density lipoprotein particle with its apo B100 component linked by a disulfide bridge to apolipoprotein (a) [apo(a)]. Apo(a) is a complex molecule that has sequence homology with plasminogen. The latter structural feature has raised the possibility that Lp(a) may inhibit endogenous fibrinolysis by competing with plasminogen for binding at the endothelial surface.

The primary determinant of Lp(a) levels is genetic[1,2]; changes in diet and physical activity have no significant impact. In addition, Lp(a) levels vary widely across racial groups and are higher in African Americans compared with whites. In several studies, Lp(a) has been shown to be an independent risk factor for vascular risk. A meta-analysis of 36 prospective studies including more than 12,000 patients found that the adjusted risk ratio of cardiovascular events is 1.13 for each standard deviation increase in Lp(a).[3] Niacin is one of the few interventions that can significantly reduce Lp(a); statin drugs do not. However, no study yet has shown that pharmacologic reduction of Lp(a) improves cardiovascular outcomes. However, pharmacologic reduction of LDL-cholesterol does significantly reduce the danger associated with Lp(a).

REFERENCES

1. Clarke R, Peden JF, Hopewell JC, et al: Genetic variants associated with Lp(a) lipoprotein level and coronary disease. N Engl J Med 361:2518, 2009.
2. Kamstrup PR, Tybjaerg-Hansen A, Steffensen R, Nordestgaard BG: Genetically elevated lipoprotein(a) and increased risk of myocardial infarction. JAMA 301:2331, 2009.
3. The Emerging Risk Factors Collaboration: Lipoprotein(a) concentration and the risk of coronary heart disease, stroke, and nonvascular mortality. JAMA 302:412, 2009.

ANSWER TO QUESTION 311

B (Braunwald, pp. 986-989)

Fibric acid derivatives (e.g., gemfibrozil, fenofibrate) are approved for use in patients with hypertriglyceridemia and in the secondary prevention of cardiovascular events in patients with low levels of high-density lipoprotein (HDL) cholesterol. These agents interact with a nuclear transcription factor (PPAR-alpha) that regulates the transcription of the lipoprotein lipase, apo CII, and apo AI

genes. Increased lipoprotein lipase augments hydrolysis of triglycerides from very low-density lipoproteins (VLDL) at peripheral tissues, which decreases VLDL and plasma triglyceride levels. However, this action may cause LDL levels to rise. A meta-analysis of fibrate trials has shown a modest reduction in rates of myocardial infarction but no reduction in mortality.[1]

Fish oils are rich in omega-3 polyunsaturated fatty acids. They *decrease* plasma triglyceride levels by reducing VLDL synthesis and have antithrombotic effects. Such therapy is recommended in cases of hypertriglyceridemia refractory to other conventional therapies.

As indicated in the Answer to Question 307, niacin (nicotinic acid, vitamin B_3) is especially effective at raising HDL and lowering triglyceride levels, but doses 200 times the recommended daily allowance are required for these effects. Niacin decreases VLDL secretion from the liver and decreases free fatty acid mobilization from peripheral tissues. Side effects include flushing, hyperuricemia, hyperglycemia, and hepatotoxicity.

Bile acid–binding resins prevent the reabsorption of bile acids from the small intestine, thereby reducing the return of cholesterol to the liver through the enterohepatic circulation with subsequent upregulation of hepatic low-density lipoprotein (LDL) receptors. The latter action increases removal of LDL from the circulation. Resins are used primarily as an adjunct to statins in patients with severe elevations of LDL cholesterol. Side effects include constipation, abdominal fullness, and hypertriglyceridemia. In addition, resins can interfere with the absorption of other medications, which therefore should be ingested at least 1 hour before or 3 hours after the resin.

Ezetimibe selectively inhibits cholesterol uptake by intestinal epithelial cells and reduces LDL cholesterol alone or in combination with statins. Clinical trials evaluating the clinical benefit of LDL lowering with ezetimibe are ongoing.

REFERENCE

1. Jun M, Foote C, Lv J, et al: Effects of fibrates on cardiovascular outcomes: A systematic review and meta-analysis. Lancet 375:1875, 2010.

ANSWER TO QUESTION 312

E (Braunwald, pp. 935, 956-959)

The seventh report of the Joint National Committee on the Detection, Evaluation and Treatment of High Blood Pressure (JNC VII) defines four levels of blood pressure: normal (systolic < 120 mm Hg and diastolic < 80 mm Hg), prehypertension (systolic 120 to 139 or diastolic 80 to 89), stage 1 hypertension (systolic 140 to 159 or diastolic 90 to 99), and stage 2 hypertension (systolic ≥ 160 or diastolic ≥ 100). By these criteria, the prevalence of hypertension rises progressively with age in both men and women.[1] Both systolic and diastolic hypertension are associated with an increased risk of coronary heart disease.

According to JNC VII, the blood pressure goal for hypertensive individuals is dependent on whether there is evidence of cardiovascular disease or other target organ damage or if there are specific risk factors, including smoking, diabetes, hyperlipidemia, or advanced age. JNC VII has set a blood pressure goal of 140/90 mm Hg for lower-risk patients but a more aggressive target of 130/80 mm Hg for those with cardiovascular disease or diabetes. Because the likelihood of coronary disease increases with the level of blood pressure, there is significant risk even among patients above the optimal level (120/80) but below the hypertensive range. Therefore, lifestyle modifications that modestly reduce blood pressure, including weight reduction, exercise, and smoking cessation, are recommended for all patients in the prehypertensive range.[1]

Drug therapy for hypertension has been shown to be of benefit in older patients, although data in the very elderly are scant. A study of 3845 individuals older than 80 years with SBP > 160 mm Hg showed that drug therapy effectively reduces stroke rates, heart failure, and mortality without causing serious adverse effects.[2] A less stringent target blood pressure of <150/80 mm Hg was used in this trial.

REFERENCES

1. Joint National Committee: The seventh report of the Joint National Committee on Prevention, Detection, Evaluation, and Treatment of High Blood Pressure (JNC-7 Express). JAMA 289:2560, 2003.
2. Beckett NS, Peters R, Fletcher AE, et al: Treatment of hypertension in patients 80 years of age or older. N Engl J Med 358:1887-1898, 2008.

ANSWER TO QUESTION 313

C (Braunwald, pp. 1359-1363)

In the United States, stroke is the third leading cause of death; only heart disease and cancer are more common. Each year approximately 700,000 strokes occur, and of these, 200,000 are recurrent events in patients with a history of stroke. Treatable risk factors for ischemic stroke include hypertension, diabetes, and cigarette smoking.[1]

Blood pressure lowering is safe and beneficial in the period after an ischemic stroke, and the American Stroke Association recommends such therapy. For example, in the PROGRESS trial,[2] 6105 stable patients with a recent stroke were randomized to placebo or antihypertensive therapy with an angiotensin-converting enzyme inhibitor and diuretic. After 4 years, the relative risk of a new stroke declines by 28% in the patients randomized to the medical regimen compared with placebo.

Although data relating hypercholesterolemia to stroke risk have been equivocal, statins have been shown to reduce the incidence of stroke in patients at increased risk of vascular disease. A meta-analysis of 90,000 patients in cholesterol-lowering trials showed that each 10% reduction in low-density lipoprotein (LDL) level reduced the risk of stroke by 15.6%. In the Heart Protection Study (see Answer to Question 327), treatment with simvastatin was associated with a highly significant reduction in stroke rates. In the SPARCL study, 4731 patients with a history of cerebrovascular disease (recent stroke or transient ischemic attack [TIA]) and baseline LDL 100 to 190 mg/dL, but no known coronary disease, were randomized to atorvastatin 80 mg daily or placebo. After a mean follow-up of 4.9 years, there was a 16% reduction in subsequent stroke rates.[3]

Aspirin, or the combination of aspirin plus dipyridamole, has been shown to be effective for secondary prevention of ischemic stroke. In the MATCH trial, the combination of aspirin plus clopidogrel was compared with aspirin alone in 7599 patients who had sustained an ischemic stroke or TIA.[4] After 18 months, there was a nonsignificant reduction in the primary outcome (a composite of ischemic stroke, TIA, myocardial infarction, or vascular death) without a difference in all-cause mortality; life-threatening bleeding was higher in the combination group. Thus, dual antiplatelet therapy with aspirin and clopidogrel is not routinely recommended for secondary prevention after ischemic stroke.

In the PRoFESS study, aspirin plus dipyridamole was comparable with clopidogrel monotherapy for secondary stroke prevention in patients with noncardioembolic stroke; however, there were more major hemorrhages in the aspirin plus dipyridamole group.[5]

In the Warfarin-Aspirin Recurrent Stroke Study there was a nonsignificant advantage of aspirin over warfarin in secondary stroke prevention.[6]

REFERENCES

1. Sacco RL, Adams R, Albers G, et al: American Heart Association; American Stroke Association Council on Stroke; Council on Cardiovascular Radiology and Intervention; American Academy of Neurology. Stroke 37:577, 2006.
2. The PROGRESS Collaborative group: Randomized trial of a perindopril-based blood pressure-lowering regimen among 6,105 individuals with previous stroke or transient ischemic attack. Lancet 358:1033, 2001.
3. Amarenco P, Bogousslavsky J, Callahan A 3rd, et al: High-dose atorvastatin after stroke or transient ischemic attack. N Engl J Med 355:549, 2006.
4. Diener HC, Bogousslavsky J, Brass LM, et al: Aspirin and clopidogrel compared with clopidogrel alone after recent ischaemic stroke or transient ischaemic attack in high-risk patients (MATCH): Randomised, double-blind, placebo-controlled trial. Lancet 364:331, 2004.
5. Sacco RL, Diener HC, Yusuf S, et al: Aspirin and extended-release dipyridamole versus clopidogrel for recurrent stroke. N Engl J Med 359:1238, 2008.
6. Mohr JP, Thompson JLP, Lazar RM, et al: Comparison of warfarin and aspirin for the prevention of recurrent ischemic stroke. N Engl J Med 345:1444, 2001.

ANSWER TO QUESTION 314

D (Braunwald, pp. 1003, 1628-1631)

Alcohol's interaction with the cardiovascular system is complex. Heavy alcohol intake is associated with increased cardiovascular and total mortality rates. However, several primary and secondary prevention studies have found that the relation between alcohol intake and cardiovascular disease is J shaped, in that moderate (1 to 2 drinks) daily intake of alcohol reduces risk compared with individuals who do not drink any alcoholic beverages.[1] Alcohol's beneficial effects may be a result of its ability to raise high-density lipoprotein levels, improve fibrinolysis, and reduce platelet aggregation. Alcohol intake is not associated with decreased low-density lipoprotein levels.

REFERENCE

1. Bagnardi V, Zatonski W, Scotti L, et al: Does drinking pattern modify the effect of alcohol on the risk of coronary heart disease? Evidence from a meta-analysis. J Epidemiol Community Health 62:615, 2008.

ANSWER TO QUESTION 315

D (Braunwald, pp. 1015-1016)

Cigarette smoking is one of the strongest risk factors for coronary artery disease but is also one of the hardest to modify. Among its deleterious effects, smoking increases platelet aggregation, serum fibrinogen, and oxidation of low-density lipoprotein cholesterol. Smoking cessation reduces coronary heart disease mortality by 36% compared with patients who continue to smoke, a benefit that does not change with age, gender, or nationality. Patients who continue to smoke after a myocardial infarction have twice the mortality rate of those who stop. However, the benefits of smoking cessation are enormous: by 1 year, the risk falls to one half of its peak value. The cardiovascular risk approaches a person who never smoked after 3 to 5 years of smoking cessation.

Addiction to nicotine can be intense. Patients who successfully quit smoking usually do so after five or more unsuccessful attempts. Physician counseling alone carries a poor success rate, with only 6% of patients achieving 1 year of abstinence.

Greater success is achieved when pharmacologic aids are included in the treatment program. Agents approved by the U.S. Food and Drug Administration for smoking cessation include (1) nicotine replacement therapy (available as patches, gums, lozenges, nasal spray, and an inhaler),[1] (2) the psychoactive drug bupropion, and (3) varenicline, a partial nicotinic acetylcholine receptor agonist. Randomized trials have shown that continuous abstinence is more likely with varenicline use than with placebo or bupropion.[2]

REFERENCES

1. Stead LF, Perera R, Bullen C, et al: Nicotine replacement therapy for smoking cessation. Cochrane Database Syst Rev (1):CD000146, 2008.
2. Tonstad S, Tonnesen P, Hajek P, et al: Effect of maintenance therapy with varenicline on smoking cessation: A randomized controlled trial. JAMA 296:64, 2006.

ANSWER TO QUESTION 316

D (Braunwald, pp. 1036-1041)

Comprehensive rehabilitation for patients with coronary disease includes physical exercise training, which benefits the cardiovascular system and skeletal muscle in ways that improve work performance. Different formats for outpatient physical activity include supervised and unsupervised programs. In supervised programs, the aerobic training goal is typically exercising to 70% to 80% of the maximum predicted heart rate; some patients may require lower intensities. In unsupervised home programs, patients are encouraged to exercise to the onset of mild dyspnea, which eliminates the need for monitoring the pulse rate.

Several meta-analyses have studied the relation between exercise-based cardiac rehabilitation and clinical outcomes and have come to similar conclusions: mortality rates are lower among exercise-program participants compared with patients who did not participate.[1] Most of the studies included in these meta-analyses were performed before the current era of aggressive revascularization and may overestimate the expected mortality results in current practice.

During exercise, an increase in heart rate accounts for a greater percentage of the augmented cardiac output than does the rise in stroke volume. In addition, at rest, the heart extracts about 75% of oxygen in the coronary flow. Because of the limited reserve, any increase in myocardial oxygen demand must be met by a more substantial augmentation of coronary blood flow. With physical training, half the improvement in exercise performance is due to increased cardiac output and half to peripheral adaptations that actually improve oxygen extraction.

REFERENCE

1. Taylor RS, Brown A, Ebrahim S, et al: Exercise-based rehabilitation for patients with coronary heart disease: Systematic review and meta-analysis of randomized controlled trials. Am J Med 116:682, 2004.

ANSWER TO QUESTION 317

E (Braunwald, p. 927)

Homocysteine is an amino acid derived from the demethylation of dietary methionine. Inherited disorders of methionine metabolism cause extremely high levels of homocysteine as well as homocystinuria. The most common cause of severe hyperhomocystinemia is cystathionine beta-synthase deficiency. Patients with this genetic defect present with atherothrombosis as early as the first decade of life. In contrast, mild to moderate elevations in homocysteine (>15 μmol/L) are common in the general population. Such elevations are often due to insufficient dietary intake of folate, use of folate antagonists such as methotrexate, polymorphisms in the methylene tetrahydrofolate reductase gene, hypothyroidism, or renal insufficiency.

A large number of epidemiologic studies have shown a link between mildly elevated homocysteine levels and atherosclerosis.[1] Folic acid supplementation can decrease homocysteine levels by approximately 25%. Additional vitamin B_{12} supplementation typically reduces levels by another 7%. Nevertheless, clinical studies that have included over 12,000 subjects have shown that reduction in plasma homocysteine concentration with B-vitamin supplements does not reduce, and may actually increase, the risk of atherothrombotic events.[2,3]

REFERENCES

1. Localzo J: Homocysteine trials: Clear outcomes for complex reasons. N Engl J Med 354:1629, 2006.
2. The Heart Outcomes Prevention Evaluation (HOPE) 2 Investigators: Homocysteine lowering with folic acid and B vitamins in vascular disease. N Engl J Med 354:1567, 2006.
3. Bønaa KH, Njølstad I, Ueland PM, et al: Homocysteine lowering and cardiovascular events after acute myocardial infarction. N Engl J Med 354:1578, 2006.

ANSWER TO QUESTION 318

D (Braunwald, pp. 919-921)

The metabolic syndrome (also termed *syndrome X*, or the *insulin resistance syndrome*) is a common constellation of risk factors that greatly increases the risk of cardiovascular disease. Insulin resistance, the underlying abnormality in the metabolic syndrome, may in part explain the association between hyperglycemia and atherosclerosis. Because it precedes overt diabetes mellitus, insulin resistance may also explain why many patients with newly diagnosed type 2 diabetes already have extensive vascular disease. The severity of insulin resistance correlates with the rates of myocardial infarction, stroke, and peripheral arterial disease, whereas decreasing insulin resistance pharmacologically may reduce vascular events.[1]

The National Cholesterol Education Program (NCEP) considers the metabolic syndrome to be present when three or more of the following are present: fasting serum glucose ≥110 mg/dL, abdominal obesity (waist circumference >40 inches in men or >35 inches in women), serum triglycerides ≥150 mg/dL, low serum high-density lipoprotein cholesterol (>40 mg/dL in men or > 50 mg/dL in women), and hypertension (≥130/≥85 mm Hg).[2]

REFERENCES

1. Opie LH: Metabolic syndrome. Circulation 115:e32, 2007.
2. Grundy SM, Brewer HB Jr, Cleeman JI, et al: Definition of metabolic syndrome: report of the National Heart, Lung, and Blood Institute/American Heart Association conference on scientific issues related to definition. Circulation 109:433, 2004.

ANSWER TO QUESTION 319

D (Braunwald, p. 1044)

Many nonpharmacologic approaches have been proposed for risk factor modification and treatment of cardiovascular disease. Among the most commonly used complementary and alternative medicine practices are hypnotherapy, relaxation, meditation, music therapy, acupuncture, yoga, and biofeedback.

A Cochrane review that included 24 randomized controlled trials concluded that acupuncture did not perform better than sham-acupuncture in helping patients achieve smoking cessation.[1] Another Cochrane review concluded that hypnotherapy had no greater effect on 6-month quit rates than no treatment.[2]

In hypertension, two clinical trials suggested that hypnotherapy may be modestly beneficial in lowering blood pressure and a meta-analysis of nine randomized controlled trials suggest a small beneficial effect of relaxation techniques in hypertension.[3] Similarly, the regular practice of qigong for 8 to 10 weeks has been shown to reduce elevated systolic and diastolic blood pressures[4] and regular adherence to yoga also has modest favorable effects in hypertension.[5]

REFERENCES

1. White AR, Rampes H, Campbell JL: Acupuncture and related interventions for smoking cessation. Cochrane Database Syst Rev (1):CD000009, 2006.
2. Barnes J, Dong CY, McRobbie H, et al: Hypnotherapy for smoking cessation. Cochrane Database of Systematic Rev (10):CD001008, 2010.
3. Ernst E, Pittler MH, Wider B, Boddy K: The Desktop Guide to Complementary and Alternative Medicine, 2nd ed. Edinburgh, Elsevier Mosby, 2006.
4. Lee MS, Pittler MH, Guo R, et al: Qigong for hypertension: A systematic review of randomized clinical trials. J Hypertens 25:1525, 2007.
5. Cohen DL, Bloedon LT, Rothman RL, et al: Iyengar yoga versus enhanced usual care on blood pressure in patients with prehypertension to stage I hypertension: A randomized controlled trial. Evid Based Complement Alternat Med 2009 Sep 4 [Epub ahead of print].

ANSWER TO QUESTION 320

D (Braunwald, pp. 999-1004)

Several clinical trials have examined the effects of diet on reducing cardiovascular events. Cholesterol-lowering diets rich in polyunsaturated fatty acids have been associated with a 25% to 50% reduction in cardiovascular disease endpoints over 5 to 12 years of follow-up.[1,2] The Lyon Diet Heart study randomized patients with coronary artery disease to either a Mediterranean-style diet (rich in fruits, legumes, vegetables, and fiber and reduced meat, butter, and cream) supplemented with alpha-linolenic acid–enriched margarine or a control diet. Despite a similar percentage of total fat in each diet and similar lipid profiles, there was a 56% reduction in all-cause mortality and a 70% reduction in nonfatal myocardial infarction (MI) in the Mediterranean-style diet group compared with the control group.[1,2]

Two large studies—the GISSI-Prevenzione and the Diet and Reinfarction Trial (DART)— randomized over 5000 patients to omega-3 fatty acid supplements (fish oil) versus placebo and found a nearly 30% reduction in total mortality and a 45% reduction in sudden death despite no significant difference in cholesterol levels.[1,2] An intense vegetarian diet with only 10% total fat (as well as aerobic exercise training and other healthful lifestyle modifications) was tested in patients with coronary artery disease in the Life-Style Heart Trial. After 5 years, patients in the low-fat diet group had angiographic evidence of disease regression and reduced rates of recurrent MI.[3]

A diet of reduced-carbohydrate, high-protein, and high-fat content was shown to result in greater weight loss at 12 months, increased high-density lipoprotein, and reduced triglycerides when compared with a low-calorie,

PREVENTIVE CARDIOLOGY; ATHEROSCLEROTIC CARDIOVASCULAR DISEASE

high-carbohydrate, low-fat diet but has not been shown in controlled trials to reduce cardiovascular events.[4]

REFERENCES

1. Sacks FM, Katan M: Randomized clinical trials on the effects of dietary fat and carbohydrate on plasma lipoproteins and cardiovascular disease. Am J Med 113:13S, 2002.
2. Hu FB, Willett WC: Optimal diets for prevention of coronary heart disease. JAMA 288:2569, 2002.
3. Ornish D, Scherwitz LW, Billings JH, et al: Intensive lifestyle changes for reversal of coronary heart disease. JAMA 280:2001, 1998.
4. Gardner CD, Kiazand A, Alhassan S, et al: Comparison of the Atkins, Zone, Ornish, and LEARN diets for change in weight and related risk factors among overweight premenopausal women: The A to Z weight loss study: A randomized trial. JAMA 297:969, 2007.

ANSWER TO QUESTION 321

C (Braunwald, pp. 1015-1021; Table 49-8)

Aspirin has proven efficacy in primary prevention, acute treatment, and secondary prevention of myocardial infarction (MI).[1] Studies support the administration of 325 mg in the acute setting and 81 to 325 mg/d in chronic usage. Beta blockers are a key strategy in the management of coronary artery disease. During infarction, beta blockers are associated with a 15% reduction in mortality. Long-term benefit for secondary prevention has also been shown, with a 30% to 40% reduction in mortality over 2 to 3 years. This improvement appears to be related to the level of beta blockade as measured by heart rate reduction.[2]

Angiotensin-converting enzyme (ACE) inhibition is a cornerstone of therapy during and after hospitalization for MI. In large clinical trials, more than 120,000 patients have been randomized to an ACE inhibitor or placebo in the setting of acute MI (regardless of left ventricular [LV] function), and the results are consistent: ACE inhibitors reduce morbidity and mortality during and after the acute event. The greatest benefit accrues during the first week post MI, especially in the highest risk patients. Putative beneficial effects include vasodilatation, increased production of nitric oxide, decreased aldosterone secretion, lowered sympathetic tone, and reduced adverse LV remodeling. In addition, in patients with documented LV dysfunction after MI, ACE inhibitor use has been associated with a 20% to 30% relative risk reduction in mortality over approximately 3 years of follow-up.[3]

Some (but not all) studies have demonstrated that ACE inhibitors reduce long-term cardiovascular mortality when prescribed to patients with chronic coronary disease, or patients with multiple coronary risk factors, despite normal or near-normal LV function.

Several studies support the use of cholesterol-lowering therapy after MI.[4] The 4S and CARE trials examined the effects of HMG-CoA reductase inhibitors (i.e., "statins") after MI among patients with elevated and average cholesterol levels, respectively. Each demonstrated a marked reduction in cardiovascular death and MI in patients randomized to the cholesterol-lowering regimen. The optimal timing and intensity of statin therapy in this setting are still unsettled, but improved outcomes have been shown with high-dose statins (e.g., atorvastatin 80 mg/d) and a target low-density lipoprotein of < 70 mg/dL.[5]

REFERENCES

1. Baigent C, Blackwell L, Collins R, et al: Aspirin in the primary and secondary prevention of vascular disease: Collaborative meta-analysis of individual participant data from randomised trials. Lancet 373:1849, 2009.
2. Bangalore S, Messerli FH, Kostis JB, et al: Cardiovascular protection using beta-blockers: A critical review of the evidence. J Am Coll Cardiol 50:563, 2007.
3. Tokmakova M, Solomon SD: Inhibiting the renin-angiotensin system in myocardial infarction and heart failure: Lessons from SAVE, VALIANT and CHARM, and other clinical trials. Curr Opin Cardiol 21:268, 2006.
4. Antman EM, Anbe DT, Armstrong PW, et al: ACC/AHA guidelines for the management of patients with ST-elevation myocardial infarction: Executive summary. A report of the American College of Cardiology/American Heart Association Task Force on Practice Guidelines (Writing Committee to Revise the 1999 Guidelines for the Management of Patients with Acute Myocardial Infarction). J Am Coll Cardiol 44:671, 2004.
5. Cannon CP, Braunwald E, McCabe CH, et al: Pravastatin or Atorvastatin Evaluation and Infection Therapy–Thrombolysis in Myocardial Infarction 22: Intensive versus moderate lipid lowering with statins after acute coronary syndromes. N Engl J Med 350:1495, 2004.

ANSWER TO QUESTION 322

C (Braunwald, pp. 982-983; Fig. 47-4; see also Answer to Question 306)

Familial hypercholesterolemia (FH) is one of the few examples of an autosomal dominant disorder in which homozygotes survive infancy. The inherited defect in FH involves the gene coding for the cell surface low-density lipoprotein (LDL) receptor. Heterozygotes inherit one mutant gene and one normal gene and therefore produce only half the normal number of receptors. Heterozygotes number about 1 in 500 persons in the population. Homozygotes inherit two copies of the mutant gene and so have virtually no LDL receptors. Physicians rarely see homozygotes, whose frequency in the population is 1 in 1 million.

FH heterozygotes commonly present with tendon xanthomas, which are nodules that may involve the Achilles tendon and various extensor tendons of the forearm and leg. They consist of deposits of cholesterol derived from LDL particles. Cutaneous planar xanthomas occur only in homozygotes and usually manifest within the first 6 years of life. These xanthomas are yellow to bright orange and occur over areas of trauma. Both the heterozygous and homozygous forms of FH are associated with an increased incidence of coronary artery disease, the homozygous form far more severely than the heterozygous form. The presence of FH may be verified by assaying the density of functional LDL receptors on circulating lymphocytes or by genetic testing, although this is rarely clinically necessary.

REFERENCE

Kwiterovich PO: Clinical implications of the molecular basis of familial hypercholesterolemia and other inherited dyslipidemias. Circulation 123:1153, 2011.

ANSWER TO QUESTION 323

D (Braunwald, pp. 983-985; Fig. 47-4)

Familial hypertriglyceridemia is a relatively common disorder in which the concentration of very low-density lipoprotein is elevated in the plasma. The prevalence is between 1 in 100 and 1 in 50. These patients do not usually exhibit hypertriglyceridemia until puberty or early adulthood, at which time plasma triglyceride levels are moderately elevated, in the range of 200 to 500 mg/dL. Both the low-density lipoprotein and high-density lipoprotein (HDL) cholesterol levels are usually low. These individuals exhibit only a slightly increased incidence of atherosclerosis, and it is unclear whether this is caused by the hypertriglyceridemia, by accompanying decreases in HDL cholesterol, or by associated illnesses. Patients with hypertriglyceridemia can experience severe exacerbations, with plasma triglyceride levels as high as 1000 mg/dL, when exposed to a variety of precipitating factors (e.g., excessive alcohol ingestion, poorly controlled diabetes, birth control pills containing estrogen, or development of hypothyroidism), or even after a meal. These high triglyceride levels may lead to pancreatitis and eruptive xanthomas.

The disorder appears to be genetically heterogeneous in that patients from different families may have different mutations. No consistent abnormalities of lipoprotein structure or receptor function have been described. Lipoprotein electrophoresis shows an increase in the prebeta fraction (type IV lipoprotein pattern). These individuals can often be treated by controlling the exacerbating conditions, such as obesity, and restricting the intake of fats and alcohol.

REFERENCE

Kolovou GD, Anagnostopoulou KK, Kostakou PM, et al: Primary and secondary hypertriglyceridaemia. Curr Drug Targets 10:336, 2009.

ANSWER TO QUESTION 324

D (Braunwald, pp. 1280, 1286; Table 58-9; see also Answer to Question 388)

Stent thrombosis is an uncommon, but potentially devastating complication of coronary stenting. Mortality rates of 20% to 45% have been reported. Stent thrombosis that occurs immediately after stent implantation is referred to as *acute thrombosis*, an occurrence within the first month is termed *subacute thrombosis*, and *late thrombosis* denotes cases that occur thereafter. Stent thrombosis is effectively prevented by the combination of aspirin and a second antiplatelet agent, currently clopidogrel or prasugrel. In the case of bare metal stents, the risk of thrombosis becomes negligible after 1 month of such therapy. However, drug-eluting stents (DES) retard the development of neointima such that there is a more prolonged exposure of the thrombogenic surface to circulating blood elements, necessitating a longer duration of antiplatelet medications. The 2005 Guidelines for Percutaneous Intervention recommended a minimum of 3 months of dual antiplatelet therapy for patients for a sirolimus-eluting stent, 6 months for a paclitaxel-eluting stent, and preferably 12 months for either in patients without high bleeding risks.[1] Whereas these recommendations were based on studies of low-risk lesions, the clinical use of drug-eluting stents has expanded to higher-risk settings. Such use has likely contributed to a greater threat of late stent thrombosis, which has been reported many months, or even years, after DES placement.

With standard dual antiplatelet regimens, the incidence of late DES thrombosis was reported to occur in 0.19% of patients in a large registry.[2] This complication likely contributed to the significantly higher rate of death or MI > 6 months in patients who received DES compared with bare metal stents in a large Swedish registry.[3]

The strongest predictor for stent thrombosis is premature cessation of antiplatelet therapies. Other factors that increase this risk include stent placement in small vessels, multiple lesions, long stents, overlapping stents, ostial or bifurcation lesions, prior brachytherapy, a suboptimal stent result (e.g., under expansion or residual dissection), low ejection fraction, diabetes mellitus, and renal failure.[4]

A 2007 Science Advisory stresses the importance of at least 12 months of aspirin plus thienopyridine therapy after DES placement,[4] and emphasizes that elective surgery should be delayed for at least 12 months after DES implantation so as to avoid interruption of these medications.

REFERENCES

1. Smith SC Jr, Feldman TE, Hirshfeld JW Jr, et al: ACC/AHA/SCAI 2005 guideline update for percutaneous coronary intervention: A report of the American College of Cardiology/American Heart Association Task Force of Practice Guidelines (ACC/AHA/SCAI Writing Committee to Update the 2001 Guidelines for Percutaneous Coronary Intervention) Circulation 113:156-175, 2006.
2. Urban P, Gershlick AH, Guagliumi G, et al: Safety of coronary sirolimus-eluting stents in daily clinical practice: One-year follow-up of the e-cypher registry. Circulation 113:1434, 2006.
3. Lagerqvist B, James SK, Stenestrand U, et al: SCAAR Study Group. Long-term outcomes with drug-eluting stents versus bare-metal stents in Sweden. N Engl J Med 356:1009, 2007.
4. Grines CL, Bonow RO, Casey DE Jr, et al: Prevention of premature discontinuation of dual antiplatelet therapy in patients with coronary artery stents: A science advisory from the American Heart Association, American College of Cardiology, Society for Cardiovascular Angiography and Interventions, American College of Surgeons, and American Dental Association, with representation from the American College of Physicians. Circulation 115:813, 2007.

ANSWER TO QUESTION 325

B (Braunwald, pp. 1354-1356; Figs. 61-20 and 61-21)

The patient described in this question has likely experienced atheroemboli to his kidneys, triggered by the catheterization procedure. Atheroemboli can be produced by mechanical manipulation of the aorta via catheters or surgery, and the kidneys are common targets for such embolism. This complication can result in acute renal failure with a stepwise decline in function. Some patients may progress to end-stage renal disease, whereas others recover full kidney function. The emboli may lodge in terminal arteries of the kidney, causing localized glomerular ischemia, or may compromise the large arteries and result in the loss of entire renal function.[1,2]

The urinalysis is often unremarkable, with only mild proteinuria and a bland sediment. Rarely, lipid droplets in the urine can be observed. Peripheral eosinophilia and low serum complement levels may be present. Livedo reticularis, the purple discoloration described in this patient and shown in the figure, occurs in 50% of patients and is due to areas of impaired perfusion, most often in the lower extremities. Other cutaneous manifestations of atheroembolic disease include purple toes, purpura, and gangrene. Often, the diagnosis of renal embolization can be made on clinical grounds alone. If there is cutaneous involvement, biopsy of the skin and muscle may be helpful. Renal biopsy may provide useful information but carries a significant complication rate.

The management of atheroemboli centers on supportive care, which may include hemodialysis. Large emboli may be amenable to surgical or catheter removal.

REFERENCES

1. Tunick PA, Kronzon I: Atheroembolism. In Creager MA, Dzau VJ, Loscalzo J (eds): Vascular Medicine: A Companion to Braunwald's Heart Disease. Philadelphia, Elsevier, 2006, pp. 677-687.
2. Molisse TA, Tunick PA, Kronzon I: Complications of aortic atherosclerosis: Atheroemboli and thromboemboli. Curr Treat Options Cardiovasc Med 9:137, 2007.

ANSWER TO QUESTION 326

B (Braunwald, p. 979; Table 47-1; Fig. 47-4)

Low-density lipoprotein (LDL) is the major cholesterol-carrying component of the plasma. It is formed mainly from metabolism of very low-density lipoprotein (VLDL) in the circulation: VLDL undergoes hydrolysis by lipoprotein lipase to form intermediate-density lipoprotein, which is then further delipidated by hepatic lipase to form LDL. The major lipid components of LDL are esterified cholesterol and triglyceride. The proportion of these components determines LDL particle size, with an increase in triglycerides and decrease in cholesterol esters leading to smaller, denser LDL particles. Apo B100 is the predominant protein present in LDL and comprises approximately 25% of LDL mass. Cells internalize LDL after it binds to cell surface LDL receptors. In familial hypercholesterolemia there is a decreased number of LDL receptors; however, over 80% of patients with elevated LDL levels do not have this single-gene disorder but rather have polygenic hypercholesterolemia.

Apo AI is the major apolipoprotein of high-density lipoprotein.

ANSWER TO QUESTION 327

C (Braunwald, p. 990, Table 47-7)

The Heart Protection Study (HPS) Collaborative Group enrolled 20,536 patients who were at increased risk of cardiovascular events and randomized them to simvastatin, 40 mg, or to placebo and follow-up for 5 years.[1] Patients were eligible for enrollment if they had a history of coronary artery disease (angina, myocardial infarction, bypass surgery, or angioplasty), known peripheral vascular disease, diabetes, or treated hypertension. Of the total, 7150 patients did not have known coronary heart disease. At baseline, the mean low-density lipoprotein (LDL) level was 132 mg/dL and the total cholesterol level was 228 mg/dL. Patients treated with simvastatin achieved a 20% reduction of total cholesterol levels and a 29% reduction of LDL. Simvastatin reduced the primary endpoint of major cardiovascular events by 24% ($P < 0.001$) with an absolute risk reduction of 5.4%. Statin therapy was beneficial across all groups, regardless of known vascular disease, baseline LDL, sex, or age. In a 2×2 factorial design, HPS also tested a combination of antioxidant vitamins (alpha-tocopherol, ascorbic acid, beta-carotene) and found no difference in outcomes between placebo and vitamin-treated patients.[2]

REFERENCES

1. Heart Protection Study Collaborative Group: MRC/BHF Heart Protection Study of cholesterol lowering with simvastatin in 20,536 high-risk individuals: A randomised placebo-controlled trial. Lancet 360:7, 2002.
2. Heart Protection Study Collaborative Group: MRC/BHF Heart Protection Study of antioxidant vitamin supplementation in 20,536 high-risk individuals: A randomised placebo-controlled trial. Lancet 360:23, 2002.

ANSWER TO QUESTION 328

D (Braunwald, p. 1353)

As reviewed in the Answer to Question 297, there are two major forms of renovascular disease—atherosclerosis and fibromuscular dysplasia. Atherosclerotic patients are older and have higher systolic blood pressure, greater target organ damage, and evidence of atherosclerotic disease elsewhere.[1] Patients with fibromuscular hyperplasia are younger, are more often female, have no family history of hypertension, and have less evidence of target organ damage. Patients with fibromuscular dysplasia are less likely to progress to complete renal artery occlusion or develop ischemic nephropathy compared with patients with atherosclerotic renal artery stenosis.

REFERENCE

1. Dworkin LD, Cooper CJ: Renal-artery stenosis. N Engl J Med 361:1972, 2009.

ANSWER TO QUESTION 329

E (Braunwald, pp. 959-961)

Hypertension frequently accompanies diabetes and greatly augments the risk of cardiovascular events in this population. Aggressive control of hypertension reduces future cardiovascular events in diabetics even more than in nondiabetics.[1] Many antihypertensive agents, including diuretics, beta blockers, calcium channel blockers, angiotensin-converting enzyme (ACE) inhibitors, and angiotensin receptor blockers (ARBs), improve blood pressure control in diabetics, and there has been much controversy about whether one group is superior to others in reducing cardiovascular morbidity and mortality. Early small studies suggested that ACE inhibitors were superior to dihydropyridine calcium channel blockers in this regard. However, the larger UKPDS, Systolic Hypertension in Europe (Sys-Eur), and HOT trials found that the degree of blood pressure control is actually more important than the agents used to achieve it; the antihypertensives captopril, atenolol, and the dihydropyridine calcium channel blockers felodipine and nitrendipine all led to beneficial reductions in cardiovascular events. As a result of such studies, current guidelines recommend that the goal blood pressure of diabetics be < 130/80 mm Hg. Achieving this goal frequently requires two or more antihypertensive agents in combination.

Drugs that interfere with the renin-angiotensin system do appear to have a special place in the treatment of diabetic patients. In patients with type 1 diabetes, ACE inhibitors slow the progression of diabetic nephropathy and end-stage renal disease, and several studies have demonstrated that ARBs provide similar benefit in patients with type 2 diabetes. In the HOPE (Heart Outcomes and Prevention Evaluation) study, the ACE inhibitor ramipril reduced cardiac events, stroke risk, and death in diabetic patients.[2] The LIFE (Losartan Intervention For Endpoint) study randomized 1195 diabetic patients with hypertension and left ventricular hypertrophy to the ARB losartan or atenolol therapy.[3] Although blood pressure control was similar in both groups, those who received the ARB had reduced all-cause mortality. Thus, ACE inhibitors and ARBs remain at the forefront in the management of hypertension in diabetics.

In the 2010 ACCORD trial, very aggressive reduction of blood pressure (BP), targeting systolic BP < 120 mm Hg, was compared with "standard" therapy (target systolic BP < 140 mm Hg) in 4733 type 2 diabetics without advanced renal dysfunction.[4] The more aggressive blood pressure lowering did *not* lead to a reduction in composite outcome of nonfatal myocardial infarction, nonfatal stroke, or death from cardiovascular causes over a mean follow-up of 4.7 years and cannot currently be recommended.

REFERENCES

1. Arauz-Pacheco C, Parrott MA, Raskin P: Hypertension management in adults with diabetes. Diabetes Care 27(Suppl 1):S65, 2004.
2. Yosuf S, Sleight P, Pogue J, et al: Effects of an angiotensin-converting enzyme inhibitor, ramipril, on cardiovascular events in high-risk patients. The Heart Outcome Prevention Evaluation Study Investigators. N Engl J Med 342:145, 2000.
3. Lindholm LH, Ibsen H, Dahlof B, et al: Cardiovascular morbidity and mortality in patients with diabetes in the Losartan Intervention For Endpoint reduction in hypertension study (LIFE): A randomised trial against atenolol. Lancet 359:1004, 2002.
4. The ACCORD Study Group. Effects of Intensive Blood-Pressure Control in Type 2 Diabetes Mellitus. N Engl J Med 362:1575, 2010.

ANSWER TO QUESTION 330

A (Braunwald, pp. 1100-1101)

Up to one half of patients with acute myocardial infarction (MI) have clear prodromal symptoms or an associated precipitant, including heavy exercise, anger, or mental stress. Of patients who have prodromal symptoms preceding the acute MI, approximately two thirds have been symptomatic for < 1 week and one third have had symptoms for 1 to 3 weeks. Nausea and vomiting occur in over half of patients with acute MI, presumably related to vagal stimulation. These symptoms are more common in inferior, compared with anterior, acute MI.

Population studies indicate that 20% to 60% of nonfatal MIs are unrecognized by the patient and are detected only by subsequent routine ECGs or by postmortem examination. Of these, one half are truly silent events; the other half of patients are able to recall some symptoms consistent with previous MI when specifically questioned. Silent MI is more common in diabetics and in individuals without a history of angina. Patients who report an increased level of stress in their life after an acute coronary syndrome have an increased risk of cardiac rehospitalization and recurrent MI.

There is a clear circadian periodicity for the time of onset of acute MI, with the peak incidence of events occurring between 6 AM and noon. This observation may be related to circadian alterations in circulating catecholamines as well as increased platelet aggregability in the early morning hours.

ANSWER TO QUESTION 331

D (Braunwald, pp. 1126-1128, Table 55-4)

Primary percutaneous coronary intervention (PCI) for acute MI has several important differences and advantages when compared with pharmacologic thrombolysis. The safety and success rate in establishing reperfusion (>90%) is clearly superior to that of thrombolytic agents, and there is less likelihood of developing complications such as reocclusion, reinfarction, and stroke with primary PCI. Multiple studies have demonstrated that primary PCI, when performed at experienced centers, results in a significant reduction in the rates of death (7% vs. 9%), reinfarction (3% vs. 9%), stroke (1% vs. 2%), and hemorrhagic stroke (0.05% vs. 1%) compared with thrombolysis.[1-3] In addition, primary angioplasty has been associated with shorter hospital stays and lower follow-up costs. Patients presenting with an acute MI and cardiogenic shock are at the highest risk of death and cardiovascular complications. The SHOCK trial randomized 302 patients with cardiogenic shock to early revascularization or medical management. Early revascularization with primary PCI or urgent bypass surgery was associated with improved survival at 6 months (49.7% vs. 36.9%, $P = 0.027$) and 1 year (46.7 vs. 33.6%, $P = 0.025$).[4]

REFERENCES

1. Keeley EC, Boura JA, Grines CL: Primary angioplasty versus intravenous thrombolytic therapy for acute myocardial infarction: A quantitative review of 23 randomised trials. Lancet 361:13, 2003.
2. Widimsky P, Budesinsky T, Vorac D, et al: Long distance transport for primary angioplasty vs immediate thrombolysis in acute myocardial infarction: Final results of the randomized national multicentre trial—PRAGUE-2. Eur Heart J 24:94, 2003.
3. Andersen HR, Nielsinsky TT, Rasmussen K, et al: A comparison of coronary angioplasty with fibrinolytic therapy in acute myocardial infarction. N Engl J Med 349:733, 2003.
4. Hochman JS, Sleeper LA, Webb JG, et al: Early revascularization and long-term survival in cardiogenic shock complicating acute myocardial infarction. JAMA 295:2511, 2006.

ANSWER TO QUESTION 332

E (Braunwald, p. 1094)

Studies have revealed that atrial infarction occurs in 7% to 17% of autopsy-proven cases of myocardial infarction.[1] Atrial infarction is often seen in conjunction with left ventricular infarction and more commonly involves the right atrium than the left. This difference may reflect the presence of well-oxygenated blood in the left atrium, which could help nourish an ischemic atrial wall. Atrial infarction is frequently accompanied by supraventricular arrhythmias, including atrial fibrillation, sinus arrhythmia, and wandering atrial pacemaker.[2] In addition, atrial infarction may be complicated by rupture of the atrial wall.

REFERENCES

1. Neven K, Crijns H, Gorgels A: Atrial infarction: A neglected electrocardiographic sign with important clinical implications. J Cardiovasc Electrophysiol 14:306, 2003.
2. Tjandrawidjaja MC, Fu Y, Kim DH, et al: Compromised atrial coronary anatomy is associated with atrial arrhythmias and atrioventricular block complicating acute myocardial infarction. J Electrocardiol 38:271, 2005.

ANSWER TO QUESTION 333

A (Braunwald, pp. 1147-1149; Table 55-12)

Free wall rupture is one of the most lethal complications of acute MI because it usually leads to hemopericardium and cardiac tamponade. Rupture typically arises after a large MI in the left anterior descending artery territory at the junction of infarcted and normal muscle. Whereas older series have quoted an incidence of free wall rupture of approximately 5%, occurring within 3 to 6 days after MI, more recent observations implicate an incidence of 1 to 2%, occurring primarily within the first 48 hours.[1] Patients with free wall rupture tend to have had greater delays to hospitalization and are more likely to have been physically active after the onset of MI. Additional risk factors include advanced age, female gender, a history of hypertension, and the *absence* of previous infarction. It is thought that patients with prior MI are "protected" against rupture, because previous scars may reduce the magnitude of the shear forces between the fresh infarct and the healthy myocardium.[1] The rate of free wall rupture is lower after primary percutaneous coronary intervention than after fibrinolytic therapy.[2]

The frequency of free wall rupture has decreased over the past 30 years, and survival has improved but remains poor.[2]

REFERENCES

1. Reynolds HR, Hochman JS. Heartbreak. Eur Heart J 31:1433, 2010.
2. Figueras J, Alcalde O, Barrabes JA , et al: Changes in hospital mortality rates in 425 patients with acute ST-elevation myocardial infarction and cardiac rupture over a 30-year period. Circulation 118:2783, 2008.

ANSWER TO QUESTION 334

B (Braunwald, pp. 1146-1272; Fig. 55-32)

Patients with right ventricular infarction (RVI) may have a hemodynamic profile that resembles that of patients with pericardial disease. For example, elevations in right atrial (RA) and RV filling pressures, as well as a rapid RA *y* descent and an early diastolic dip-and-plateau ("square root sign") may occur. In addition, Kussmaul's sign may be present in patients with RVI and is highly predictive for RV involvement in the setting of inferior wall infarction.[1] Patients who present with inferior wall infarction who are suspected of having RV involvement should have an ECG obtained with precordial leads placed on the right side of the chest: most patients with RVI demonstrate ST-segment elevation of 1 mm or more in lead V_4R (not standard lead V_4).[2] Echocardiography can confirm the presence of RV dilatation and depression of systolic function and can distinguish RVI from other hemodynamically similar conditions, including pericardial tamponade, constrictive pericarditis, and pulmonary embolism.

From a hemodynamic standpoint, treatment is typically aimed at increasing RA and RV filling pressures through administration of intravenous fluids, so as to maintain normal left-sided preload. A marked hypotensive response to nitroglycerin may be a clinical clue to the presence of RVI, reflecting the significance of the RV filling pressure in this condition. Similarly, the contribution of atrial contraction to RV filling is important in patients with RVI. Thus, patients who require pacemaker therapy benefit from atrioventricular sequential pacing, which has been shown to improve the hemodynamic parameters in this condition.

REFERENCES

1. Pfisterer M: Right ventricular involvement in myocardial infarction and cardiogenic shock. Lancet 362:392, 2003.
2. Zimetbaum PJ, Josephson ME: Use of the electrocardiogram in acute myocardial infarction. N Engl J Med 348:933, 2003.

ANSWER TO QUESTION 335

C (Braunwald, pp. 1149-1150)

The progressive development of mitral regurgitation (MR) in this 60-year-old patient after an inferior myocardial infarction (MI) is most consistent with infarction of the posterior papillary muscle. Because papillary muscles are perfused via terminal portions of the coronary vascular bed, they are particularly vulnerable to ischemia. The posterior papillary muscle, supplied usually by only the posterior descending branch of the right coronary artery, is more susceptible to ischemia and infarction than the anterolateral papillary muscle, which has a dual blood supply from the diagonal branches of the left anterior descending artery and the marginal branches from the left circumflex artery. Although necrosis of a papillary muscle is a potential complication of MI, particularly of inferior infarction, frank rupture of a papillary muscle is far less common. Total papillary muscle rupture is usually fatal because of the extremely severe and rapid-onset MR that it produces. MR may also develop later after MI, in which case it usually results from left ventricular dilatation. In that case, dyskinesis of the left ventricle results in an abnormal spatial relationship between the papillary muscles and the chordae tendineae, hence promoting MR.

Rupture of chordae tendineae is also an important cause of MR, although such an event bears no special relation to MI. Common causes of chordal rupture include congenitally abnormal chordae, infective endocarditis, trauma, rheumatic fever, and myxomatous degeneration. The posterior chordae rupture spontaneously more frequently than do the anterior chordae.

REFERENCE

Wilansky S, Moreno CA, Lester SJ: Complications of myocardial infarction. Crit Care Med 35:S348, 2007.

ANSWER TO QUESTION 336

B (Braunwald, pp. 1157-1158)

Post–myocardial infarction (MI) pericarditis has become uncommon in the era of acute coronary reperfusion therapies, likely related to the improved pharmacologic and mechanical interventions that limit infarct size. The incidence of early post-MI pericarditis in 743 patients with acute ST segment elevation myocardial infarctions treated with primary percutaneous coronary intervention was 4.2%, with an increasing prevalence in patients with longer delays to hospital presentation.[1] Pericarditis can develop as early as the first day after the infarction. The diagnosis is often based on the presence of a pericardial friction rub; typical ECG changes are less common. Post-MI pericardial effusions are found most often in patients with larger infarcts, when congestive heart failure is present, and in the setting of an anterior MI.

The Dressler, or post-MI, syndrome typically occurs between 2 and 10 weeks after infarction, although some overlap between this syndrome and post-MI pericarditis exists. The Dressler syndrome has also been observed less commonly in recent years. Treatment of the syndrome typically includes high-dose salicylates. Other nonsteroidal anti-inflammatory agents are relatively contraindicated for the first month after MI owing to their association with impaired infarct healing.[2]

REFERENCES

1. Imazio M, Negro A, Belli R, et al: Frequency and prognostic significance of pericarditis following acute myocardial infarction treated by primary percutaneous coronary intervention Am J Cardiol 103:1525, 2009.
2. Jugdutt BI: Cyclooxygenase inhibition and adverse remodeling during healing after myocardial infarction. Circulation 115:288, 2007.

ANSWER TO QUESTION 337

E (Braunwald, pp. 1153-1155; Table 55-14)

A variety of conduction disturbances can occur in acute myocardial infarction (MI). In almost all patients with first-degree atrioventricular (AV) block, the disturbance is intranodal (above the bundle of His) and generally does not require specific treatment. First-degree AV block may also be a manifestation of increased vagal tone in the setting of acute MI. Other manifestations of increased vagal tone include sinus bradycardia and hypotension that are generally responsive to atropine.

Approximately 90% of patients with second-degree AV admitted to coronary care units have Mobitz type I (Wenckebach) block. Mobitz type I block occurs most commonly in patients with inferior MI, is usually transient, and rarely progresses to complete AV block. It usually resolves within 72 hours after infarction and does not require specific therapy. In contrast, Mobitz type II block typically reflects conduction disease below the bundle of His, is associated with a widened QRS complex, and almost always occurs in the setting of anterior infarction. Mobitz type II block may progress to complete heart block and therefore generally justifies pacemaker placement.

Complete AV block (third-degree AV block) may occur in either anterior or inferior infarction. Its prognosis relates to the location of the inciting infarction. In inferior infarction, complete heart block usually evolves from first-degree and type I second-degree AV block, usually has a stable escape rhythm, and is usually transient, with spontaneous resolution. Patients with anterior infarction may develop third-degree AV block without warning; however, it is usually preceded by less advanced conduction abnormalities such as Mobitz type II block. In general, patients in this setting have unstable escape rhythms, wide QRS complexes, and a high mortality rate.

REFERENCE

Hreybe H, Saba S: Location of acute myocardial infarction and associated arrhythmias and outcome. Clin Cardiol 32:274, 2009.

ANSWER TO QUESTION 338

C (Braunwald, pp. 1119-1126)

Overall, fibrinolytic therapy in ST-segment elevation myocardial infarction is associated with a 15% to 20% reduction in mortality at 35 days. The Fibrinolytic Therapy Trialists' (FTT) Collaborative Group performed an overview of nine major fibrinolytic trials that each randomized more than 1000 patients. Among patients stratified by presenting ECG, patients with bundle branch block (BBB) had the highest overall mortality, followed by patients with anterior ST-segment elevations, and then patients with inferior ST-segment elevations.[1] The relative risk reductions with fibrinolytic therapy in patients with BBB and anterior ST-segment elevation were both approximately 21%. Compared with patients with anterior ST-segment elevation, patients with inferior ST-segment elevation had less of a risk reduction.

The benefits of fibrinolysis are time dependent, and there is a stepwise decrease in improvement with later therapy over the first 24 hours. Two trials (LATE and EMERAS) showed a mortality reduction in patients treated with fibrinolytic therapy 6 to 12 hours after the onset of ischemic symptoms. However, there was no benefit for individuals treated beyond that time. Patients treated within 1 to 2 hours after onset of symptoms gained the most benefit.

Fibrinolytic trials have also demonstrated that patients older than 75 years have a more modest relative risk reduction compared with individuals younger than 55 years. However, because the risk of adverse outcomes is so high for older patients, the absolute risk reductions are comparable between the age groups.[2]

REFERENCES

1. Stenestrand U, Tabrizi F, Lindback J, et al: Comorbidity and myocardial dysfunction are the main explanations for the higher 1-year mortality in acute myocardial infarction with left bundle-branch block. Circulation 110:1896, 2004.
2. Stenestrand U, Wallentin L: Fibrinolytic therapy in patients 75 years and older with ST-segment-elevation myocardial infarction: One-year follow-up of a large prospective cohort. Arch Intern Med 163:965, 2003.

ANSWER TO QUESTION 339

C (Braunwald, pp. 1088-1090)

Plaque rupture is the typical pathophysiologic substrate that leads to acute coronary syndromes.[1] When the resulting intracoronary thrombus is only partially occlusive, ST-segment depressions or T wave inversions (or both) commonly develop. When the thrombus is completely occlusive, ST-segment elevations typically occur. In the latter setting, Q waves subsequently form in approximately 75% of patients who are not treated with fibrinolysis or acute mechanical coronary revascularization.[2] In the remaining 25%, other ECG manifestations may develop, including reduction of the R wave height or notching of the QRS complex.

In the pre-fibrinolytic era, it was common to divide patients with myocardial infarction (MI) into those experiencing either a "Q wave MI" (now called "ST-segment elevation MI") or a "non–Q wave" MI (now called "non–ST-segment elevation MI") based on the evolution of the ECG over several days. Q wave infarction was considered to be synonymous with the pathology of a transmural infarction, whereas non–Q wave infarctions were considered to involve only the subendocardial layer. However,

contemporary studies using cardiac magnetic resonance imaging indicate that the development of a Q wave on the ECG is determined more by the size of the infarct than the depth of mural involvement.[3]

REFERENCES

1. Libby P, Theroux P: Pathophysiology of coronary artery disease. Circulation 111:3481, 2005.
2. Goodman SG, Langer A, Ross AM, et al: Non–Q-wave versus Q-wave myocardial infarction after thrombolytic therapy: Angiographic and prognostic insights from the Global Utilization of Streptokinase and Tissue Plasminogen Activator for Occluded Coronary Arteries–I angiographic substudy. GUSTO-I Angiographic Investigators. Circulation 97:444, 1998.
3. Moon JC, De Arenaza DP, Elkington AG, et al: The pathologic basis of Q-wave and non–Q-wave myocardial infarction: A cardiovascular magnetic resonance study. J Am Coll Cardiol 44:554, 2004.

ANSWER TO QUESTION 340

D (Braunwald, pp. 1126-1128; Fig. 55-16)

Primary angioplasty in acute MI, when performed by experienced operators, has been shown in large registries and randomized trials to result in higher patency rates (93% to 98% vs. 54%) and lower 30-day mortality rates (5% vs. 7%) than fibrinolytic therapy. An additional advantage of primary angioplasty over fibrinolysis is a significant reduction in bleeding complications and strokes.

The use of primary stenting versus primary angioplasty does not result in a mortality advantage but correlates with a reduced need for subsequent target vessel revascularization. A meta-analysis of trials comparing primary stenting with angioplasty found no difference in the rates of death (3.7% vs. 3.6%) or recurrent MI (2.1% vs. 2.9%).

REFERENCES

Huynh T, Perron S, O'Loughlin J, et al: Comparison of primary percutaneous coronary intervention and fibrinolytic therapy in ST-segment-elevation myocardial infarction: Bayesian hierarchical meta-analyses of randomized controlled trials and observational studies. Circulation 119:3101, 2009.
Stone GW: Angioplasty strategies in ST-segment-elevation myocardial infarction: I. Primary percutaneous coronary intervention. Circulation 118:538, 2008.

ANSWER TO QUESTION 341

C (Braunwald, p. 1285; Fig. 51-42)

Left ventricular (LV) aneurysms arise in <5% of patients who survive acute ST-segment elevation myocardial infarction (MI). Formation of the aneurysm is presumed to occur when intraventricular tension leads to expansion of the noncontracting, infarcted myocardial tissue. An anterior MI complicated by LV aneurysm occurs due to total occlusion of a poorly collateralized left anterior descending artery. The presence of multivessel disease, extensive collateral vessels, or a nonoccluded left anterior descending artery makes the development of an aneurysm much less likely. Aneurysms occur approximately four times more often at the apex and in the anterior wall than in the inferoposterior wall and, in general, range from 1 to 8 cm in diameter.

True LV aneurysms, in contrast to pseudoaneurysms, rarely rupture. However, even when compared with mortality in patients having comparable LV ejection fractions, the presence of LV aneurysm leads to a mortality that is up to six times higher than that of patients without aneurysm. Death in such patients is often sudden and presumed to be secondary to a high incidence of ventricular tachyarrhythmias that originate from the aneurysmal tissue itself. Diagnosis of aneurysm is best made by echocardiography, magnetic resonance imaging, or at the time of cardiac catheterization by left ventriculography. Interestingly, the "classic" evidence of aneurysm on the ECG—persistent ST-segment elevation in the area of the infarction—actually indicates a large infarct but does not necessarily imply an aneurysmal segment.[1]

REFERENCE

1. Napodano M, Tarantini G, Ramondo A, et al: Myocardial abnormalities underlying persistent ST-segment elevation after anterior myocardial infarction. J Cardiovasc Med (Hagerstown) 10:44, 2009.

ANSWER TO QUESTION 342

D (Braunwald, p. 1156)

The ECG demonstrates atrial fibrillation with a rapid ventricular rate. Atrial fibrillation in acute myocardial infarction (MI) is usually transient and occurs more commonly in patients with left ventricular failure, infarct-associated pericarditis, or ischemic injury to the atria. Atrial fibrillation is more common during the first 24 hours after infarction than later. It is associated with increased mortality, in part because it occurs more frequently with extensive anterior wall infarctions.[1,2] The rapid ventricular response and loss of atrial contribution to ventricular filling may lead to an important reduction in cardiac output.

In patients who are hemodynamically stable, the use of negative chronotropic drugs to slow ventricular response is an appropriate first step in management. However, electrical cardioversion is the treatment of choice in patients with evidence of hemodynamic decompensation. Treatment with an angiotensin-converting enzyme inhibitor has been associated with a reduced rate of atrial fibrillation in acute MI.[3]

REFERENCES

1. Kober L, Swedberg K, McMurray JJ, et al: Previously known and newly diagnosed atrial fibrillation: a major risk indicator after a myocardial infarction complicated by heart failure or left ventricular dysfunction. Eur J Heart Fail 8:591, 2006.
2. Saczynski JS, McManus D, Zhou Z, et al: Trends in atrial fibrillation complicating acute myocardial infarction. Am J Cardiol 104:169, 2009.
3. Levy S: Drug Insight: Angiotensin-converting-enzyme inhibitors and atrial fibrillation—indications and contraindications. Nat Clin Pract Cardiovasc Med 3:220, 2006.

ANSWER TO QUESTION 343

A (Braunwald, p. 1152)

The rhythm displayed is accelerated idioventricular rhythm (AIVR), which is defined as a ventricular escape rhythm with a rate between 60 and 100 beats/min. This rhythm is frequently referred to as "slow ventricular tachycardia" and may be seen in up to 20% of patients with acute myocardial infarction (MI), most commonly in the first 2 days after the infarction. In addition, AIVR is the most common arrhythmia noted after reperfusion of an occluded coronary artery by fibrinolytic therapy. Approximately 50% of all episodes of AIVR are initiated by a premature beat; the rest emerge during periods of sinus slowing. In general, episodes of AIVR are of short duration and may show variation in rate. Unlike more rapid forms of ventricular tachycardia, episodes of AIVR have not been found to affect prognosis in acute MI. If AIVR is accompanied by hemodynamic compromise, treatment with atropine or atrial pacing will often suppress the rhythm.

REFERENCE

Antman EM, Anbe DT, Armstrong PW, et al: ACC/AHA guidelines for the management of patients with ST-elevation myocardial infarction: Executive summary. A report of the American College of Cardiology/American Heart Association Task Force on Practice Guidelines (Writing Committee to Revise the 1999 Guidelines for the Management of Patients with Acute Myocardial Infarction). J Am Coll Cardiol 44:671, 2004.

ANSWER TO QUESTION 344

E (Braunwald, pp. 1180, 1183-1185; Table 56-3)

Several cardiac biomarkers have been found to have prognostic value in patients with acute coronary syndrome (ACS), independent of more established markers of cardiac necrosis such as cardiac-specific troponins and creatine kinase. The level of C-reactive protein (CRP), an acute-phase reactant, is approximately five times higher in patients with an ACS compared with those with stable coronary disease, and patients with the highest levels of CRP have an increased risk of death, even if cardiac troponin levels are not elevated.[1] The white blood cell count is a simpler but nonspecific marker of inflammation. Patients with unstable angina/non–ST segment elevation MI and elevated white blood cell counts have *higher* mortality and recurrent MI rates. This association is independent of CRP levels.[2]

Myeloperoxidase, a hemoprotein expressed by neutrophils, is a potent pro-oxidant that is associated with the presence of angiographic coronary artery disease. In patients with an ACS, myeloperoxidase levels have been associated with increased rates of death or recurrent MI, independent of other cardiac markers.[3]

Elevated levels of B-type natriuretic peptide, a neurohormone released in response to ventricular wall stress, are associated with a twofold to threefold higher risk of death by 10 months.[4]

PREVENTIVE CARDIOLOGY; ATHEROSCLEROTIC CARDIOVASCULAR DISEASE

REFERENCES

1. James SK, Armstrong P, Barnathan E, et al: Troponin and C-reactive protein have different relations to subsequent mortality and myocardial infarction after acute coronary syndrome: A GUSTO-IV study. J Am Coll Cardiol 41:916, 2003.
2. Sabatine MS, Morrow DA, Cannon CP, et al: Relationship between baseline white blood cell count and degree of coronary artery disease and mortality in patients with acute coronary syndromes: A TACTICS-TIMI 18 substudy. J Am Coll Cardiol 40:1761, 2002.
3. Morrow DA: Appraisal of myeloperoxidase for evaluation of patients with suspected acute coronary syndromes. J Am Coll Cardiol 49:2001, 2007.
4. Morrow DA, Cannon CP, Jesse RL, et al: National Academy of Clinical Biochemistry Laboratory Medicine Practice Guidelines: Clinical characteristics and utilization of biochemical markers in acute coronary syndrome. Clin Chem 53:552, 2007.

ANSWER TO QUESTION 345

D (Braunwald, pp. 986-990, 1016-1017; Table 47-7)

This patient is at high risk for coronary artery disease and his low-density lipoprotein (LDL) cholesterol remains above the recommended targets. In a patient with two or more atherosclerotic risk factors, the target LDL cholesterol is <130 mg/dL or, optimally, <100 mg/dL in this man's case, given his high 10-year Framingham risk score.[1]

Because each doubling of statin dosage results in only another approximately 6% decline in LDL cholesterol, he would not likely achieve the target LDL even with simvastatin 80 mg daily. Furthermore, in 2011 the U.S. Food and Drug Administration (FDA) issued an advisory against augmenting simvastatin to 80 mg daily because (1) there is an increased risk of muscle injury compared with patients taking lower doses of simvastatin, or other available statins, especially during the first year of 80 mg dosage, and (2) in the 7-year prospective, randomized, double-blinded SEARCH trial, the incidence of major vascular events was no lower in those randomized to simvastatin 80 mg daily compared with patients receiving 20 mg daily.[2]

Simvastatin is metabolized primarily by the cytochrome P-450 CYP3A4 isozyme, which if inhibited by other medications leads to an augmented serum simvastatin level and the potential for increased toxicity, including myositis and rhabdomyolysis. Among commonly used cardiovascular medications, such impaired simvastatin metabolism can result from verapamil, diltiazem, gemfibrozil, and amiodarone.[3] The 2011 FDA notice advises that gemfibrozil *not* be prescribed concurrently with simvastatin, and the dosage of simvastatin should not exceed 10 mg daily for patients who also take verapamil, diltiazem, or amiodarone.[4]

As a reasonable next step, this patient could be switched to an alternate, high-potency statin that is not metabolized by CYP3A4, such as rosuvastatin.

REFERENCES

1. Third Report of the National Cholesterol Education Program (NCEP) Expert Panel on Detection, Evaluation, and Treatment of High Blood Cholesterol in Adults (Adult Treatment Panel III) final report. Circulation 106:3143, 2002.
2. Armitage J, Bowman L, Wallendszus K, et al: Intensive lowering of LDL cholesterol with 80 mg versus 20 mg simvastatin daily in 12,064 survivors of myocardial infarction: A double-blind randomised trial. Lancet 376:1658, 2010.
3. Bellosta S, Paoletti R, Corsini A: Safety of statins: Focus on clinical pharmacokinetics and drug interactions. Circulation 109(Suppl 1): III50, 2004.
4. U.S. Food and Drug Administration: FDA Drug Safety Communication: New restrictions, contraindications, and dose limitations for Zocor (simvastatin) to reduce the risk of muscle injury. Available at www.fda.gov/Drugs/DrugSafety/ucm256581.htm. Accessed June 20, 2011.

ANSWER TO QUESTION 346

D (Braunwald, p. 1240)

Venous graft occlusion occurs in 8% to 12% of patients before they leave the hospital, and by 1 year post CABG 15% to 30% of vein grafts have become occluded.[1] Graft occlusion within the first year usually involves vessel thrombosis, with or without intimal hyperplasia. After the first year, atherosclerotic changes begin to accumulate in saphenous grafts. The histologic appearance of atherosclerosis in venous bypass grafts is indistinguishable from that seen in arterial vessels. The annual occlusion rate for vessels after the first year is 2%, although in grafts that are between 6 and 10 years old an increased annual attrition rate of 4% is observed. The overall occlusion rate by 10 years is 40% to 50%. Internal mammary artery grafts have much longer durability than vein grafts, with patency rates of 95%, 88%, and 83% at 1, 5, and 10 years, respectively.[2] Aspirin (80-325 mg daily, started preoperatively and continued indefinitely) and lipid-lowering therapy have favorable impacts on the development of graft disease.[3]

Historically, atherosclerotic progression in nongrafted arteries has occurred at a rate of 18% to 38% over the first decade, although this may potentially be lessened by aggressive lipid-lowering regimens. The risk of disease progression in the native circulation is three to six times higher in those vessels to which a graft is placed, as compared with ungrafted native arteries. In general, this progression in the native vessel usually occurs proximal to the site of graft insertion. These data are the basis for the recommendation that arteries with minimal disease not receive a bypass graft.

REFERENCES

1. Eagle KA, Guyton RA, Davidoff R, et al: ACC/AHA 2004 guideline update for coronary artery bypass graft surgery: Summary article. A report of the American College of Cardiology/American Heart Association Task Force on Practice Guidelines (Committee to Update the 1999 Guidelines for Coronary Artery Bypass Graft Surgery). Circulation 110:1168, 2004.
2. Dabal RJ, Goss JR, Maynard C, Aldea GS: The effect of left internal mammary artery utilization on short-term outcomes after coronary revascularization. Ann Thorac Surg 76:464, 2003.
3. Smith SC Jr, Allen J, Blair SN, et al: AHA/ACC guidelines for secondary prevention for patients with coronary and other atherosclerotic vascular disease: 2006 update: Endorsed by the National Heart, Lung, and Blood Institute. Circulation 113:2363, 2006.

ANSWER TO QUESTION 347

A (Braunwald, pp. 1066, 1068-1073; Figs. 52-24 and 52-25; Table 52-2)

Myocardial stunning represents prolonged myocardial dysfunction that follows a brief episode of severe ischemia, with gradual return of contractile activity. *Myocardial hibernation*, on the other hand, is the term applied to myocardial dysfunction resulting from chronic hypoperfusion.[1]

Myocardial stunning affects both systolic and diastolic function and may occur in globally as well as regionally ischemic myocardium. Clinically, stunning is most frequently seen in patients recovering from ischemic arrest during cardiopulmonary bypass. It is also observed in ischemic regions adjacent to infarcted zones and in territories that are severely ischemic in patients with unstable angina. There are three likely mechanisms of myocardial stunning: (1) generation of oxygen-derived free radicals, (2) calcium overload, and (3) reduced sensitivity of myofilaments to calcium.[2]

REFERENCES

1. Camici PG, Prasad SK, Rimoldi OE: Stunning, hibernation, and assessment of myocardial viability. Circulation 117:103, 2008.
2. Depre C, Vatner SF: Mechanisms of cell survival in myocardial hibernation. Trends Cardiovasc Med 15:101, 2005.

ANSWER TO QUESTION 348

E (Braunwald, pp. 1185-1191; Figs. 56-8 and 56-10)

Unstable angina is typically caused by atherosclerotic plaque rupture with formation of a platelet-rich intracoronary nonocclusive thrombus. Aspirin, presumably because of its antithrombotic effect, reduces the risk of cardiovascular death and nonfatal myocardial infarction (MI) by approximately 50%. The addition of unfractionated heparin (UFH) improves clinical outcomes more than aspirin alone, resulting in an additional 33% reduction in death and nonfatal MI.[1]

Clopidogrel inhibits platelet activity via blockage of the platelet ADP receptor. The CURE trial demonstrated that the addition of clopidogrel to standard acute coronary syndrome (ACS) therapy resulted in a 20% reduction in death, MI, or stroke. Further analysis of this trial showed that the beneficial effects became apparent within 24 hours of treatment initiation and persisted for 12 months.[2]

Low-molecular-weight heparins (LMWHs) have also been studied in the setting of unstable angina. Enoxaparin is the preferred LMWH for ACS on the basis of several clinical trials that demonstrate its efficacy, whereas the experience with other LMWHs has not been as convincing.[3]

The factor Xa inhibitor fondaparinux was studied in patients with unstable angina/non–ST-segment elevation MI in the OASIS-5 trial and was associated with a *lower* risk of risk of major bleeding and of mortality at 30 days when compared with enoxaparin.[4]

REFERENCES

1. Anderson JL, Adams CD, Antman EM, et al: ACC/AHA 2007 Guidelines for the Management of Patients with Unstable Angina/Non–ST-Elevation Myocardial Infarction: Executive Summary: A report of the American College of Cardiology/American Heart Association Task Force on Practice Guidelines. Circulation 116:803, 2007.
2. Yusuf S, Mehta SR, Zhao F, et al: Early and late effects of clopidogrel in patients with acute coronary syndromes. Circulation 107:966, 2003.
3. Petersen JL, Mahaffey KW, Hasselblad V, et al: Efficacy and bleeding complications among patients randomized to enoxaparin or unfractionated heparin for antithrombin therapy in non–ST-segment elevation acute coronary syndromes: A systematic overview. JAMA 292:89, 2004.
4. Yusuf S, Mehta SR, Chrolavicius S, et al: Comparison of fondaparinux and enoxaparin in acute coronary syndromes. N Engl J Med 354:1464-76, 2006.

ANSWER TO QUESTION 349

D (Braunwald, pp. 1064-1066)

Preexisting collateral vessels are small (20 to 200 μm) vascular channels that interconnect epicardial coronary arteries. They are normally closed and nonfunctional, because there is no pressure gradient between the arteries they connect. However, with an acute coronary occlusion, the distal pressure drops suddenly and any preexisting collateral vessels open instantaneously. The increased flow through these rudimentary collateral vessels triggers a maturation process that includes three stages. In the first 24 hours there is passive widening due to the increased flow. Over the next several weeks, increased flow and shear stress trigger endothelial cell activation, with subsequent inflammation and cellular proliferation with fragmentation of the basement membrane and dissolution of the extracellular matrix, and recruitment of leukocytes. Over the next several months, the collateral vessel wall thickens as a result of deposition of extracellular matrix. The resultant blood vessel is a three-layer structure that is nearly indistinguishable from a normal coronary artery, with a luminal diameter as large as 1 mm.[1]

Growth of the collateral circulation is triggered primarily by the severity of coronary obstruction. There is no clear evidence that exercise by itself triggers collateral formation. The reduction of myocardial ischemia in the setting of exercise training is more likely to be related to improved conditioning. Conditions that reduce endothelial production of nitric oxide, such as diabetes mellitus, may reduce the ability of collateral vessels to develop.

In angioplasty studies, collateral vessels typically provide < 50% of normal coronary blood flow. Nonetheless, in the setting of an acute MI, they have been shown to decrease infarct size and contribute to improved survival. In patients with stable coronary disease, those with well-developed collateral circulations have a significantly lower rate of ischemic events.[2]

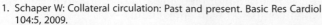
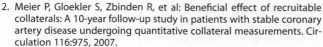

REFERENCES

1. Schaper W: Collateral circulation: Past and present. Basic Res Cardiol 104:5, 2009.
2. Meier P, Gloekler S, Zbinden R, et al: Beneficial effect of recruitable collaterals: A 10-year follow-up study in patients with stable coronary artery disease undergoing quantitative collateral measurements. Circulation 116:975, 2007.

ANSWER TO QUESTION 350

C (Braunwald, pp. 1236-1239; Figs. 57-11 and 57-12)

Several trials have compared pharmacologic therapy to percutaneous coronary intervention (PCI) for patients with chronic stable angina. In most of these, PCI has resulted in greater symptomatic relief as measured by severity of angina, the need for antianginal medications, and improved quality of life.[1,2] However, with respect to major cardiac events (e.g., myocardial infarction [MI] or cardiac death), the two strategies appear equivalent. In the largest of the trials, COURAGE, 2287 patients with moderately severe chronic angina were randomized to PCI and optimal medical therapy (including aspirin, lipid lowering to a low-density lipoprotein (LDL) goal of 60 to 85 mg/dL, antianginal drugs and angiotensin-converting enzyme [ACE] inhibitors) or optimal medical therapy alone. Bare metal stents were used for PCI in the majority of patients in the PCI group. After 4.6 years of follow-up, there was no reduction in death and/or myocardial infarction in patients randomized to PCI.

The AVERT trial compared an aggressive pharmacologic lipid-lowering strategy with PCI in stable patients with one- to two-vessel coronary disease, originally referred for coronary angioplasty.[3] Those randomized to atorvastatin achieved a 46% decrease in serum low-density lipoprotein cholesterol (to 77 mg/dL), compared with 18% in the angioplasty plus usual care group (to 119 mg/dL). The group randomized to aggressive lipid lowering had nearly half the rate of ischemic events (13% vs. 21%, P = 0.048) of the individuals who underwent PCI.

REFERENCES

1. Katritsis DG, Ioannidis JP: Percutaneous coronary intervention versus conservative therapy in nonacute coronary artery disease: A meta-analysis. Circulation 111:2906, 2005.
2. Boden WE, O'Rourke RA, Teo KK, et al: Optimal medical therapy with or without PCI for stable coronary disease. N Engl J Med 356:1503, 2007.
3. Pitt B, Waters D, Brown WV, et al: Aggressive lipid-lowering therapy compared with angioplasty in stable coronary artery disease. Atorvastatin versus Revascularization Treatment Investigators. N Engl J Med 341:70, 1999.

ANSWER TO QUESTION 351

B (Braunwald, pp. 1310-1313)

Although the average rate of expansion of abdominal aortic aneurysms (AAAs) is 0.4 cm per year, larger aneurysms tend to expand faster than smaller ones, as a consequence of Laplace's law (wall tension is proportional to the radius of the aneurysm). Once aneurysmal rupture has occurred, mortality is extremely high: 60% of patients die before they reach the hospital, and 50% of those who are successfully hospitalized die perioperatively. Approximately 20% of aneurysms >5 cm in diameter will rupture within 2 years. Almost all vascular surgeons would electively repair aneurysms >6 cm, and most would operate on aneurysms >5 cm if surgical risk is acceptable. Few would operate on aneurysms <4 cm in diameter. Of note, women have a higher rate of rupture of AAAs than men and at a smaller aneurysm diameter. Rupture is also more common among current smokers and those with hypertension.

Two trials have examined the value of immediate repair of aneurysms 4.0 to 5.5 cm in diameter versus serial surveillance ultrasound or computed tomographic scanning. Each found no mortality difference between the two strategies.[1,2] Important limitations of these studies were that they enrolled almost exclusively men and follow-up was much more intense than in general practice.

The consensus guidelines recommend repair of AAAs ≥5.5 cm in diameter.[3]

REFERENCES

1. The United Kingdom Small Aneurysm Trial Participants: Long-term outcomes of immediate repair compared with surveillance of small abdominal aortic aneurysms. N Engl J Med 346:1445, 2002.
2. Lederle FA, Wilson ES, Johnson GR, et al: Immediate repair compared with surveillance of small abdominal aortic aneurysms. N Engl J Med 346:1437, 2002.
3. Chaikof EL, Brewster DC, Dalman RL, et al: The care of patients with an abdominal aortic aneurysm: The Society for Vascular Surgery practice guidelines. J Vasc Surg 50 (Suppl):S2, 2009.

ANSWER TO QUESTION 352

D (Braunwald, pp. 1326-1332; Figs. 60-18 and 60-20; Table 60-4)

The figure displays a contrast-enhanced chest computed tomogram showing an intimal flap ("I") due to aortic dissection. Acute aortic dissection is a medical and surgical emergency. Mortality in untreated cases exceeds 25% in the first 24 hours and 50% in the first week after presentation. Immediate medical management should focus on reduction of blood pressure, reduction of arterial dP/dt (the force of left ventricular ejection), fluid resuscitation if necessary, and preparation of the patient for operative intervention if indicated. Beta blockers are the agents of choice for lowering blood pressure; nitroprusside can be added for additional blood pressure control. Labetalol is an appropriate initial choice of beta blocker because it combines blood pressure–lowering effects (alpha and beta blockade) with reduction in dP/dt (beta blockade).

Surgical therapy for type A (proximal) acute dissection improves survival.[1] This is because progression of proximal dissection can (1) compromise flow to one of the major vessels, including the coronary arteries, (2) rupture into the pericardium, resulting in tamponade and death, or (3) lead to severe aortic valve regurgitation.[1] Uncomplicated type B (distal) dissections, however, can be managed with initial pharmacologic therapy alone, with a 30-day survival rate of 92%. For patients with complicated type B dissections (e.g., intractable pain or visceral ischemia), invasive intervention is necessary. Although open surgical repair in such patients is fraught with high mortality rates, the results of newer endovascular repair procedures have been encouraging.[2]

A small percentage of patients present with chronic dissections. By surviving the acute stage, these patients represent a select subset of lower risk patients who can be managed conservatively with medical therapy regardless of the location of the dissection, unless the dissection is complicated by aneurysm, rupture, vascular compromise, or aortic regurgitation.

When aortic regurgitation complicates acute dissection, decompression of the false lumen may be all that is required to correct the geometry of the aortic valve and restore valve competence. If abnormalities of the aortic valve leaflets prevent such repair, aortic valve and root replacement are usually necessary instead.

REFERENCES

1. Rampoldi V, Trimarchi S, Eagle KA, et al: Simple risk models to predict surgical mortality in acute type A aortic dissection: The International Registry of Acute Aortic Dissection score. Ann Thorac Surg 83:55, 2007.
2. Nienaber CA, Rousseau H, Eggbrecht H, et al: Randomized comparison of strategies for type B aortic dissection. The INvestigation of STEnt grafts in Aortic Dissection (INSTEAD) Trial. Circulation 120:2519, 2009.

ANSWER TO QUESTION 353

D (Braunwald, pp. 1231-1232; Fig. 57-9)

Ranolazine is an antianginal agent that may be used in combination with beta blockers, nitrates and calcium channel blockers. Unlike beta blockers, nitrates, and calcium channel blockers, ranolazine exerts its anti-ischemic effect without significant effect on heart rate or blood pressure. Ranolazine inhibits the slowly inactivating component of the cardiac sodium current (late I_{NA+}) and is therefore believed to reduce the deleterious effects of intracellular sodium and calcium overload that accompany, and may promote, myocardial ischemia.[1]

Clinical trials have shown that ranolazine is effective as monotherapy, or in combination with traditional antianginal agents. In studies of patients with moderate angina, ranolazine decreased the frequency of angina and need for sublingual nitroglycerin.[2,3]

Ranolazine is generally well tolerated; its most common side effects are dizziness, headache, and constipation. Because ranolazine produces a concentration-dependent prolongation of repolarization and the QT interval there has been concern that it may precipitate arrhythmias such as torsades de pointes. However, in the MERLIN-TIMI 36 study of 6560 patients with acute coronary syndromes there was no difference in the rates of documented dysrhythmias or sudden cardiac death in patients receiving ranolazine compared with placebo.[1]

Ranolazine is metabolized in the liver (primarily by CYP3A), and its use is contraindicated in patients with hepatic impairment.

REFERENCES

1. Morrow DA, Scirica BM, Karwatowska-Prokopczuk E, et al, for the MERLIN-TIMI 36 Trial Investigators: Effects of ranolazine on recurrent cardiovascular events in patients with non–ST-elevation acute coronary syndromes: The MERLIN-TIMI 36 Randomized Trial. JAMA 297:1775, 2007.
2. Chaitman BR, Pepine CJ, Parker JO, et al: Effects of ranolazine with atenolol, amlodipine, or diltiazem on exercise tolerance and angina frequency in patients with severe chronic angina: CARISA: A randomized controlled trial. JAMA 291:309, 2004.
3. Stone PH, Gratsiansky NA, Blokhim A, et al: Antianginal efficacy of ranolazine when added to treatment with amlodipine: The ERICA (Efficacy of Ranolazine in Chronic Angina) trial. J Am Coll Cardiol 48:566, 2006.

ANSWER TO QUESTION 354

D (Braunwald, pp. 1310-1312; Fig. 60-2)

The figure is an axial contrast-enhanced computed tomographic (CT) scan demonstrating a 6.6-cm abdominal aortic aneurysm (AAA). The majority of AAAs are asymptomatic. On physical examination, such an aneurysm may be appreciated as a pulsatile mass extending variably from the xiphoid process to the umbilicus. The size of an aneurysm tends to be overestimated by physical examination, owing to the difficulty in distinguishing the aorta from adjacent structures. AAAs may be sensitive to palpation, especially if they are rapidly expanding.[1]

Ultrasonography and CT are both highly accurate means to diagnose and quantitate the size of AAAs. Each technique has a measurement accuracy within ± 0.3 cm. However, ultrasonography is not sufficient for planning operative repair because it cannot define associated mesenteric and renal artery anatomy. Spiral CT with three-dimensional reconstruction provides a more comprehensive evaluation of the aortic tree but tends to measure aneurysms as slightly larger than by ultrasonography. Aortography, historically the "gold standard" for preoperative aneurysm evaluation, may actually underestimate the size of an AAA if nonopacified mural thrombus lines the wall. Magnetic resonance angiography is an alternative to angiography that is highly accurate in determining aneurysm size and, with three-dimensional reconstruction, can define the proximal extent of disease and iliofemoral involvement in more than 80% of cases.

Serial imaging studies suggest that aneurysms expand at a mean rate of 0.4 cm per year. However, this is highly variable and larger aneurysms tend to expand more rapidly than smaller ones.

REFERENCE

1. Chaikof EL, Brewster DC, Dalman RL, et al: The care of patients with an abdominal aortic aneurysm: The Society for Vascular Surgery practice guidelines. J Vasc Surg 50 (Suppl):S2, 2009.

ANSWER TO QUESTION 355

D (Braunwald, pp. 1282-1283)

The use of platelet GP IIb/IIIa inhibitors in the setting of percutaneous coronary intervention (PCI) has been tested in multiple randomized trials, involving the full spectrum of coronary disease, from stable angina to ST-segment elevation myocardial infarction (MI). Excluding studies that used inadequate doses, the trials are remarkably consistent in demonstrating a 35% to 55% reduction in the composite endpoint of death, MI, and need for urgent revascularization over 30 days of follow-up. Most of this benefit is realized by patients experiencing acute coronary syndrome (ACS) and relates to reductions in periprocedural MI and the need for urgent revascularization. Several studies have concluded that patients who sustain a periprocedural MI have a worse long-term prognosis. The disadvantage of GP IIb/IIIa inhibitors is an increased risk of bleeding complications during their use.

The reduction in clinical events with GP IIb/IIIa inhibition is typically achieved in the first 48 hours, with little separation of the event rate curves after that time. They do not appear to have any long-term effects on rates of restenosis.[1]

There is clinical trial evidence that for patients with acute ST-segment elevation MI who have received aspirin plus clopidogrel there is no significant benefit of routine GP IIb/IIIa inhibitor administration before transport to the catheterization laboratory.[2,3]

REFERENCES

1. Smith SC Jr, Feldman TE, Hirshfeld JW Jr, et al: ACC/AHA/SCAI 2005 Guideline Update for Percutaneous Coronary Intervention—summary article: A report of the American College of Cardiology/American Heart Association Task Force on Practice Guidelines (ACC/AHA/SCAI Writing Committee to Update the 2001 Guidelines for Percutaneous Coronary Intervention). Circulation 113:156, 2006.
2. Mehilli J, Kastrati A, Schulz S, et al: Abciximab in patients with acute ST-segment-elevation myocardial infarction undergoing primary percutaneous coronary intervention after clopidogrel loading: A randomized double-blind trial. Circulation 119:1933, 2009.
3. Wright RS, Anderson JL, Adams CD, et al: 2011 ACCF/AHA focused update of the guidelines for the management of patients with unstable angina/non–ST-elevation myocardial infarction (updating the 2007 guideline): A report of the American College of Cardiology Foundation/American Heart Association Task Force on Practice Guidelines. J Am Coll Cardiol 57:1920-1959, 2011.

ANSWER TO QUESTION 356

D (Braunwald, pp. 1195-1198; Fig. 56-20)

Prinzmetal angina is caused by transient coronary artery vasospasm. Although the site of vasospasm may not appear to contain a significant plaque on angiography, intravascular ultrasound studies have shown that nearly all such sites have underlying atherosclerosis.[1] Both nitrates and calcium channel blockers have been shown to be efficacious in treating and preventing attacks of Prinzmetal angina.[2] Provocative testing with ergonovine or acetylcholine is indicated only when Prinzmetal angina is suspected and ECG evidence of transient ST segment elevation is lacking, because these agents can sometimes cause severe prolonged coronary spasm, resulting in myocardial infarction or arrhythmias. Patients with Prinzmetal angina generally have an excellent prognosis, with a sudden cardiac death rate of only 3.6% at 7 years.

REFERENCES

1. Kawano H, Motoyama T, Yasue H, et al: Endothelial function fluctuates with diurnal variation in the frequency of ischemic episodes in patients with variant angina. J Am Coll Cardiol 40:266, 2002.
2. Anderson JL, Adams CD, Antman EM, et al: ACC/AHA 2007 Guidelines for the Management of Patients with Unstable Angina/Non–ST-Elevation Myocardial Infarction—executive summary: A report of the American College of Cardiology/American Heart Association Task Force on Practice Guidelines. Circulation 116:803, 2007.

ANSWER TO QUESTION 357

C (Braunwald, pp. 1354-1356; see also Answer to Question 325)

The figure shows atheroemboli to the left foot resulting in "blue toe syndrome." Showers of microemboli that arise from atherosclerotic plaques in the aortic or major arterial trunks lead to clinical and pathologic changes as the particulate material lodges in small arterial branches. Atheromatous embolism (also called "cholesterol embolism") occurs most often after surgery involving manipulation of an atherosclerotic aorta, such as major abdominal vascular procedures, especially resection of abdominal aortic aneurysms. Showers of atherosclerotic emboli may also be provoked by cardiac catheterization, cardiopulmonary bypass, and intra-arterial cannulations of any type and may occasionally occur spontaneously as well. Clinical findings in this disorder may include bilateral lower extremity pain, livedo reticularis, and purpuric and ecchymotic lesions in the lower extremities. In addition, abdominal pain may occur.

Two important recognized complications of cholesterol emboli after abdominal aortic surgery are pancreatitis and renal failure due to diffuse microinfarction of the affected organ. The resulting renal failure may be severe and irreversible. Hepatitis is not part of the clinical syndrome. Because showers of cholesterol emboli may be widely scattered, cerebral involvement may occur; and, in some instances, visualization of cholesterol particles in the retinal arteries is possible. Unfortunately, there is no specific therapy for cholesterol emboli; treatment of the resulting complications of the disorder is the cornerstone of management. The use of anticoagulants to prevent further episodes of embolization remains controversial. Antiplatelet and antilipid agents should be considered in affected patients because these therapies may prevent other cardiovascular events in this high-risk population.

REFERENCE

Molisse TA, Tunick PA, Kronzon I: Complications of aortic atherosclerosis: Atheroemboli and thromboemboli. Curr Treat Options Cardiovasc Med 9:137, 2007.

ANSWER TO QUESTION 358

D (Braunwald, pp. 1050-1052; Fig. 52-7)

Nitric oxide (NO) is formed in endothelial cells by the action of NO synthase on L-arginine. In this reaction, the terminal nitrogen from the guanidino group of L-arginine forms NO, and L-citrulline is produced as a by-product, which is recycled back to L-arginine. NO diffuses to neighboring smooth muscle cells, where it activates guanylate cyclase, causing an increase in cyclic *guanosine* monophosphate and smooth muscle relaxation.

Hypoxia, thrombin, and adenosine diphosphate all stimulate endothelial NO production. Acetylcholine (ACh) induces both endothelium-dependent (i.e., NO-mediated) vasodilatation and direct smooth muscle constriction. As a result, ACh induces vasodilatation in healthy vessels but vasoconstriction predominates in atherosclerotic vessels in which there is dysfunctional endothelium. Some vasodilators (e.g., nitroglycerin, nitroprusside, and prostacyclin) act independently of endothelial NO production and continue to produce vascular smooth muscle relaxation even in the setting of a dysfunctional endothelium.

REFERENCE

Forstermann U, Munzel T: Endothelial nitric oxide synthase in vascular disease: From marvel to menace. Circulation 113:1708, 2006.

ANSWER TO QUESTION 359

A (Braunwald, pp. 1132-1333)

Intramural hematoma is a condition closely related to aortic dissection. It consists of a hematoma contained within the medial layer of the aortic wall. Although the pathogenesis remains uncertain, rupture of the vasa vasorum has been postulated to be the initiating event. The hemorrhage occurs in the outer media and may extend into the adventitia. As opposed to classic aortic dissection, there is no associated tear in the intima; therefore, this condition is sometimes called "aortic dissection without intimal rupture." Pathologic studies have indicated that intramural hematoma comprises 3% to 13% of what were previously classified as aortic dissections. In the International Registry of Aortic Dissection, 10% of patients with the clinical diagnosis of aortic dissection were found to have an intramural hematoma, and two thirds of these were localized to the descending aorta. These patients were elderly, had a history of hypertension, and had extensive atherosclerotic disease. Their signs and symptoms were essentially indistinguishable from those of classic aortic dissection.

The diagnosis of intramural hematoma is best made by computed tomography (CT) or magnetic resonance imaging (MRI). Non–contrast-enhanced CT typically demonstrates a crescentic, high-attenuation area along the aortic wall without evidence of an intimal tear. Subsequent contrast CT demonstrates failure of the intramural hematoma to enhance. On MRI, an intramural hematoma is identified as a crescent-shaped area of high intensity along the aortic wall. Because there is lack of communication with the aorta, aortography actually has very low sensitivity for this diagnosis.

REFERENCE

Evangelista A, Mukherjee D, Mehta RH, et al: Acute intramural hematoma of the aorta. Circulation 111:1063, 2005.

ANSWER TO QUESTION 360

B (Braunwald, pp. 1190-1191)

Low-molecular-weight heparins (LMWHs) are derived from unfractionated heparin (UFH) through chemical or enzymatic depolymerization. The shorter molecules still contain the critical pentasaccharide sequence necessary for binding to and activating antithrombin, but the anti-Xa activity is much greater.[1] They do not cause a significant rise in the activated partial thromboplastin time, and that test is not useful for clinical monitoring. Although the anticoagulation effect of LMWHs can be determined by measuring anti-Xa activity, the stable pharmacokinetics of these drugs usually renders such measurement unnecessary.

Clearance of LMWH is reduced in patients with renal impairment, and dosage reduction is appropriate if used in such patients. LMWHs are not neutralized by platelet factor 4. Compared with UFH, treatment with LMWHs is less likely to result in type II heparin-induced thrombocytopenia (HIT). However, HIT antibodies can cross react with LMWHs, and the latter should not be used when type II HIT has occurred.[1,2]

REFERENCES

1. Hirsh J, Raschke R: Heparin and low-molecular-weight heparin. Chest (Suppl) 26:188S, 2004.
2. Arepally GM, Ortel TL: Heparin-induced thrombocytopenia. N Engl J Med 355:809, 2006.

ANSWER TO QUESTION 361

D (Braunwald, pp. 1183-1185; Table 56-2)

Unstable angina is a heterogeneous condition with a range of possible outcomes. For some patients, minor pharmacologic alterations result in clinical stability, whereas in others the risk of myocardial infarction (MI) or death is very high. Clinical trials have identified subgroups of patients who are at greater risk and who are more likely to accrue benefit from therapeutic interventions. High-risk individuals include those with acute rest pain or post-MI unstable angina and those who are of advanced age or who have diabetes, cerebrovascular disease, or peripheral vascular disease.[1,2] In addition, patients who present with unstable angina despite having been on prior chronic aspirin therapy appear to be at particularly high risk.

The presence of ST segment deviations of as little as 0.05 mV is associated with an adverse prognosis in unstable angina, and the greater the ST-segment deviation, the

PREVENTIVE CARDIOLOGY; ATHEROSCLEROTIC CARDIOVASCULAR DISEASE

worse the outcome.[3] Similarly, an elevated cardiac troponin level confers a higher risk of death.[4] Increased levels of C-reactive protein (CRP) have also related to an augmented risk of MI and death. Although CRP, as a marker of inflammation, is often elevated in acute coronary syndromes, those patients with the highest levels have worse short- and long-term outcomes.[4]

REFERENCES

1. Donahoe SM, Steward GC, McCabe CH, et al: Diabetes and mortality following acute coronary syndromes. JAMA 298:765, 2007.
2. Eagle KA, Lim MJ, Dabbous OH, et al: A validated prediction model for all forms of acute coronary syndrome: Estimating the risk of 6-month postdischarge death in an International Registry. JAMA 291:2727, 2004.
3. Mueller C, Neumann FJ, Perach W, et al: Prognostic value of the admission electrocardiogram in patients with unstable angina/non–ST-segment elevation myocardial infarction treated with very early revascularization. Am J Med 117:145, 2004.
4. James SK, Armstrong P, Barnathan E, et al: Troponin and C-reactive protein have different relations to subsequent mortality and myocardial infarction after acute coronary syndrome: A GUSTO-IV substudy. J Am Coll Cardiol 41:916, 2003.

ANSWER TO QUESTION 362

B (Braunwald, pp. 1138-1342; Fig. 61-1; Tables 61-1 and 61-4)

The prevalence of peripheral artery disease (PAD) varies depending on the population studied and the diagnostic methods used but ranges from 4.6% to 19.1%.[1] The prevalence increases with age and is >20% in patients 75 years and older.[2] The same risk factors that contribute to coronary artery disease are also associated with PAD, including cigarette smoking, diabetes mellitus, dyslipidemia, hypertension, and hyperhomocystinemia. Of these, however, dyslipidemia is not one of the strongest predictors, conveying only a 1.2- to 1.4-fold increased risk. Rather, cigarette smoking and diabetes mellitus are more significantly associated, with relative risks of 2.0 to 5.0.

Evidence of PAD has been observed even in young individuals. Data from the Pathobiological Determinants of Atherosclerosis in Youth Study indicated that, in patients younger than 35 years, fatty streaks and atheroma form first in the dorsal portion of the abdominal aorta, later followed by similar lesions in the descending thoracic aorta.

The lack of symptoms is not a reliable way to exclude the presence of PAD, because only 10% to 30% of patients with PAD experience claudication.

REFERENCES

1. Murabito JM, Evans JC, Nieto K, et al: Prevalence and clinical correlates of peripheral arterial disease in the Framingham Offspring Study. Am Heart J 143:961, 2002.
2. Norgren L, Hiatt WR, Dormandy JA, et al: Inter-Society consensus for the management of peripheral arterial disease (TASC II). J Vasc Surg 45:S5, 2007.

ANSWER TO QUESTION 363

C (Braunwald, pp. 1321-1323)

Aortic dissection affects twice as many men as women and is seen most commonly in the sixth and seventh decades of life. Over 90% of patients presenting with aortic dissection complain of severe pain. The pain is usually sudden in onset and most intense at its inception and may be unbearable; words such as "tearing" and "ripping" are frequently used to describe it. The discomfort tends to migrate in association with dissection of the hematoma into the aortic wall. The diagnosis is often confirmed by physical examination. Although patients may appear to be in shock, the measured blood pressure is often elevated, especially in patients with distal dissection. The characteristic physical findings associated with aortic dissection, such as pulse defects and aortic regurgitation, are more commonly seen in proximal dissection. For example, approximately 30% of patients with a proximal dissection display some form of a pulse deficit, often a decrease or loss of pulse associated with the brachiocephalic vessels. Similarly, aortic regurgitation is most commonly seen in association with proximal dissection.

Several conditions may mimic the pain of aortic dissection, including myocardial infarction, acute aortic regurgitation without dissection, thoracic nondissecting aneurysm, mediastinal tumors, musculoskeletal pains, and pericarditis.

REFERENCE

Tsai TT, Trimarchi S, Neinaber CA: Acute aortic dissection: Perspectives from the International Registry of Acute Aortic Dissection (IRAD). Eur J Vasc Endovasc Surg 37:149, 2009.

ANSWER TO QUESTION 364

A (Braunwald, pp. 1340-1346)

Intermittent claudication due to peripheral artery disease (PAD) is characterized by pain or a sense of fatigue during exercise that resolves with rest. In contrast, neurogenic pseudoclaudication (e.g., due to spinal stenosis) is associated with pain with both walking and standing. Classic physical examination findings include diminished or absent distal pulses, bruits over regions of stenosis, and coolness and signs of chronic low-grade ischemia such as hair loss, smooth shiny skin, and brittle nails of the affected extremity.

Among the simpler noninvasive diagnostic tests for PAD are systolic blood pressure measurements along select segments of each extremity. A pressure gradient of >20 mm Hg between successive segments in the lower extremities or >10 mm Hg in the upper extremities is evidence of significant stenosis. A sensitive office-based screening method for the diagnosis of PAD is the ankle/brachial index (ABI), the ratio between the ankle and brachial systolic blood pressures. An ABI value <1 is consistent with arterial insufficiency of the measured lower extremity and is 95% sensitive for that diagnosis. The ABI of patients with symptoms of leg claudication is typically 0.5 to 0.8, and in those with critical limb ischemia it is usually <0.5. Contrast angiography is the invasive "gold standard" for the identification of arterial stenoses. However, the resolution of gadolinium-enhanced magnetic resonance angiography (MRA) approaches that of conventional digital subtraction angiography. MRA is 95% sensitive and 97% specific for anatomic resolution of the aorta, iliac, femoral-popliteal, and tibial-peroneal arteries.

REFERENCES

Lau JF, Weinberg MD, Olin JW: Peripheral artery disease: I. Clinical evaluation and non-invasive diagnosis. Nat Rev Cardiol 8:1-14, 2011.

ANSWER TO QUESTION 365

A (Braunwald, pp. 1283-1284)

Intravenous unfractionated heparin (UFH) has been the standard anticoagulant administered during percutaneous coronary interventions (PCIs) to prevent arterial thrombus formation on the percutaneous guidewires and catheters. Use of lower, weight-adjusted heparin dosing of 50 to 70 IU/kg has been shown to result in similar clinical outcomes and earlier sheath removal.[1] The routine use of intravenous heparin *after* the procedure is not recommended because that approach does not reduce ischemic complications but does increase the risk of bleeding.

In the ISAR-REACT 3 trial, which compared the intravenous direct thrombin inhibitor bivalirudin to UFH in patients pretreated with clopidogrel (600 mg), there were no differences in the rates of ischemic complications in patients undergoing PCI.[2] However, the incidence of major bleeding was lower in patients who received bivalirudin.

In the EPILOG trial, in which GP IIb/IIIa inhibition was used, standard-dose UFH (10,000-U bolus, activated clotting time [ACT] goal >300 seconds) resulted in similar rates of ischemic events but a greater number of hemorrhagic complications compared with low-dose UFH (70-U/kg bolus, ACT goal >200 seconds). Therefore, when used in combination with a GP IIb/IIIa inhibitor, low-dose UFH is preferred.

The low-molecular-weight heparin enoxaparin is efficacious as an anticoagulant during PCI but cannot be monitored by the ACT test. However, the pharmacokinetics of this agent are so stable that patients who received their last dose within 8 hours of the procedure do not require any further anticoagulation. An intravenous bolus of 0.3 mg/kg is appropriate if the last dose was 8 to 12 hours before the procedure.[3] If the last dose was more than 12 hours earlier, then standard heparin anticoagulation during PCI is appropriate.

REFERENCES

1. Chew D, Bhatt D, Lincoff A, et al: Defining the optimal activated clotting time during percutaneous coronary intervention: Aggregate results from 6 randomized, controlled trials. Circulation 103:961, 2001.
2. Kastrati A, Neumann FJ, Mehilli J, et al: Bivalirudin versus unfractionated heparin during percutaneous coronary intervention. N Engl J Med 359:688, 2008.
3. Gurm HS, Eagle KA: Use of anticoagulants in ST-segment elevation myocardial infarction patients: A focus on low-molecular-weight heparin. Cardiovasc Drugs Ther 22:59, 2008.

ANSWER TO QUESTION 366

E (Braunwald, pp. 1223-1225; Fig. 57-4; Table 57-5)

Nitrates are important agents for treatment of ischemic heart disease. They directly relax vascular smooth muscle by activating intracellular guanylate cyclase, thus causing an increase in cyclic guanosine monophosphate, which triggers smooth muscle relaxation. Nitrates act directly on smooth muscle and therefore do not require an intact endothelium to secrete nitric oxide (NO) as a secondary messenger. The vasodilating effect of nitrates is manifest in both arteries and veins but predominates in the venous circulation. The decrease in venous tone lessens the return of blood to the heart and reduces preload and ventricular dimensions, which in turn diminishes wall tension. As well as decreasing wall tension and myocardial oxygen demand, nitrates may also increase oxygen supply by dilating coronary arteries.[1] Such dilatation can be effected in vessels containing atherosclerosis, presumably because the pathologic atherosclerotic changes are eccentric and normal vascular smooth muscle, which can respond to nitrates, is present in a portion of the plaque.[2] Sulfhydryl groups (SH) are necessary as a cofactor for transformation of nitroglycerin to the active molecule NO. N-acetylcysteine increases the amount of SH available and therefore may reverse the tolerance that develops with long-term nitroglycerin use.[3]

REFERENCES

1. Gori T, Parker JD: Long-term therapy with organic nitrates: The pros and cons of nitric oxide replacement therapy. J Am Coll Cardiol 44:632, 2004.
2. Jansen R, Cleophas TJ, Zwinderman AH, et al: Chronic nitrate therapy in patients with angina with comorbidity. Am J Ther 13:188, 2006.
3. Munzel T, Daiber A, Mulsch A: Explaining the phenomenon of nitrate tolerance. Circ Res 97:618, 2005.

ANSWER TO QUESTION 367

A (Braunwald, p. 1282)

The GP IIb/IIIa inhibitors represent a powerful class of antiplatelet agents.[1] By impairing the final common pathway of platelet aggregation, they greatly limit thrombus formation. There are significant differences between the three agents of this class currently approved for use. Abciximab is a monoclonal antibody that has high affinity but relatively low specificity for the GP IIb/IIIa receptor. Although the original murine monoclonal antibody (7E3) was chimerized with human immunoglobulin to minimize antibody formation, antichimeric antibodies develop in 5% to 6% of patients treated with abciximab.

Although there has been no evidence of severe allergic reactions after the re-administration of abciximab to previously exposed patients, thrombocytopenia has been reported.

Eptifibatide and tirofiban are small-molecule GP IIb/IIIa inhibitors that have lower affinity but higher specificity for the GP IIb/IIIa receptor. Eptifibatide is a cyclic heptapeptide related to pygmy rattlesnake venom, whereas tirofiban is a nonpeptide molecule based on the structure of fibrinogen. Both have half-lives of about 2 hours. Current evidence suggests that the long-term benefits of GP IIb/IIIa inhibitors are greater when they are administered in conjunction with heparin.[1]

The upstream administration of a GP IIb/IIIa inhibitor before transport to the catheterization laboratory in acute ST-segment elevation myocardial infarction has not been shown to benefit patients pretreated with dual antiplatelet therapy (aspirin plus clopidogrel 600 mg).[2]

REFERENCES

1. King SB 3rd, Smith SC Jr, Hirshfeld JW Jr, et al: 2007 Focused Update of the ACC/AHA/SCAI 2005 Guideline Update for Percutaneous Coronary Intervention: A report of the American College of Cardiology/American Heart Association Task Force on Practice Guidelines: 2007 Writing Group to Review New Evidence and Update the ACC/AHA/SCAI 2005 Guideline Update for Percutaneous Coronary Intervention, Writing on Behalf of the 2005 Writing Committee. Circulation 117:261, 2008.
2. Mehilli J, Kastrati A, Schulz S, et al: Abciximab in patients with acute ST-segment-elevation myocardial infarction undergoing primary percutaneous coronary intervention after clopidogrel loading: A randomized double-blind trial. Circulation 119:1933, 2009.

ANSWER TO QUESTION 368

C (Braunwald, pp. 1374-1380; Fig. 63-12; Tables 63-6, 63-7, and 63-8)

Renovascular disease is common and can contribute to hypertension and progressive deterioration of kidney function. Renal artery stenosis (RAS) can be managed with percutaneous renal artery angioplasty and stenting, and the technical success rate of these procedures exceeds 95%. The use of stents has greatly improved the procedural outcome even for ostial lesions and reduces restenosis rates.[1] Clinical trial data of patients with unilateral RAS have demonstrated that surgical revascularization and percutaneous angioplasty lead to similar degrees of blood pressure improvement and stabilization of renal function.

Although successful percutaneous treatment of atherosclerotic RAS commonly improves blood pressure, at least modestly, complete resolution of hypertension is unusual because many affected patients have accompanying essential hypertension or intrinsic renal disease. As a result, only about two thirds of patients who undergo successful intervention have a reduced requirement of antihypertensive medications. Furthermore, recent data have not demonstrated superior benefit of percutaneous intervention compared with medical antihypertensive therapy alone. The ASTRAL trial prospectively randomized 806 patients with atherosclerotic renal artery disease to either percutaneous revascularization or medical therapy and the revascularization group did not experience superior clinical effect as measured by progression of renal dysfunction, blood pressure levels, or cardiovascular events. Moreover, among the patients assigned to percutaneous revascularization there were serious periprocedural complications, including cholesterol embolism leading to gangrene and toe or limb amputation.[2]

REFERENCES

1. Dworkin LD, Cooper CJ: Clinical practice: Renal-artery stenosis. N Engl J Med 361:1972, 2009.
2. The ASTRAL Investigators. Revascularization versus Medical Therapy for Renal-Artery Stenosis. N Engl J Med 361:1953, 2009.

ANSWER TO QUESTION 369

B (Braunwald, pp. 1249-1250)

Syndrome X refers to angina or angina-like chest pain in the presence of a normal coronary arteriogram.[1] This syndrome encompasses a heterogeneous population that includes patients with true heart disease as well as those with noncardiac chest pain. Although most studies have failed to reveal consistent biochemical evidence of ischemia, such as an elevation of myocardial lactate with exercise, evidence of decreased perfusion may be found in many of these patients by exercise testing or scintigraphy using single-photon emission computed tomography or positron emission tomography. The incidence of coronary calcification on multislice computed tomography is higher than that of normal subjects but lower than that of patients with obstructive coronary artery disease (CAD). Some patients with this syndrome have evidence of microvascular dysfunction with inadequate vasodilator reserve and an exaggerated response to vasoconstrictor stimuli.[2] Increased sensitivity to pain and a high prevalence of psychiatric disorders have also been associated with this condition.

Largely because of the heterogeneous population, studies of potential treatments have given varying and often contradictory results.[3] Nitrates have been shown to both improve and reduce exercise tolerance. Calcium channel blockers and estrogen therapy in women may be more effective, perhaps by enhancing endothelial-dependent vasodilatation. In addition, some patients appear to benefit from antidepressant drugs. Overall, the cardiac prognosis of patients with syndrome X is very good and better than that of patients with obstructive CAD. However, in the Women's Ischemic Syndrome Evaluation (WISE) study, women with angina and no obstructive CAD who had persistent symptoms demonstrated more than a twofold increase in cardiovascular events.[4]

REFERENCES

1. Johnson BD, Shaw LJ, Buchthal SD, et al: Prognosis in women with myocardial ischemia in the absence of obstructive coronary disease: Results from the National Institutes of Health-National Heart, Lung, and Blood Institute-Sponsored Women's Ischemia Syndrome Evaluation (WISE). Circulation 109:2993, 2004.

2. Sun H, Mohri M, Shimokawa H, et al: Coronary microvascular spasm causes myocardial ischemia in patients with vasospastic angina. J Am Coll Cardiol 39:847, 2002.
3. Bugiardini R, Bailey Merz CN: Angina with "normal" coronary arteries: A changing philosophy. JAMA 293:477, 2005.
4. Bugiardini R: Women, "non-specific" chest pain, and normal or near-normal coronary angiograms are not synonymous with favourable outcome. Eur Heart J 27:1387, 2006.

ANSWER TO QUESTION 370

E (Braunwald, p. 1313)

For patients with an abdominal aortic aneurysm (AAA) and suitable anatomy, endovascular aortic aneurysm repair (EVAR) is a less invasive approach than standard open surgery. The endograft is introduced percutaneously or via arterial cutdown into the femoral artery and maneuvered to the involved aortic segment. Anatomic constraints limit the use of EVAR, but reported primary success rates for aneurysm exclusion in carefully chosen patients have ranged from 78% to 99%. An endoleak (persistent flow into the aneurysmal sac external to the endograft after it has been deployed) is a serious complication of EVAR and leaves the patient at risk for aneurysm rupture.

Randomized trials have shown a lower 30-day mortality for endovascular repair of abdominal aortic aneurysm compared with an open surgical procedure.[1] Recent trials have begun to define the long-term outcomes of EVAR. In the United Kingdom Endovascular Aneurysm Repair 1 trial,[2] 1252 patients with a large AAA ($\geq$5.5 cm) were randomized to endovascular or open operative repair. The 30-day mortality rate favored endovascular repair, but there was no difference in mortality over the long-term (median follow up of 6 years), and the endovascular procedure was associated with higher rates of complications (including fatal endograft rupture), need for re-intervention, and increased cost.

REFERENCES

1. Lederle FA, Freischlag JA, Kyriakides TC, et al: Outcomes following endovascular vs open repair of abdominal aortic aneurysm: A randomized trial. JAMA 302:1535, 2009.
2. The United Kingdom EVAR Trial Investigators. Endovascular versus open repair of abdominal aortic aneurysm. N Engl J Med 362:1863, 2010.

ANSWER TO QUESTION 371

B (Braunwald, pp. 1349-1351, 1369-1370; Figs. 61-15, 61-16, and 61-17)

Treatment of symptomatic peripheral arterial disease (PAD) is multidisciplinary.[1] Currently available drug therapy is not as effective as agents used to treat chronic CAD. Pentoxifylline is a xanthine derivative, and its beneficial effects in PAD are believed to be mediated by its hemorheologic properties, including an increase in red blood cell flexibility, as well as by its anti-inflammatory and antiproliferative effects. Several studies have shown that pentoxifylline increases both the walking distance to initial claudication symptoms and the absolute distance able to be traveled. Cilostazol is a quinolinone derivative that inhibits phosphodiesterase III, thereby enhancing vasodilatation and inhibition of platelet aggregation. Clinical trials have demonstrated that cilostazol improves walking distances and quality of life. It should not be prescribed to patients with heart failure, since other drugs with similar mechanisms of action decrease survival in that population.[2]

Supervised exercise rehabilitation significantly improves symptoms of claudication. Meta-analyses have found that walking programs increase maximum walking distances in patients with PAD by 50% to 200%.[3]

Revascularization options in patients with PAD include percutaneous transluminal angioplasty (PTA) and bypass surgery. PTA of the iliac artery results in patency rates of 60% to 80% at 4 years. This figure improves further with the use of stenting.[4] Aortobifemoral bypass surgery results in 10-year patency rates of nearly 90%.

REFERENCES

1. White C: Intermittent claudication. N Engl J Med 356:1241, 2007.
2. Hankey GJ, Norman PE, Eikelboom JW: Medical treatment of peripheral arterial disease. JAMA 295:547, 2006.
3. Watson L, Ellis B, Leng GC: Exercise for intermittent claudication. Cochrane Database Syst Rev (4):CD000990, 2008.
4. Hirsch AT, Haskal ZJ, Hertzer NR, et al: ACC/AHA 2005 guidelines for the management of patients with peripheral arterial disease (lower extremity, renal, mesenteric, and abdominal aortic): Executive summary. J Am Coll Cardiol 47:1239, 2006.

ANSWER TO QUESTION 372

D (Braunwald, pp. 1326-1330; see also Answer to Question 352)

The immediate therapeutic goals in the management of aortic dissection are reduction of systolic arterial pressure to decrease stress on the vascular wall and elimination of pain. The most common pharmacologic approach is the simultaneous use of the vasodilator sodium nitroprusside to lower arterial pressure and of an intravenous beta-adrenoreceptor blocking agent, such as labetalol or esmolol, to reduce wall stress acutely. Such lowering of arterial pressure and reduction of left ventricular ejection force allows for temporary stabilization in appropriate surgical candidates and is the treatment of choice for those patients in whom surgery is not indicated. The appearance of a life-threatening complication such as aortic rupture, aortic regurgitation, cardiac tamponade, or compromise of a vital organ mandates immediate surgical intervention.

As indicated in the Answer to Question 352, surgical repair is the standard of therapy for type A (proximal) acute dissection because it has been shown to improve survival. Conversely, patients with type B (distal) aortic dissection can be safely managed with initial pharmacologic therapy alone.

REFERENCES

Rampoldi V, Trimarchi S, Eagle KA, et al: Simple risk models to predict surgical mortality in acute type A aortic dissection: The International Registry of Acute Aortic Dissection score. Ann Thorac Surg 83:55, 2007.

ANSWER TO QUESTION 373

E (Braunwald, pp. 1392, 1405; Fig. 64-1; Table 64-1)

Diabetes is a major risk factor for atherosclerosis of the coronary, cerebral, and peripheral arteries, and the prevalence of this condition is increasing in both developed and developing countries.[1] According to the American Diabetes Association, diagnostic criteria for the presence of diabetes include a fasting plasma glucose concentration >126 mg/dL or a hemoglobin A1c level ≥ 6.5%.[2]

Aggressive and comprehensive risk factor modification reduces adverse cardiovascular outcomes in diabetic patients. In addition to glycemic control, targets for intervention include hypertension (treatment goal < 130/80 mm Hg), cigarette smoking, and modification of abnormal lipid levels. A strategy of antilipidemic therapy in diabetic patients without markedly increased cholesterol levels has been tested in several important trials. In the CARDS study,[3] diabetic subjects without established coronary disease or high cholesterol levels were randomized to atorvastatin 10 mg daily or placebo. The median low-density lipoprotein (LDL) concentration of participants was 118 mg/dL at the time of randomization. After 4 years, LDL decreased to 82 mg/dL in the atorvastatin group compared with 122 mg/dL in the placebo cohort. Atorvastatin reduced major cardiovascular events by 37% ($P = 0.001$) and total mortality by 27% ($P = 0.059$) compared with placebo. Baseline lipid levels did not predict benefit from statin therapy: patients with lower than median LDL at entry received the same advantage from statin therapy as did patients with higher cholesterol levels.

Patients with type 2 diabetes often display reduced serum high-density lipoprotein (HDL), increased triglycerides, and near-normal LDL cholesterol levels. Fibrate therapy (e.g., gemfibrozil or fenofibrate) is effective at reducing triglycerides and raising HDL cholesterol, but the impact of such therapy has not been shown to be beneficial on cardiovascular outcomes in diabetics. In the FIELD study, 9795 middle-aged type 2 diabetics were randomized to placebo or fenofibrate.[4] Over 5 years, fenofibrate did not significantly reduce the risk of the primary outcome of coronary events and there was a trend toward higher total mortality. Similarly, in the ACCORD trial, the addition of fenofibrate to statin therapy did not improve cardiovascular outcomes in type 2 diabetics over 4.7 years of follow-up.[5]

The rate of diabetes development can be reduced by interventions that target undesired lifestyles. In the Diabetes Prevention Program, 3234 nondiabetic persons with impaired glucose tolerance were randomized to an intense lifestyle-modification program (with goals of ≥ 7% weight loss and at least 150 minutes of physical activity per week), to standard lifestyles, or to metformin. After an average follow-up of 2.8 years, the incidence of diabetes was significantly reduced in both the intense lifestyle group and those taking metformin, but more so in the intense lifestyle group (reductions of 58% and 31%, respectively).[6]

REFERENCES

1. Wild S, Roglic G, Green A, et al: Global prevalence of diabetes: Estimates for the year 2000 and projections for 2030. Diabetes Care 27:1047, 2004.
2. American Diabetes Association: Diagnosis and classification of diabetes mellitus. Diabetes Care 33 (Suppl 1):S62, 2010.
3. Colhoun HM, Betteridge DJ, Durrington PN, et al: Primary prevention of cardiovascular disease with atorvastatin in type 2 diabetes in the Collaborative Atorvastatin Diabetes Study (CARDS): Multicentre randomised placebo-controlled trial. Lancet 364:685, 2004.
4. Keech A, Simes RJ, Barter P, et al: Effects of long-term fenofibrate therapy on cardiovascular events in 9795 people with type 2 diabetes mellitus (the FIELD study): Randomised controlled trial. Lancet 366:1849, 2005.
5. The ACCORD Study Group: Effects of combination lipid therapy in type 2 diabetes mellitus. N Engl J Med 362:1563-1574, 2010.
6. Diabetes Prevention Program Research Group: Reduction in the incidence of type 2 diabetes with lifestyle intervention or metformin. N Engl J Med 346:393, 2002.

ANSWER TO QUESTION 374

D (Braunwald, pp. 1049-1050; Fig. 52-4)

Blood flow to the myocardium is determined by the perfusion pressure gradient and the vascular resistance of the myocardial bed. This is influenced by extrinsic factors (particularly compressive forces within the myocardium) and by intrinsic metabolic, neural, and humoral factors. Intramyocardial pressure is determined primarily by the ventricular pressure throughout the cardiac cycle. Because the ventricular pressure is so much higher in systole than it is in diastole, myocardial compressive forces acting on intramyocardial vessels are much greater during this phase. Therefore, the subendocardium, which is subject to higher systolic pressures, has less systolic flow than the subepicardium. However, *total* flow is greater in the subendocardium than the subepicardium because there is enhanced basal vasodilatation in the former. Interventions that reduce the perfusion gradient during diastole, when the majority of subendocardial flow occurs, lower the ratio of subendocardial to subepicardial flow and may cause the subendocardium to become ischemic. Thus, an increase in ventricular end-diastolic pressure (as occurs with aortic stenosis) or a decrease in diastolic time (e.g., during tachycardia) can reduce subendocardial flow disproportionately. Because the subendocardium has higher metabolic demands and hence lower basal vascular tone, the reserve for vasodilatation is less than in the subepicardium. Therefore, as perfusion is reduced, the deeper layers of the myocardium become ischemic sooner than the more superficial ones.

The subendocardium is susceptible to ischemia owing to the combination of limited reserve of vasodilatation, intrinsic compression from the higher wall stress to which it is subjected, and the increased metabolic demands.

ANSWER TO QUESTION 375

C (Braunwald, pp. 1067-1072)

As described in the Answer to Question 347, *myocardial stunning* is defined as myocardial dysfunction that persists after a period of severe ischemia, with gradual return of contractile activity. Molecular mechanisms include the generation of oxygen-derived free radicals, calcium overload, and reduced sensitivity of myofilaments to calcium.[1] Stunned myocardium does respond to inotropic therapy, hence the need for transient inotropic support in some patients after myocardial infarction until the adjacent stunned myocardium recovers contractile function.

In contrast, *hibernating* myocardium refers to myocardial dysfunction that results from chronically decreased coronary blood flow, a condition that can be reversed with revascularization.[2] Histopathologic studies reveal both myocyte dedifferentiation and apoptosis, suggesting that irreversible changes may occur if revascularization is not undertaken.

REFERENCES

1. Kloner RA, Jennings RB: Consequences of brief ischemia: Stunning, preconditioning, and their clinical implications: II. Circulation 104:3158, 2001.
2. Heusch G, Schulz R, Rahimtoola SH: Myocardial hibernation: A delicate balance. Am J Physiol Heart Circ Physiol 288:H984, 2005.

ANSWER TO QUESTION 376

C (Braunwald, pp. 1178-1179, 1182)

About 15% of patients who present with symptoms consistent with unstable angina are found to have no significant coronary artery disease on angiography. Approximately one third of such patients present with impaired coronary flow, suggesting the presence of microvascular dysfunction. The short-term prognosis is excellent in this situation.

For patients with a clear culprit lesion, the responsible plaque typically is eccentric, with overhanging edges consistent with a disrupted atherosclerotic locus. On intravascular angioscopy, superimposed thrombus in unstable angina tends to be "white" (platelet rich), rather than the "red" (red blood cell–rich) thrombus typical of ST-segment elevation myocardial infarction. Intravascular ultrasonography in patients with unstable angina often demonstrates more soft echolucent lesions (thin fibrous cap and lipid-rich core) and fewer calcified lesions compared with patients with chronic stable angina.

ANSWER TO QUESTION 377

B (Braunwald, pp. 1245-1248)

Comparison of outcomes of coronary artery bypass grafting (CABG) with those of percutaneous coronary intervention (PCI) is a "moving target" because continued new technologies for both strategies have improved outcomes and reduced complications. Nonetheless, randomized trials comparing the two strategies have yielded consistent results.[1] For the majority of patients, there is no difference in the rates of subsequent death or myocardial infarction between the two interventions. The similar outcomes are observed in patients with single-vessel coronary artery disease (including left anterior descending coronary artery disease) as well as in patients with multivessel disease.[2] There is, however, consistent evidence that patients who undergo PCI are more likely to have recurrent angina or require additional subsequent interventional procedures.

There are populations for which bypass surgery has been shown to offer improved survival compared with PCI. For example, the Bypass Angioplasty Revascularization Investigation (BARI) trial was a large comparison of the two treatment strategies among symptomatic patients with angina whose coronary anatomy was deemed suitable for revascularization by either technique (i.e., two- or three-vessel disease, but not left main stenosis). In this study, patients with diabetes and multivessel disease showed significantly improved survival with CABG compared with coronary angioplasty. These findings were confirmed in the Arterial Revascularization Therapy Study (ARTS), which included patients who received more modern percutaneous strategies (e.g., coronary stents and the antiplatelet therapies clopidogrel and glycoprotein IIb/IIIa antagonists).[3,4]

REFERENCES

1. Gibbons RJ, Abrams J, Chatterjee K, et al: ACC/AHA 2002 guideline update for the management of patients with chronic stable angina: Summary article. A report of the American College of Cardiology/American Heart Association Task Force on Practice Guidelines (Committee on the Management of Patients with Chronic Stable Angina). J Am Coll Cardiol 41:159, 2003.
2. Diegeler A, Thiele H, Falk V, et al: Comparison of stenting with minimally invasive bypass surgery for stenosis of the left anterior descending coronary artery. N Engl J Med 347:561, 2002.
3. Legrand VM, Serruys PW, Unger F, et al, for the Arterial Revascularization Therapy Study (ARTS) Investigators: Three-year outcome after coronary stenting versus bypass surgery for the treatment of multivessel disease. Circulation 109:1114, 2004.
4. King SB III, Dangas G, Moses JW, et al: Surgery is preferred for the diabetic with multivessel disease. Circulation 112:1500, 2005.

ANSWER TO QUESTION 378

C (Braunwald, pp. 1193-1194)

Multiple studies have demonstrated the benefits of statin therapy in primary and secondary prevention of coronary disease. Most of the early studies compared a moderate dose of statin with placebo therapy. Subsequent trials examined the role of high-dose statins and more aggressive lipid lowering in patients with established coronary artery disease. For example, the Myocardial Ischemia Reduction with Aggressive Cholesterol Lowering (MIRACL) trial found that treatment with high-dose atorvastatin (80 mg/d) over 4 months reduced cardiac events by 16% compared with placebo.[1]

The Pravastatin or Atorvastatin Evaluation and Infection Therapy–Thrombolysis in Myocardial Infarction

(PROVE IT-TIMI) 22 trial compared high-dose atorvastatin (80 mg/d) versus moderate-dose pravastatin (40 mg/d) begun within 10 days of an ACS and found that the risk of death, nonfatal myocardial infarction, or revascularization was reduced by 25%, with a significant difference seen within 30 days of randomization.[2] The Reversal of Atherosclerosis with Aggressive Lipid Lowering (REVERSAL) study compared similar doses of pravastatin and high-dose atorvastatin and, using intravascular ultrasound, demonstrated reduction in atheroma size in the patients randomized to the high-dose atorvastatin over 18 months of therapy.[3]

Not all studies have demonstrated an advantage of high-dose statin therapy over less intense regimens. In the Aggrastat to Zocor (A to Z; TIMI 21) trial, patients with ACS were randomized to an initial therapy of moderate-dose simvastatin (40 mg/d) for 1 month followed by high-dose (80 mg/d) therapy versus placebo for 4 months, followed by low-dose simvastatin (20 mg/d). After 2 years of follow-up, there was no difference in the composite endpoint of cardiovascular events. However, myopathy (creatine kinase > 10 times the upper limit of normal) occurred in nine patients receiving high-dose simvastatin versus one patient receiving the less intensive regimen ($P = 0.02$). Three patients developed rhabdomyolysis while taking the high-dose simvastatin regimen.[4] Furthermore, as indicated in the Answer to Question 345, the SEARCH trial showed that the incidence of major vascular events was no lower in those randomized to simvastatin 80 mg daily compared with patients receiving 20 mg daily.[5]

REFERENCES

1. Schwartz GG, Olsson AG, Ezekowitz MD, et al: Effects of atorvastatin on early recurrent ischemic events in acute coronary syndromes. The MIRACL study: A randomized controlled trial. JAMA 285:1711, 2001.
2. Nissen SE, Tuzcu EM, Schoenhagen P, et al: Effect of intensive compared with moderate lipid-lowering therapy on progression of coronary atherosclerosis: A randomized controlled trial. JAMA 291:1071, 2004.
3. Cannon CP, Braunwald E, McCabe CH, et al: Intensive versus moderate lipid lowering with statins after acute coronary syndromes. N Engl J Med 350:1495, 2004.
4. de Lemos JA, Blazing MA, Wiviott SD, et al: Early intensive vs a delayed conservative simvastatin strategy in patients with acute coronary syndromes: Phase Z of the A to Z trial. JAMA 292:1307, 2004.
5. Armitage J, Bowman L, Wallendszus K, et al: Intensive lowering of LDL cholesterol with 80 mg versus 20 mg simvastatin daily in 12,064 survivors of myocardial infarction: A double-blind randomised trial. Lancet 376:1658, 2010.

ANSWER TO QUESTION 379

B (Braunwald, pp. 1133, 1365)

Antiplatelet agents act at a variety of sites to inhibit platelet aggregation. Aspirin is an irreversible inhibitor of cyclooxygenase (COX), thereby blocking the formation of thromboxane A_2, a potent mediator of platelet aggregation and vasoconstriction. Because platelets are incapable of new COX synthesis, the effect is permanent for the 7- to 10-day lifetime of the affected platelet.[1] Other nonsteroidal anti-inflammatory drugs (NSAIDs) may prevent acetylation of COX by aspirin. For example, there is evidence that concomitant administration of some nonselective NSAIDs, such as ibuprofen, may inhibit the effects of aspirin on COX and reduce aspirin's antiplatelet efficacy.[2]

Clopidogrel and prasugrel are thienopyridine derivatives that block the adenosine diphosphate–dependent pathway of platelet activation. Both result in *irreversible* blockade of the $P2Y_{12}$ ADP receptor and therefore have long effective half-lives.[1] Prasugrel is a more potent inhibitor of the $P2Y_{12}$ receptor and has favorable pharmacokinetics with a more rapid onset of action than clopidogrel. In the TRITON-TIMI 38 trial of patients with moderate-to-high risk acute coronary syndromes, patients who received prasugrel had a lower composite rate of death from cardiovascular causes, nonfatal myocardial infarction, or nonfatal stroke compared with those who received clopidogrel, but at an increased risk of major bleeding.[3]

Cilostazol is a potent inhibitor of platelet phosphodiesterase-3 that has vasodilator properties. It has been shown to benefit individuals with intermittent claudication due to peripheral arterial disease (see Answer to Question 371).

REFERENCES

1. Meadows TA, Bhatt DL: Clinical aspects of platelet inhibitors and thrombus formation. Circ Res 100:1261, 2007.
2. Antman EM, Bennett JS, Daugherty A, et al: Use of nonsteroidal anti-inflammatory drugs: An update for clinicians: A scientific statement from the American Heart Association. Circulation 115:1634, 2007.
3. Wiviott SD, Braunwald E, McCabe CH, et al: Prasugrel versus clopidogrel in patients with acute coronary syndromes. N Engl J Med 357:2001, 2007.

ANSWER TO QUESTION 380

B (Braunwald, pp. 1136-1138; Figs. 55-26, 55-27, and 55-28; see also Answer to Question 321)

The SAVE study was the first trial to demonstrate that angiotensin-converting enzyme (ACE) inhibitor therapy reduces mortality in patients with ST-segment elevation myocardial infarction (STEMI). Many subsequent studies have demonstrated a similar and consistent benefit of these agents at reducing cardiovascular endpoints after MI. This has been shown with short-term use in all patients with MI and in long-term treatment of patients with depressed left ventricular systolic function after MI. Analysis of short-term trials indicates that one third of the mortality benefit occurs within the first 2 days of ACE inhibitor therapy.[1]

Two studies, OPTIMAAL and VALIANT, evaluated the efficacy of the angiotensin receptor blockers (ARBs) losartan and valsartan, respectively, versus the ACE inhibitor captopril in MI patients. In OPTIMAAL, losartan was better tolerated but there was a nonsignificant trend toward improved survival with captopril. In the VALIANT trial, captopril and valsartan resulted in similar clinical outcomes. The combination of valsartan plus captopril did not offer any advantage of either drug used alone.[2] Thus, in patients intolerant of ACE inhibitors, an ARB is an adequate substitute, but there does not appear to be an advantage of combining the two together in post-MI patients.

The EPHESUS trial examined the role of the selective aldosterone inhibitor eplerenone in patients with MI complicated by left ventricular dysfunction. During 16 months of follow-up, this agent resulted in a 15% relative risk reduction in mortality compared with standard treatment. Such therapy must be prescribed with care, because significant hyperkalemia was more common among the patients treated with eplerenone in this study.[3]

REFERENCES

1. ACE Inhibitor Myocardial Infarction Collaborative Group: Indications for ACE inhibitors in the early treatment of acute myocardial infarction: Systematic overview of individual data from 100,000 patients in randomized trials. Circulation 97:2202, 1998.
2. Pfeffer MA: Effects of valsartan relative to captopril in patients with myocardial infarction complicated by heart failure and/or left ventricular dysfunction. N Engl J Med 349:1843, 2003.
3. Pitt B, Remme W, Zannad F, et al: Eplerenone, a selective aldosterone blocker, In patients with left ventricular dysfunction after myocardial infarction. N Engl J Med 348:1309, 2003.

ANSWER TO QUESTION 381

B (Braunwald, pp. 1351-1352)

This history and angiogram are consistent with thrombo-angiitis obliterans (TAO), also known as Buerger disease. This disease of small and medium arteries of the arms and legs predominantly affects young individuals (onset usually <age 45) and is almost always associated with tobacco use.[1] TAO is more prevalent in Asia than in North America and Europe, and >75% of affected patients are men. The most common presentation includes resting pain of the feet, calves, hands, or forearms, and digital ulcerations are frequently observed. The Raynaud phenomenon and superficial thrombophlebitis are common.

Angiography of affected limbs in patients with TAO demonstrates segmental occlusion of small and medium vessels, the absence of atherosclerosis, and corkscrew collateral vessels bypassing the occlusions.

Smoking cessation is the most important therapy for this condition. Patients who continue to smoke face a 40% to 45% risk of future amputation. There is no evidence that statin therapy is beneficial in this setting. There is usually no role for vascular surgery because of the diffuse nature of the disease and the generally poor distal vasculature.

REFERENCE

1. Olin JW, Shih A: Thromboangiitis obliterans (Buerger's disease). Curr Opin Rheumatol 18:18, 2006.

ANSWER TO QUESTION 382

C (Braunwald, pp. 952-953, 970-971)

The incidence of hypertensive emergencies is falling as a result of widespread treatment of chronic hypertension. In addition to a marked rise in blood pressure, a hypertensive crisis is associated with end-organ damage. Acute retinal effects include hemorrhages, exudates, or papilledema (termed *accelerated-malignant hypertension*). *Hypertensive encephalopathy* is manifest by headache, irritability, confusion, somnolence, stupor, focal neurologic deficits, seizures, and eventually coma. In previously normotensive individuals, encephalopathy may occur at a lower blood pressure than in those with a history of chronic hypertension. The pathogenesis of hypertensive encephalopathy is thought to involve failure of cerebral autoregulation, with *dilatation* of cerebral arterioles leading to excessive cerebral blood flow and damage to the arteriolar wall with *increased* vascular permeability.[1]

Other clinical features of hypertensive crises include renal insufficiency with proteinuria, microangiopathic hemolytic anemia, congestive heart failure, and nausea and vomiting. Patients who have elevated blood pressure and any end-organ manifestations of hypertensive emergency require rapid therapeutic intervention, usually with parenteral drug therapy.[2]

REFERENCES

1. Preston RA, Jy W, Jimenez JJ, et al: Effects of severe hypertension on endothelial and platelet microparticles. Hypertension 41:211, 2003.
2. Feldstein C: Management of hypertensive crises. Am J Ther 14:135, 2007.

ANSWER TO QUESTION 383

A (Braunwald, pp. 1319-1321)

The transesophageal echocardiogram shows the proximal ascending aorta in long-axis view in a patient with proximal aortic dissection. The aortic valve (AV), left atrium (LA), and true (T) and false (F) lumina are identified. The linear shadow (labeled "I") is an intimal flap. The major predisposing factor for aortic dissection is cystic medial degeneration. Of the conditions that promote cystic medial degeneration, age and hypertension are the two most common. The hereditary abnormalities of connective tissue—Marfan syndrome, Loeys-Dietz syndrome, and Ehlers-Danlos syndrome—are all associated with cystic medial degeneration, as is bicuspid aortic valve.

Pregnancy, for reasons that have not been elucidated, accounts for about half of all dissections in women younger than 40 years. Dissection associated with pregnancy occurs most commonly in the third trimester or early postpartum period.[1] Cocaine, but not heroin use, has also been associated with aortic dissection.[2]

REFERENCES

1. Tsai TT, Trimarchi S, Neinaber CA: Acute aortic dissection: Perspectives from the International Registry of Acute Aortic Dissection (IRAD). Eur J Vasc Endovasc Surg 37:149, 2009.
2. Eagle KA, Isselbacher EM, DeSanctis W: Cocaine-related aortic dissection in perspective. Circulation 105:1529, 2002.

ANSWER TO QUESTION 384

B (Braunwald, pp. 1144-1146; Fig. 55-31)

Cardiogenic shock is defined as persistent hypotension with systolic arterial pressure <80 mm Hg and a marked reduction of the cardiac index (<1.8 L/mm/m^2) with an elevated left ventricular (LV) filling pressure (pulmonary capillary wedge pressure >18 mm Hg). Mechanical causes, such as acute mitral regurgitation or ventricular septal rupture, should be excluded in order to attribute cardiogenic shock to LV dysfunction. The SHOCK trial randomized patients with cardiogenic shock due to LV failure to either medical therapy or urgent revascularization by percutaneous coronary intervention or bypass surgery. At 30 days there was no significant difference in cardiovascular outcomes between the medical and revascularization groups. However, after 1 year, survival rates were higher in the patients who had undergone revascularization therapies.[1]

From this evidence, urgent revascularization, not fibrinolysis, is recommended for patients with cardiogenic shock. Vasopressors, percutaneous left ventricular assist devices,[2] and intra-aortic balloon counterpulsation can improve hemodynamics in cardiogenic shock and are often useful as temporizing measures but have not been shown to improve survival in randomized trials.

REFERENCES

1. Sanborn TA, Sleeper LA, Webb JG, et al: Correlates of one-year survival in patients with cardiogenic shock complicating acute myocardial infarction: Angiographic findings from the SHOCK trial. J Am Coll Cardiol 42:1373, 2003.
2. Seyfarth M, Sibbing D, Bauer I, et al: A randomized clinical trial to evaluate the safety and efficacy of a percutaneous left ventricular assist device versus intra-aortic balloon pumping for treatment of cardiogenic shock caused by myocardial infarction. J Am Coll Cardiol 52:1584, 2008.

ANSWER TO QUESTION 385

D (Braunwald, pp. 1146-1147; Fig. 55-32; see also Answer to Question 334)

Right ventricular infarction (RVI) frequently accompanies inferior left ventricular infarction and may be recognized by a characteristic clinical and hemodynamic pattern.[1] Hypotension or a marked hypotensive response to low-dose nitroglycerin in patients with inferior infarction suggests the diagnosis of RVI. The hemodynamic picture of this condition is similar to that of pericardial disease and may include an elevated RV filling pressure, a steep right atrial *y* descent, and a "square root sign" in the RV pressure tracing. Kussmaul's sign may also be present. The presence of unexplained systemic hypoxemia in the setting of RVI suggests the possibility of right-to-left shunting through a patent foramen ovale because of the elevated right-sided pressures.

The placement of right-sided precordial ECG leads may be quite helpful in establishing the diagnosis of RVI.[2] ST-segment elevation in lead V$_4$R is specific and sensitive for the diagnosis of RVI.

Because left-sided filling pressures are dependent on the compromised right-sided transport of blood, loss of left ventricular preload in patients with RVI may lead to a marked reduction in stroke volume and systemic arterial hypotension. Thus, initial therapy for hypotension in RVI should usually include volume expansion, and diuretics should generally be avoided.

REFERENCES

1. Pfisterer M: Right ventricular involvement in myocardial infarction and cardiogenic shock. Lancet 362:392, 2003.
2. Zimetbaum PJ, Josephson ME: Use of the electrocardiogram in acute myocardial infarction. N Engl J Med 348:933, 2003.

ANSWER TO QUESTION 386

A (Braunwald, pp. 1342-1343; Fig. 61-4)

Segmental pressure measurements and determination of the ankle/brachial index (ABI) are simple and very useful noninvasive methods to evaluate symptoms of peripheral arterial disease. To measure segmental pressures, pneumatic cuffs are placed over the upper and lower thigh, calf, and ankle and above the metatarsal area of the foot, and then systolic pressures are measured using a Doppler flow probe. In the iliac and femoral arteries, a 70% to 90% decrease in the cross-sectional area of the artery must be present to create a pressure gradient. A gradient >20 mm Hg between successive levels of the cuffs is evidence of a significant stenosis.

Measurement of the ABI is an even simpler screening tool that represents the ratio of the systolic pressure at the ankle to that of the brachial artery, typically measured using a Doppler flow probe. A normal ABI is >1.0. An ABI of <0.9 is very sensitive for angiographic evidence of an arterial stenosis. Patients with critical limb ischemia typically have an ABI of <0.5. The sensitivity of the ABI is decreased in severely calcified arteries because such vessels do not compress and therefore have spuriously high systolic pressure readings.

This patient in this case has segmental pressure measurements consistent primarily with significant stenoses in the right iliac and common femoral arteries.

REFERENCE

Gerhard-Herman M, Gardin JM, Jaff M, et al: Guidelines for noninvasive vascular laboratory testing: A report from the American Society of Echocardiography and the Society for Vascular Medicine and Biology. Vasc Med 11:183, 2006.

ANSWER TO QUESTION 387

C (Braunwald, pp. 1270, 1277-1280; Table 58-6; Fig. 58-7)

Restenosis after percutaneous coronary intervention is due to the local proliferation of neointimal tissue. Factors that affect rates of restenosis include coronary lesion diameter and length, vessel size, and the presence of diabetes. Original plain balloon angioplasty was associated with a high (30% to 40%) rate of restenosis. The introduction of bare metal stents reduced the rate of restenosis on repeat angiography to 20% to 30%.[1]

There is no evidence that treatment of in-stent restenosis with either direct coronary atherectomy or rotational atherectomy improves recurrences of in-stent restenosis compared with balloon angioplasty using a cutting balloon. Brachytherapy, using gamma radiation, prevents neointimal proliferation and greatly reduces the rate of this complication.[2] The introduction of drug-eluting stents has been the most effective means to suppress local neointimal proliferation and restenosis rates, as discussed in the Answer to Question 388.

REFERENCES

1. Smith SC Jr, Dove JT, Jacobs AK, et al: ACC/AHA guidelines for percutaneous coronary intervention: A report of the American College of Cardiology/American Heart Association Task Force on Practice Guidelines (Committee to Revise the 1993 Guidelines for Percutaneous Transluminal Coronary Angioplasty). J Am Coll Cardiol 37:2215, 2001.
2. Popma J, Suntharalingam M, Lansky A, et al: Randomized trial of ^{90}Sr/^{90}Y beta-radiation versus placebo control for treatment of in-stent restenosis. Circulation 106:1090, 2002.

ANSWER TO QUESTION 388

D (Braunwald, pp. 1280-1282; see also Answer to Question 324)

A drug-eluting stent (DES), which releases a pharmaceutical agent that suppresses neointimal proliferation, is very effective at preventing restenosis after percutaneous coronary intervention. Currently available systems include those that slowly release sirolimus, paclitaxel, or everolimus. *Sirolimus* is a cytostatic inhibitor of neointimal growth. In the RAVEL study, the first large study comparing a DES with a bare metal stent, there was no angiographic evidence of restenosis in the patients randomized to the sirolimus-eluting group.[1] The larger SIRIUS trial demonstrated a 4.1% restenosis rate compared with 16.6% in the bare-metal stent group.[2] *Paclitaxel* stabilizes microtubules and prevents cell division. The TAXUS-IV trial, a large randomized study of bare metal versus paclitaxel-eluting stents, found that the latter exhibited a marked reduction of subsequent in-stent stenosis. The target vessel revascularization at 9 months was reduced from 11.3% to 3%.[3] *Everolimus*, a rapamycin analogue with immunosuppressive and antiproliferative properties, was compared with paclitaxel in the SPIRIT III trial of patients with coronary artery disease undergoing percutaneous coronary intervention. Those who received the everolimus-eluting stent had reduced angiographic late loss and fewer major adverse cardiac events over 1 year of follow up.[4]

Because a DES impairs endothelial regrowth after balloon expansion, extended use of aspirin plus an oral thienopyridine antiplatelet drug (clopidogrel or prasugrel) is required after implantation. Rare cases of life-threatening late stent thrombosis have been reported many months or years after DES implantation, particularly when dual antiplatelet therapy has been discontinued prematurely. Current guidelines recommend at least 12 months of dual antiplatelet therapy after DES implantation.[5]

DES has been shown to result in superior outcomes compared with brachytherapy in the treatment of in-stent restenosis within bare metal stents.[6]

REFERENCES

1. Morice M, Serruys P, Sousa J, et al: A randomized comparison of a sirolimus-eluting stent with a standard stent for coronary revascularization. N Engl J Med 346:1773, 2002.
2. Moses J, Leon M, Popma J, et al: Angiographic and clinical outcomes after a sirolimus-eluting stent compared to a standard stent in patients with complex coronary stenoses. N Engl J Med 349:1315, 2003.
3. Stone C, Ellis SG, Cox DA, et al: A polymer-based, paclitaxel-eluting stent in patients with coronary artery disease. N Engl J Med 350:221, 2004.
4. Stone GW, Midei M, Newman W, et al: Comparison of an everolimus-eluting stent and a paclitaxel-eluting stent in patients with coronary artery disease: A randomized trial. JAMA 299:1903-1913, 2008.
5. Pinto Slottow TL, Waksman R: Overview of the 2006 Food and Drug Administration Circulatory System Devices Panel meeting on drug-eluting stent thrombosis. Cathet Cardiovasc Interv 69:1064, 2007.
6. Holmes DR Jr, Teirstein P, Satler L, et al: Sirolimus-eluting stents vs vascular brachytherapy for in-stent restenosis within bare-metal stents: The SISR randomized trial. JAMA 295:1264, 2006.

ANSWER TO QUESTION 389

B (Braunwald, pp. 1037-1038)

A program of regular exercise is associated with reduced cardiovascular risk presumably because of its beneficial effects on traditional risk factors such as hypertension, dyslipidemia, and diabetes. Regular exercise also appears to contribute to a less prothrombotic state by improving the activity of the fibrinolytic system: exercise reduces plasma fibrinogen and plasminogen activator inhibitor-1 levels and increases tissue plasminogen activator levels.[1] In addition, although sudden exercise in chronically sedentary individuals may increase platelet activation, a program of regular exercise has the beneficial opposite effect.

Heart rate variability is a measure of autonomic function that is dependent on the relation between parasympathetic and sympathetic tone. Reduced heart rate variability is associated with an elevated risk of coronary artery disease and mortality. Regular exercise reduces parasympathetic tone and *increases* (i.e., improves) heart rate variability.[2]

Exercise has been shown to improve the impaired endothelial-dependent vasodilatation typical of patients with coronary artery disease or coronary risk factors, likely because of increased expression of nitric oxide (NO) synthase and NO production.[3] Exercise also tends to produce beneficial changes in the lipid profile, including higher levels of high-density lipoprotein and lower levels of low-density lipoprotein and triglycerides.[4]

REFERENCES

1. Wannamethee SG, Lowe GD, Whincup PH, et al: Physical activity and hemostatic and inflammatory variables in elderly men. Circulation 105:1785, 2002.

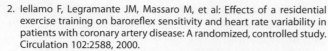

2. Iellamo F, Legramante JM, Massaro M, et al: Effects of a residential exercise training on baroreflex sensitivity and heart rate variability in patients with coronary artery disease: A randomized, controlled study. Circulation 102:2588, 2000.
3. Hambrecht R, Wolf A, Gielen S, et al: Effect of exercise on coronary endothelial function in patients with coronary artery disease. N Engl J Med 342:454, 2000.
4. Kraus WE, Houmard JA, Duscha BD, et al: Effects of the amount and intensity of exercise on plasma lipoproteins. N Engl J Med 347:1483, 2002.

ANSWER TO QUESTION 390

B (Braunwald, p. 1049)

The three major components of myocardial oxygen demand (MVO_2) are heart rate, the myocardial contractile state, and wall tension.[1] In turn, wall tension during systole is proportional to the aortic pressure and intraventricular volume. An increase in any of these parameters results in augmented myocardial oxygen consumption.

Heart rate is generally the most important determinant of MVO_2 and the balance between myocardial oxygen supply and demand. For example, during tachycardia, MVO_2 increases and, at the same time, coronary oxygen supply may suffer because the shortened diastolic filling period tends to reduce subendocardial coronary blood flow.

The circulating content of hemoglobin is an important determinant of myocardial oxygen supply, not MVO_2.

REFERENCE

1. Braunwald E: Myocardial oxygen consumption: The quest for its determinants and some clinical fallout. J Am Coll Cardiol 35:45B, 2000.

ANSWER TO QUESTION 391

D (Braunwald, p. 1404)

Diabetes and hypertension frequently coexist and augment the risk of coronary events. Diabetics with mild chronic renal disease are particularly prone to develop the syndrome of hyporeninemic hypoaldosteronism because they are affected by a combination of low renin production and impaired insulin secretion, both of which increase the serum potassium concentration. With progressive renal insufficiency there is loss of the renin-producing juxtaglomerular apparatus in the nephron. Thus, supplemental potassium and potassium-sparing diuretics must be used with caution in such patients. Calcium channel blockers have also been reported to impair the adrenal secretion of aldosterone.

Although tomatoes and bananas are rich sources of potassium, it would be unusual for a normal diet to cause such a marked rise in potassium. Urinary tract infections may increase potassium in the setting of worsened renal function (which was not observed in this patient). Primary hyperaldosteronism and Cushing syndrome are more likely to cause hypokalemia than hyperkalemia.

REFERENCE

Palmer B: Managing hyperkalemia caused by inhibitors of the renin-angiotensin-aldosterone system. N Engl J Med 351:58, 2004.

ANSWER TO QUESTION 392

C (Braunwald, pp. 1188-1189; Fig. 56-12)

Prasugrel, like clopidogrel, is a thienopyridine drug that impairs platelet aggregation through irreversible inhibition of the $P2Y_{12}$ receptor.[1] Active metabolites of prasugrel render it 10 times more potent an antiplatelet agent than clopidogrel. In the TRITON-TIMI 38 trial, 13,608 patients with acute coronary syndromes for whom PCI was planned were randomized to either prasugrel (60 mg loading dose, followed by 10 mg daily) or clopidogrel (300 mg loading dose, followed by 75 mg daily).[2] Over 15 months of follow-up, prasugrel reduced the outcomes of cardiovascular death, myocardial infarction, or stroke by 19%. In patients who received stents, prasugrel also reduced the risk of stent thrombosis by half. However, prasugrel was associated with an increased rate of fatal bleeding compared with clopidogrel (0.4 vs. 0.1%, $P = 0.002$). Bleeding complications were greatest in the elderly (≥75 years), patients with prior stroke or transient ischemic attack, and those who weighed <60 kg, so that prasugrel should be avoided in such patients.[3]

REFERENCES

1. Wallentin L: P2Y 12 inhibitors: Differences in properties and mechanisms of action and potential consequences for clinical use. Eur Heart J 30:1964, 2009.
2. Wiviott SD, Braunwald E, McCabe CH, et al: Prasugrel versus clopidogrel in patients with acute coronary syndromes. N Engl J Med 357:2001, 2007.
3. Bhatt DL: Prasugrel in clinical practice. N Engl J Med 361:940, 2009.

ANSWERS TO QUESTIONS 393 TO 396

393–B, 394–C, 395–A, 396-D (Braunwald, pp. 900-906)

Each of the cell types listed is involved in the process of atherogenesis. *Endothelial cells*, which represent a large and extensive lining of the entire vascular tree, form a highly selective, permeable barrier to the bloodstream and maintain a nonthrombogenic surface. They also actively manufacture and secrete several important vasoactive substances. Endothelial cells have a surface coat of heparan sulfate, which helps maintain nonthrombogenicity, and produce prostaglandin derivatives, in particular prostacyclin. The latter is a vasodilator that inhibits platelet aggregation. In addition, endothelial cells secrete tissue plasminogen activator, which may contribute to lysis of fibrin clots and regulation of the local hemostatic milieu, and nitric oxide, which causes vasodilatation and inhibits platelet aggregation. Thus, endothelial cells regulate or provide protection against the development of inappropriate thrombus formation through several mechanisms.

The *smooth muscle cell* is originally derived from the media of the blood vessel and proliferates in the arterial intima to form atherosclerotic plaques. The principal physiologic role of this cell in the media is presumably to maintain arterial wall tone by its capacity to alter contractile state in response to a variety of substances. Thus, prostacyclin may induce relaxation and vasodilatation whereas other vasoactive agents such as epinephrine and angiotensin may cause smooth muscle contraction. During atheroma formation, smooth muscle cells migrate into the intima, likely attracted by platelet-derived growth factor and other chemoattractants. Extensive proliferation of smooth muscle cells in the intima contributes significantly to the development of the mature atherosclerotic lesion.

Macrophages, derived from circulating blood monocytes, are capable of secreting a large number of biologically active substances that participate in inflammatory and immune responses. Macrophages become foam cells by extensive, non–low-density lipoprotein receptor–mediated, accumulation of cholesteryl ester and as such form the principal cells in the fatty streak. The macrophage foam cells provide a major source of proinflammatory mediators, which are thought to play a critical role in atherogenesis.

Platelets interact in an important manner with both the endothelium and developing atherosclerotic plaque. Although platelets are capable of little or no protein synthesis, they contain numerous protein substances in their granules that are released on platelet activation. These include factors that participate in the coagulation cascade as well as several potent growth factors or mitogens. Growth factors may play an important role in stimulating both vasoconstriction and subsequent proliferation in the injured vessel wall. In addition, the factors released that participate in the coagulation cascade contribute to thrombus formation and as such are important in the sequelae of atherosclerotic disease.

REFERENCE

Libby P, Ridker PM, Hansson GK: Inflammation in atherosclerosis: From pathophysiology to practice. J Am Coll Cardiol 54:2129, 2009.

ANSWERS TO QUESTIONS 397 TO 400

397–B, 398–A, 399–D, 400–C (Braunwald, pp. 1225-1227; Table 50-8)

Beta blockers inhibit the beta-adrenergic receptor, which is part of the adenylate cyclase system.[1] Inhibition results in lower levels of cyclic adenosine monophosphate and cytosolic calcium. Beta blockers can be divided into three general groups. First-generation agents are nonselective, inhibiting both $beta_1$- and $beta_2$-adrenergic receptors (e.g., propranolol); second-generation agents are relatively $beta_1$ selective, although this selectivity diminishes with higher doses (e.g., metoprolol or atenolol); and

third-generation agents have additional vasodilatation properties (e.g., carvedilol, which has alpha- and beta-receptor blocking activities).

In addition to these pharmacodynamic properties, there are also important pharmacokinetic differences among beta blockers. For example, propranolol is very lipophilic, is readily absorbed from the gastrointestinal tract, is metabolized by the liver, and has a short half-life. In contrast, atenolol is very hydrophilic, is not as readily absorbed from the gastrointestinal tract, is metabolized by the kidney, and has a longer half-life so that it can be administered less frequently.

Some beta blockers (e.g., pindolol, acebutolol) have partial beta-agonist activity. These agents produce low-grade beta stimulation when sympathetic tone is low (e.g., at rest) but behave like more conventional beta blockers when sympathetic activity is high, such as during exercise.

REFERENCE

1. Gorre F, Vandekerckhove H: Beta-blockers: Focus on mechanism of action. Which beta-blocker, when and why? Acta Cardiol 65:565, 2010.

ANSWERS TO QUESTIONS 401 TO 405

401–A, 402–B, 403–B, 404–C, 405–B (Braunwald, pp. 1147-1150, 1158-1159)

Both aneurysms and pseudoaneurysms can complicate acute myocardial infarction. A true aneurysm is a discrete dyskinetic region of the ventricular wall that results from expansion and dilatation of a segment of scarred, thinned myocardium. The wall always contains some myocardial elements. The base of a true aneurysm is wide and the risk of free wall rupture is low. Mural thrombus may form along the wall of the aneurysmal segment, and anticoagulation is usually appropriate, at least temporarily. Surgical repair is sometimes indicated, for example, if the aneurysm results in intractable heart failure or uncontrolled ventricular arrhythmias.

In contrast, pseudoaneurysms represent an incomplete rupture of the ventricular free wall that is sealed by organizing thrombus and pericardium, rather than myocardial elements. Pseudoaneurysms can become very large and communicate with the left ventricle through a narrow neck. Although the base is narrow, the risk of progressive rupture is high and surgical repair is indicated. The distinction between true aneurysms and pseudoaneurysms can usually be readily discerned by echocardiography.

REFERENCE

Cheitlin MD, Armstrong WF, Aurigemma GP, et al: ACC/AHA/ASE 2003 guideline update for the clinical application of echocardiography: A report of the American College of Cardiology/American Heart Association Task Force on Practice Guidelines (ACC/AHA/ASE Committee to Update the 1997 Guidelines on the Clinical Application of Echocardiography). Circulation 108:1146, 2003.

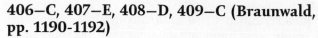

ANSWERS TO QUESTIONS 406 TO 409

406–C, 407–E, 408–D, 409–C (Braunwald, pp. 1190-1192)

Unfractionated heparin (UFH) is a glycosaminoglycan with a high binding affinity for antithrombin. When bound to heparin, antithrombin undergoes a conformational change that results in greater inactivation of factor IIa (thrombin) and factor Xa, thus interfering with clot formation.

Low-molecular-weight heparins (LMWHs) are derived from UFH via chemical or enzymatic depolymerization. The shorter molecules still activate antithrombin but have greater anti–factor Xa than anti–factor IIa activity. This feature causes LMWHs to inhibit thrombin generation more effectively, and the high bioavailability permits subcutaneous, rather than intravenous, administration. The reduced binding of LMWHs to plasma proteins allows a predictable drug effect such that routine monitoring of anticoagulant activity is not usually necessary. If the anticoagulant effect does need to be assessed (e.g., in obese individuals or patients with renal impairment), anti-Xa activity, not the activated partial thromboplastin time (aPTT), should be measured. LMWHs are less likely to trigger type II heparin-induced thrombocytopenia (HIT) but are still contraindicated in patients with this syndrome, because HIT antibodies can cross react with LMWH.

Bivalirudin is a synthetic peptide that is a direct thrombin inhibitor—it binds directly to thrombin without requiring antithrombin. Because it is cleaved once bound to thrombin, bivalirudin has a very short half-life. It appears to be safe in patients with a history of HIT. Its anticoagulant effect can be followed by measuring the aPTT. The doses of both bivalirudin and LMWH require adjustment in the setting of advanced renal insufficiency.

REFERENCE

Sakhuja R, Yeh RW, Bhatt DL: Anticoagulant agents in acute coronary syndromes. Curr Probl Cardiol 36:127, 2011.

ANSWERS TO QUESTIONS 410 TO 414

410–B, 411–C, 412–D, 413–C, 414–A (Braunwald, pp. 897-904)

Experimental data suggest that the initial stages of atherogenesis include extracellular lipid accumulation and leukocyte recruitment.[1] The latter process is mediated by several groups of adhesion molecules.[2] The first group includes members of the immunoglobulin superfamily, including vascular cell adhesion molecule (VCAM)-1 and intercellular adhesion molecule (ICAM)-1. The second group includes selectins such as P-selectin and E-selectin. Expression of these adhesion molecules on the surface of endothelial cells regulates the adherence of monocytes and T cells to the arterial wall. Entry of leukocytes into the intima is then mediated by chemoattractant cytokines such as monocyte chemoattractant protein-1.

Once recruited into the arterial intima, monocytes imbibe lipid particles to become lipid-laden macrophages, termed *foam cells*. Although other cells in the body express surface low-density lipoprotein (LDL) receptors that regulate LDL uptake, this is not true of foam cells. In these cells, scavenger uptake receptors allow unregulated lipid accumulation.[3] The precursor atherosclerotic lesion composed of foam cells is known as the fatty streak.

A subsequent step in formation of an atherosclerotic lesion involves smooth muscle cell migration and proliferation in the intima. Many of the smooth muscle cells in atherosclerotic lesions derive from the arterial medial layer.[4] The chemoattractants responsible for migration into the intima include platelet-derived growth factor, which is secreted by activated macrophages. With the addition of extracellular matrix consisting of collagen and proteoglycans secreted by the smooth muscle cells, the fibrous plaque is formed.

REFERENCES

1. Hansson GK: Inflammation, atherosclerosis, and coronary artery disease. N Engl J Med 352:1685, 2005.
2. Ley K: The role of selectins in inflammation and disease. Trends Mol Med 9:263, 2003.
3. van Berkel TJ, Out R, Hoekstra M, et al: Scavenger receptors: Friend or foe in atherosclerosis? Curr Opin Lipidol 16:525, 2005.
4. Hoofnagle MH, Thomas JA, Wamhoff BR, Owens GK: Origin of neointimal smooth muscle: We've come full circle. Arterioscler Thromb Vasc Biol 26:2579, 2006.

ANSWERS TO QUESTIONS 415 TO 419

415–B, 416–D, 417–D, 418–A, 419–A (Braunwald, pp. 1125-1126; Table 55-6)

Each of the available fibrinolytic drugs for use in acute ST-segment elevation myocardial infarction (MI) possesses unique characteristics. The first-generation fibrinolytic agent was *streptokinase* (SK), which is an indirect plasminogen activator and therefore relatively nonspecific for fibrin. In comparative trials, it had the lowest rate of intracranial hemorrhage. Produced by beta-hemolytic streptococci, SK is antigenic and allergic reactions occur in 5% to 6% of patients. *Alteplase* (tissue plasminogen activator [tPA]) represents a second-generation, more fibrin-specific fibrinolytic. It has the shortest half-life (4 to 8 minutes) of all current fibrinolytics and therefore is administered as a bolus followed by an infusion over 90 minutes or longer.

Modifications to the basic structure of tPA have yielded a series of third-generation fibrinolytics with more prolonged plasma clearance rates, including *reteplase* (RPA) and *tenecteplase* (TNK-tPA). RPA is a deletion mutant of tPA with a longer half-life (15 minutes) but reduced fibrin specificity.[1] It is administered as a double intravenous bolus, 30 minutes apart. TNK-tPA is a triple mutant with resultant increased fibrin specificity, a longer half-life, and reduced sensitivity to plasminogen activation inhibitor-1. It is administered as a single intravenous bolus.

The third-generation fibrinolytics result in 30-day post-MI mortality rates similar to tPA administered in the standard accelerated (90-minute infusion) fashion. However, they offer the convenience of bolus administration.

REFERENCE

1. Van de Werf FJ, Topol EJ, Sobel BE: The impact of fibrinolytic therapy for ST-segment-elevation acute myocardial infarction. J Thromb Haemost 7:14, 2009.

ANSWERS TO QUESTIONS 420 TO 423

420–C, 421–C, 422–B, 423–A (Braunwald, pp. 1147-1151; Table 55-12)

Rupture of the interventricular septum after acute myocardial infarction (MI) usually occurs in the setting of anterior wall infarction and in patients with poor collateral circulation.[1] In fibrinolytic trials, it developed in only 0.8% of patients, with an associated 30-day mortality of 74%. Septal defects in patients with anterior infarction tend to be apical in location, whereas inferior infarctions are associated with perforation of the basal septum (a more difficult area to surgically repair).[2] Partial or total rupture of a papillary muscle (as shown in the figure) in the setting of acute MI is usually due to ischemic damage to the posteromedial papillary muscle in inferior wall infarction. Papillary muscle rupture occurs with relatively small infarctions in approximately half of the cases, in contrast to rupture of the ventricular septum, which almost always results from large infarcts.[3]

Clinically, patients with both lesions develop a new holosystolic murmur. The murmur of interventricular septal rupture is often louder and accompanied by a systolic thrill. In both lesions, the murmur may decrease or disappear as arterial blood pressure (and therefore systemic afterload) falls. The distinction between acute ventricular septal rupture and mitral regurgitation can be made readily by echocardiography.

At heart catheterization, patients with either lesion may demonstrate tall v waves in the pulmonary capillary wedge tracing; therefore, this finding is not useful in differentiating between the two. However, measurement of oxygen saturation via a pulmonary artery catheter can distinguish them: in ventricular septal rupture there is a "step-up" in oxygen saturation in the right ventricle (compared with the right atrium) as a result of oxygenated blood entering the right ventricle from the left ventricle.

REFERENCES

1. Birnbaum Y, Fishbein MC, Blanche C, Siegel RJ: Ventricular septal rupture after acute myocardial infarction. N Engl J Med 347:1426, 2002.
2. Bursi F, Enriquez-Sarano M, Jacobsen SJ, Roger VL: Mitral regurgitation after myocardial infarction: A review. Am J Med 119:103, 2006.
3. Stout KK, Verrier ED: Acute valvular regurgitation. Circulation 119:3232, 2009.

ANSWERS TO QUESTIONS 424 TO 427

424–C, 425–C, 426–A, 427–C (Braunwald, pp. 989-990; Tables 47-7; Fig. 47-6)

The 4S was a secondary prevention trial that examined the effect of simvastatin over 5.4 years in 4444 individuals with known coronary disease and very high serum cholesterol. Treatment with simvastatin was associated with highly significant reductions in nonfatal myocardial infarction (MI) and cardiovascular death (34%) and overall mortality (30%).[1]

The HPS study compared the benefit of simvastatin (40 mg/day) with placebo in over 20,000 patients at risk for vascular events who would not have met criteria for lipid lowering at the time of enrollment. The study included patients with established atherosclerotic disease and those with multiple risk factors. Randomization to simvastatin was associated with a 24% reduction in major vascular events and 13% reduction in all-cause mortality. Subgroup analysis showed there was equal benefit for women, the elderly, and diabetic patients.[2]

The ASCOT-LLA investigators randomized 10,305 hypertensive patients with total cholesterol <250 mg/dL to either atorvastatin 10 mg daily or placebo. Patients with a history of myocardial infarction, cerebrovascular disease, or current angina were excluded. After 3.3 years, atorvastatin was associated with a 27% reduction in stroke and a 21% reduction in total cardiovascular events, but overall mortality was not significantly impacted.[3]

The JUPITER trial examined the effects of rosuvastatin 20 mg daily versus placebo over 1.9 years in 17,802 apparently healthy men and women who had LDL cholesterol <130 mg/dL but high-sensitivity C-reactive protein (hsCRP) >2.0 mg/L. Treatment with rosuvastatin was associated with a significant 44%% reduction of the composite outcome of MI, stroke, revascularization, unstable angina or cardiovascular death. The individual components of the primary outcome were also significantly reduced, as was overall mortality. There was a higher incidence of physician-reported diabetes in the rosuvastatin-treated group.[4]

REFERENCES

1. Randomised trial of cholesterol lowering in 4444 patients with coronary heart disease: The Scandinavian Simvastatin Survival Study (4S). Lancet 344:1383-1389, 1994.
2. Heart Protection Study Collaborative Group. MRC/BHF Heart Protection Study of cholesterol lowering with simvastatin in 20,536 high-risk individuals: A randomised placebo-controlled trial. Lancet 360:7, 2002.
3. Server PS, Dahlof B, Poulter NR, et al: Prevention of coronary and stroke events with atorvastatin in hypertensive patients who have average or lower-than-average cholesterol concentrations, in the Anglo-Scandinavian Cardiac Outcomes Trial-Lipid Lowering Arm (ASCOT-LLA): A multicentre randomised controlled trial. Lancet 361:1149, 2003.
4. Ridker PM, Danielson E, Fonseca FAH, et al: Rosuvastatin to Prevent Vascular Events in Men and Women with Elevated C-Reactive Protein (JUPITER). N Engl J Med 359:2195, 2008.

PREVENTIVE CARDIOLOGY; ATHEROSCLEROTIC CARDIOVASCULAR DISEASE

ANSWERS TO QUESTIONS 428 TO 431

428–D, 429–D, 430–B, 431–C (Braunwald, p. 986; Table 47-5)

Prescription medications can contribute to abnormal serum lipids. Many beta blockers (excluding those with intrinsic sympathomimetic activity and those with concurrent alpha-blocking properties) have been shown to lower serum high-density lipoprotein (HDL) cholesterol. Second-generation antipsychotic medications (e.g., clozapine, olanzapine) can contribute to weight gain, insulin resistance, and increased low-density lipoprotein cholesterol and triglyceride levels.[1] Corticosteroids raise triglyceride levels and lower serum HDL levels.

Examples of cardiovascular drugs that have no significant effect on plasma lipoproteins include calcium channel antagonists, angiotensin-converting enzyme inhibitors, and angiotensin receptor blockers.

REFERENCE

1. Perez-Iglesias R, Crespo-Facorro B, Amado JA, et al. 12-Week randomized clinical trial to evaluate metabolic changes in drug-naive, first-episode psychosis patients treated with haloperidol, olanzapine, or risperidone. J Clin Psychiatry 68:1733, 2007.

ANSWERS TO QUESTIONS 432 TO 435

432–A, 433–A, 434–C, 435–B (Braunwald, pp. 982-984, Table 47-4)

Familial hypercholesterolemia (FH) is associated with specific dermatologic lesions. Heterozygotes may develop nodular swellings of the tendons around the knee, elbow, dorsum of the hand, and ankle, known as *tendon xanthomas*, as shown in part B of the figure. Microscopically, these consist of large deposits of cholesterol, both extracellularly and within scavenger macrophage cells.

Although deposition of cholesterol in the tissues of the eyelid and within the cornea, known respectively as *xanthelasma* (part C in the figure) and *arcus corneae*, may be observed in FH, they can also occur in adults with other lipid disorders and even in those with normal plasma lipid levels.

Patients with homozygous FH have dramatic elevations in plasma low-density lipoprotein from birth, with levels typically sixfold to eightfold higher than normal. In addition, they demonstrate a unique cutaneous finding, the *planar xanthoma*. The latter may be present at birth but always develops within the first 6 years of life. Planar xanthomas are yellow and occur at points of trauma over the knees, elbows, and buttocks. In addition, they may be found in the interdigital webs of the hands, especially between the thumb and index finger (part A in the figure). Tendon xanthomas, xanthelasma, and arcus corneae also occur in homozygotes.

Type III hyperlipoproteinemia, or familial dysbetalipoproteinemia, is a single-gene disorder that requires both the presence of a mutation in the gene for apolipoprotein E and contributory environmental or genetic factors. In this disorder, the plasma concentrations of both cholesterol and triglycerides are elevated because of the accumulation of remnant-like particles derived from the partial metabolism of both very low-density lipoprotein and chylomicrons. Two specific dermatologic lesions are characteristic of type III hyperlipoproteinemia. *Xanthoma striatum palmare* appears as orange or yellow discolorations of the palmar and digital creases, as illustrated in part D in the figure. In addition, *tuberoeruptive xanthomas* are characteristically located over the elbows and knees in this disorder (not shown).

DISEASES OF THE HEART, PERICARDIUM, AND PULMONARY VASCULAR BED

DIRECTIONS: For each question below, select the ONE BEST response.

QUESTION 436

A 65-year-old man with a history of radiation therapy to the chest for lymphoma presents with worsening exertional dyspnea. On physical examination the heart rate is 120 beats/min, blood pressure 90/55 mm Hg with a pulsus paradoxus of 15 mm Hg. The jugular venous pressure is 10 cm H_2O with a prominent x descent. He is found by echocardiography to have a large pericardial effusion, which is drained by pericardiocentesis. After the procedure in the cardiac catheterization laboratory the intrapericardial pressure normalizes but the initially elevated right atrial pressure fails to decline and displays a prominent y descent. This scenario is most consistent with:

A. Persistence of pericardial tamponade
B. Cor pulmonale
C. Effusive-constrictive pericarditis
D. Restrictive cardiomyopathy
E. Uremic pericarditis

QUESTION 437

A 55-year-old previously healthy man is brought to the emergency department because of left-sided chest pain over the past 3 hours. He denies shortness of breath or cough. The discomfort is less intense when he sits forward. The chest radiograph is unremarkable; the ECG is shown in Figure 4-1. Which of the following statements regarding this patient's condition is TRUE?

A. Thrombolytic therapy is indicated if cardiac catheterization is not immediately available
B. Nitrates will substantially relieve the chest pain
C. Aspirin should be administered
D. Glucocorticoid therapy should be started immediately
E. Measurement of serum cardiac biomarkers can quickly differentiate the cause of his chest pain

QUESTION 438

Which of the following statements about localized coarctation of the aorta is TRUE?

A. After successful repair, systemic hypertension frequently persists

B. Coarctation is more common in females
C. Chest pain and palpitations are common symptoms in older children and adults
D. Atrial septal defect is the most common associated cardiac finding
E. A midsystolic murmur over the mid anterior abdomen is common

QUESTION 439

An 80-year-old man presents with syncope. During evaluation a murmur is detected and an echocardiogram is obtained. A continuous-wave Doppler recording through the aortic valve is shown in Figure 4-2. True statements in this disorder include all of the following EXCEPT:

A. A gradual decrease in exercise tolerance or dyspnea on exertion are the earliest manifestations
B. Patients who describe typical angina may not have significant coronary arterial obstruction
C. Syncope commonly occurs without significant change in systemic vascular tone
D. Orthopnea, paroxysmal nocturnal dyspnea, and pulmonary edema are late manifestations
E. Gastrointestinal bleeding has been associated with this disorder

QUESTION 440

A 28-year-old man presents to the emergency department because of severe chest pain and dyspnea after cocaine use. His medical history is notable for several years of intermittent cocaine use, alcohol abuse, and cigarette smoking. He has no other known cardiac risk factors. Each of the following statements about cocaine use and the cardiovascular system is true EXCEPT:

A. The concomitant use of cocaine with alcohol increases cardiovascular morbidity and mortality compared with cocaine alone
B. The risk of myocardial infarction after cocaine is related to the amount ingested and the frequency of its use
C. Left ventricular systolic dysfunction can occur both acutely and after long-term cocaine use
D. Mechanisms of cocaine-related myocardial ischemia and infarction include coronary arterial vasoconstriction and enhanced platelet aggregation

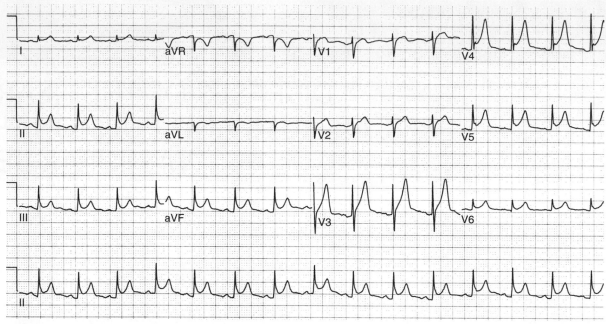

FIGURE 4-1

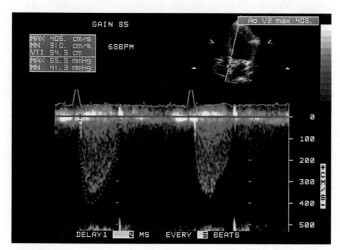

FIGURE 4-2

D. Children with ASDs typically experience easy fatigability and exertional dyspnea

E. Atrial arrhythmias are uncommon in children with ASDs

QUESTION 442

True statements about the ECG in congenital heart disease include all of the following EXCEPT:

A. First-degree atrioventricular (AV) block is often present in patients with AV septal defects, congenitally corrected transposition of the great arteries, or Ebstein anomaly

B. Atrial fibrillation is the most common atrial arrhythmia in young patients with congenital heart disease

C. The presence of right ventricular hypertrophy suggests pulmonary hypertension or right ventricular outflow tract obstruction

D. In infants the electrocardiographic pattern of myocardial infarction is associated with anomalous origin of a coronary artery

E. Deep Q waves in the left chest leads can be caused by left ventricular volume overload in a young person with aortic or mitral regurgitation

E. Approximately 25% of nonfatal myocardial infarctions in individuals 18 to 45 years of age are associated with cocaine use

QUESTION 443

All of the following statements regarding ventricular septal defects (VSDs) are true EXCEPT:

A. Muscular VSDs are bordered entirely by myocardium

B. Small VSDs pose a high risk of endocarditis

C. A restrictive VSD does not cause significant hemodynamic derangement and may close spontaneously during childhood

QUESTION 441

True statements about atrial septal abnormalities include all of the following EXCEPT:

A. The sinus venosus type atrial septal defect (ASD) is almost always accompanied by anomalous pulmonary venous connections

B. A patent foramen ovale can be found in approximately 25% of healthy adults

C. The most common presenting symptoms of ASDs in adults are exercise intolerance and palpitations

D. Infants with large, nonrestrictive VSDs come to medical attention at an earlier age than those with restrictive defects

E. The ECG after VSD repair usually demonstrates right bundle branch block

QUESTION 444

Which of the following statements regarding atrial septal defects (ASDs) is TRUE?

A. Percutaneous device closure of ASDs improves functional status in symptomatic patients and exercise capacity in both asymptomatic and symptomatic patients

B. Children with successful repair of an isolated secundum defect require lifelong endocarditis prophylaxis

C. Murmurs are not typically present in patients with ASD

D. Left-axis deviation on the ECG suggests the presence of a sinus venosus ASD

E. Surgical or device closure is not indicated in patients with pulmonary:systemic shunt ratios <2.5:1.0

QUESTION 445

A 34-year-old woman presents with recurrent syncope. In recent months she has noted a 10-lb unintentional weight loss, fatigue, and mild diffuse arthralgias. She denies dyspnea, palpitations, or chest pain. A two-dimensional echocardiogram (subcostal view) is shown in Figure 4-3. All of the following statements are true about this patient's condition EXCEPT:

A. This is an example of the most common type of primary cardiac tumor

B. This lesion is equally likely to develop in the right atrium as in the left atrium

C. Distal embolism is a common complication

D. Fever is commonly present

E. Operative excision of this lesion is indicated

QUESTION 446

A 42-year-old woman underwent a mitral valve replacement with a St. Jude prosthesis. She was maintained on warfarin therapy and was documented to have adequate anticoagulation. Two years after the operation she had recurrent transient ischemic attacks; a work-up was undertaken. Transthoracic echocardiography proved unrevealing. A transesophageal echocardiogram was performed (Fig. 4-4). True statements include each of the following EXCEPT:

A. Large vegetations are seen on the left atrial surface of the St. Jude valve

B. *Streptococcus viridans* is the most likely organism to be cultured in this setting

C. Methicillin resistance is present in the majority of patients with this complication

D. The prosthetic mitral valve is seated in a normal position

E. Transesophageal echocardiography is consistently more sensitive than transthoracic studies for establishing this diagnosis

QUESTION 447

True statements about the percutaneous treatment of valvular stenosis include all of the following EXCEPT:

A. Balloon valvuloplasty has essentially replaced surgical repair for valvular pulmonic stenosis

B. Mitral stenosis due to rheumatic fever does not typically allow for successful balloon valvuloplasty

C. The development of moderate or severe mitral regurgitation after balloon mitral valvuloplasty is uncommon

D. Systemic embolization rarely results from mitral valvuloplasty in patients without documented left atrial thrombus

E. Balloon valvuloplasty for calcific aortic stenosis in adults is much less effective than balloon mitral valvuloplasty for mitral stenosis

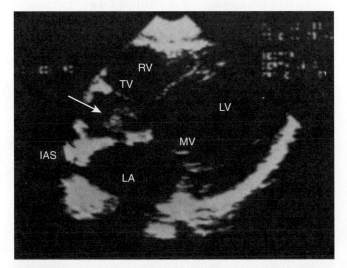

FIGURE 4-3 From Panadis IP, Kotler MN, Mintz GS, et al: Clinical and echocardiographic features of the right atrial masses. Am Heart J 107:745, 1984.

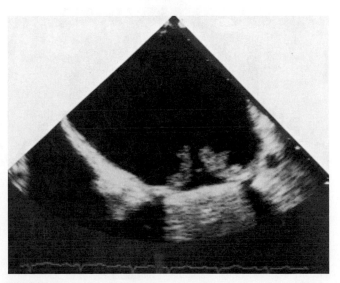

FIGURE 4-4

QUESTION 448

A 9-month-old infant is found to have a well-circumscribed mass in the left ventricle. Histology of the mass demonstrates enlarged cells with clear cytoplasm and occasional "spider cells." Which of the following cardiac tumors is most likely?

A. Lipoma
B. Papillary fibroelastoma
C. Angiosarcoma
D. Atrial myxoma
E. Rhabdomyoma

QUESTION 449

A 3-month-old infant is referred for evaluation because of failure to thrive and cardiomegaly. Gestation and delivery were normal. The physical examination shows evidence of congestive heart failure and poor skeletal muscle tone. Chest radiography shows cardiomegaly and mild pulmonary edema. The ECG reveals tall, broad QRS complexes consistent with left ventricular hypertrophy and a PR interval of 0.08 second. An endomyocardial biopsy was obtained and the histopathology is shown in Figure 4-5. The most likely diagnosis is:

A. Endocardial fibroelastosis
B. Coarctation of the aorta
C. Shone syndrome
D. Type II glycogen storage disease (Pompe disease)
E. Friedreich ataxia

QUESTION 450

A 53-year-old woman with ischemic cardiomyopathy presents for percutaneous ablation of ventricular

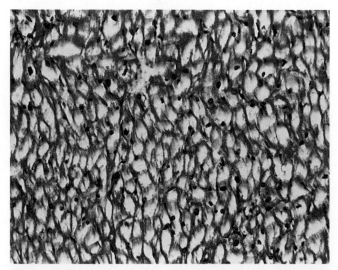

FIGURE 4-5 From Cotran RS, Kumar V, Collins T: Robbins Pathologic Basis of Disease. 6th ed. Philadelphia, WB Saunders, 1999.

tachycardia. She tolerates the procedure well; however, a few hours after the procedure she develops sinus tachycardia and hypotension. An emergent echocardiogram reveals a large circumferential pericardial effusion with findings consistent with tamponade physiology. Each of the following statements about the pathophysiology of cardiac tamponade is correct EXCEPT:

A. Cardiac tamponade occurs when the intrapericardial pressure is equal to the mean right atrial and right ventricular diastolic pressures
B. In the presence of hypovolemia, the rise in intrapericardial and right atrial pressures is less dramatic; thus cardiac tamponade may be more difficult to detect
C. Equalization of intrapericardial and ventricular filling pressures leads to an inspiratory increase in left ventricular stroke volume
D. Sinus bradycardia may occur during severe cardiac tamponade

QUESTION 451

A 57-year-old woman comes to your office because of 6 months of fatigue, weight loss, and periods of tachycardia, flushing and diarrhea. She also describes vague fullness in her neck. Examination discloses clear lungs, an irregular pulse, distended jugular veins with a prominent v wave, a holosystolic murmur at the lower left sternal border that intensifies with inspiration, and peripheral edema. She is afebrile. The likely cause of her illness is:

A. Subacute bacterial endocarditis
B. Carcinoid syndrome
C. Ebstein anomaly
D. Chronic pulmonary emboli
E. Pheochromocytoma

QUESTION 452

A 32-year-old woman with a history of IV drug abuse presents to the emergency department with fatigue and night sweats. Physical examination reveals a temperature of 38.4°C, scattered rhonchi and wheezes in the lung fields, tachycardia without heart murmurs, and needle tracks on her arms. Chest radiograph reveals several small infiltrates in the left lung field. A transthoracic echocardiogram is obtained and an apical four-chamber view showing the right-sided chambers is displayed in Figure 4-6. Each of the following statements about this case is true EXCEPT:

A. The vegetation displayed occupies the most common endocardial site of infection in IV drug abusers
B. The site of involvement displayed is associated with a higher mortality than other endocardial sites
C. The most likely associated organism is *Staphylococcus aureus*
D. Gram-negative bacilli are a prominent cause of such lesions
E. The majority of patients with this presentation are found to have pneumonia or multiple septic emboli on a chest radiograph

QUESTION 453

A 27-year-old man with no significant past medical history is involved in a head-on automobile collision as an unrestrained driver. He sustains blunt chest trauma as a result of impact with the steering wheel. An urgent echocardiogram is performed in the emergency department. Of the following choices, which is the LEAST likely complication of blunt cardiac trauma?
A. Ventricular septal defect
B. Atrial septal defect
C. Cardiac free wall rupture
D. Coronary artery thrombosis
E. Papillary muscle rupture

QUESTION 454

A 54-year-old man with a history of hypertension, heart failure with preserved ejection fraction, and human immunodeficiency virus (HIV) infection presents with worsening shortness of breath. The chest radiograph shows diffuse bilateral infiltrates consistent with *Pneumocystis jiroveci* pneumonia. An echocardiogram is performed to assess left ventricular function, and the study is notable for a small posterior pericardial effusion without cardiac chamber compression. Which one of the following statements regarding pericardial effusion in patients with HIV infection is TRUE?
A. Pericardial effusion is one of the least common cardiac manifestations of HIV infection
B. Progression to a symptomatic effusion and/or cardiac tamponade is likely
C. The presence of a pericardial effusion in HIV patients is a marker for increased mortality
D. Direct HIV infection of the pericardium is almost always the cause of such effusions

E. Most effusions of this type require glucocorticoid therapy for resolution

QUESTION 455

True statements about the clinical findings in patients with atrial septal defect (ASD) include all of the following EXCEPT:
A. A midsystolic ejection murmur and a diastolic rumbling murmur at the lower left sternal border are common features on cardiac examination
B. Patients with ostium primum defects usually show right ventricular hypertrophy, a small rSR′ pattern in the right precordial levels, and rightward axis on the ECG
C. Tall R or R′ waves in V_1 may signal the development of pulmonary hypertension
D. Echocardiographic features of ASD include right ventricular and pulmonary arterial dilatation and paradoxical intraventricular septal motion
E. Radiographic features include cardiomegaly, dilated central pulmonary arteries, and pulmonary plethora

QUESTION 456

A 54-year-old African-American man presents with dyspnea on exertion. He had been routinely exercising four or five times a week, but over the past few months he has noted a decline in exertional capacity. His blood pressure has been consistently <130/85 mm Hg at his physician's office. An apical four-chamber view image from his echocardiogram is shown in Figure 4-7. Which of the following statements regarding this condition is TRUE:
A. This variant represents <10% of hypertrophic cardiomyopathy (HCM) in Japan

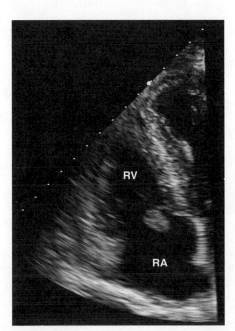

FIGURE 4-6

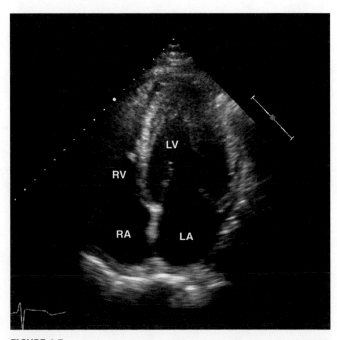

FIGURE 4-7

B. Tall peaked precordial T waves are typically present on the ECG
C. The risk of sudden cardiac death is higher than that of other forms of HCM
D. A subaortic dynamic pressure gradient is typically present
E. Magnetic resonance imaging would show a spade-like deformity of the ventricle

QUESTION 457

A 36-year-old man from the Dominican Republic presents to the emergency department with shortness of breath. A grade III/VI systolic murmur is auscultated at the apex. The chest radiograph demonstrates pulmonary vascular congestion. Echocardiography in the emergency department confirms the presence of mitral regurgitation and vigorous left ventricular contractile function. Each of the following findings would suggest the *acute* onset of mitral regurgitation EXCEPT:
A. Absence of cardiomegaly on the chest radiograph
B. Lack of left atrial or ventricular hypertrophy on the ECG
C. Acute pulmonary edema
D. The systolic murmur extends beyond S_2
E. Jugular venous distention

QUESTION 458

The hemodynamic tracing in Figure 4-8 is most consistent with:
A. Constrictive pericarditis
B. Mitral stenosis
C. Mitral regurgitation
D. Restrictive cardiomyopathy
E. None of the above

QUESTION 459

A 45-year-old woman is evaluated by her physician because of the new onset of pleuritic, positional left anterior chest pain that radiates to the left trapezius ridge. Three weeks earlier she had been evaluated for a viral respiratory tract infection. Cardiac auscultation reveals evanescent coarse scratching sounds at the lower left sternal border with components in both systole and diastole. Each of the following statements about expected electrocardiographic findings are correct EXCEPT:
A. ST-segment elevations likely have a concave upward configuration
B. PR-segment depression may be the only electrocardiographic manifestation
C. Reciprocal ST-segment depressions are typically present
D. Sinus tachycardia is common
E. T wave inversions develop weeks later, after ST-segment elevations have returned to the baseline

QUESTION 460

Which of the following statements regarding post–myocardial infarction (post-MI) pericarditis is TRUE?
A. Thrombolytic therapy increases the incidence of early post-MI pericarditis
B. Post-MI pericarditis is more common after non–ST-segment elevation MI compared with ST-segment elevation MI
C. A pericardial friction rub is not detectable until 24 hours after infarction
D. The use of heparin is associated with an increased risk of pericarditis
E. The incidence of early post-MI pericarditis is related to infarct size

QUESTION 461

The hemodynamic tracing in Figure 4-9 is characteristic of which of the following disorders?
A. Aortic stenosis
B. Mitral regurgitation
C. Dilated cardiomyopathy
D. Hypertrophic cardiomyopathy
E. Infiltrative cardiomyopathy

QUESTION 462

Each of the following statements about congenital valvular aortic stenosis (AS) in children is true EXCEPT:
A. This anomaly occurs more frequently in males than in females
B. Most children with congenital AS grow and develop normally and are asymptomatic
C. In children with hemodynamically significant AS, the electrocardiogram is usually notable for left ventricular hypertrophy
D. Any child with clinical evidence of AS should undergo cardiac catheterization
E. Aortic valvulotomy by balloon dilation is an effective initial treatment

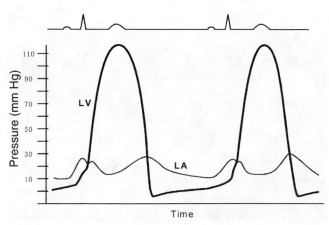

FIGURE 4-8

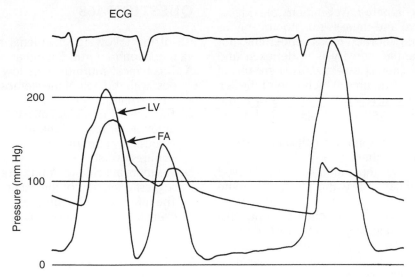

ECG

200

Pressure (mm Hg)

100

0

LV

FA

FIGURE 4-9 ECG, electrocardiogram; LV, left ventricle; FA, femoral artery. From Baim D, Grossman W (eds): Cardiac Catheterization, Angiography and Intervention. Baltimore, Williams & Wilkins, 1996, p 794.

QUESTION 463

True statements about congenital heart disease in infancy and childhood include all of the following EXCEPT:
A. Extracardiac anomalies occur in about 25% of infants with significant congenital heart disease
B. Patent ductus arteriosus is found more commonly in females
C. Approximately one third of infants with both cardiac and extracardiac congenital anomalies have an established syndrome
D. The rubella syndrome may be accompanied by patent ductus arteriosus or pulmonic valvular stenosis
E. Maternal systemic lupus erythematosus is associated with congenital cardiac malformations, including ventricular septal defect and pulmonic stenosis

FIGURE 4-10

QUESTION 464

According to the 2007 update to the American Heart Association guidelines for the prevention of infective endocarditis, antibiotic prophylaxis is appropriate for each of the following cardiac conditions before invasive dental procedures EXCEPT:
A. Presence of a prosthetic cardiac valve
B. Unrepaired cyanotic congenital heart disease
C. Cardiac transplantation recipients with cardiac valvulopathy
D. Mitral valve prolapse with murmur of severe mitral regurgitation
E. Previous episode of infective endocarditis

QUESTION 465

A 50-year-old man with long-standing hypertension and chronic aortic regurgitation presented to his physician with daily fevers for the past 3 weeks and new dyspnea.

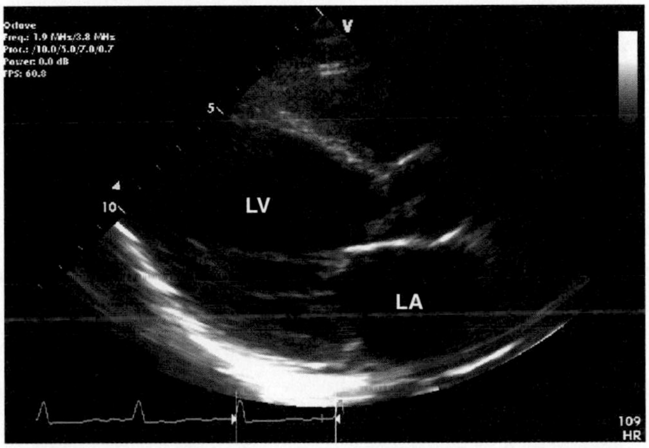

Physical examination revealed basilar crackles in both lung fields, the patient's prior murmur of aortic regurgitation, and bilateral pitting edema of the ankles. The ECG revealed sinus rhythm and unifocal ventricular premature beats. A transthoracic echocardiogram was obtained, and a parasternal long-axis view from that study is shown in Figure 4-10. True statements about this patient include all of the following EXCEPT:
A. The left ventricle is dilated
B. The posterior mitral valve leaflet is prolapsing into the left atrium
C. No pericardial effusion is visualized
D. The left atrium is enlarged
E. A vegetation is present

QUESTION 466

A 45-year-old man presents with fevers, chills, and shortness of breath. His chest radiograph shows pulmonary edema. Echocardiography reveals vigorous left ventricular contractile function. Vegetations are identified on the aortic valve and there is non-homogeneous thickening within the aortic root concerning for abscess formation. Cardiac surgery is undertaken and an aortic valve homograft is selected as a means of replacing the diseased structures. Which one of the following statements is TRUE regarding the use of aortic valve homografts in the surgical management of aortic valve disease?

A. Homografts have high thrombogenicity and require chronic anticoagulation therapy
B. The rate of structural degeneration of cryopreserved homografts is significantly less than that of porcine xenograft valves
C. Homografts are the prostheses of choice for patients in need of urgent cardiac surgery for infective endocarditis of the aortic valve
D. Homografts offer a less favorable hemodynamic profile than mechanical valves
E. The operative mortality of aortic homograft placement is higher than that of mechanical valve replacement surgery

QUESTION 467

True statements concerning the auscultatory findings of the valvular abnormality depicted in Figure 4-11 include all of the following EXCEPT:

A. In patients with leaflets that are still flexible, S_1 is accentuated
B. In patients with heavily calcified leaflets, the intensity of S_1 is diminished
C. As the severity of this condition increases, the A_2-OS interval (the interval between A_2 and the mitral opening sound) shortens
D. The intensity of the diastolic murmur is closely related to the severity of this condition
E. P_2 (the pulmonic valve closure sound) is commonly accentuated

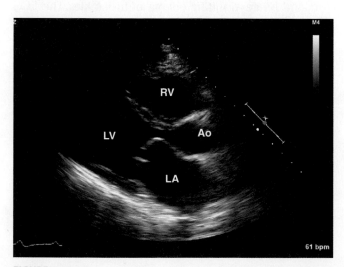

FIGURE 4-11

QUESTION 468

All of the following statements regarding the physical examination in aortic regurgitation are true EXCEPT:

A. The typical murmur is of low frequency and heard best with the bell of the stethoscope placed along the left sternal border
B. The severity of regurgitation correlates better with the duration rather than the intensity of the murmur
C. A musical murmur ("cooing dove" murmur) usually signifies eversion or perforation of a cusp
D. Murmurs auscultated on the right side of the sternum suggest dilatation of the ascending aorta
E. The intensity of the murmur is increased by isometric exercise (e.g., strenuous handgrip)

QUESTION 469

A 75-year-old woman with chronic obstructive pulmonary disease presents with fever, rigors, productive cough, and worsening shortness of breath. She was recently admitted with a left lower lobe infiltrate. On physical exam she is overtly dyspneic, the temperature is 102.1°F, heart rate 120 beats/min, blood pressure 82/50 mm Hg. The chest radiograph shows a dense left lower lobe infiltrate and symmetric enlargement of the cardiac silhouette. Echocardiography demonstrates a large circumferential pericardial effusion. She is admitted to the intensive care unit for suspected bacterial pericarditis. Which of the following statements is TRUE?

A. Uremic pericarditis with a preexisting pericardial effusion predisposes to bacterial pericarditis
B. Direct extension into the pericardium of bacterial pneumonia accounts for only a minority of cases of purulent pericarditis
C. Bacterial pericarditis is most often a subacute illness
D. The modern survival rate of this condition is excellent
E. Antibiotics administered intravenously do not achieve high concentrations in the pericardial space

QUESTION 470

A 16-year-old boy undergoes a physical examination before competing in high school athletics. His mother states that a first cousin died suddenly while playing in a basketball game and she recalls that there was something wrong with his heart. The boy has no symptoms. His vital signs are heart rate 64 beats/min, respirations 12 breaths/min, and blood pressure 120/75 mm Hg. His cardiac examination is remarkable for a grade 2/6 systolic ejection murmur along the left sternal border, which decreases with squatting and increases with sudden standing. An ECG shows left ventricular hypertrophy with prominent septal forces. Your recommendations regarding participation in athletics are:

A. No competitive sports
B. Noncontact competitive sports
C. Noncontact competitive sports with beta-blocker therapy
D. High-intensity competitive sports

E. High-intensity competitive sports with beta-blocker therapy

QUESTION 471

Abnormalities of left ventricular (LV) function and hemodynamics in isolated moderate to severe aortic stenosis include all of the following EXCEPT:
A. Normal cardiac output at rest
B. Elevated LV end-diastolic pressure
C. Elevated LV end-diastolic volume
D. Increased *a* wave in the left atrial pressure curve
E. Normal LV stroke volume

QUESTION 472

A 76-year-old man presents to the emergency department with aphasia and a dense right hemiplegia. His wife reports that he had experienced intermittent fevers and chills over the previous 2 weeks. Cardiac examination is notable for a grade 2/6 systolic ejection murmur at the upper right sternal border and grade 1/4 early diastolic murmur at the same position. Four sets of blood cultures grow *Staphylococcus aureus*. A transthoracic echocardiogram demonstrates normal left ventricular contractile function and mild aortic stenosis. No vegetations are seen. Computed tomography of the head shows an acute nonhemorrhagic stroke in the territory of the left middle cerebral artery. Which of the following statements is TRUE?
A. Endocarditis is not present because valvular vegetations are absent by echocardiography
B. Endocarditis caused by *S aureus* is an absolute indication for surgery
C. In patients with endocarditis, a vegetation >10 mm in diameter represents an immediate indication for surgery
D. The likelihood of subsequent embolic events will decrease with appropriate antibiotic therapy
E. Even if intractable heart failure develops, corrective valve surgery should be postponed until well after blood cultures have become sterile

QUESTION 473

True statements about tuberculous pericarditis include all of the following EXCEPT:
A. Tuberculous pericarditis usually develops by retrograde spread from adjacent lymph nodes or by early hematogenous spread from the primary infection
B. Tuberculous pericardial effusions usually accumulate slowly
C. Measurement of adenosine deaminase in pericardial fluid is a highly sensitive and specific test for the diagnosis of tuberculous pericarditis
D. It is often difficult to isolate the organism from pericardial fluid
E. The addition of corticosteroids to a three-drug antibacterial regimen consistently reduces mortality in patients with tuberculous pericarditis

QUESTION 474

A 42-year-old previously healthy insurance salesman presents to his physician with a complaint of lower extremity edema. On further questioning, he says he has also experienced "flushing" episodes over the past several months, intermittent wheezing, and episodic diarrhea. On physical examination, there is jugular venous distention, a prominent holosystolic murmur at the lower left sternal border, a pulsatile liver, and peripheral edema. The urinary 5-hydroxyindoleacetic acid level is markedly elevated. True statements about this patient's condition include all of the following EXCEPT:
A. The underlying disorder has invaded the liver
B. Echocardiography would demonstrate thickened tricuspid and/or pulmonary valve leaflets with right ventricular dilatation
C. Involvement of the left-sided heart valves is common in this disorder
D. The symptoms are associated with elevated levels of circulating serotonin
E. The primary disease does not invade the myocardium

QUESTION 475

A 65-year-old woman, who is originally from Puerto Rico, presents for evaluation of known mitral stenosis. Over the past few months she has developed worsening exertional dyspnea, atrial fibrillation, and moderate pulmonary hypertension. Which of the following statements regarding percutaneous balloon mitral valvuloplasty for this condition is TRUE?
A. The risk of stroke during the procedure is 10%
B. Transthoracic echocardiography is the appropriate imaging study before the procedure to exclude the presence of left atrial thrombus
C. Balloon mitral valvuloplasty is the treatment of choice for patients with hemodynamically significant mitral stenosis, without left atrial thrombus and an echo score of ≤8
D. A small atrial septal defect can normally be detected in 25% of patients after the procedure
E. Approximately 10% of patients develop severe mitral regurgitation as a result of the procedure

QUESTION 476

A 25-year-old man is an unrestrained driver in a head-on motor vehicle accident. He is brought into the trauma bay where he is unconscious and is noted to have multiple head lacerations, a large contusion on his anterior chest, and abdominal enlargement. Each of the following statements regarding the acute evaluation of a patient with blunt cardiac trauma is true EXCEPT:
A. Chest radiography should be obtained urgently
B. Serum cardiac-specific troponin measurements correlate with the presence and prognosis of blunt myocardial injury
C. Common consequences of blunt cardiac trauma can be readily identified by transesophageal echocardiography

D. Arrhythmias and conduction blocks frequently occur after blunt cardiac trauma

E. Traumatic ventricular septal defect formation is a recognized complication

QUESTION 477

Each of the following statements regarding patients with sarcoid heart disease is true EXCEPT:

A. Fewer than 5% of patients with pulmonary sarcoidosis have clinical manifestations of sarcoid heart disease

B. Granulomatous involvement of the cardiac valves is found in most patients

C. Percutaneous endomyocardial biopsy for the diagnosis has a substantial false-negative rate

D. Conduction disturbances and ventricular arrhythmias are common manifestations

E. Imaging with ^{99m}Tc-sestamibi typically demonstrates segmental myocardial perfusion defects

QUESTION 478

True statements about the natural history of untreated ventricular septal defect (VSD) include all of the following EXCEPT:

A. The natural history of VSD differs depending on the size of the defect and the magnitude of the pulmonary vascular resistance

B. Regardless of size, the presence of a VSD confers an increased risk for endocarditis

C. Progressive pulmonary vascular disease with reversal of shunting (Eisenmenger complex) most often becomes manifest in the fifth or sixth decade

D. Women with VSDs and ratios of pulmonary to systemic flow <2:1 generally tolerate pregnancy well

QUESTION 479

Each of the following statements regarding endomyocardial fibrosis (EMF) is correct EXCEPT:

A. This condition is characteristically found in tropical and subtropical Africa

B. It is predominantly a disease of children and young adults

C. Involvement of the mitral valve apparatus typically results in mitral stenosis

D. EMF involves the left ventricle, alone or in combination with the right ventricle, in 90% of patients

E. Echocardiographic features include increased endocardial reflectivity, fibrotic obliteration of the apex, atrial enlargement, and pericardial effusion

QUESTION 480

Each of the following statements regarding risk factors for sudden cardiac death (SCD) in hypertrophic cardiomyopathy (HCM) is true EXCEPT:

A. The severity of the outflow tract gradient correlates linearly with the risk of SCD

B. A family history of HCM with SCD identifies a high-risk patient

C. Specific mutations have been identified that portend a higher risk of SCD

D. The presence of nonsustained ventricular tachycardia on an ambulatory event monitor is associated with the risk of SCD

E. The diagnosis of HCM before age 30 is a risk factor for SCD

QUESTION 481

An 8-month-old boy is evaluated because of cyanosis that was first noted at 2 months of age, and that worsens with physical activity or crying. A systolic thrill is present at the left sternal border, and there is a loud systolic murmur across the precordium. Echocardiography is diagnostic for tetralogy of Fallot. Each of the following statements about tetralogy of Fallot is correct EXCEPT:

A. Classic tetralogy of Fallot is composed of a large ventricular septal defect (VSD), infundibular or valvular pulmonic stenosis or both, right ventricular (RV) hypertrophy, and an overriding aorta

B. In some cases, the VSD in tetralogy of Fallot communicates with the right ventricle distal to the level of outflow tract obstruction

C. Survival of patients with tetralogy of Fallot into adult life usually reflects mild to moderate obstruction of RV outflow

D. Pseudotruncus arteriosus is a variant of tetralogy of Fallot in which complete ventricular outflow tract obstruction occurs

E. Congestive heart failure is unusual in patients with tetralogy of Fallot

QUESTION 482

A 54-year-old man with a known bicuspid aortic valve presents with a 1-week history of fevers and chills. Initial blood cultures are negative, but echocardiography reveals a large vegetation on the aortic valve. On the fifth hospital day, blood cultures become positive for gram-negative bacteria. All of the following are members of the fastidious, slow-growing group of HACEK organisms that may be the cause of this patient's endocarditis EXCEPT:

A. *Haemophilus parainfluenzae*

B. *Aggregatibacter* (formerly *Actinobacillus*) *actinomycetemcomitans*

C. *Cardiobacterium hominis*

D. *Escherichia coli*

E. *Kingella kingae*

QUESTION 483

Which of the following statements regarding endocardial fibroelastosis (EFE) is TRUE?

A. Symptoms of EFE first manifest in early adolescence
B. Myocardial involvement is characteristic
C. The clinical course is usually benign
D. Hypereosinophilia is typically present
E. There is an association with maternal mumps during pregnancy

QUESTION 484

True statements regarding long-term complications after the Fontan procedure include all of the following EXCEPT:
A. It is a palliative, not curative operation
B. Physical examination typically reveals an elevated, nonpulsatile jugular venous pulse
C. A widely split S_2 is expected
D. Atrial arrhythmias are common
E. Protein-losing enteropathy is a recognized complication

QUESTION 485

A 27-year-old woman presents with 2 days of shortness of breath. The plasma D-dimer level is elevated. A high-resolution chest CT scan reveals a segmental pulmonary embolism, and deep vein thrombosis is found in the right femoral vein. She denies any recent travel, immobility, or surgery. Which of the following primary hypercoagulable states is most frequent among patients who present with deep vein thrombosis?
A. Protein C deficiency
B. Activated protein C resistance
C. Antithrombin deficiency
D. Prothrombin 20210 mutation
E. Protein S deficiency

QUESTION 486

A 48-year-old man comes to the office because of episodic palpitations. His other symptoms include paroxysmal nocturnal dyspnea, nocturnal enuresis, and mild angina. His wife adds that he snores loudly. He has a history of several recent automobile accidents. On examination, his blood pressure is elevated at 190/100 mm Hg and he is moderately overweight. Laboratory evaluation reveals a hematocrit of 58%. The most likely cardiac finding would be:
A. Mitral valve stenosis
B. Aortic valve stenosis
C. Right ventricular hypertrophy
D. Pulmonary valve stenosis
E. Atrial septal defect

QUESTION 487

Each of the following constitutes a major criterion for the diagnosis of infective endocarditis by the modified Duke criteria EXCEPT:

A. Two separate blood cultures positive for *Streptococcus bovis* drawn more than 12 hours apart
B. New partial dehiscence of an aortic bioprosthesis
C. Single blood culture positive for *Coxiella burnetii*
D. Detection of a mycotic aneurysm
E. New mitral regurgitation

QUESTION 488

A 20-year-old woman is brought to the hospital because of extreme fatigue and exertional dyspnea over the past month. Past medical history is unremarkable except for an upper respiratory tract infection 4 weeks earlier. There is no family history of cardiac illness. On examination in the emergency department, the patient's blood pressure is 90/60 mm Hg and the heart rate is 110 beats/min. The jugular veins are distended to 10 cm H_2O, the chest examination reveals bilateral rales, and on cardiac examination there is a prominent apical S_3 gallop. An echocardiogram demonstrates dilatation of both ventricles with diffuse hypokinesia; the left ventricular ejection fraction is 15%. Each of the following statements regarding this patient's disorder is true EXCEPT:
A. The most likely etiology of this patient's disorder is viral
B. Myocardial biopsy will not likely reveal a specific etiology
C. Corticosteroids will slow progression of the illness
D. Acute and convalescent serologic tests are generally unhelpful in management
E. Myocardial biomarker elevation may occur in the absence of coronary artery disease

QUESTION 489

A 28-year-old man is referred for echocardiography after his brother was diagnosed with a cardiac condition that caused recurrent syncope. An M-mode panel of the echocardiogram is shown in the Figure 4-12. Important aspects of this patient's management include all of the following EXCEPT:
A. Endocarditis prophylaxis is not recommended before dental procedures
B. Beta blockers are helpful in reducing symptoms and improving hemodynamics
C. He should refrain from competitive sports
D. Digitalis glycosides are beneficial
E. Diuretics should be avoided or prescribed with great caution

QUESTION 490

True statements about peripheral pulmonary artery stenosis include all of the following EXCEPT:
A. Pulmonary artery stenosis may occur anywhere from the main pulmonary trunk to the smallest peripheral arterial branches

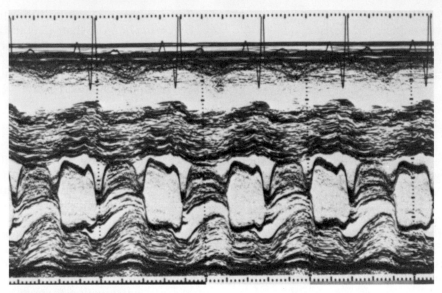

FIGURE 4-12

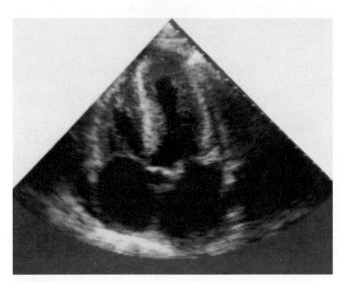

FIGURE 4-13

B. Peripheral pulmonary artery stenosis is most often an isolated finding; only occasionally are other cardiovascular defects present
C. Intrauterine rubella infection is an important cause
D. Most children with peripheral pulmonary artery stenosis are asymptomatic
E. Percutaneous transcatheter balloon angioplasty is an effective treatment for this disorder

QUESTION 491

A 70-year-old man with multiple myeloma presented with new biventricular heart failure. An apical four-chamber view from a transthoracic echocardiographic study is shown in Figure 4-13. All of the following statements about this case are true EXCEPT:
A. Biventricular increased wall thickness and enlarged atria are present
B. The ECG likely demonstrates low lead voltage

C. Cardiac involvement is rare in the primary (AL) form of this disorder
D. The most common clinical presentation of this disorder is restrictive cardiomyopathy
E. Patients with this disorder may present with orthostatic hypotension

QUESTION 492

The M-mode echocardiogram in Figure 4-14 was recorded from an asymptomatic 24-year-old woman. Valvular regurgitation is absent by Doppler interrogation. Which of the following statements is TRUE?
A. The patient should undergo repeat echocardiography every 6 months to follow this disorder
B. She should receive antibiotic prophylaxis to prevent infective endocarditis prior to invasive dental procedures
C. She is at increased risk of sudden cardiac death
D. She is at increased risk of thromboembolism and requires chronic oral anticoagulation therapy
E. Advanced age and male gender are risk factors for progression of this disorder and the need for surgical intervention

QUESTION 493

A 75-year-old woman presented to her physician with severe fatigue and intermittent cyanosis. Initial evaluation revealed that cyanosis had been present for approximately 1 year and occurred chiefly during mild to moderate exertion. Transthoracic echocardiography (TTE) yielded images that were suboptimal; therefore, transesophageal echocardiography (TEE) was peformed. Part A in Figure 4-15 shows a basal image from the TEE, and part B shows an image obtained after injection of agitated saline into the right antecubital vein. True statements about this patient and the echocardiographic images displayed include all of the following EXCEPT:

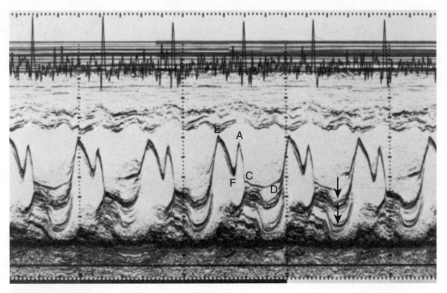

FIGURE 4-14

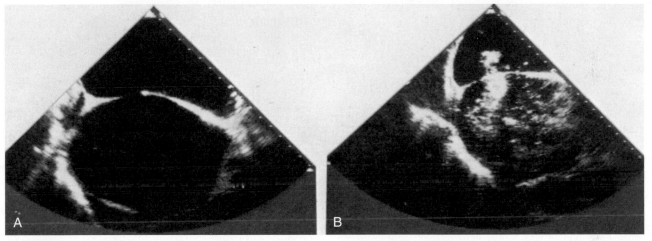

FIGURE 4-15

A. The saline contrast image demonstrates right-to-left interatrial flow
B. The images verify a secundum-type atrial septal defect
C. An anomalous pulmonary vein is demonstrated
D. In TTE, the subcostal position is most useful for studying the lesion displayed
E. When left atrial pressure exceeds right atrial pressure in this condition, echocardiography with IV saline contrast injection may demonstrate a negative contrast effect within the right atrium

QUESTION 494

A 29-year-old man is referred by his family practitioner for evaluation of a heart murmur that was first heard during childhood. He is asymptomatic. Part of his evaluation included an echocardiogram. An M-mode panel from that study is displayed in Figure 4-16. True statements about this case include all of the following EXCEPT:

A. A vegetation is present on the anterior leaflet of the mitral valve

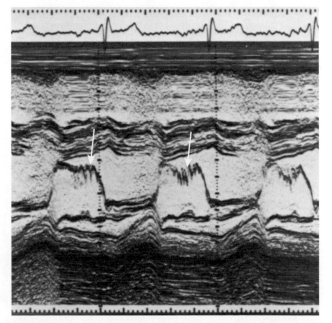

FIGURE 4-16

B. The aortic valve in this disorder may be bicuspid

C. Infective endocarditis of the aortic valve may lead to the lesion present in this case

D. This disorder can be associated with ankylosing spondylitis

E. The M-mode finding may be present even in mild forms of this condition

QUESTION 495

A 34-year-old woman presents with dyspnea and is found to be in atrial fibrillation. Following conversion to normal sinus rhythm, an echocardiographic study is obtained. Figure 4-17 displays a continuous-wave Doppler recording through the mitral valve. True statements about this condition include all of the following EXCEPT:

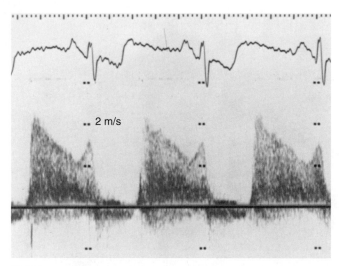

2 m/s

FIGURE 4-17

A. Two-dimensional echocardiography would demonstrate thickening of the valve leaflets and chordal apparatus

B. The peak velocity of transmitral flow in this case is decreased

C. In early diastole, the posterior leaflet of the mitral valve commonly moves in an anterior direction in patients with this condition

D. Mitral orifice size can be accurately determined by Doppler pressure half-time measurement

E. Elevation of the pulmonary artery systolic pressure, as estimated by the tricuspid regurgitant jet, would likely be present in this patient

QUESTION 496

A 34-year-old man with known human immunodeficiency virus (HIV) infection presented with the recent onset of fever and dyspnea. Physical examination revealed fever, tachycardia, jugular venous distention, a pericardial friction rub, and hepatomegaly. The chest radiograph shown in part A of Figure 4-18 was obtained. A diagnosis was ascertained by obtaining pericardial fluid and a pericardial biopsy specimen. The pericardial fluid was notable for an elevated level of adenosine deaminase. The chest radiograph in part B was obtained 3 weeks after the initiation of appropriate therapy. True statements about this case include all of the following EXCEPT:

A. In industrialized nations, the incidence of this disorder has decreased markedly in recent decades

B. This condition is the most common cause of pericardial disease in African HIV-infected patients

C. Clinical detection of this disorder usually occurs either in the effusive stage or after the development of constrictive pericarditis

D. The acute onset of characteristic severe pericardial pain is common

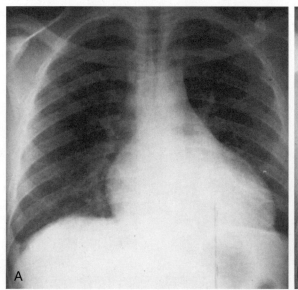

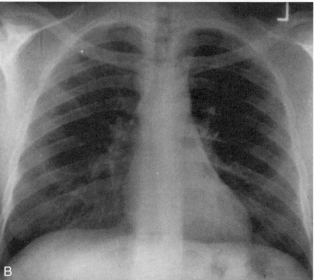

FIGURE 4-18 From Jay M: Plain Film in Heart Disease. Boston, Blackwell Scientific Publishing, 1992.

E. This disorder is most likely to be diagnosed if both pericardial fluid and a pericardial biopsy specimen are obtained

QUESTION 497

Each of the following statements about ostium primum atrial septal defects (ASDs) is true EXCEPT:

A. Ostium primum ASDs often displace and cause a "cleft" appearance of both the anterior and posterior leaflets of the mitral valve
B. The clinical features of ostium primum ASDs are similar to those of the ostium secundum type
C. Imaging usually reveals both right atrial and right ventricular enlargement
D. The presence of an ostium primum ASD accompanied by a ventricular septal defect comprises a complete atrioventricular canal malformation
E. Left ventriculography may demonstrate a "gooseneck" deformity

QUESTION 498

Surgical reconstruction (in distinction to replacement) of the mitral valve is likely to be successful in each of the following patients EXCEPT:

A. A 33-year-old man with mitral valve prolapse
B. A 62-year-old man with severe mitral regurgitation due to annular dilatation after myocardial infarction
C. A 40-year-old woman with mitral regurgitation due to ruptured chordae tendineae with active infective endocarditis
D. A 70-year-old woman with rheumatic heart disease, calcified mitral valve with deformed leaflets, and combined mitral stenosis and regurgitation
E. A 23-year-old man with a congenitally cleft mitral valve

QUESTION 499

A 53-year-old man with chronic mitral regurgitation underwent echocardiographic examination, which demonstrated a mildly enlarged left ventricular (LV) diastolic chamber size, a normal end-systolic dimension (38 mm), and an LV ejection fraction of 60%. He is asymptomatic and has not experienced unusual dyspnea on exertion, orthopnea, or lower extremity edema. For this patient, each of the following statements is correct regarding the timing of mitral valve surgery EXCEPT:

A. Surgical correction is not mandatory at present
B. The risk of postoperative heart failure is heightened when the preoperative ejection fraction falls below 60%
C. His postoperative prognosis will be worse if he undergoes valve surgery after the LV end-systolic diameter has enlarged to >45 mm
D. Chronic administration of an angiotensin-converting enzyme inhibitor would delay the need for surgery
E. Signs of pulmonary hypertension should prompt corrective mitral valve surgery

QUESTION 500

A 23-year-old women delivers a baby boy at 36 weeks' gestation. Soon after delivery the neonate is noted to be cyanotic with a physical exam notable for a right ventricular impulse and a systolic thrill along the left sternal border. An echocardiogram reveals obstruction to right ventricular outflow, an outlet ventricular septal defect, overriding of the aorta, and right ventricular hypertrophy. With regard to the management of this condition, each of the following statements is correct EXCEPT:

A. Early definitive repair is indicated
B. Postoperative increases in pulmonary venous return often leads to right ventricular decompensation
C. The size of the pulmonary arteries is the single most important determinant in assessing candidacy for primary repair
D. If early corrective operation is not possible, a palliative procedure that leads to increased pulmonary blood flow is usually recommended
E. Bleeding complications are common in the postoperative period after repair

QUESTION 501

A 62-year-old man presents with the acute onset of shortness of breath 2 weeks after prostate surgery. A high-resolution contrast chest computed tomographic (CT) scan is shown in Figure 4-19. Which of the following statements is correct?

A. Echocardiography is useful for further risk stratification of this patient
B. Pulmonary angiography is required to make a definitive diagnosis

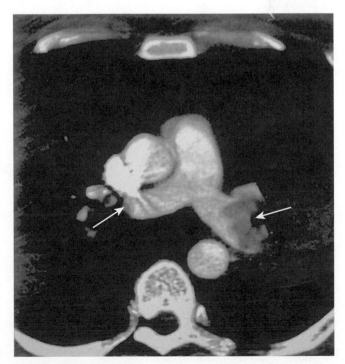

FIGURE 4-19

C. Pulmonary radionuclide perfusion scintigraphy is the best imaging test to establish the diagnosis of this disorder

D. New-generation multidetector CT scanners are more expensive but offer no superior imaging of subsegmental pulmonary arteries compared with earlier-generation machines

E. The majority of patients with this disorder have evidence of deep vein thrombosis in the systemic venous system

QUESTION 502

Each of the following conditions is associated with elevated right ventricular diastolic pressures with the pattern shown in Figure 4-20 EXCEPT:

A. Cardiac tamponade

B. Acute right ventricular infarction

C. Massive pulmonary embolism

D. Constrictive pericarditis

E. Restrictive cardiomyopathy

QUESTION 503

A 54-year-old man presented with increasing dyspnea on exertion. He was initially treated for an upper respiratory tract infection; however, his symptoms persisted. A subsequent echocardiogram revealed an intracardiac mass suggestive of a malignant tumor. Regarding primary malignancies of the heart, which of the following statements is TRUE?

A. The left ventricle is the most common site of involvement

B. Most patients already have metastases at the time of diagnosis

C. Malignant tumors account for half of primary cardiac tumors

D. Lymphomas are the most common primary malignancies of the heart

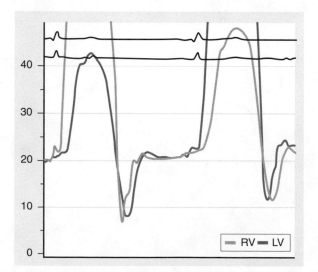

FIGURE 4-20 From Vaitkus PT, Cooper KA, Shuman WP, Hardin NJ: Images in cardiovascular medicine. Circulation 93:834, 1996.

E. Tumors confined to the myocardial wall may be asymptomatic

QUESTION 504

A 63-year-old man presented with a 4-month history of dyspnea on exertion and lower extremity edema. Echocardiography revealed a normal LV ejection fraction with no significant valvular disease. A chest CT showed a dense rim of calcium around the heart. Coronary angiography showed no significant coronary disease. Hemodynamic evaluation demonstrated elevation and equalization of right and left ventricular diastolic pressures with a "dip and plateau" configuration. Each of the following statements about the management of this condition is correct EXCEPT:

A. The therapy of choice is complete resection of the pericardium

B. Pericardiectomy should be performed early in the course of disease in symptomatic patients

C. Nearly all patients develop a low-output syndrome immediately after pericardiectomy

D. Symptomatic improvement is reported in approximately 80% of surgical survivors

E. The operative mortality of pericardiectomy is 5% to 15%

QUESTION 505

A 25-year-old woman presents to her primary care doctor with fatigue and a rash. She recently returned from a New England vacation during which she hiked at least 6 miles daily. On physical examination she has a well-demarcated erythematous rash with central clearing on her chest. A Lyme titer is positive. Which of the following statements regarding cardiac involvement in Lyme disease is TRUE?

A. Cardiac manifestations of Lyme disease typically occur within days of the development of erythema chronicum migrans

B. Ten percent of patients with Lyme disease develop cardiac manifestations

C. Supraventricular and ventricular tachyarrhythmias are the most common cardiac manifestations of Lyme disease

D. Cardiomegaly and congestive heart failure are common among patients who develop Lyme carditis

E. Antibiotic therapy shortens the course of active Lyme carditis

QUESTION 506

Which of the following statements regarding idiopathic pulmonary arterial hypertension is TRUE?

A. The prevalence is equal in males and females

B. Chest pain related to right ventricular ischemia is the most common manifesting symptom

C. Sudden cardiac death is a potential complication, but only in patients with Class IV symptoms

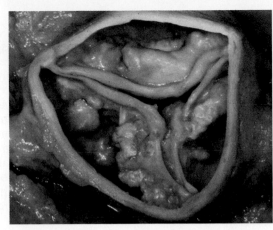

FIGURE 4-21 From Salem DN, Isner JM: Chest 92:326, 1987.

A. The left ventricular (LV) cavity is typically enlarged
B. The mitral valve area can be accurately determined by direct planimetry or by Doppler measurements
C. A flattened E-F slope on M-mode tracings is characteristic of MS
D. Diastolic "doming" of the mitral valve leaflets on two-dimensional echocardiography suggests true stenosis of the mitral valve rather than decreased motion of the valve associated with a low-output state
E. Using Doppler measurements of transmitral LV inflow, the time interval between the peak diastolic pressure and one half of its initial value (the pressure half-time) is directly related to the severity of MS

D. Increased intensity of S_1 is the most common physical finding
E. Electrocardiographic evidence of right ventricular hypertrophy is present in a small minority of patients

QUESTION 507

Which of the following statements is TRUE about the heart valve abnormality shown in Figure 4-21?
A. The abnormality is most likely congenital
B. Cardiac auscultation is almost certainly normal
C. Endocarditis frequently leads to this abnormality
D. Diabetes mellitus and hypercholesterolemia are risk factors for its development
E. A loud diastolic blowing murmur is likely

QUESTION 508

Each of the following statements about hemodynamic findings in constrictive pericarditis and restrictive cardiomyopathy is correct EXCEPT:
A. A diastolic "dip-and-plateau" pattern is seen on the right ventricular (RV) waveform in both conditions
B. Discordance of left ventricular (LV) and RV systolic pressures during respiration is suggestive of constrictive pericarditis
C. In constrictive pericarditis, an intravenous fluid challenge typically separates the LV diastolic pressure tracing from that of the right ventricle
D. RV systolic pressure >50 mm Hg is more consistent with restrictive cardiomyopathy than with constrictive pericarditis
E. In restrictive cardiomyopathy, the ratio of RV systolic pressure to RV end-diastolic pressure is usually >3

QUESTION 509

Each of the following statements regarding the echocardiographic features of mitral stenosis (MS) is correct EXCEPT:

QUESTION 510

A 54-year-old man presents to his physician with a 1-week history of dyspnea on exertion, cough, and pleuritic chest pain. His examination is notable for an elevated jugular venous pressure, distant heart sounds, and mild bilateral lower extremity edema. The chest radiograph reveals an enlarged cardiac silhouette. Echocardiography demonstrates a large circumferential pericardial effusion. An echocardiographic-guided pericardiocentesis is performed, removing most of the fluid; cytologic evaluation reveals adenocarcinoma. Each of the following statements is correct EXCEPT:
A. The most likely primary malignancy in this patient is in the lung
B. The prognosis is poor despite aggressive surgery or chemotherapy
C. Pericardial sclerotherapy would not significantly improve the long-term prognosis
D. Total surgical pericardiectomy should be performed urgently
E. Echocardiography should be repeated within 72 hours

QUESTION 511

A 34-year-old man presents to the emergency department with pleuritic chest pain after a recent upper respiratory tract infection. The pain is positional, relieved by sitting up. The ECG demonstrates diffuse ST-segment elevations. Each of the following statements about the evolution of the ECG in acute pericarditis is correct EXCEPT:
A. Four sequential stages of abnormalities of the ST segments and T waves are typical
B. Initial ST-segment elevation is usually most prominent in lead aVR
C. The ratio of the height of ST-segment elevation to the height of the T wave in acute pericarditis is typically >0.25 in lead V_6
D. In acute pericarditis, the ST segment usually returns to baseline before the appearance of T wave inversion
E. T wave inversion may persist for months after the acute presentation

QUESTION 512

Which of the following statements regarding the natural history of untreated aortic stenosis (AS) is TRUE?
A. Average survival from the onset of syncopal symptoms is approximately 6 months
B. Average survival from the onset of congestive heart failure is approximately 2 years
C. Syncope due to AS usually occurs at rest
D. Sudden death in patients with AS usually occurs in previously asymptomatic individuals
E. Development of atrial fibrillation is usually well tolerated in patients with AS

QUESTION 513

Sudden cardiac death due to ventricular tachyarrhythmias is a complication of each of the following EXCEPT:
A. Sarcoidosis
B. Giant cell myocarditis
C. Chagas disease
D. Idiopathic dilated cardiomyopathy
E. Hyperthyroidism

QUESTION 514

A 45-year-old man is transported to the emergency department, a victim of a stab wound to the chest that occurred during a robbery attempt at his convenience store. Which of the following statements about penetrating cardiac trauma is correct?
A. The left ventricle is the cardiac chamber most commonly injured by penetrating trauma
B. Penetrating injuries to the atria are associated with better survival than wounds to the ventricles
C. Rupture of the interventricular septum is a potential late complication
D. In penetrating cardiac injury with suspected tamponade, urgent pericardiocentesis is a mandatory intervention

QUESTION 515

Each of the following statements regarding persistent patent ductus arteriosus (PDA) in adults is correct EXCEPT:
A. Patients with small shunts and no audible murmur are at negligible risk of endovascular infection
B. Patients with a moderate-sized PDA typically present with dyspnea or palpitations
C. Patients with a moderate-sized PDA typically have a loud continuous "machinery" murmur and a narrow pulse pressure
D. Patients with a large PDA may develop enlarged central pulmonary arteries with peripheral pruning on chest radiograph
E. Transcatheter devices result in successful closure rates of >95%

QUESTION 516

A 46-year-old man is admitted to the hospital because of worsening shortness of breath. His history is notable for hypertension, treated with an angiotensin-converting enzyme inhibitor. Social history reveals that he has consumed one-half pint of liquor daily for the past 10 years. Physical examination reveals an elevated jugular venous pressure (14 cm), bibasilar rales on pulmonary examination, a laterally displaced cardiac apical impulse, a grade II/VI holosystolic murmur and an S_3 gallop at the apex, and pitting edema of both lower extremities. Echocardiography demonstrates a dilated left ventricle with an ejection fraction of 25% and moderate mitral regurgitation. Each of the following statements regarding the cardiac effects of alcohol is true EXCEPT:
A. Alcohol abuse is the leading cause of nonischemic dilated cardiomyopathy in industrialized countries
B. The likelihood of developing dilated cardiomyopathy correlates with the amount of alcohol consumed over a lifetime
C. Women are less susceptible than men to alcohol-associated cardiomyopathy
D. In the absence of known coronary artery disease, moderate alcohol consumption is associated with a reduction in sudden death
E. Dilated cardiomyopathy due to alcohol is reversible

QUESTION 517

Common clinical manifestations of amyloidosis of the cardiovascular system include all of the following EXCEPT:
A. Pericardial constriction
B. Right-sided heart failure
C. Orthostatic hypotension
D. Systolic dysfunction
E. Restrictive cardiomyopathy

QUESTION 518

Which of the following statements regarding endocarditis caused by *Staphylococcus aureus* is correct?
A. Central nervous system complications are rare, occurring in fewer than 5% of patients
B. *Staphylococcus aureus* native valve endocarditis is an absolute indication for surgical debridement
C. The prognosis of right-sided *S. aureus* native valve endocarditis is similar to that of left-sided involvement
D. Empirical initial therapy with oxacillin or cefazolin is appropriate for suspected *S. aureus* endocarditis
E. Prosthetic valve endocarditis with *S. aureus* is associated with a high mortality rate in patients treated medically

QUESTION 519

Each of the following is associated with Ebstein anomaly of the tricuspid valve EXCEPT:

A. Atrial septal defect
B. Paradoxical splitting of S_2
C. Ventricular preexcitation
D. A widely split S_1
E. Atrial flutter

QUESTION 520

A 42-year-old man presents with Löffler endocarditis. Expected findings include all of the following EXCEPT:
A. Eosinophilia
B. Signs and symptoms of heart failure
C. Asthma and nasal polyposis
D. Right ventricular pressure tracing showing a "dip-and-plateau" pattern
E. Normal left ventricular ejection fraction

QUESTION 521

Each of the following statements concerning cyanosis and cyanotic heart disease are correct EXCEPT:
A. Bleeding tendencies occur in patients with cyanotic heart disease and erythrocytosis
B. Peripheral cyanosis is due to increased oxygen extraction from normally saturated arterial blood
C. Cyanosis often worsens with physical exertion
D. Differential cyanosis results when aortic coarctation is accompanied by a left-to-right shunt
E. In cyanotic heart disease, cyanosis is sometimes improved by the squatting posture

QUESTION 522

A 55-year-old woman seeks medical attention because of progressive exertional dyspnea and rapid heart action. At age 12 she suffered from rheumatic fever, and a heart murmur has been subsequently noted. She has had intermittent episodes of atrial fibrillation over the past 2 years with good rate control on metoprolol succinate. Her vital signs include a heart rate of 80 beats/min, blood pressure 130/80 mm Hg, and respirations 16/min. She has inspiratory rales at the lung bases. Her cardiac impulse is displaced laterally. There is a loud S_1, a single S_2, an apical opening snap, a holodiastolic rumbling murmur at the apex, and a soft diastolic blowing murmur along the left sternal border. Isometric handgrip augments the diastolic murmurs. She has mild peripheral edema. Her ECG is illustrated in Figure 4-22. The most likely valve lesions are:
A. Mitral regurgitation and tricuspid stenosis
B. Mitral stenosis and mitral regurgitation
C. Mitral stenosis and aortic regurgitation
D. Mitral stenosis and pulmonic regurgitation
E. Tricuspid stenosis and pulmonic regurgitation

QUESTION 523

Each of the following statements regarding the medical management of mitral stenosis (MS) is correct EXCEPT:
A. According to the 2007 American Heart Association guidelines, antibiotic prophylaxis is not recommended for patients with MS undergoing dental surgery
B. Diuretic therapy is an appropriate measure for relieving symptoms of dyspnea
C. In pure MS with normal left ventricular function, digoxin is useful only if atrial fibrillation is present
D. The benefits of beta blocker therapy in MS include heart rate reduction and improved exercise tolerance
E. Anticoagulation has been shown to prevent thromboembolism in patients with MS regardless of the

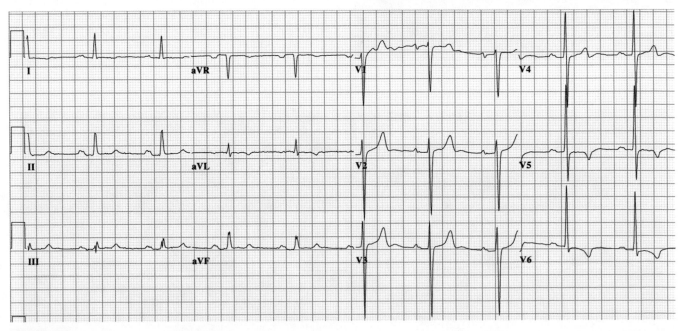

FIGURE 4-22

heart rhythm or history of previous thromboembolic events

QUESTION 524

Each of the following statements regarding the infectious causes of pericarditis is correct EXCEPT:
A. Enteroviruses are among the most common causes of viral pericarditis
B. The most common organisms that cause bacterial pericarditis are streptococci and staphylococci
C. The prognosis of patients with bacterial pericarditis is poor even with appropriate antibiotic therapy
D. Tuberculosis is the leading cause of constrictive pericarditis in Western nations
E. Antifungal therapy is generally not necessary in pericarditis caused by histoplasmosis

QUESTION 525

A 25-year-old graduate student presents to your office for physical examination. Several years ago, while growing

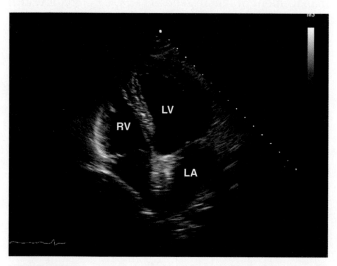

FIGURE 4-23

up in Ecuador, he was diagnosed with Chagas disease when he had presented with fever, malaise, myalgias and unilateral eyelid edema. Each of the following statements regarding Chagas disease is correct EXCEPT:
A. The level of parasitemia does not correspond to the severity of chronic Chagas disease
B. The disease is transmitted to humans by the reduviid bug
C. An asymptomatic phase typically lasts for many years between initial infection and chronic manifestations of the disease
D. The most common ECG abnormality in chronic Chagas disease is left bundle branch block
E. The classic echocardiographic findings are those of a dilated cardiomyopathy with an apical aneurysm

QUESTION 526

A 29-year-old woman was diagnosed with a congenital heart defect 6 years ago. At a routine office visit she describes occasional single palpitations during periods of emotional stress. An echocardiogram is obtained; the apical four-chamber view is shown in Figure 4-23. Which of the following is demonstrated?
A. Bilateral atrial myxomas
B. Lipomatous hypertrophy of the interatrial septum
C. Normal position of an atrial septal closure device
D. Infiltrative disease, most likely amyloidosis
E. Normal echocardiogram

QUESTION 527

A 42-year-old woman, originally from Thailand, presents for evaluation because of exertional dyspnea. As part of her evaluation an echocardiographic study is performed; a parasternal long-axis view and a Doppler recording from the apical long-axis view are displayed in Figure 4-24. Which of the following statements is TRUE?
A. This abnormality results from myxomatous valvular degeneration
B. The Doppler profile in part B in the figure is essentially normal

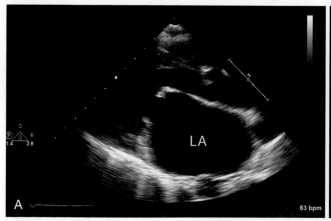
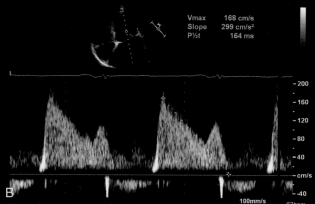

FIGURE 4-24

C. The severity of this abnormality correlates with the likelihood of developing endocarditis
D. The risk of systemic embolism related to this condition correlates with age
E. Chest pain accompanies this condition in the majority of patients

QUESTION 528

A premature infant is found to have bounding peripheral pulses, a continuous murmur in the infraclavicular and interscapular regions, and precordial hyperactivity. An echocardiogram demonstrates a left-to-right shunt between the proximal descending aorta and the pulmonary artery. Which of the following statements about this condition is TRUE?
A. Most preterm infants with a birth weight <1500 g have this condition
B. Cardiopulmonary deterioration occurs in nearly all such infants
C. Chest radiography likely shows a decreased size of the cardiac silhouette
D. Surgical ligation is the only effective treatment
E. Noninvasive imaging typically shows right ventricular enlargement with normal left ventricular size

QUESTION 529

A 17-year-old boy has a syncopal event while playing soccer. He is noted to have a systolic ejection murmur on examination. An echocardiogram is obtained and a parasternal long-axis view is shown in Figure 4-25. Correct statements regarding hemodynamic findings in patients with this condition include each of the following EXCEPT:
A. Systolic function is usually impaired to a greater extent than diastolic function
B. The majority of ventricular emptying is more rapid than usual
C. Left ventricular end-diastolic pressure is usually increased
D. Left ventricular ejection fraction is usually normal

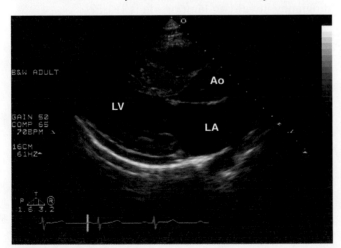

FIGURE 4-25

E. The associated murmur may vary in intensity from one day to another

QUESTION 530

A 46-year-old man is admitted with fever, dyspnea, hypotension and a new murmur of aortic regurgitation. Which of the following is typical of acute aortic regurgitation?
A. A widened systemic pulse pressure
B. A long, decrescendo diastolic murmur
C. Delayed closure of the mitral valve on echocardiography
D. Diastolic mitral regurgitation on echocardiography
E. An enlarged left ventricle

QUESTION 531

True statements concerning tetralogy of Fallot include each of the following EXCEPT:
A. Tetralogy of Fallot accounts for approximately 10% of all forms of congenital heart disease
B. It is one of the most common causes of cardiac cyanosis in children after 1 year of age
C. Anomalous coronary circulation is present in approximately 5% of patients with tetralogy of Fallot
D. The degree of right-to-left shunting in tetralogy of Fallot depends on the severity of pulmonary obstruction
E. The aortic root in this disorder is located to the left of the origin of the pulmonary artery

QUESTION 532

A 68-year-old man presents for evaluation of progressive dyspnea. He has an extensive smoking history. Pulmonary function testing is consistent with severe airway obstruction. An echocardiogram shows normal left ventricular systolic function, right ventricular hypertrophy and dilation, and an elevated calculated pulmonary artery systolic pressure. Which of the following therapies improves survival in patients with chronic obstructive lung disease with pulmonary hypertension?
A. Digoxin
B. Oxygen
C. Beta-adrenergic agonists
D. Theophylline
E. Hydralazine

QUESTION 533

True statements regarding coarctation of the aorta include each of the following EXCEPT:
A. It is more common in males than females
B. Most infants and children with coarctation are symptomatic
C. It is associated with a bicuspid aortic valve in the majority of cases identified in the adult
D. Mean survival time in the presence of uncorrected coarctation is 35 years

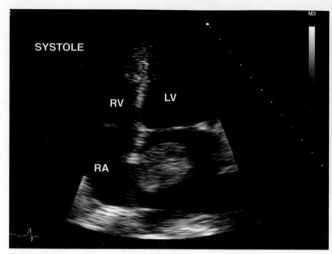
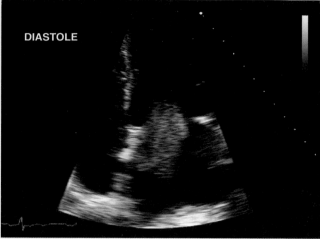

FIGURE 4-26

E. Recoarctation and aneurysm formation at the site of repair are common complications after corrective surgery

QUESTION 534

A 30-year-old woman presented to the hospital after a recent transient neurologic event consistent with a small cerebral embolism. During her evaluation, a transthoracic echocardiogram was performed. An apical four-chamber view from the study is displayed in Figure 4-26, with panels from both systole and diastole. Which of the following statements is TRUE?
A. The echocardiographic appearance is most consistent with intracardiac thrombus formation
B. Systemic symptoms associated with this condition include fever, malaise and an elevated erythrocyte sedimentation rate
C. Surgery is indicated only if there is hemodynamic compromise
D. The majority of such lesions are familial
E. Unlike this patient, this condition most commonly arises in the right atrium

QUESTION 535

A 24-year-old previously healthy woman presents to the emergency department because of sudden shortness of breath and right-sided pleuritic chest pain. She has been using oral contraceptives for several years. Physical examination demonstrates a tachypneic, normotensive, and tachycardic woman. Which of the following results would be most useful in EXCLUDING the diagnosis of pulmonary embolism?
A. Normal PaO_2 by arterial blood gas determination
B. Normal cardiopulmonary examination
C. Intermediate probability $\dot{V}/\dot{Q}$ (ventilation/perfusion) lung scan
D. Normal plasma level of D-dimer
E. Absence of right-sided heart strain on ECG

QUESTION 536

True statements regarding primary tumors of the heart include each of the following EXCEPT:
A. Benign tumors are more common than malignant tumors
B. The most common malignant cardiac tumors are angiosarcomas and rhabdomyosarcomas
C. The presence of a hemorrhagic pericardial effusion is more consistent with a malignant tumor
D. Malignant tumors are more likely to occur on the left side of the heart
E. Precordial pain occurs more commonly with malignant tumors compared with benign ones

QUESTION 537

A 67-year-old man with adenocarcinoma of the lung presents with dyspnea and weakness. Physical examination is notable for hypotension with pulsus paradoxus and jugular venous distention. An echocardiogram is ordered. Which of the following statements regarding echocardiography in cardiac tamponade is TRUE?
A. On inspiration, there is augmentation of transmitral flow velocities and reduction in transtricuspid flow velocities
B. The absence of right ventricular diastolic collapse ensures that the pericardial pressure is not elevated
C. Right ventricular diastolic collapse is more specific than right atrial collapse in the diagnosis of tamponade
D. Cardiac tamponade is associated with normal inferior vena caval collapse with inspiration
E. A small volume pericardial effusion observed on echocardiography excludes the presence of tamponade

QUESTION 538

A 64-year-old woman with a remote history of chest irradiation presents with gradually progressive symptoms of

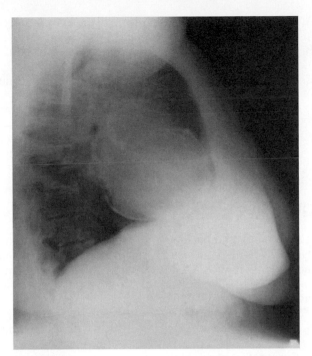

FIGURE 4-27

fatigue, abdominal bloating, and lower extremity edema over the past 4 months. Her lateral chest radiograph is shown in Figure 4-27. Which of the following findings would be inconsistent with the likely diagnosis?

A. Kussmaul sign
B. Hepatomegaly
C. Early diastolic pericardial knock
D. Right and left ventricular systolic pressure concordance during inspiration
E. Elevation and equalization of intracardiac diastolic pressures

QUESTION 539

Which of the following statements regarding the causes of aortic stenosis (AS) is TRUE?

A. A congenitally bicuspid valve accounts for 20% of patients requiring surgical treatment for AS in the United States
B. In patients >age 70, rheumatic deformity is the most common cause of AS that leads to surgical valve replacement
C. There are no established risk factors for the development of calcific AS of a trileaflet valve other than age
D. Age-related calcification of a congenitally bicuspid, or normal trileaflet valve, is the most common cause of AS in adults in the United States
E. Rheumatic deformity of the aortic valve, without mitral valve involvement, occurs commonly in adults

QUESTION 540

An 68-year-old man with chronic aortic regurgitation presents for routine office follow up. He describes reduced stamina, progressive symptoms of exertional dyspnea, and occasional orthopnea. His echocardiogram shows severe aortic regurgitation, a left ventricular (LV) end-systolic diameter of 48 mm, and an LV ejection fraction of 45%. Each of the following statements regarding valve replacement for chronic aortic regurgitation (AR) is true EXCEPT:

A. Asymptomatic patients with advanced AR who have normal LV function and end-systolic diameter <50 mm have an excellent prognosis such that surgery can be safely postponed
B. A left ventricular (LV) end-systolic diameter >55 mm before surgical intervention portends a worse postoperative prognosis than does a smaller ventricular diameter
C. Angiotensin-converting enzyme inhibitors delay the need for aortic valve replacement in chronic AR
D. Patients with chronic AR who have symptoms of congestive heart failure accompanied by reduced LV ejection fraction should be referred for aortic valve replacement
E. A preoperative ejection fraction <50% increases the risk of postoperative death from LV dysfunction

QUESTION 541

A 44-year-old man, recently diagnosed with human immunodeficiency virus (HIV) infection, presents to your office for evaluation of shortness of breath. He reports 2 months of progressive fatigue and dyspnea on exertion. His CD4 count is 500 cells/mm³ (normal = 500 to 1500 cells/mm³), and he remains on highly active antiretroviral therapy. Transthoracic echocardiography reveals a dilated heart with a left ventricular (LV) ejection fraction of 15% and a small pericardial effusion. Which of the following statements is TRUE?

A. Fifty percent of HIV-infected individuals will ultimately develop symptomatic LV dysfunction
B. Pericardial tamponade is the most common cardiac manifestation of HIV infection
C. In HIV-infected individuals, LV dysfunction has little bearing on 1-year mortality rates
D. Accelerated coronary artery disease is uncommon in HIV-infected individuals
E. Protease inhibitor therapy is associated with an increased risk of myocardial infarction

QUESTION 542

True statements regarding the cardiovascular consequences of Turner syndrome include all of the following EXCEPT:

A. Cardiovascular defects are seen in fewer than 5% of patients
B. Coarctation of the aorta is the most commonly associated congenital cardiovascular abnormality
C. There is an increased risk of aortic dissection
D. Bicuspid aortic valve occurs at a higher frequency than in the general population
E. Partial anomalous venous drainage occurs more frequently than in the general population

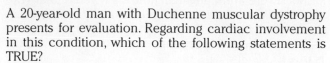

QUESTION 543

A 20-year-old man with Duchenne muscular dystrophy presents for evaluation. Regarding cardiac involvement in this condition, which of the following statements is TRUE?

A. Fewer than 25% of patients with Duchenne muscular dystrophy >age 18 develop a dilated cardiomyopathy

B. The ECG typically shows tall R waves and increased R/S amplitude in V_1 and deep narrow Q waves in the left precordial leads

C. There is a direct association between the presence of dilated cardiomyopathy and electrocardiographic abnormalities

D. Early cardiac involvement typically manifests as global left ventricular dysfunction

E. The most common rhythm disturbance is ventricular tachycardia

QUESTION 544

A 34-year-old man is receiving doxorubicin chemotherapy for lymphoma. Each of the following statements is true regarding the risk of doxorubicin-induced cardiotoxicity EXCEPT:

A. Previous or concurrent mediastinal irradiation increases the risk of cardiotoxicity

B. The age groups most at risk are the very young and the very old

C. Cardiomyopathy does not develop unless the total cumulative dose exceeds 700 mg/m²

D. Concurrent use of cyclophosphamide increases the risk of cardiotoxicity

E. A baseline LV ejection fraction of 45% increases the risk of cardiotoxicity

QUESTION 545

A 63-year-old man with metastatic colon cancer is prescribed therapy targeting vascular endothelial growth factor (VEGF). Which of the following statements is correct about the use of the monoclonal antibody/VEGF antagonist bevacizumab (Avastin)?

A. The LV ejection fraction tends to increase with use of this drug

B. Hypotension is a common side effect

C. The risk of arterial, but not venous, thromboembolic events is increased

D. Vasoconstriction and acute coronary syndromes may be precipitated

E. Hemorrhagic pericardial effusion is associated with continuous use of this agent

QUESTION 546

A 2-year-old boy with Down syndrome and a heart murmur is brought to the pediatrician's office because of poor weight gain. The most likely finding on cardiac auscultation is:

A. An early diastolic opening sound at the apex followed by a diastolic rumbling murmur

B. A midsystolic murmur at the upper left sternal border and wide, fixed splitting of S_2

C. A midsystolic click followed by a late systolic murmur at the apex

D. A blowing diastolic murmur at the right upper sternal border

E. A late-peaking systolic ejection murmur heard best at the upper right sternal border with a diminished S_2

QUESTION 547

A 35-year-old man presents with complaints of exertional dyspnea. His medical history is significant for mediastinal radiation therapy as a teenager for treatment for a hematologic malignancy. Regarding cardiovascular effects of radiation therapy, which of the following statements is TRUE?

A. Most complications develop within 5 years of radiation exposure

B. Constrictive pericarditis is typically an acute reaction to radiation therapy

C. The conduction system is typically spared from adverse effects of radiation

D. Dilated cardiomyopathy is the most common manifestation of mediastinal radiation therapy

E. Cancer survivors who received head and neck radiation are at a heightened risk of stroke

QUESTION 548

Which of the following statements is correct regarding familial forms of dilated cardiomyopathy (DCM)?

A. Familial forms account for less than 3% of cases of DCM

B. Most inherited forms of dilated cardiomyopathy fit an autosomal recessive pattern

C. Familial DCM most commonly results from mutations in genes that encode sarcolemmal surface receptors

D. In symptomatic patients, histologic examination of the heart typically demonstrates extensive areas of interstitial and perivascular fibrosis

E. Familial cardiomyopathy can be readily identified as the cause of DCM by specific immunologic markers

QUESTION 549

A 68-year-old woman with metastatic breast cancer presents with pleuritic chest pain, dyspnea, and tachycardia. Regarding the diagnostic approach for pulmonary embolism (PE), which of the following statements is TRUE?

A. Arterial blood gas measurement is the first step in the contemporary diagnostic algorithm for the diagnosis of acute PE

B. The most common electrocardiographic finding in patients with acute PE is an S1Q3T3 pattern
C. It would be reasonable to proceed directly to PE protocol chest CT angiography without D-dimer testing
D. Reduced intensity of the pulmonic component of S_2 is typical in patients with large PE
E. Elevated fibrin degradation products (e.g., D-dimer) are highly specific for PE

DIRECTIONS: Each group of questions below consists of lettered headings followed by a set of numbered questions. For each question, select the ONE lettered heading with which it is most closely associated. Each lettered heading may be used once, more than once, or not at all.

QUESTIONS 550 TO 553

For each statement below, match the appropriate lesion:
A. Osler nodes
B. Janeway lesions
C. Roth spots
D. Subungual hemorrhages
E. Bracht-Wächter bodies

550. Small (1- to 4-mm diameter), irregular, erythematous, nontender macules present on the thenar and hypothenar eminences of the hands
551. Small, raised red (or purple) tender lesions present in the pulp spaces of the terminal phalanges of the fingers
552. Collections of lymphocytes in the nerve layer of the retina
553. Linear or flame-shaped streaks

QUESTIONS 554 TO 558

For each cardiac condition, match the electrocardiographic finding that is most closely associated with it:
A. Low QRS voltage
B. Atrioventricular nodal block
C. Right bundle branch block
D. Diffuse ST-segment elevation
E. Deeply inverted precordial T waves

554. Chronic Chagas disease
555. Sarcoidosis
556. Apical hypertrophic cardiomyopathy
557. Amyloidosis
558. Lyme carditis

QUESTIONS 559 TO 562

For each statement, match the appropriate prosthetic valve type:
A. Starr-Edwards valve
B. Hancock valve
C. St. Jude valve
D. Omniscience valve

559. Single pivoting-disc valve
560. Lowest profile mechanical valve
561. Least thrombogenic mechanical prosthesis for the mitral position
562. Porcine heterograft mounted on a Dacron cloth–covered strut

QUESTIONS 563 TO 566

For each description, match the related cardiac condition(s):
A. Constrictive pericarditis
B. Restrictive cardiomyopathy
C. Both
D. Neither

563. Atrial fibrillation, low QRS voltage
564. Right and left ventricular systolic pressure discordance with respiration during cardiac catheterization
565. Abnormality can usually be diagnosed by chest computed tomography or magnetic resonance imaging
566. Doppler tissue imaging E′ velocity is usually reduced

QUESTIONS 567 TO 571

For each statement listed below, match the most appropriate condition:
A. Cardiac myxoma
B. Large papillary fibroelastoma
C. Both
D. Neither

567. Familial predilection
568. Risk of distal embolism
569. Surgical excision is management of choice
570. May undergo malignant transformation
571. Typically attaches to valves and subvalvular structures

QUESTIONS 572 TO 575

Match the description with the associated form of therapy for pulmonary embolism:
A. Unfractionated heparin or low-molecular-weight heparin
B. Fibrinolytic therapy
C. Both
D. Neither

572. May be effective in pulmonary embolism even 1 to 2 weeks after the onset of symptoms
573. Dissolution of recently formed thrombus is a major action
574. Should be administered along with an antiplatelet agent
575. May suppress aldosterone secretion

QUESTIONS 576 TO 580

Match each description with the associated condition:
A. Hemochromatosis
B. Amyloidosis
C. Both
D. Neither

576. Results in restrictive cardiomyopathy
577. Early-stage disease is reversible with chelating agents
578. Ventricular tachyarrhythmia is the most common initial presentation
579. Autosomal recessive inheritance may be responsible
580. Low-voltage QRS on ECG

QUESTIONS 581 TO 585

Match each description with the associated condition:
A. Tricuspid stenosis
B. Pulmonic stenosis
C. Both
D. Neither

581. Usually rheumatic in origin
582. Typical of carcinoid heart disease
583. Most adults are asymptomatic
584. Ascites is common on physical examination
585. Balloon valvuloplasty is the treatment of choice

QUESTIONS 586 TO 589

Match each description with the associated drug therapy in patients with idiopathic pulmonary arterial hypertension (IPAH):
A. Calcium channel blockers
B. Epoprostenol (prostacyclin)
C. Both
D. Neither

586. Studies have shown a survival benefit in patients with IPAH
587. Should be started empirically in all patients with IPAH
588. Require(s) intravenous infusion
589. Exert(s) an antithrombotic effect

QUESTIONS 590 TO 593

Match each hemodynamic scenario with the associated condition:
A. Chronic constrictive pericarditis
B. Cardiac amyloidosis
C. Both
D. Neither

590. Right ventricular (RV) pressure tracing shows a deep and rapid early decline at the onset of diastole, with a rapid rise to a plateau in early diastole ("dip and plateau" configuration)
591. Left ventricular end-diastolic pressure exceeds right ventricular end-diastolic pressure (RVEDP) by 10 mm Hg
592. Peak RV systolic pressure = 35 mm Hg, RVEDP = 18 mm Hg
593. Pulmonary artery systolic pressure = 68 mm Hg, RVEDP = 15 mm Hg

QUESTIONS 594 TO 597

Match the following descriptions with the appropriate symptom in aortic stenosis:
A. Palpitations
B. Angina
C. Syncope
D. Exertional dyspnea as a manifestation of heart failure

594. Most significant clinical marker for adverse outcome in aortic stenosis, predictive of a 1- to 2-year survival if the valve lesion is not surgically corrected
595. Associated with reduced survival in untreated aortic stenosis of 3 to 5 years
596. Associated with reduced survival in untreated aortic stenosis of 2 to 3 years
597. Not a marker of reduced survival in patients with aortic stenosis

QUESTIONS 598 TO 601

For each type of procedure below, match the appropriate prophylactic antibiotic regimen:
A. No antibiotic prophylaxis required
B. Amoxicillin, 2 g orally, taken 30 to 60 minutes before the procedure
C. Clindamycin 600 mg orally, taken 30 to 60 minutes before the procedure
D. Ampicillin, 2 g IM or IV 30 to 60 minutes before the procedure

598. Elective colonoscopy in a patient with a mechanical mitral valve
599. Dental extraction in a patient with a bioprosthetic aortic valve
600. Dental extraction in penicillin-allergic patient with a mechanical aortic valve
601. Elective cholecystectomy in a patient with mitral stenosis

QUESTIONS 602 TO 606

Match the following descriptions with the appropriate condition:
A. Complete atrioventricular septal defect
B. Complete transposition of the great arteries
C. Both
D. Neither

602. Presents with cyanosis
603. Right-axis deviation on the ECG
604. An interatrial communication is almost always present
605. On echocardiography, the AV valves appear abnormally aligned at the same level
606. A high-pitched, blowing, decrescendo diastolic murmur is common at the left sternal border

QUESTIONS 607 TO 611

Match the following descriptions with the appropriate condition:
A. Kartagener syndrome
B. Holt-Oram syndrome
C. LEOPARD syndrome
D. Noonan syndrome

607. Webbed neck, pulmonic stenosis, left anterior fascicular block
608. Deafness, pulmonic stenosis, complete heart block
609. Lentigines, pulmonic stenosis, PR prolongation
610. Sinusitis, dextrocardia, bronchiectasis

611. Abnormal scaphoid bone, atrial septal defect, right bundle branch block

QUESTIONS 612 TO 615

Match each photograph in Figure 4-28 with the condition it represents:
A. Part A
B. Part B
C. Part C
D. Part D

612. Fabry disease
613. Infective endocarditis
614. Amyloidosis
615. Scleroderma

QUESTIONS 616 TO 619

Match the following descriptions with the appropriate association:
A. Turner syndrome
B. Noonan syndrome

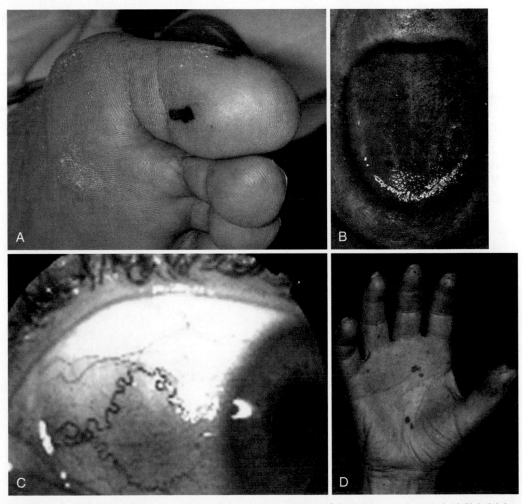

FIGURE 4-28 A Courtesy of Alan J. Lesse, MD; **B** from duVivier A: Atlas of Clinical Dermatology. 3rd ed. Philadelphia, Elsevier, 2002; **C** from Samiy N: Surv Ophthalmol 53:416-423, 2008; **D** from Habif TP: Clinical Dermatology. 5th ed. Philadelphia, Mosby Elsevier, 2009.

DISEASES OF THE HEART, PERICARDIUM, AND PULMONARY VASCULAR BED

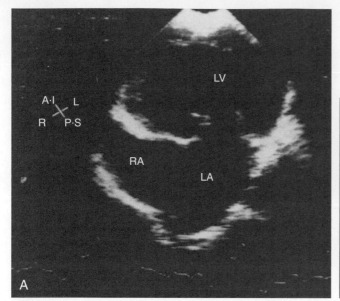

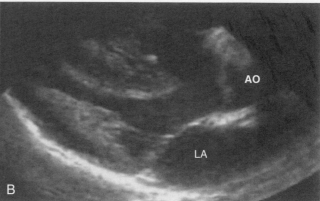

FIGURE 4-29

C. Both
D. Neither

616. Coarctation of the aorta
617. Normal karyotype
618. Pulmonic stenosis
619. Short stature, webbing of the neck, skeletal anomalies, and renal anomalies

QUESTIONS 620 TO 624

Match the following descriptions with the appropriate part of Figure 4-29:
A. Part A
B. Part B
C. Both
D. Neither

620. A ventricular septal defect typically accompanies this anomaly
621. d-Transposition of the great arteries is known to sometimes accompany this anomaly
622. Coronary variations in this disorder include the abnormal origin of the anterior descending artery from the right coronary artery

623. Cyanosis and an electrocardiographic finding of left ventricular hypertrophy are typical
624. The Fontan procedure may be a useful intervention for this condition

QUESTIONS 625 TO 629

Match the following descriptions with the associated antineoplastic therapy:
A. Thoracic radiation therapy
B. Anthracycline therapy
C. Both
D. Neither

625. Pericarditis is the most common cardiac complication
626. Premature coronary atherosclerosis
627. Left ventricular systolic dysfunction
628. Ventricular arrhythmias
629. Aortic dissection

DISEASES OF THE HEART, PERICARDIUM, AND PULMONARY VASCULAR BED

ANSWER TO QUESTION 436

C (Braunwald, p. 1665)

The clinical scenario is most consistent with effusive-constrictive pericarditis, which indicates the simultaneous presence of a hemodynamically significant pericardial effusion and visceral pericardial constriction. This pathophysiology leads to the hemodynamic hallmark of the condition, which is continued elevation of the right atrial pressure following aspiration of the pericardial fluid despite the return of intrapericardial pressure to normal. The causes of this entity are the same as those for chronic constrictive pericarditis. The most common include idiopathic or postviral pericarditis, tuberculosis, neoplastic infiltration of the pericardium, and mediastinal radiation therapy. The physical findings on initial presentation are most consistent with cardiac tamponade, including pulsus paradoxus and jugular venous distention with a prominent x descent.

The diagnosis of effusive-constrictive pericarditis is made at cardiac catheterization, with careful hemodynamic monitoring of intrapericardial and right atrial pressures before and after pericardiocentesis. Although intrapericardial pressure returns to baseline (i.e., ~0 mm Hg) after pericardiocentesis, intracardiac pressures do not normalize. Rather, hemodynamic tracings convert to a form more consistent with constrictive pericarditis, with a prominent y descent in the atrial pressure tracings as well as a "dip-and-plateau" pattern in the right ventricular pressure tracing. As might be expected from the pathophysiology, pericardiocentesis provides only partial and transient symptomatic relief; definitive therapy for this condition requires total pericardiectomy.

REFERENCE

Sagrist-Sauleda J, Angel J, Sanchez A, et al: Effusive-constrictive pericarditis. N Engl J Med 350:469, 2004.

ANSWER TO QUESTION 437

C (Braunwald, pp. 1652-1655)

The ECG demonstrates diffuse ST-segment elevations and PR-segment depressions that are most consistent with acute pericarditis.[1] ST-segment elevations in all leads except aVR develop in the majority of patients with acute pericarditis, and PR-segment depression is found in up to 80%.

Although chest pain is the most common symptom in acute pericarditis, its location and quality are variable. The pain is often positional in that it improves by sitting upright or leaning forward and is often aggravated with coughing, deep inspiration, or lying supine. Fever is common, but the cardinal physical finding is the pericardial friction rub. The three components of the complete pericardial rub correspond to atrial systole, ventricular systole, and the early filling phase of ventricular diastole.

Cardiac serum biomarkers and other markers of infarction can be elevated in acute pericarditis because of irritation of the adjacent myocardium. As a result, an initial determination of such markers cannot reliably differentiate between acute pericarditis and myocardial infarction.[2]

Thrombolytic therapy is of potential harm if errantly administered to a patient with acute pericarditis, because hemorrhagic tamponade could follow. Initial therapy for patients with acute viral or idiopathic pericarditis should include aspirin or other nonsteroidal anti-inflammatory drugs. For truly refractory symptoms, glucocorticoids may be beneficial, but they should not be used as initial therapy. The results of an open label randomized trial show that the drug colchicine reduces the duration of acute symptomatology and recurrent episodes of pericarditis.[3] Nitrates have no role in the management of pericardial symptoms.

REFERENCES

1. Khandaker M, Espinoza R, Nishimura R, et al: Pericardial disease: Diagnosis and management. Mayo Clin Proc 85:772, 2010.
2. Imazio M, Demichelis B, Cecchi E, et al: Cardiac troponin I in acute pericarditis. J Am Coll Cardiol 42:2144, 2003.
3. Imazio M, Bobbio M, Cecchi E, et al: Colchicine in addition to conventional therapy for acute pericarditis: Results of the Colchicine for Acute Pericarditis (COPE) trial. Circulation 112:2012, 2005.

ANSWER TO QUESTION 438

A (Braunwald, pp. 1452-1454)

Localized coarctation of the aorta consists of a shelf in the posterolateral aortic wall opposite the ductus arteriosus. It is more common in males and there is a high degree of association with bicuspid aortic valve and Turner syndrome. Other associated congenital cardiac malformations include patent ductus arteriosus, ventricular septal defect, and mitral valve abnormalities. Young patients with coarctation are usually asymptomatic. In older children or adults, symptoms may include headache, leg fatigue, and intermittent claudication. Patients may also come to medical attention because of symptoms associated with left ventricular failure, infective endarteritis, or aortic rupture or dissection.

Simultaneous palpation of the upper and lower extremities in patients with coarctation often reveals diminished and delayed femoral pulses compared with the radial pulse. Exercise typically accentuates this finding. A midsystolic murmur over the chest and back is often present. In addition, auscultation may demonstrate the ejection click and systolic murmur of a co-existent bicuspid aortic valve.

Persistent systemic hypertension after repair of the coarctation occurs in up to one third of patients, even in the absence of recoarctation. Risk factors include older age at repair and higher blood pressure at the time of repair.[1,2]

REFERENCES

1. De Divitiis M, Pilla C, Kattenhorn M, et al: Ambulatory blood pressure, left ventricular mass, and conduit artery function late after successful repair of coarctation of the aorta. J Am Coll Cardiol 41:2259, 2003.
2. Vohra HA, Adamson L, Haw MP: Does surgical correction of coarctation of the aorta in adults reduce established hypertension. Interact Cardiovasc Thorac Surg 8:127, 2009.

ANSWER TO QUESTION 439

C (Braunwald, pp. 1468-1478)

The Doppler recording displays an elevated transaortic valve systolic velocity of 4 m/sec, which corresponds to a peak instantaneous systolic gradient of 64 mm Hg across the aortic valve. This patient thus presents with symptomatic aortic stenosis (AS). Angina pectoris, syncope, and heart failure are the cardinal symptoms of this condition.[1] The onset of symptoms in patients with AS is an ominous sign: natural history survival trends show that the time of death following symptom occurrence is approximately 5 years for patients with angina, 3 years for those with syncope, and 2 years for patients with heart failure. Angina is present in approximately two thirds of patients with critical AS. It arises in the absence of significant coronary artery obstruction in up to half of patients, owing to both increased oxygen demand and impaired coronary vasodilatory reserve with microcirculatory dysfunction.[2] Whereas the most common early symptom in patients with AS is a decrease in exercise tolerance or dyspnea on exertion (due to left ventricular diastolic dysfunction or the limited ability to increase cardiac output with exercise), symptoms of advanced heart failure (orthopnea, paroxysmal nocturnal dyspnea and pulmonary edema) occur late in the course.

Syncope in AS is usually due to systemic vasodilation in the setting of a fixed cardiac output.

An association between calcific aortic stenosis and gastrointestinal hemorrhage, particularly due to angiodysplasia, has been observed. Bleeding is thought to arise from shear stress–induced platelet aggregation by the stenotic valve with reduction of high-molecular-weight multimers of von Willebrand factor and an increased number of proteolytic fragments.[3] This abnormality is correctable by aortic valve replacement.

REFERENCES

1. Maganti K, Rigolin VH, Sarano ME, et al: Valvular heart disease: Diagnosis and management. Mayo Clin Proc 85:483, 2010.
2. Rajappan K, Rimoldi OE, Dutka DP, et al: Mechanisms of coronary microcirculatory dysfunction in patients with aortic stenosis and angiographically normal coronary arteries. Circulation 105:470, 2002.
3. Vincentelli A, Susen S, Le Tourneau T, et al: Acquired von Willebrand syndrome in aortic stenosis. N Engl J Med 349:343, 2003.

ANSWER TO QUESTION 440

B (Braunwald, pp. 1631-1634)

Cocaine is the most commonly used illicit drug among patients presenting to emergency departments, and associated cardiovascular consequences include ischemia and infarction, myocardial diastolic and/or systolic dysfunction, and arrhythmias.[1,2] In a survey of young adults aged 18 to 45 years old, approximately one in four nonfatal myocardial infarctions was attributable to cocaine use.[3] The mechanisms of myocardial ischemia and infarction include (1) increased myocardial oxygen demand in the setting of limited oxygen supply, (2) intense coronary arterial vasoconstriction, and/or (3) enhanced platelet aggregation and thrombogenicity. In addition, the vascular injury caused by cocaine may lead to increased endothelial permeability and accelerated atherogenesis. The occurrence of myocardial infarction after cocaine use is not associated with the amount ingested, route of administration, or frequency of use.

Mechanisms of myocardial dysfunction after long-term cocaine use include (1) myocardial ischemia or infarction, (2) cardiomyopathy due to repeated sympathetic stimulation, and (3) altered myocardial and endothelial cytokine production. Myocardial dysfunction can also occur acutely after cocaine use, likely reflecting drug-associated metabolic disturbances or direct toxic effects of the drug. The co-ingestion of other toxins with cocaine can amplify the former's deleterious effects. For example, the combination of cocaine and ethanol is associated with a higher rate of cardiovascular complications than the use of either agent alone.

REFERENCES

1. Schwarts BG, Rezkalla S, Kloner RA: Cardiovascular effects of cocaine. Circulation 122:2558, 2010.
2. Maraj S, Figueredo VM, Lynn Morris D: Cocaine and the heart. Clin Cardiol 33:264, 2010.
3. Quereshi AI, Suri MF, Guterman LR, et al: Cocaine use and the likelihood of nonfatal myocardial infarction and stroke: Data from the Third National Health and Nutrition Examination Survey. Circulation 103:502, 2001.

ANSWER TO QUESTION 441

D (Braunwald, pp. 1426-1428)

The common anatomic types of ASD include the sinus venosus or "high" ASD, the ostium secundum ASD, and the ostium primum ASD. The sinus venosus defect is often accompanied by anomalous pulmonary venous return. The ostium secundum type of ASD, which appears in the mid-interatrial septum, should be distinguished from patent foramen ovale, which occurs in up to 25% of adults. Ostium primum ASDs are a type of atrioventricular septal defect, discussed in a subsequent question.

Patients with ASDs are usually asymptomatic in early life, and only rare children with this disorder experience exertional dyspnea and easy fatigability. Children with ASDs do tend to be underdeveloped physically and prone to respiratory tract infections. The diagnosis of ASD in the young is most often prompted by detection of a heart murmur on routine physical examination. In adults, the most common manifesting symptoms are exercise intolerance and palpitations.

REFERENCES

Kharouf R, Luxenerg DM, Khalid O, et al: Atrial septal defect: Spectrum of care. Pediatr Cardiol 29:271, 2008.

Webb G, Gatzoulis MA: Atrial septal defects in the adult: Recent progress and overview. Circulation 114:1645, 2006.

ANSWER TO QUESTION 442

B (Braunwald, p. 1421)

The ECG is helpful in the assessment of congenital heart disease. In particular, evaluation for right-axis deviation and right ventricular hypertrophy, and rhythm and conduction disturbances, is frequently important. For example, right ventricular hypertrophy may be a sign of pulmonary hypertension or right ventricular outflow tract obstruction or other disorders causing right-sided pressure or volume overload, including septal defects.

Atrial arrhythmias commonly accompany congenital heart disease. Atrial flutter is much more frequent in young patients than atrial fibrillation. It often arises in patients with a history of surgical repair and can be challenging to treat. Pharmacologic agents are generally ineffective, and catheter ablation therapy is usually necessary; recurrence is common. Conduction disturbances, such as first-degree atrioventricular (AV) block, are often evident in patients with AV septal defects, congenitally corrected transposition of the great arteries, and Ebstein anomaly.

The electrocardiographic findings of myocardial infarction in an infant suggest the presence of an anomalous origin of a coronary artery. Left ventricular volume overload due to aortic or mitral regurgitation can result in deep Q waves in the left precordial leads.

REFERENCES

Abadair S, Khairy P: Electrophysiology and adult congenital heart disease: Advances and options. Prog Cardiovasc Dis 53:281, 2011.

Triedman JK: Arrhythmias in adults with congenital heart disease. Heart 87:383, 2002.

ANSWER TO QUESTION 443

D (Braunwald, pp. 1430-1432)

Ventricular septal defects (VSDs) may be classified by their locations and margins. Muscular VSDs are bordered entirely by myocardium and may be found in the trabecular septum, inlet septum, or outlet septum. Membranous VSDs are bordered in part by fibrous continuity between an atrioventricular valve and an arterial valve. Doubly committed subarterial VSDs, which are more common in Asian patients, are situated in the outlet septum and bordered by fibrous continuity of the aortic and pulmonary valves.

The size of a VSD relates to the consequent pathophysiology and potential complications. A restrictive VSD is small ($Q_p/Q_s < 1.4$) and thus produces a significant pressure gradient between the left and right ventricles. It typically does not cause hemodynamic impairment and may eventually spontaneously close, but the turbulence of the high-pressure jet across the defect presents a high risk of endocarditis. Because of the high gradient, infants with a restrictive VSD demonstrate a loud murmur and often present at an early age. Conversely, infants with large nonrestrictive defects present at a later age because the equalization of pressures across the defect attenuates the systolic murmur. A large, nonrestrictive VSD ($Q_p/Q_s > 2.2$) is accompanied by a large left-to-right shunt, with subsequent development of an elevated pulmonary artery systolic pressure. Such patients may eventually develop left ventricular volume overload, heart failure, and Eisenmenger syndrome (related to the progressive rise in pulmonary artery pressure). Closure of the defect, either surgically or by transcatheter device placement, is the treatment of choice for those with a significant VSD in the absence of contraindications (e.g., irreversible pulmonary hypertension). After repair, the ECG is usually notable only for right bundle branch block.

REFERENCE

Minette MS, Sahn DJ: Ventricular septal defects. Circulation 114:2190, 2006.

ANSWER TO QUESTION 444

A (Braunwald, pp. 1426-1428)

Although atrial septal defects (ASDs) are frequently asymptomatic, children may experience exertional dyspnea or frequent chest infections. Physical examination usually reveals the diagnostic wide fixed splitting of the second heart sound. Other findings may include a systolic murmur of increased flow across the pulmonic valve or a mid-diastolic rumble due to increased flow through the tricuspid valve. The ECG may be helpful in determining the type of ASD. Secundum ASD patients often exhibit right-axis deviation on the ECG, whereas those with primum ASD characteristically exhibit left-axis deviation. Patients with sinus venosus ASD exhibit left-axis deviation of the P wave, and PR prolongation can be seen with all types of ASD.

Repair of the defect is advised for patients with Q_p/Q_s ≥ 1.5:1.0, particularly if the anatomy is suitable for percutaneous transcatheter device closure. Repair of a significant (i.e., Q_p/Q_s ≥ 1.5:1.0) ASD improves New York Heart Association functional class in symptomatic patients. For adults who are asymptomatic or mildly symptomatic, device closure improves exercise capacity, indicating that even those with seemingly minimal symptoms may benefit from such a procedure.[1,2] In patients who undergo successful repair of an isolated secundum defect (by surgery or by transcatheter device), lifelong endocarditis prophylaxis is not required.

REFERENCES

1. Rao PS: When and how should atrial septal defects be closed in adults. J Invasive Cardiol 21:76, 2009.
2. Brochu MC, Baril JF, Dore A, et al: Improvement in exercise capacity in asymptomatic and mildly symptomatic adults after atrial septal defect percutaneous closure. Circulation 106:1821, 2002.

ANSWER TO QUESTION 445

B (Braunwald, pp. 1640-1641)

The echocardiogram demonstrates a pedunculated mass in the right atrium that is most suggestive of an atrial myxoma. Features that suggest myxoma include (1) attachment of the mass to the interatrial septum (the most common site of attachment is in the region of the fossa ovalis) and (2) a mass that is pedunculated and heterogeneous in appearance. Other cardiac tumors, including lipomas and rhabdomyomas, would be within the differential diagnosis. However, these other tumors are rarely pedunculated and more often infiltrate into the myocardium itself. The echocardiographic appearance would also prompt consideration of an intracardiac thrombus. However, atrial thrombi tend to be located in the posterior portion of the atrium and have more of a layered appearance than the heterogeneous mottling apparent in this example.

Atrial myxoma is the most common primary tumor of the heart, and 75% to 80% of such tumors arise in the left atrium. The clinical presentation of myxomas is often part of the triad of intracardiac obstruction, embolization, and constitutional symptoms. Nearly 70% of patients with left atrial myxomas have cardiac symptoms, typically related to obstructive heart failure and syncope. Embolic events occur in approximately 30% of patients, with left atrial myxomas causing strokes and transient ischemic attacks and with right atrial myxomas leading to pulmonary emboli. Myxomas may secrete interleukin-6, an inflammatory cytokine associated with systemic symptoms such as fever, malaise, and weight loss. Surgical resection of myxomas is warranted to relieve systemic or intracardiac obstructive symptoms and to prevent embolic complications.

REFERENCE

McCoskey EH, Mehta JB, Krishnan K, Roy TM: Right atrial myxoma with extracardiac manifestations. Chest 118:547, 2000.

ANSWER TO QUESTION 446

C (Braunwald, pp. 1541-1542, 1552-1556; Table 67-3)

Prosthetic valve endocarditis (PVE) may occur "early," within the first 60 days after placement of the valve, or "late," in subsequent months or years.[1] Whereas this distinction is somewhat arbitrary, differences in both the clinical features and microbial patterns have been documented. Cases of early PVE usually are due to contamination in the immediate operative or perioperative setting. *Staphylococcus epidermidis* is the most common organism isolated in this group, occurring in over 30% of cases. *Staphylococcus aureus* is found in 20% to 25%. In the first year after surgery, the incidence of methicillin-resistant organisms is high.

In late cases, as in this question, the source of infection is often difficult to identify but is presumed to be seeding of the valve by a transient bacteremia. The bacteriology in late PVE is thus similar to that of native valvular endocarditis. The most common organism isolated in this setting is *Streptococcus viridans*.

The transesophageal echocardiographic image displayed demonstrates that the mitral valve prosthesis is well seated in the appropriate position. The prominent vegetations seen on the atrial side of the valve are well delineated by the technique and provide an excellent example of the increased sensitivity of this form of echocardiography as compared with transthoracic studies (as described later in the Answer to Question 472).[2]

REFERENCES

1. Nataloni M, Pergolini M, Rescigno G, et al: Prosthetic valve endocarditis. J Cardiovasc Med 11:869, 2010.
2. Evangelista A, Gonzalez-Alujas MT: Echocardiography in infective endocarditis. Heart 90:614, 2004.

ANSWER TO QUESTION 447

B (Braunwald, pp. 1304-1305, 1462-1463, 1476, 1495-1498, 1518-1519)

Balloon valvuloplasty for valvular pulmonic stenosis (PS) has proved highly successful and has essentially replaced open surgical repair for valvular pulmonic stenosis. This procedure is recommended in PS when the right ventricular outflow gradient is > 50 mm Hg or if the patient is symptomatic.

In 1985, successful balloon valvuloplasty using a transseptal approach was first reported in young adult patients with rheumatic mitral stenosis, and this technique is now the mainstay of interventional therapy for this condition. Mitral valvuloplasty is especially useful in patients without mitral valvular calcification or thickening.[1] Moderate or severe mitral regurgitation occurs rarely after balloon valvuloplasty. One minor complication without significant hemodynamic consequence is that approximately 5% of patients show evidence of a persistent, left-to-right shunt at the site of atrial septal puncture, owing to the necessary transseptal left-sided heart catheterization. Systemic embolization in the absence of a left atrial thrombus is uncommon.[1]

Balloon aortic valvuloplasty is used as an alternative to aortic valvotomy in young patients with congenital, noncalcific aortic stenosis (AS). However, the usefulness of this technique is very limited in adults with calcific AS. Although the initial relief of critical stenosis can be achieved in most patients, the rates of serious complications and restenosis are very high.[2] Thus, for adults with critical AS, balloon aortic valvuloplasty is reserved for select patients who are not cardiac surgical candidates and who require immediate improvement in the aortic valve gradient (e.g., preceding an urgent noncardiac operation). Percutaneous prosthetic aortic valve *implantation* is undergoing active clinical investigation as an alternative to surgical valve replacement in suitable patients whose comorbidities place them are at excessive risk of standard surgical replacement.

REFERENCES

1. Carabello BA: Modern management of mitral stenosis. Circulation 112:432, 2005.
2. Hara H, Pederson WR, Ladich E, et al: Percutaneous aortic valvuloplasty revisited: Time for a renaissance? Circulation 115:e334, 2007.

ANSWER TO QUESTION 448

E (Braunwald, pp. 1638-1640, 1644-1646)

Primary tumors of the heart are quite rare—autopsy series indicate a prevalence of 0.001% to 0.03%. Metastatic tumors to the heart are far more common. Approximately three fourths of primary cardiac tumors are benign.[1] The most common benign primary cardiac tumor in children is rhabdomyoma, and 80% of such tumors appear before the age of 1 year. The most common malignant cardiac tumor in children is rhabdomyosarcoma.[2] In adults, the most common benign primary cardiac tumor is the atrial myxoma, which accounts for 30% to 50% of cases. Lipomas and papillary fibroelastomas are the next most common benign primary tumors. The most frequent malignant primary tumor of the heart in adults is angiosarcoma, accounting for 30% to 37% of cases.

REFERENCES

1. Butany J, Nair V, Naseemuddin A, et al: Cardiac tumours: Diagnosis and management. Lancet Oncol 6:219, 2005.
2. Becker AE: Primary heart tumors in the pediatric age group: A review of salient pathologic features relevant for clinicians. Pediatr Cardiol 21:317, 2000.

ANSWER TO QUESTION 449

D (Braunwald, p. 1575)

The patient described has the classic clinical signs and findings of type II glycogen storage disease.[1] This disease is a consequence of the deficiency of alpha-1,4-glucosidase (acid maltase), a lysosomal enzyme that hydrolyzes glycogen into glucose. The condition commonly manifests in the neonatal period. Characteristic symptoms include failure to thrive, progressive hypotonia, lethargy, and a weak cry. Of all the glycogen storage diseases, type II (or Pompe disease) is the most likely to cause cardiac symptoms. The ECG shows extremely tall, broad QRS complexes with a short PR interval (commonly < 0.09 second). The chest radiograph frequently shows cardiomegaly with pulmonary vascular redistribution. The diagnosis is confirmed by demonstrating the enzymatic deficiency in lymphocytes, skeletal muscle, or liver. The displayed myocardial biopsy (Fig. 4-30B) shows prominent vacuoles within

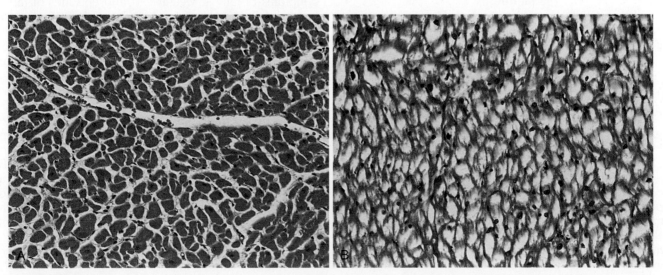

FIGURE 4-30 From Cotran RS, Kumar V, Collins T: Robbins Pathologic Basis of Disease. 6th ed. Philadelphia, WB Saunders, 1999.

the myocardial fibers, which contain glycogen. Normal myocardial histology is shown in part A of the figure for comparison.

Cardiac glycogenosis may be confused with other entities that cause cardiac failure, particularly in association with cardiomegaly in the early months of life. Endocardial fibroelastosis, a disease of unknown etiology, differs from Pompe disease in lacking the short PR interval and the fact that symptoms are limited to the cardiac system, whereas in Pompe disease skeletal muscle hypotonia is prominent. Furthermore, in endocardial fibroelastosis, mitral regurgitation and abnormalities of the cardiac valves, especially mitral and aortic, are frequent. Coarctation of the aorta, another common cause of congestive heart failure in infants, can readily be distinguished by the presence of pulse and blood pressure discrepancies between the upper and lower extremities. Myocarditis, yet another cause of congestive heart failure, is usually of abrupt onset and is not associated with hypotonia. Anomalous pulmonary origin of the left coronary artery can cause cardiomegaly but usually has a distinctive electrocardiographic pattern of anterolateral myocardial infarction.

Shone syndrome is a developmental complex that consists of four obstructive anomalies: (1) a supravalvular ring of the left atrium; (2) a parachute mitral valve; (3) subaortic stenosis; and (4) coarctation of the aorta. It typically manifests with findings of mitral stenosis, because flow from the left atrium must pass through the abnormal intrachordal spaces of the mitral valve, which poses functional obstruction. Pulmonary venous hypertension is a common finding in this condition because of left ventricular inflow and outflow obstruction. Shone syndrome manifests more often in early childhood than in infancy and lacks the skeletal muscle changes of Pompe disease.

Friedreich ataxia is a hereditary autosomal recessive disease that manifests during late childhood with progressive ataxia. The limbs, in addition to being ataxic, generally show considerable weakness. About 50% of patients with Friedreich ataxia have cardiac involvement, typically hypertrophic cardiomyopathy.

REFERENCE

1. Kishani PS, Hwu WL, Mandel H, et al: A retrospective, multinational, multicenter study on the natural history of infantile-onset Pompe disease. J Pediatr 148:671, 2006.

ANSWER TO QUESTION 450

C (Braunwald, pp. 1655-1661)

Cardiac tamponade occurs when the accumulation of pericardial fluid causes significant cardiac chamber compression.[1] It is characterized by an increase in intrapericardial pressure and impedance to diastolic filling of the ventricles, with a consequent fall in cardiac output. Normal intrapericardial pressure is several millimeters of mercury lower than right ventricular (RV) and left ventricular (LV) diastolic pressures. As fluid accumulates in the pericardial space, intrapericardial pressure rises to

the level of right atrial (RA) and RV diastolic pressures. At that point, the transpericardial pressure distending the cardiac chambers declines to zero, and tamponade physiology occurs.

Although the rise of RA and intrapericardial pressures may be less dramatic in the presence of hypovolemia, cardiac tamponade can occur during this state and may be masked because the pressures in these two spaces equalize at a lower absolute value.[2]

As intrapericardial and RV diastolic pressures rise toward the level of LV diastolic pressure, all three pressures equalize, leading to a marked decrease in transmural distending pressures and, eventually, to a fall in stroke volume. Cardiac output in this setting may initially be maintained by reflex tachycardia and the blood pressure maintained by increased vascular tone. However, as pericardial fluid continues to accumulate, compensatory mechanisms are no longer able to maintain cardiac output and blood pressure falls.

Whereas tachycardia is the usual response to falling stroke volume, bradycardia can be seen in severe cases. Both the cardiac depressor branches of the vagus nerve and sinoatrial node ischemia are believed to contribute to this phenomenon. Echocardiographic features of tamponade include RA inversion and RV diastolic collapse. Conversely, left atrial and/or LV diastolic collapse are more variable findings.

REFERENCES

1. Spodick DH: Acute cardiac tamponade. N Engl J Med 349:684, 2003.
2. Sagristà-Sauleda J, Angel J, Sambola A, et al: Low-pressure cardiac tamponade: Clinical and hemodynamic profile. Circulation 114:945, 2006.

ANSWER TO QUESTION 451

B (Braunwald, pp. 1516-1518)

This woman presents with physical findings and symptoms of tricuspid regurgitation (TR). By history, the course of her illness is relatively rapid and includes systemic symptoms of fatigue, weight loss, and episodes of rapid heartbeat, flushing, and diarrhea. The most likely diagnosis is the carcinoid syndrome. Carcinoid is a slowly growing tumor that leads to focal or diffuse deposits of fibrous tissue in the endocardium of the valvular cusps and cardiac chambers. The white fibrous carcinoid plaques are most extensive on the right side of the heart because vasoactive substances are released from hepatic metastases and drain through the inferior vena cava into the right atrium. This results in endocardial damage and fibrosis and causes the cusps of the tricuspid valve to adhere to the underlying right ventricle, producing TR (often accompanied by pulmonic valve disease on a similar basis, as described in later questions). Carcinoid syndrome is suggested by the coexistence of TR with flushing and diarrhea, which result from the release of vasoactive amines by the tumor cells.

Other causes of isolated TR may be divided into those involving an anatomically abnormal valve (*primary* TR) and those with an anatomically normal valve (*functional*

TR). The latter, in which TR is due to dilatation of the right ventricle and tricuspid annulus, is more common. The most frequent cause of functional TR is right ventricular (RV) hypertension, especially as a result of mitral valve disease, congenital heart disease, primary pulmonary hypertension, or cor pulmonale. RV infarction may also cause functional TR.

Many disease processes may affect the tricuspid valve directly, leading to primary TR. Among these are (1) congenital abnormalities of the tricuspid valve (e.g., Ebstein anomaly or an atrioventricular canal defect); (2) rheumatic tricuspid valve disease (which is much less common than rheumatic mitral or aortic disease); (3) connective tissue disorders, including myxomatous redundancy of the leaflets; and (4) infective endocarditis. Other less common causes include endomyocardial fibroelastosis, trauma, cardiac tumors (particularly right atrial myxomas), transvenous pacemaker leads, repeated endomyocardial biopsies in a transplanted heart, or exposure to certain drugs, such as methysergide or the appetite suppressant dexfenfluramine.

REFERENCE

Bhattacharyya S, Davar J, Dreyfus G, et al: Carcinoid heart disease. Circulation 116:2860, 2007.

ANSWER TO QUESTION 452

B (Braunwald, pp. 1541-1542)

This patient has right-sided endocarditis in the setting of illicit IV drug use. The echocardiographic image shows a large vegetation on the atrial surface of the septal leaflet of the tricuspid valve (arrow in Fig. 4-31). Injection drug users with endocarditis most frequently demonstrate right-sided valvular involvement (the tricuspid valve in 46% to 78%), with less common

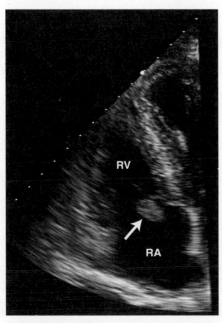

FIGURE 4-31

involvement of the left-sided valves (mitral valve involvement in 24% to 32% and aortic valve involvement in 8% to 19%), however the latter group displays greater mortality. *Staphylococcus aureus* infections account for more than 50% of IV drug user endocarditis (and for 60% to 70% of those with tricuspid valve involvement), with the remainder caused by streptococcal species, gram-negative bacilli, and fungi. Pulmonary findings are frequent in those with right-sided endocarditis, with 65% to 75% displaying evidence of septic pulmonary emboli on chest radiograph. Other pulmonary complications include pulmonary infarction, abscess formation, and empyema. Serious cardiac complications include destruction of the tricuspid valve apparatus, with consequent severe regurgitation and right-sided heart failure.

REFERENCE

Murdoch DR, Corey GR, Hoen B, et al: Clinical presentation, etiology, and outcome of infective endocarditis in the 21st century. Arch Intern Med 169:463, 2009.

ANSWER TO QUESTION 453

B (Braunwald, pp. 1672-1675)

Blunt cardiac trauma is a form of nonpenetrating injury of the heart. The most common causes of blunt chest trauma in the United States are motor vehicle accidents, usually involving impact against the steering wheel. Other causes include blows to the chest from a kick, a fall, or a projectile object. Clinical presentations of blunt cardiac injuries include free wall rupture (ventricular or atrial), ventricular septal defect, coronary artery trauma with thrombosis, arrhythmias, rupture of chordae tendineae or papillary muscles, or pericardial rupture with cardiac herniation. Less dramatically, a myocardial contusion may result in a regional wall motion abnormality visualized by echocardiography, with or without an associated pericardial effusion. In some patients, initial myocardial contusion can lead to delayed wall rupture. Atrial septal defects are not a commonly recognized consequence of blunt cardiac injury.

REFERENCE

Cook CC, Gleason TG: Great vessel and cardiac trauma. Surg Clin North Am 89:797, 2009.

ANSWER TO QUESTION 454

C (Braunwald, pp. 1621-1622)

In a recent autopsy study, pericardial effusion was the most common cardiac manifestation of human immunodeficiency virus (HIV) infection. Such effusions tend to occur in patients with lower CD4 counts and more advanced disease and have been shown to be a marker for increased mortality. However, the effusions tend to be small, rarely cause symptoms, and many spontaneously resolve without specific therapy. Cardiac tamponade is a rare complication.

The causes of pericardial effusions in HIV infection include opportunistic infections and malignancy (e.g., Kaposi sarcoma or lymphoma); however, a definite etiology is often not found. In some cases, the development of effusions (pericardial and pleural) may occur as a result of a capillary leak phenomenon induced by elevated cytokine levels in patients with advanced HIV disease.

REFERENCE

Ho JE, Hsue PY: Cardiovascular manifestations of HIV infection. Heart 95:1193, 2009.

ANSWER TO QUESTION 455

B (Braunwald, pp. 1426-1428; see also Answer to Question 444)

There are several diagnostically helpful clinical features in patients with atrial septal defects (ASDs). On physical examination, common findings include a prominent right ventricular (RV) impulse, palpable pulmonary artery pulsations, accentuation of the tricuspid valve closure sound leading to splitting of S_1, and a midsystolic pulmonary ejection murmur due to increased flow across the pulmonic valve. If the shunt is large, a middiastolic rumbling murmur may be audible at the lower left sternal border. This murmur results from increased blood flow across the tricuspid valve.

The ECG may be helpful in the diagnostic evaluation of a patient with suspected ASD. The ECG in ostium secundum ASD usually shows right-axis deviation and an rSR′ or rsR′ pattern in the right precordial leads with a normal QRS complex duration. The presence of negative P waves in the inferior leads (indicating a low atrial pacemaker) suggests the presence of a sinus venosus type ASD. Left-axis deviation and superior orientation of the QRS complex in the frontal plane is consistent with

either an ostium primum defect or, less commonly, a secundum atrial defect combined with mitral valve prolapse. Tall R or R′ waves in V_1 may indicate the presence of pulmonary hypertension and concomitant RV hypertrophy.

The chest radiograph may reveal enlargement of the right atrium and right ventricle, pulmonary arterial dilatation, and increased pulmonary vascular markings. Echocardiographic evaluation of ASD commonly shows pulmonary arterial and RV dilatation as well as anterior systolic (paradoxical) intraventricular septal motion, reflecting RV volume overload. The defect itself may sometimes be visualized by two-dimensional echocardiography, particularly using the subcostal view. Doppler interrogation reveals the presence and direction of the transatrial shunt and allows calculation of the Q_p/Q_s ratio.

ANSWER TO QUESTION 456

E (Braunwald, p. 1583)

This patient has the apical variant of hypertrophic cardiomyopathy (HCM), evidenced on this echocardiographic apical long-axis view. This variant is marked by predominant hypertrophy of the left ventricular apex, which causes the chamber to display a "spade-like" deformity on cardiac imaging. This is even more clearly demonstrated on this patient's subsequent cardiac magnetic resonance imaging study (see arrows in Fig. 4-32). The disorder is rare in other parts of the world, but in Japan it accounts for 25% of patients with HCM. The ECG in this condition is frequently striking for deep, *inverted* T waves in the apical precordial leads. Intraventricular pressure gradients are usually *absent*. Symptoms associated with the apical variant tend to be more mild and the risk of sudden death is *lower* than in the traditional septal form of HCM.

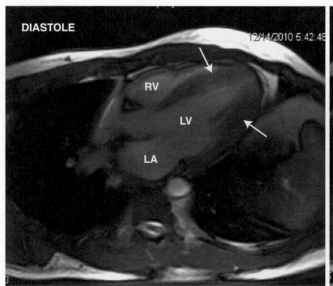
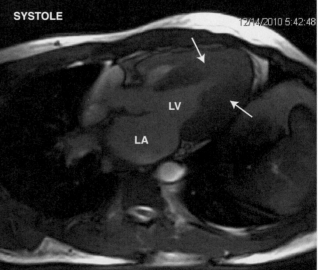

FIGURE 4-32

REFERENCE

Fattori R, Biagini E, Lorenzini M et al: Significance of magnetic resonance imaging in apical hypertrophic cardiomyopathy. Am J Cardiol 105:1592, 2010.

ANSWER TO QUESTION 457

D (Braunwald, pp. 1499-1505)

Physical findings in mitral regurgitation (MR) are influenced by the compliance of the left atrium. In patients with severe, *acute* mitral regurgitation (e.g., due to rupture of chordae tendineae), the regurgitant volume encounters an unprepared, relatively noncompliant left atrium. As a result, the left atrial pressure quickly rises, which serves to limit the pressure gradient between the left ventricle and left atrium late in systole, causing the systolic murmur to shorten and end *before* the second heart sound. However, the acutely elevated left atrial pressure also augments the pulmonary venous pressure and commonly results in acute pulmonary edema as well as findings of right-sided heart failure (e.g., jugular venous distention).

In contrast, the more gradual development of *chronic* MR allows the left atrium to gradually dilate and increase its compliance, such that the chamber is able to accommodate larger volumes without a substantial increase in pressure. As a result, in compensated chronic MR, substantial elevation in pulmonary venous and capillary pressures is avoided. However, the mitral regurgitant volume returns to the left ventricle during diastole, resulting in gradual left ventricular enlargement. Thus, in distinction to acute MR, patients with chronic MR commonly demonstrate left ventricular and left atrial enlargement on the chest radiograph and ECG.[1]

REFERENCE

1. Enriquez-Sarano M, Akins CW, Vahanian A: Mitral regurgitation. Lancet 373:1382, 2009.

ANSWER TO QUESTION 458

B (Braunwald, pp. 1491-1492, 1663-1664; Fig. 66-20)

The tracing shows the simultaneous recording of left atrial (LA) and left ventricular (LV) pressures and depicts the hemodynamic profile of mitral stenosis. The left atrial pressure is elevated (mean ~ 20 mm Hg) with a prominent atrial contraction (*a*) wave and an abnormally gradual pressure decline in diastole after mitral valve opening (*y* descent). There is a persistent gradient between left atrial and left ventricular pressure throughout diastole, in contrast to the normal situation, in which there is rapid equilibration of left atrial and left ventricular pressures in diastole.

Mitral regurgitation would be associated with prominent *v* waves on the left atrial pressure tracing but no persistent diastolic atrioventricular pressure gradient.

In constrictive pericarditis and restrictive cardiomyopathy, the atrial pressure decline in early diastole is typically brisk (prominent *y* descent), the converse of this example.

ANSWER TO QUESTION 459

C (Braunwald, pp. 1653-1654)

This patient has typical symptoms and signs of acute pericarditis. The vast majority of patients with pericarditis manifest electrocardiographic abnormalities. The most common early finding is global ST-segment elevation, particularly in the inferior, lateral, and apical leads. The ST-segment elevations are believed to represent a current of injury caused by superficial inflammation of the adjacent myocardium. In contrast to the acute ST-segment abnormalities of myocardial infarction (MI), the elevations in pericarditis tend to be oriented in a concave upward direction and reciprocal ST-segment depressions in the opposite leads are not present. In later stages of pericarditis (days or weeks after presentation), the ST segment returns to baseline, and thereafter the T waves may deeply invert.[1]

The PR segment is found to be depressed (or elevated in lead aVR) in 75% to 80% of patients with acute pericarditis.[2] This finding may be the result of abnormal atrial repolarization due to atrial inflammation and is not typical of other conditions such as acute MI. PR-segment depression may occur even in the absence of ST-segment elevation and can be the initial, or only, electrocardiographic manifestation of acute pericarditis. Sinus tachycardia is also a common finding in acute pericarditis, related to pericardial inflammation, pain, or fever.

REFERENCES

1. Khandaker MH, Espinosa RE, Nishimura RA, et al: Pericardial disease: Diagnosis and management. Mayo Clin Proc 85:572, 2010.
2. Lange RA, Hillis LD: Clinical practice: Acute pericarditis. N Engl J Med 351:2195, 2004.

ANSWER TO QUESTION 460

E (Braunwald, p. 1668)

Two forms of pericarditis can follow acute MI: early and delayed. Early acute fibrinous pericarditis develops within the first few days. The incidence and degree of such pericardial inflammation are associated with the size of the infarct. The use of thrombolytic therapy, which limits infarct size, reduces the incidence of this complication, and the earlier reperfusion therapy is delivered, the lower is the incidence of pericarditis. In addition, pericarditis is less common after non–ST-segment elevation infarction. The use of heparin has *not* been associated with increased risk of pericarditis or tamponade. Clinical evidence of pericarditis can be found as early as 12 hours after MI, and the earliest sign may be a pericardial friction rub. In about 70% of patients, the rub may be accompanied by pleuritic chest pain.

The appearance of symptoms and signs of pericarditis more than 10 days after MI suggests the second type of post-MI pericarditis, termed the *Dressler syndrome*. This delayed phenomenon is believed to be autoimmune, arising from the sensitization to myocardial cells at the time of infarction. Typical diagnostic electrocardiographic changes of pericarditis are uncommon in post-MI pericarditis or Dressler syndrome. Instead, atypical T wave changes have been described, consisting of persistently upright T waves or premature reversal of initially inverted T waves after the infarction.

REFERENCE

Imazio M, Negro A, Belli R, et al: Frequency and prognostic significance of pericarditis following acute myocardial infarction treated by primary percutaneous coronary intervention. Am J Cardiol 103:1525, 2009.

ANSWER TO QUESTION 461

D (Braunwald, pp. 1585-1586)

The tracing demonstrates simultaneous recordings of left ventricular (LV) and systemic pressure in a patient in normal sinus rhythm. The second electrocardiographic complex is a ventricular premature beat (VPB). The beat following the VPB demonstrates a rise in LV pressure due to post-extrasystolic potentiation. However, the aortic systolic pressure and the pulse pressure decline in the post-VPB beat. This is an example of the Brockenbrough-Braunwald phenomenon that is typical of hypertrophic cardiomyopathy (HCM) and is a reliable sign of dynamic LV outflow tract obstruction.

In normal subjects, and even in those with valvular abnormalities such as aortic stenosis or mitral regurgitation, a post-VPB contraction is associated with an increased systolic aortic pressure and pulse pressure. Conversely, in HCM, the premature contraction increases the force of contraction and the degree of outflow obstruction of the subsequent beat, with a decline in the pulse pressure. While increased ventricular filling during the post-VPB compensatory pause would be expected to reduce the outflow gradient in HCM, that effect is outweighed by the increased contractility associated with post-extrasystolic potentiation. In addition to the narrowed pulse pressure, the peripheral arterial waveform may show a "spike-and-dome" configuration, reflecting the attenuation of LV output due to dynamic outflow obstruction.

REFERENCES

Fifer MA, Vlahakes GJ: Management of symptoms in hypertrophic cardiomyopathy. Circulation 117:429, 2008.

Gersh BJ, Maron BJ, Bonow RO, et al: 2011 ACCF/AHA guideline for the diagnosis and treatment of hypertrophic cardiomyopathy: Executive summary. J Am Coll Cardiol 58:2703, 2011.

ANSWER TO QUESTION 462

D (Braunwald, pp. 1456-1457)

Valvular aortic stenosis (AS) is a relatively common congenital anomaly. It has been estimated to occur in 3% to 6% of patients with congenital cardiovascular defects and is seen more frequently in males than in females, with a sex ratio of approximately 4:1. Up to 20% of individuals with congenital valvular AS have associated cardiovascular anomalies, of which patent ductus arteriosus and coarctation of the aorta are most frequent. The majority of children with congenital AS develop and grow in a normal manner and are asymptomatic. The diagnosis is therefore usually suspected when a murmur is detected on physical examination. When symptoms do occur, the most common include fatigability, exertional dyspnea, syncope, and angina pectoris. In general, the presence of symptoms suggests critical stenosis.

Findings on physical examination of children with congenital valvular AS depend on the age of the patient. In newborns, a murmur may be difficult to hear despite significant obstruction. Rather, the examination is notable for weak pulses and signs of heart failure. In older children, the signs can include an ejection click, followed by a systolic murmur along the left sternal border.

The ECG in congenital AS is generally notable for left ventricular hypertrophy with or without "strain." Echocardiography with continuous-wave Doppler flow analysis is accurate in diagnosing the morphology and severity of congenital AS, as well as the presence of associated left-sided lesions.

Cardiac catheterization in infants and young children with valvular AS is rarely indicated to determine the site or severity of the lesion, given the established reliability of noninvasive evaluation. Rather, cardiac catheterization is performed when interventional balloon valvuloplasty is considered.

Participation in competitive sports is usually restricted in patients with milder degrees of obstruction, and strict avoidance of strenuous physical activity is advisable if advanced AS is present.[1] Aortic valvulotomy is a safe, effective initial treatment for congenital valvular AS in children. Because the leaflets remain deformed, subsequent degeneration and calcification may ensue, leading to valve replacement surgery in approximately 35% of patients within 15 to 20 years of the original operation.[2]

REFERENCES

1. Graham TP, Driscoll DJ, Gersony WM, et al: Task Force 2: Congenital heart disease. J Am Coll Cardiol 45:1326, 2005.
2. Detter C, Fischlein T, Feldmeier C, et al: Aortic valvotomy for congenital valvular aortic stenosis: A 37-year experience. Ann Thorac Surg 71:1564, 2001.

ANSWER TO QUESTION 463

E (Braunwald, pp. 1411-1412)

Whereas the true incidence of congenital cardiovascular malformations is difficult to determine, it has been estimated that approximately 0.8% of live births are complicated by such a disorder. The most common significant malformation is ventricular septal defect, followed in frequency by atrial septal defect (ASD) and patent ductus arteriosus. These data do not take into account the common anomalies of a congenital, functionally normal bicuspid aortic valve and mitral valve prolapse.

Specific defects show a sex predilection. For example, patent ductus arteriosus and ASDs are more common in females, whereas valvular aortic stenosis, congenital aneurysms of the sinus of Valsalva, coarctation of the aorta, tetralogy of Fallot, and transposition of the great arteries are seen more frequently in males. Extracardiac anomalies occur in approximately 25% of infants born with significant cardiac disease and often are multiple.

Approximately one third of infants with both cardiac and extracardiac anomalies have an established syndrome. For example, maternal rubella during pregnancy is associated with the rubella syndrome, which consists of cataracts, deafness, microcephaly, and some combination of patent ductus arteriosus, pulmonic valvular or arterial stenosis or both, and ASD. Maternal systemic lupus erythematosus during pregnancy has been linked to congenital complete heart block but not to any specific anatomic abnormality.

REFERENCE

Hoffman JI, Kaplan S: The incidence of congenital heart disease. J Am Coll Cardiol 39:1890, 2002.

ANSWER TO QUESTION 464

D (Braunwald, pp. 1556-1557; Table 67G-1)

In 2007 the American Heart Association published updated guidelines for the prevention of infective endocarditis (IE), which significantly reduced the number of patients for whom antibiotic prophylaxis is recommended. The statement recognizes that (1) infective endocarditis is more likely to occur after random bacteremias (e.g., after daily tooth brushing) than from dental and/or genitourinary or gastrointestinal procedures; and (2) because prophylaxis may prevent only a small number of cases of IE, the risk of antibiotic use in many cases may outweigh the benefit.

According to the revised guidelines, prophylaxis is only recommended for those patients with cardiac conditions associated with the highest risk of endocarditis, including the presence of (1) prosthetic cardiac valves, (2) previous infective endocarditis, (3) cardiac transplantation recipients who develop cardiac valvulopathy, and (4) specific types of congenital heart disease (unrepaired cyanotic lesions, repaired congenital lesions with residual defects, or during the first 6 months after repair with prosthetic material or device). Prophylaxis is not recommended for native valvular abnormalities such as mitral valve prolapse with murmur.

REFERENCE

Wilson W, Taubert KA, Gewitz M, et al: Prevention of infective endocarditis—recommendations by the American Heart Association. Circulation 115:1656, 2007.

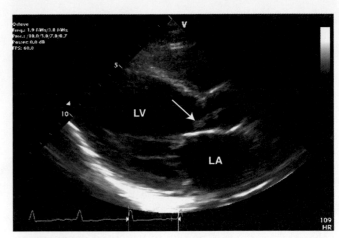

FIGURE 4-33

ANSWER TO QUESTION 465

B (Braunwald, p. 1548)

This patient has endocarditis, with an aortic valve vegetation on the noncoronary cusp as indicated by the arrow in Figure 4-33. The vegetation prolapses into the left ventricular (LV) outflow tract in the diastolic image displayed. The left ventricle is enlarged (>6-cm diameter in this figure, referencing the 1-cm markers on the left side of the figure) and the left atrial diameter is increased at 4.5 cm. There are no signs of mitral valve prolapse on this diastolic image.

Echocardiography is helpful in the diagnosis and assessment of infective endocarditis by virtue of its ability to identify vegetations and evaluate valvular dysfunction and complications. The sensitivity of transthoracic echocardiography (TTE) for this diagnosis is limited and depends on the size of the vegetation. For example, the sensitivity of TTE is 25% for vegetations <5 mm in diameter and 70% for vegetations between 6 to 10 mm in diameter. In contrast, transesophageal echocardiography has reported sensitivity of 85% to 95% for the detection of vegetations. Echocardiography is also very useful in identifying the complications of endocarditis, such as leaflet perforation, valvular regurgitation, and the development of a myocardial or aortic abscess.

REFERENCE

Kini V, Logani S, Ky B, et al: Transthoracic and transesophageal echocardiography for the indication of suspected infective endocarditis: Vegetations, blood cultures and imaging. J Am Soc Echocardiogr 23:396, 2010.

ANSWER TO QUESTION 466

C (Braunwald, pp. 1523-1525)

Homograft (also known as allograft) aortic valves are harvested from cadavers, sterilized, cryopreserved, and then placed directly into the recipient's heart without the use of a prosthetic stent. The popularity of aortic homografts has increased because this type of valve provides potential advantages over bioprosthetic (xenograft) and mechanical prostheses. The rate of thromboembolism is very low, similar to that of bioprosthetic valves, and therefore lifelong anticoagulation is not necessary. In addition, homografts appear to be more resistant to infection than other prostheses, so they are often chosen for patients with infective endocarditis of the aortic valve who are in need of an urgent operation. They provide a more physiologic hemodynamic profile than mechanical valves, and, because a prosthetic support stent is not used, they are also hemodynamically superior to stented porcine tissue valves.

In experienced hands, the surgical mortality related to homograft placement is 1% to 2%, similar to that of other valve replacements.[1] The rate of structural degeneration of cryopreserved homografts is similar to that of porcine xenografts. Valve dysfunction develops in 20% of patients by 10 years postoperatively, and in over 50% of patients 15 years postoperatively, although rates may be lower in those who undergo complete aortic root homograft replacement.[1,2]

REFERENCES

1. Melina G, De Robertis F, Gaer JA, et al: Mid-term pattern of survival, hemodynamic performance and rate of complications after Medtronic Freestyle versus homograft full aortic root replacement: Results from a prospective randomized trial. J Heart Valve Dis 13:973, 2004.
2. Palka P, Harrocks S, Lange A, et al: Primary aortic valve replacement with cryopreserved aortic allograft: An echocardiographic follow-up study of 570 patients. Circulation 105:61, 2002.

ANSWER TO QUESTION 467

D (Braunwald, pp. 1492-1493)

The echocardiographic image demonstrates diastolic doming of the mitral valve leaflets, typical of rheumatic mitral stenosis (MS). Patients with preserved flexibility of the leaflets in MS (i.e., fusion confined to the valve commissures) demonstrate an accentuated S_1. This is thought to occur because the persistent pressure gradient between the left atrium and left ventricle at the end of diastole keeps the flexible portion of the leaflets in a maximally separated position prior to ventricular contraction. Contraction then forces the leaflets together from a relatively wide position, causing the intensity of S_1 to be loud. If, however, the valve is markedly calcified, there is little movement of the leaflets during the cardiac cycle, such that S_1 becomes abnormally soft.

The opening snap occurs when the left ventricular diastolic pressure falls below that of the left atrium and the stenotic mitral leaflets open. The more severe the mitral stenosis, the higher the left atrial pressure becomes, such that mitral opening occurs earlier and therefore the interval between A_2 and the opening snap shortens. In patients with long standing MS, pulmonary hypertension develops, in part because of chronically elevated left atrial pressure. As a result, P_2 becomes accentuated. The intensity of the diastolic murmur is not a good guide to the severity of mitral stenosis. A more reliable sign is the duration of the murmur: increasing severity of stenosis causes greater persistence of the gradient between the left atrium and left ventricle, and therefore the murmur lasts longer in diastole.

REFERENCE

Chandrashekhar Y, Westaby S, Narula J: Mitral stenosis. Lancet 374:1271, 2009.

ANSWER TO QUESTION 468

A (Braunwald, p. 1481)

The murmur of aortic regurgitation (AR) is of high frequency and begins immediately after A_2. It is best heard with the diaphragm of the stethoscope applied firmly while the patient is sitting up and leaning forward, with the breath held in expiration. The severity of regurgitation correlates better with the duration rather than severity of the murmur, and in cases of severe AR, a holodiastolic murmur with a "rough" quality may be heard. However, with the development of heart failure, equilibration of aortic and left ventricular diastolic pressures abolishes the late diastolic component and the murmur becomes shorter. When the murmur is musical ("cooing dove" murmur), it usually signifies eversion or perforation of a cusp, and when it is louder on the right side of the sternum, it usually indicates the presence of a dilated ascending aorta, which may be the underlying cause of the valvular insufficiency. In general, maneuvers that increase afterload, such as a strenuous handgrip, augment aortic regurgitation and the associated murmur.

ANSWER TO QUESTION 469

A (Braunwald, p. 1666)

Bacterial (purulent) pericarditis tends to occur via one of several mechanisms, including hematogenous seeding during bacteremia, contiguous spread of infection after thoracic surgery or after rupture of a perivalvular abscess in endocarditis. The majority of occurrences, however, are attributable to direct extension from an adjacent pulmonary infection. Several factors may predispose to the development of purulent pericarditis, including a preexisting pericardial effusion in uremic pericarditis, or in immunosuppressed states such as that seen in burns, hematologic malignancies, or human immunodeficiency virus infection/acquired immunodeficiency syndrome. Bacterial pericarditis is usually an acute fulminant illness of rapid onset that is characterized by high spiking fevers, shaking chills, night sweats, and dyspnea. Typical symptoms of pericarditis may be absent, and the process may be heralded by new jugular venous distention and pulsus paradoxus as a result of cardiac tamponade.

Despite the lower incidence of purulent pericarditis in the antibiotic era, overall survival continues to be very poor, with a mortality of approximately 30% in most series. The poor prognosis is in large part due to delayed diagnosis, as well as disease severity and comorbidities. Early complete surgical drainage and appropriate parenteral antibiotic therapy are important parts of the treatment of this devastating disorder. High concentrations of antibiotics may be achieved in pericardial fluid with parenteral therapy; therefore, instillation of antibiotics directly into the pericardial space is not warranted.

REFERENCE

Imazio M, Brucato A, Mayosi BM, et al: Medical therapy of pericardial diseases: I. Idiopathic and infectious pericarditis. J Cardiovasc Med (Hagerstown) 11:712, 2010.

ANSWER TO QUESTION 470

A (Braunwald, p. 1590)

This 16-year-old youth has an examination and ECG consistent with hypertrophic cardiomyopathy, which could be confirmed by echocardiography. Current recommendations are that competitive sports not be allowed in this condition if high-risk clinical features are present, including marked ventricular hypertrophy, evidence of significant outflow gradient, supraventricular or ventricular arrhythmias, history of exertional syncope or hypotension, or history of sudden death in close relatives. Low-intensity sports may be allowed if none of these conditions is present. This boy has evidence of left ventricular hypertrophy on the ECG and a history of sudden death in a first cousin. Thus, competitive sports should be restricted.

REFERENCE

Maron BJ, Haas TS, Doerer JJ, et al: Comparison of U.S. and Italian experiences with sudden cardiac deaths in young competitive athletes and implications for preparticipation screening strategies. Am J Cardiol 104:276, 2009.

ANSWER TO QUESTION 471

C (Braunwald, pp. 1469-1472)

The left ventricle responds to *sudden* obstruction to outflow by dilatation and reduction of stroke volume. However, in most adults with aortic stenosis the obstruction develops slowly over a long period of time, resulting in significant compensatory measures. Fundamentally, left ventricular (LV) output is maintained by development of LV hypertrophy. This enables the heart to sustain a large pressure gradient across the aortic valve without reduction in cardiac output, LV dilatation, or symptoms. The compensation is contributed to by coexisting left atrial (LA) hypertrophy; the more forceful atrial contraction helps to maintain appropriate LV filling. This is expressed by the development of a large *a* wave in the LA pressure curve and an elevated LV end-diastolic pressure. The latter is also augmented by the reduced LV diastolic compliance due to the ventricular hypertrophy. However, it is only the patient with LV contractile dysfunction in whom dilatation and an increase in LV end-diastolic volume occur.

ANSWER TO QUESTION 472

D (Braunwald, pp. 1547-1549)

Although helpful, the observation of vegetations by echocardiography is not mandatory to establish the diagnosis of endocarditis. In addition, although the sensitivity of transesophageal echocardiography to detect vegetations in suspected endocarditis is 85% to 95%, the sensitivity of transthoracic echocardiography is substantially less (see Answer to Question 465). *Staphylococcus aureus* is a particularly aggressive organism that results in rapid destruction of valves and perivalvular tissue. Nonetheless, antibiotic therapy alone is often curative for native valve endocarditis caused by this organism. Recent studies have found that vegetations > 10 mm in diameter have a greater risk of thromboembolism than smaller vegetations, but it has not been proved that early surgical intervention in patients with larger vegetations improves the long-term outcome. Therefore, a vegetation size > 10 mm is considered a relative indication for surgery. Although cerebral embolism can be a devastating complication of endocarditis, the rate of recurrence declines during the course of appropriate antibiotic treatment. Patients with endocarditis and intractable heart failure due to valve dysfunction have a 55% to 85% mortality rate when treated medically; the mortality falls to 10% to 30% with early surgical intervention.

REFERENCE

Ansari A, Rigolin VH: Infective endocarditis: An update on the role of echocardiography. Curr Cardiol Rep 12:265, 2010.

ANSWER TO QUESTION 473

E (Braunwald, pp. 1666-1667)

Although tuberculous pericarditis is now uncommon in industrialized nations, the disease continues to be an important problem is developing nations and in immunosuppressed patients. Tuberculous pericarditis usually develops by retrograde spread from peritracheal, peribronchial, or mediastinal lymph nodes or by early hematogenous spread from the primary tuberculous infection. The process is usually chronic, with gradual development of pericardial effusion. Symptoms may be systemic and nonspecific, and clinical detection of tuberculous pericarditis often does not occur until the effusive or late constrictive pericarditic stages are reached. The typical pericardial chest pain of acute viral or idiopathic pericarditis is uncommon in tuberculous pericarditis. In addition, typical signs or symptoms of cavitary pulmonary tuberculosis are usually absent.

Examination of patients with tuberculous pericarditis may reveal evidence of chronic cardiac compression, which can mimic heart failure. Common symptoms include cough, dyspnea, orthopnea, weight loss, and peripheral edema. Definitive diagnosis of tuberculous pericarditis is usually difficult because of the low yield of the bacillus in pericardial fluid, failure of the bacillus to grow on an appropriate medium, and/or the need to observe cultures for a minimum of 8 weeks. The probability of a definitive diagnosis is greatest if both pericardial fluid and a pericardial biopsy are obtained in the effusive stage of the disease. Polymerase chain reaction amplification of pericardial specimens offers the potential to obtain results much more rapidly than standard cultures. Measurement of pericardial fluid adenosine deaminase is diagnostically useful, with reported sensitivity and specificity for tuberculous pericarditis of 88% and 83%, respectively.

Initial therapy for tuberculous pericarditis includes a three-drug regimen ordinarily consisting of isoniazid, rifampin, and streptomycin or ethambutol. The role of corticosteroids in this setting remains unclear. Studies have failed to show that the early use of corticosteroids affects mortality or progression to constriction, although such therapy may shorten the duration of symptoms.

REFERENCE

Syed FF, Mayosi BM: A modern approach to tuberculous pericarditis. Prog Cardiovasc Dis 50:218, 2007.

ANSWER TO QUESTION 474

C (Braunwald, p. 1578; see also Answer to Question 451)

This patient has findings of carcinoid syndrome, characterized by episodic flushing, diarrhea, and bronchoconstriction. The vast majority of carcinoid tumors originate in the appendix and other areas of the gastrointestinal tract, with the remainder arising in the respiratory tract. Carcinoid tumors secrete large amounts of vasoactive substances, including serotonin and bradykinin, which are usually inactivated by the liver, lungs, and brain. However, in the presence of large hepatic metastases, these vasoactive substances reach the systemic circulation and heart. Cardiovascular involvement occurs in up to two thirds of patients with carcinoid syndrome and includes the formation of fibrous plaques in the right heart endocardium, which can lead to fixation and retraction of the tricuspid and pulmonic valves.[1] This results in tricuspid and/or pulmonic valve dysfunction and eventual right-sided heart failure. Higher circulating serotonin levels are associated with greater severity and progression of cardiac disease.[2] Left-sided heart involvement is not common (occurring in <10% of patients) presumably because of pulmonary inactivation of the vasoactive hormones.[2] Patients who do develop left-sided disease may have a right-to-left intracardiac shunt or a primary pulmonary carcinoid tumor. It is rare for carcinoid tumor to metastasize to the heart.

REFERENCES

1. Fox DJ, Chattar RS: Carcinoid heart disease: Presentation, diagnosis, and management. Heart 90:1224, 2004.
2. Gustafsson BI, Hauso O, Drozdov I, et al: Carcinoid heart. Int J Cardiol 129:318, 2008.

ANSWER TO QUESTION 475

C (Braunwald, pp. 1495-1497; see also Answer to Question 447)

Percutaneous balloon mitral valvuloplasty (BMV) is the treatment of choice for patients with mitral stenosis who require mechanical intervention. Surgical valve repair or replacement is now reserved for patients who are not candidates for the percutaneous procedure. In the most commonly practiced form of BMV, a catheter is maneuvered across the interatrial septum through a small puncture and a balloon device is advanced across the mitral valve. Balloon inflation separates and fractures the calcified valve commissures, improving the transmitral gradient, valve area, and cardiac output. Selection of patients for this approach is usually determined by echocardiographic features including (1) mitral valve rigidity, (2) leaflet thickening, (3) valve calcification, and (4) subvalvular apparatus thickening and calcification. In a commonly used scoring system, each of these factors is assigned a score from 0 to 4, with 0 representing the absence of each abnormality and 4 representing the most severe form (Table 4-1). A total score ≤8 is associated with excellent results after balloon valvuloplasty. Transesophageal echocardiography is usually performed before the procedure to exclude the presence of left atrial thrombus, a potential source of embolism during catheter manipulation.

The major complications of BMV include death (1% to 2%), thromboembolism (1% to 2%), cardiac perforation (1%), and severe mitral regurgitation requiring surgical repair (approximately 2%). A small residual iatrogenic atrial septal defect persists in approximately 5% of patients and is rarely hemodynamically significant.

REFERENCE

Nobuyoshi M, Arita T, Shirai S, et al: Percutaneous balloon mitral valvuloplasty: A review. Circulation 119:211, 2009.

ANSWER TO QUESTION 476

B (Braunwald, pp. 1672-1673)

The incidence of cardiac injury after blunt chest trauma varies by mode of injury and criteria for diagnosis but ranges between 10% and 50%. The diagnosis of cardiac injury after blunt chest trauma requires a high index of suspicion. Immediate evaluation should include assessment for cardiac tamponade (e.g., hypotension, pulsus paradoxus, distended jugular veins, and muffled heart sounds). Chest radiography is an important part of this evaluation that can identify pneumothorax, bony fractures, or an enlarged cardiac silhouette suggesting pericardial effusion. Echocardiography can confirm the presence of traumatic blood in the pericardial space, but a transthoracic study often has limited value in identifying other consequences of blunt trauma as the accompanying chest wall injuries render the study technically limited. Conversely, transesophageal

TABLE 4-1 ECHOCARDIOGRAPHIC SCORE USED TO PREDICT OUTCOME OF MITRAL BALLOON VALVULOPLASTY*

GRADE	MOBILITY	SUBVALVULAR THICKENING	THICKENING	CALCIFICATION
1	Highly mobile valve with only leaflet tips restricted	Minimal thickening just below the mitral leaflets	Leaflets nearly normal in thickness (4-5 mm)	A single area of increased echo brightness
2	Leaflet mid and base portions have normal mobility	Thickening of chordal structures extending up to one third of the chordal length	Mid leaflets normal, considerable thickening of margins (5-8 mm)	Scattered areas of brightness confined to leaflet margins
3	Valve continues to move forward in diastole, mainly from the base	Thickening extending to the distal third of the chords	Thickening extending through the entire leaflet (5-8 mm)	Brightness extending into the midportion of the leaflets
4	No or minimal forward movement of the leaflets in diastole	Extensive thickening and shortening of all chordal structures extending down to the papillary muscles	Considerable thickening of all leaflet tissue (>8-10 mm)	Extensive brightness throughout much of the leaflet tissue

*The total echocardiographic score was derived from an analysis of mitral leaflet mobility, valvular and subvalvular thickening, and calcification, which were graded from 0 (normal) to 4 according to the above criteria. This gave a total score of 0 to 16.

Modified from Oh JK, Seward JB, Tajik AJ: The Echo Manual. 3rd ed. Philadelphia, Lippincott Williams & Wilkins, 2006. Used with permission of Mayo Foundation for Medical Education and Research.

echocardiography is more sensitive in identifying the effects of blunt injury, including traumatic ventricular septal defects, rupture of chordae tendineae or portions of papillary muscle with valvular insufficiency, and wall motion abnormalities.

The most common electrocardiographic abnormality in blunt cardiac trauma is sinus tachycardia. Other common findings include ST-segment abnormalities, atrioventricular blocks, right bundle branch blocks (with or without left anterior fascicular block), atrial fibrillation, and ventricular dysrhythmias. Although debate exists over the role of cardiac-specific biomarker elevations after chest trauma, studies have not shown a consistent correlation between cardiac troponin I or T levels and the presence and prognosis of blunt cardiac injury.

REFERENCES

Cook CC, Gleason TG: Great vessel and cardiac trauma. Surg Clin North Am 89:797, 2009.

Elie MC: Blunt cardiac injury. Mt Sinai J Med 73:542, 2006.

ANSWER TO QUESTION 477

B (Braunwald, pp. 1575-1576)

Clinical cardiac involvement occurs in fewer than 5% of patients with pulmonary sarcoidosis, although at autopsy granulomas are found in the myocardium of 20% to 30% of patients with this condition.[1]

The typical pathologic feature of sarcoidosis is the presence of noncaseating granulomas that infiltrate the myocardium and eventually become fibrotic scars. The granulomas may involve any region of the heart, but the left ventricular (LV) free wall and interventricular septum are the most common sites. The extensive granular scar tissue in the septum leads to conduction system abnormalities. Involvement of cardiac valves is unusual. The murmur of mitral regurgitation is common; however, it appears to be caused by LV dilatation rather than by direct sarcoid involvement of either papillary muscles or the valve.[2]

The diagnosis of sarcoid heart disease may be suspected in patients with bilateral hilar adenopathy on chest radiography, in whom there is clinical or echocardiographic evidence of myocardial dysfunction. Percutaneous myocardial biopsy may be useful in establishing the diagnosis; however, cardiac involvement tends to be patchy such that a negative biopsy does not exclude the diagnosis. Cardiac imaging with thallium-201 or technetium-99m sestamibi typically demonstrates segmental perfusion defects resulting from granulomatous infiltration. Magnetic resonance imaging (MRI) has emerged as a useful modality for diagnosis of this condition. On contrast-enhanced MRI, focal areas of increased signal intensity demarcate disease foci.

Sudden death is the most common cause of mortality in sarcoid heart disease, likely resulting from paroxysmal arrhythmias or high-grade atrioventricular block. Because the risk of sudden death appears to be greatest in patients with extensive myocardial involvement, it is reasonable to administer glucocorticosteroids to such patients, although the benefit of this approach has not been confirmed in prospective trials. Arrhythmias in this condition may be refractory to standard therapy, and insertion of an implantable cardiac defibrillator should be considered in those deemed at high risk of sudden death. In other cases, permanent pacing may be appropriate for those with advanced heart block.[3]

REFERENCES

1. Fasano R, Rimmerman CM, Jaber WA: Cardiac sarcoidosis: A cause of infiltrative cardiomyopathy. Cleve Clin J Med 781:483, 2004.
2. Dubrey SW, Falk RH: Diagnosis and management of cardiac sarcoidosis. Prog Cardiovasc Dis 52:33, 2010.
3. Kim JS, Judson MA, Donnino R, et al: Cardiac sarcoidosis. Am Heart J 157:21, 2009.

ANSWER TO QUESTION 478

C (Braunwald, pp. 1430-1432)

The size of a VSD and the degree to which pulmonary vascular resistance is altered lead to varied clinical presentations in adults with this lesion. In general, patients with small defects are asymptomatic and are not at risk for the development of pulmonary vascular obstructive disease. However, all patients with ventricular septal defects are at increased risk for infective endocarditis, which arises in up to 4% of individuals with VSDs.[1] This complication usually occurs by the third or fourth decade of life. The infection usually develops in the right ventricle at the site where shunted blood impacts against the ventricular wall.

In an asymptomatic individual, a VSD with a normal pulmonary artery pressure and a pulmonary:systemic flow ratio < 1.5:1 generally does not require surgical closure. Women with VSDs that lead to pulmonary: systemic flow ratios < 2:1 and only modest pulmonary hypertension generally tolerate pregnancy very well. In women with larger left-to-right shunts, however, LV failure may occur during pregnancy. In those who have Eisenmenger complex, pregnancy is extremely poorly tolerated, with a maternal mortality between 40% and 45%.[2] The development of Eisenmenger complex due to progressive pulmonary vascular disease is one of the most dreaded complications in patients with VSD. This usually occurs in early adulthood, at the end of the second or during the third decade of life,[3] and may be complicated by heart failure, hemoptysis, chest pain, cerebral abscess, thromboembolism, and sudden death.

REFERENCES

1. Gabriel HM, Heger M, Innerhofer P, et al: Long-term outcome of patients with ventricular septal defect considered not to require surgical closure during childhood. J Am Coll Cardiol 39:1066, 2002.
2. Minette MS, Sahn DJ: Ventricular septal defects. Circulation 114:2190, 2006.
3. Brickner ME, Hillis LD, Lange RA: Congenital heart disease in adults. N Engl J Med 342:334, 2000.

ANSWER TO QUESTION 479

C (Braunwald, pp. 1576-1578)

Endomyocardial fibrosis (EMF) is found primarily in tropical and subtropical Africa, although it has been increasingly recognized in tropical regions in South America, Asia, and the Middle East. It is most common in children and young adults and only occasionally manifests in older individuals. It results in fibrous obliteration of the apex of the affected ventricle(s) and typically involves the papillary muscles and chordae tendineae. EMF affects both ventricles in approximately 50% of patients, purely the left ventricle in 40%, and solely the right ventricle in 10%.

Echocardiographic features include increased endocardial reflectivity, fibrotic obliteration of the affected ventricular apex, atrial enlargement, and pericardial effusion. Fibrotic lesions of the papillary muscles and chordae tendineae distort the valve apparatus and, in the case of the left ventricle, lead to mitral *regurgitation*.

Clinical features of EMF depend on which of the ventricles is involved: left-sided disease manifests as pulmonary congestion and right-sided involvement may manifests as symptoms and signs similar to restrictive cardiomyopathy or constrictive pericarditis. The clinical course of EMF tends to be progressive and complications include heart failure and thromboemboli, because the fibrotic tissue provides a site for thrombus formation. Up to 50% of patients with advanced disease die within 2 years.

REFERENCE

Hassan WM, Fawzy ME, Al Helaly S, et al: Pitfalls in diagnosis and clinical, echocardiographic, and hemodynamic findings in endomyocardial fibrosis: A 25-year experience. Chest 128:3985, 2005.

ANSWER TO QUESTION 480

A (Braunwald, p. 1590)

Clinical features that have been most consistently associated with a high risk of sudden death in HCM include prior cardiac arrest or sustained ventricular tachycardia, presence of nonsustained ventricular tachycardia (NSVT) on ambulatory Holter monitoring, unexplained syncope, young age (<30 years) at diagnosis, family history of HCM with SCD, an abnormal hypotensive blood pressure response to exercise, and an extreme degree of hypertrophy (left ventricular wall thickness ≥ 3.0 cm). The specific genetic defect, although not always identifiable, may also provide prognostic information. For example, certain mutations in genes that encode troponin T confer a higher risk of sudden death.[1] Approximately 25% to 30% of patients with HCM demonstrate dynamic left ventricular outflow tract obstruction, and although patients with a gradient have an overall higher incidence of death than those without a gradient, the risk of sudden death does not increase above a threshold of 30 mm Hg.[2] The presence of NSVT on a 48-hour ambulatory Holter monitor portends an increased risk of sudden death, particularly in younger patients.[3]

REFERENCES

1. Braunwald E, Seidman CE, Sigwart U: Contemporary evaluation and management of hypertrophic cardiomyopathy. Circulation 106:1312, 2002.
2. Maron MS, Olivetto I, Betocchi S, et al: Effect of left ventricular outflow tract obstruction on clinical outcome in hypertrophic cardiomyopathy. N Engl J Med 348:295, 2003.
3. Monserrat L, Elliott PM, Gimeno JR, et al: Non-sustained ventricular tachycardia in hypertrophic cardiomyopathy: An independent marker of sudden death risk in young patients. J Am Coll Cardiol 42:873, 2003.

ANSWER TO QUESTION 481

B (Braunwald, pp. 1435-1436)

Classic tetralogy of Fallot is marked by a large ventricular septal defect (VSD) in association with infundibular or valvular pulmonic stenosis or both, right ventricular (RV) hypertrophy, and an overriding aorta. In all cases, the VSD is located proximal to the level of the RV outflow tract obstruction and is therefore associated with elevated RV systolic pressure and right-to-left shunting. This is in contrast to the situation in patients who have a double-chambered right ventricle and a membranous VSD, in whom the septal defect communicates with the low-pressure distal portion of the right ventricle and leads to simple VSD physiology rather than the right-to-left shunting and cyanosis that mark tetralogy of Fallot.

Symptoms and clinical findings of tetralogy of Fallot depend on the severity of RV outflow tract obstruction. With only mild obstruction, a left-to-right shunt through the VSD is predominant and the patient may remain acyanotic. The condition in patients with RV obstruction severe enough to cause cyanosis usually is recognized during infancy or early childhood; such patients may then undergo palliative or total surgical repair. Patients with uncorrected tetralogy of Fallot who survive into adult life usually have at most moderate obstruction to RV outflow, in association with relatively well-preserved pulmonary blood flow. At the other end of the spectrum, if obstruction to RV outflow is complete, a large obligatory right-to-left shunt will be present, and the lungs are then perfused through collateral vessels that arise from systemic vessels. In these patients there is severe cyanosis, absence of the typical systolic heart murmur, and the presence of a continuous murmur that originates from bronchial collateral vessels. This variant of tetralogy of Fallot is termed *pseudotruncus arteriosus*.

Because the large VSD allows for decompression of the right ventricle in tetralogy of Fallot, the RV systolic pressure does not exceed that in the aorta, even in the presence of severe obstruction to RV outflow. Congestive heart failure is unusual in patients with tetralogy of Fallot. Instead, a decrease in cardiac reserve in adults with this condition is more typical, with symptoms of dyspnea and limited exercise tolerance.

REFERENCES

Bashore TM: Adult congenital heart disease: Right ventricular outflow tract lesions. Circulation 115:1933, 2007.

Kalra N, Klewer SE, Raasch H, Sorrell VL: Update on tetralogy of Fallot for the adult cardiologist including a brief historical and surgical perspective. Congenit Heart Dis 5:208, 2010.

ANSWER TO QUESTION 482

D (Braunwald, p. 1544)

The HACEK group of organisms refers to a number of gram-negative bacilli that are among the less common causes of endocarditis. The E in HACEK stands for *Eikenella corrodens*, not *Escherichia coli*. Although they are fastidious and slow growing, HACEK organisms can usually be detected in blood cultures within 5 days. Native valve endocarditis with HACEK organisms have been associated with large vegetations and a high frequency of systemic emboli. All of these organisms share common antibiotic sensitivities.

ANSWER TO QUESTION 483

E (Braunwald, p. 1578)

Endocardial fibroelastosis (EFE) is a rare disorder of fetuses and infants in which there is thickening of the endocardium due to deposition of collagen and elastin. This entity is distinct from endomyocardial fibrosis (see Answer to Question 479), a tropical and subtropical condition in which there is prominent myocardial involvement and, commonly, eosinophilia. EFE does not appear to be a specific disease but rather a reaction in the first 1 to 2 years of life to stressors that include viral infections (including mumps exposure during fetal life), metabolic disorders, and congenital left-sided obstructive lesions.[1] Recent reports also implicate mitochondrial disorders and placental insufficiency as causative.[2] EFE predominantly involves the left ventricle and usually progresses to severe congestive heart failure and death.

The echocardiographic finding of a highly reflective endocardial surface of the ventricular myocardium suggests the presence of endocardial fibroelastosis.

REFERENCES

1. Lurie PR: Changing concepts of endocardial fibroelastosis. Cardiol Young 20:115, 2010.
2. Perez MH, Boulos T, Stucki P, et al: Placental immaturity, endocardial fibroelastosis and fetal hypoxia. Fetal Diagn Ther 26:107, 2009.

ANSWER TO QUESTION 484

C (Braunwald, pp. 1441-1443)

The Fontan procedure, developed originally for tricuspid atresia, involves surgical diversion of systemic venous return directly to the pulmonary arteries without passing through a subpulmonary ventricle. It is a palliative, not curative, operation. The majority of patients (~90%) are in functional Class I or II 5 years after the operation, but progressive deterioration over time is typical. The most common causes of death are due to congestive heart failure and arrhythmias.

Physical findings after the Fontan procedure include an elevated nonpulsatile jugular venous pulse and a *single* S_2 (the pulmonary artery is typically tied off).

Supraventricular arrhythmias are common (especially atrial fibrillation and flutter), observed in 15% to 20% of patients by 5 years after the operation, and the development of such arrhythmias can lead to hemodynamic deterioration and heart failure. Thromboemboli occur in 6% to 25% of patients, sources of which include the atrial arrhythmias, right atrial dilatation with blood stasis, and the potentially thrombogenic material used to construct the circuit.

Protein-losing enteropathy (PLE) develops in 4% to 13% of patients, and 5-year survival in this subgroup is approximately 50%. This complication is diagnosed by the finding of low plasma alpha$_1$-antitrypsin levels and high alpha$_1$-antitrypsin stool clearance. Chronically elevated systemic venous pressure with resultant intestinal lymphangiectasia and protein leakage has been implicated in the pathogenesis of PLE.

REFERENCE

Driscoll DJ: Long-term results of the Fontan operation. Pediatr Cardiol 28:438, 2007.

ANSWER TO QUESTION 485

B (Braunwald, p. 1681; Table 77-2)

A primary hypercoagulable state should be suspected when a patient presents with deep vein thrombosis (DVT) in the absence of a predisposing condition such as trauma, prolonged bed rest, or malignancy. Activated protein C (aPC) resistance is a hypercoagulable state in which aPC cannot cleave and inactivate coagulation factor V. This is caused by a single amino acid mutation of glutamine for arginine, known as the factor V Leiden mutation, which abolishes a protein C cleavage site in factor V. Because factor V is important in the conversion of prothrombin to thrombin and subsequent clot formation, the inability to inactivate it leads to a hypercoagulable state. This mutation has been found in nearly 20% of unselected patients with DVT. In contrast, the prothrombin 20210 mutation (a G-to-A substitution at nucleotide position 20210) has been identified in 5% to 8% of patients with DVT, whereas protein C deficiency has been found in 2% to 4%, protein S deficiency in 2% to 5%, and antithrombin deficiency in 1% to 3%.

REFERENCE

Anderson JA, Weitz JI: Hypercoagulable states. Clin Chest Med 37:659, 2010.

ANSWER TO QUESTION 486

C (Braunwald, pp. 1719-1723)

This man has classic findings of the sleep apnea syndrome. Such patients often present with daytime sleepiness, nighttime snoring with apnea, nocturnal awakenings, difficulties in their jobs, and automobile accidents due to falling asleep at the wheel. Specific symptoms include paroxysmal nocturnal dyspnea, morning headaches, cardiac arrhythmias, truncal obesity, pulmonary hypertension, nocturnal enuresis, peripheral edema, hypertension, and an elevated hematocrit on laboratory examination.

Although the precise cause of the sleep apnea syndrome is unclear, three types of patterns have been recorded: central apnea, obstructive apnea, and mixed apnea. In *central apnea,* there appears to be a decrease in central nervous system sympathetic outflow to the respiratory effort. Conversely, in *obstructive apnea,* the upper airway becomes transiently obstructed, causing airflow to stop despite continuing efforts of the respiratory muscles. Affected patients experience apneic periods, which can occur between 40 and 100 times per hour. During prolonged periods of apnea, the Po_2 can fall to values of 20 to 25 mm Hg with oxygen saturation < 50%. Sustained hypoxemia of this type leads to arrhythmias, including sinus bradycardia, sinus arrest, long asystoles, frequent atrial premature beats, and ventricular arrhythmias. Pulmonary hypertension may develop with secondary right ventricular hypertrophy.

An effective therapy for many patients with sleep apnea is continuous positive airway pressure (CPAP), applied during sleep via mask or nasal prongs. Patients treated with CPAP demonstrate improved neuropsychiatric function and reduced daytime somnolence. Nocturnal desaturation, pulmonary hypertension, and right-sided heart failure findings can all improve with this technique.

More severe forms of sleep apnea may require palatal corrective surgery or, in the most difficult cases, tracheostomy.

REFERENCE

Bradley TD, Floras JS: Obstructive sleep apnoea and its cardiovascular consequences. Lancet 373:82, 2009.

ANSWER TO QUESTION 487

D (Braunwald, pp. 1547-1549; Table 67-4)

The modified Duke criteria provide a framework for the systematic diagnostic evaluation of patients with suspected infective endocarditis, integrating clinical, laboratory, and imaging data. The clinical criteria are divided into major and minor, and the details of each criterion are listed in Table 67-4. The major criteria include (1) positive blood cultures of typical microorganisms for infective endocarditis acquired in appropriate fashion and (2) evidence of endocardial involvement, by echocardiographic findings of vegetation, abscess, new dehiscence of prosthetic valve, or new clinical valvular regurgitation.

Minor criteria include predisposing factors (e.g., predisposing structural cardiac condition or intravenous drug use), fever, vascular phenomena (including arterial or pulmonary septic emboli, mycotic aneurysm and Janeway lesions), and immunologic phenomena (e.g., Osler nodes and Roth spots). The definitive clinical diagnosis of infective endocarditis is established by identifying two major criteria, one major criterion and three minor criteria, or five minor criteria.

REFERENCE

Murdoch DR, Corey GR, Hoen B, et al: Clinical presentation, etiology, and outcome of infective endocarditis in the 21st century. Arch Intern Med 169:463, 2009.

ANSWER TO QUESTION 488

C (Braunwald, pp. 1597-1598, 1602-1606)

This patient presents with symptoms of a dilated cardiomyopathy of rapid onset. In North America, the majority of new dilated cardiomyopathies are not found to have a specific cause and the cause is presumed to be related to viral myocarditis. The most common viruses that have been implicated are the enteroviruses and adenovirus. Myocardial biopsy is rarely helpful in identifying the etiology of dilated cardiomyopathy because the findings are often nonspecific. Furthermore, a negative biopsy does not rule out active viral myocarditis, because the myocardial damage may be focal and not included in the biopsy specimen. Conversely, modern cardiac magnetic resonance imaging protocols have a high diagnostic accuracy for the presence of global or focal myocarditis.

Acute and convalescent serologic testing can be obtained to confirm a viral cause, but the findings are not available sufficiently rapidly to affect management. Myocardial damage in viral myocarditis is believed to be due to cell-mediated immunologic recognition of new antigens expressed on myocardial cells by the infecting virus, although direct invasion of the myocardium and production of a myocardial toxin may play a role. Because of myocardial cell destruction, serum myocardial markers, including CK-MB and the cardiac troponins, can be elevated in active myocarditis even in the absence of coronary artery disease. Because of the immunologic nature of cell death, it stands to reason that corticosteroid therapy would be beneficial in the treatment of acute myocarditis. However, randomized trial data to date indicate that immunosuppressive therapy for acute idiopathic/viral myocarditis does not significantly affect left ventricular function or survival.

REFERENCE

Blauwet LA, Cooper LT: Myocarditis. Prog Cardiovasc Dis 52:274, 2010.

ANSWER TO QUESTION 489

D (Braunwald, pp. 1588-1592)

The M-mode echocardiogram demonstrates marked left ventricular (LV) hypertrophy with severe asymmetric septal hypertrophy (ASH). The septal thickness is 26 mm (normal, ≤11 mm). There is normal contractile wall movement, but the motion of the mitral valve is abnormal: the anterior leaflet moves anteriorly during systole, toward the interventricular septum. The findings of ASH and systolic anterior motion of the mitral valve are consistent with the diagnosis of hypertrophic cardiomyopathy (HCM) with dynamic outflow obstruction. The patient should be advised to refrain from competitive sports, because such activity may increase the likelihood of syncope and sudden death. Medical therapy for this disorder includes beta blockers and/or calcium channel antagonists. These agents reduce myocardial oxygen consumption and may lower the outflow gradient in patients with dynamic obstruction.

Diuretics are generally avoided in patients with HCM to prevent intravascular volume depletion and intensification of the outflow gradient. However, recent experience has demonstrated that cautious use of diuretics in this condition can reduce pulmonary congestion

without adverse effect. Digoxin *should* be avoided in HCM in the absence of systolic dysfunction; any increased inotropic effect could exacerbate the LV outflow gradient. Per the 2007 updated American Heart Association guidelines for the prevention of endocarditis, HCM is no longer an indication for routine antibiotic prophylaxis before dental procedures (see Answer to Question 464).

REFERENCE

Ho CY: Hypertrophic cardiomyopathy. Heart Fail Clin 6:59, 2010.

ANSWER TO QUESTION 490

B (Braunwald, pp. 1461-1462)

Stenoses of the pulmonary artery (PA) may be single or multiple and may be found from the main PA trunk to the smaller peripheral arterial branches. PA stenosis is usually associated with other cardiovascular defects, including ventricular septal defect, tetralogy of Fallot, supravalvular aortic stenosis, and pulmonic valvular stenosis. An important cause of PA stenosis in the newborn is intrauterine rubella infection. Associated cardiovascular malformations in that syndrome include patent ductus arteriosus, pulmonic valve stenosis, and atrial septal defect. Other general findings include cataracts, microphthalmia, thrombocytopenia, hepatitis, deafness, and blood dyscrasias.

The clinical features vary, but most infants and children with peripheral PA stenosis remain asymptomatic. Auscultation is notable for a systolic ejection murmur at the upper left sternal border, although a continuous murmur may be present if there is significant branch stenosis. The ECG demonstrates right ventricular hypertrophy when obstruction is severe.

The presence of peripheral PA stenosis may be confirmed by detecting pressure gradients within the PA at cardiac catheterization. Mild to moderate stenoses do not require intervention, and multiple stenoses may not be amenable to correction. Percutaneous balloon angioplasty is used to treat more advanced forms.

ANSWER TO QUESTION 491

C (Braunwald, pp. 1571-1572)

The provided apical four-chamber view demonstrates biventricular increased wall thickness, enlarged atria, and a small pericardial effusion, all of which are typical findings of cardiac amyloidosis. Systemic amyloidosis represents a collection of pathologic disorders that result in the extracellular deposition of insoluble fibrillar proteins in organs and tissues. The most common form is primary (AL) amyloidosis, which is associated with plasma cell dyscrasias such as multiple myeloma. Cardiac involvement occurs in approximately 50% of patients with AL amyloidosis, and the most common presentation is that of restrictive cardiomyopathy. In such cases, right-sided findings predominate on physical examination.

Another presentation of cardiac amyloidosis is congestive heart failure due to systolic dysfunction, generally a later finding. In approximately 10% of patients with amyloidosis, orthostatic hypotension occurs and is presumed to be a result of amyloid infiltration of the autonomic nervous system or of the blood vessels themselves. A fourth, rare presentation of cardiac amyloidosis infiltration is impaired cardiac impulse formation and conduction. Such patients present with arrhythmias and conduction disturbances and sudden death may occur.

Although not obvious in this example, the echocardiographic findings in cardiac amyloidosis may include a distinctive granular, sparkling appearance of the thickened cardiac walls, representative of the infiltrative process. Despite the thickened ventricular walls, the ECG in cardiac amyloidosis typically demonstrates low limb lead voltage, often accompanied by ventricular conduction delay and pseudoinfarction patterns.

REFERENCE

Falk RH, Dubrey SW: Amyloid heart disease. Prog Cardiovasc Dis 52:347, 2010.

ANSWER TO QUESTION 492

E (Braunwald, pp. 1510-1514)

The figure is an M-mode panel obtained at the midventricular level demonstrating prominent late-systolic mitral valve prolapse (MVP). Point C represents coaptation of the anterior and posterior mitral valve leaflets at the onset of systole. The posterior displacement (the U-shaped deformity) of the C-D segment represents prolapse of the leaflets into the left atrium in late systole.

By using standardized echocardiographic criteria the prevalence of MVP in the population is 2.4%. MVP is twice as common in women as in men, and there appears to be a strong hereditary component. The majority of affected people are asymptomatic, and moderate or severe mitral regurgitation (MR) is found in only 10%. For asymptomatic patients who do not have significant MR, reassurance is appropriate, with follow-up every few years, including repeat echocardiographic evaluation if there is a clinical change. For patients with significant MR, more frequent (e.g., yearly) clinical and echocardiographic evaluations are recommended. Patients with MVP do not routinely require predental antibiotic prophylaxis to prevent endocarditis (see Answer to Question 464).

The risk of sudden death in patients with MVP in the absence of significant MR is very low. Extensive evaluation for arrhythmias is not warranted for asymptomatic patients but should be pursued in those with a history of sustained palpitations, lightheadedness, or syncope. Cerebral embolic events have been reported to be more common in patients with MVP. However, a large case-controlled study showed no association between this disorder and ischemic neurologic events in patients < age 45 years. The most common serious complication of MVP is progressive MR. Those at the highest risk are men and individuals >50 years of age.

REFERENCE

Shah PM: Current concepts in mitral valve prolapse: Diagnosis and management. J Cardiol 56:125, 2010.

ANSWER TO QUESTION 493

C (Braunwald, pp. 1426-1427)

These images reveal an ostium secundum atrial septal defect (ASD). Two-dimensional echocardiography, especially from the subcostal position, allows direct examination of the interatrial septum. Some types of ASDs, such as the sinus venosus defect, may be difficult to identify by transthoracic esophagography and can be more easily resolved by a transesophageal study. Both color flow Doppler and saline contrast echocardiography (part B) may be used to evaluate the direction of flow across an ASD. In the uncomplicated situation, in which flow is directed predominantly from the left to the right atrium, left atrial (noncontrast) blood passes through the ASD and produces a negative contrast effect within the right atrium. Conversely, when Eisenmenger syndrome has developed, as in the case described, the shunt reverses (i.e., right-to-left direction) and contrast medium passes from the right atrium into the left-sided chambers after a peripheral vein saline injection. Anomalous pulmonary venous return (not demonstrated in this case) is most commonly associated with the sinus venosus type of ASD and is best visualized by transesophageal esophagography.

REFERENCE

Rigatelli G, Cardaioli P, Hijazi ZM: Contemporary clinical management of atrial septal defects in the adult. Expert Rev Cardiovasc Ther 5:1135, 2007.

ANSWER TO QUESTION 494

A (Braunwald, pp. 1478-1481)

This M-mode panel displays high-frequency vibration of the anterior leaflet of the mitral valve in diastole, which is characteristic of aortic regurgitation (AR). This sign is an echocardiographic correlate of the Austin Flint murmur, although unlike the auscultatory finding it may occur even in cases of mild AR.

AR develops due to abnormalities of the aortic valve itself and/or because of dilatation of the aortic root. In recent decades, primary aortic root pathology has become the most common cause of pure AR in the United States, reflecting the decline of rheumatic heart disease. AR due to dilatation of the ascending aorta is typically degenerative in origin (annuloaortic ectasia), and it may also be associated with specific disorders, including systemic hypertension, cystic medial necrosis of the aorta (isolated or in association with Marfan syndrome), giant cell arteritis, ankylosing spondylitis, rheumatoid arthritis, and syphilis. Causes of valvular AR include rheumatic fever, endocarditis, traumatic injury, and congenitally bicuspid aortic valve. Regardless of the underlying disorder that leads to AR, enlargement and eccentric hypertrophy of the left ventricle are common sequelae.

REFERENCES

Maurer G: Aortic regurgitation. Heart 92:994, 2006.
Stout KK, Verrier ED: Acute valvular regurgitation. Circulation 119:3232, 2009.

ANSWER TO QUESTION 495

B (Braunwald, p. 1493)

The transmitral Doppler pattern is typical of mitral stenosis (MS). Echocardiographic study in a patient with MS provides a wealth of information about the presence and severity of the lesion. Typical findings include leaflet thickening, decreased leaflet separation in diastole, and anterior movement of the posterior mitral valve leaflet during early diastole. The chordae are variably thickened, fused, and shortened.

Accurate determination of mitral orifice size can be obtained from two-dimensional and Doppler echocardiography (see Answer to Question 26). Planimetry of the mitral orifice in the parasternal short-axis view permits an accurate determination of the valve area. Doppler echocardiography is especially useful in quantifying the severity of MS. The peak velocity of transmitral flow is *increased* in MS, as in this case, and the rate of decline is reduced during early diastole. In the continuous-wave Doppler flow velocity signal illustrated, the peak velocity exceeds 2 m/sec, yielding a peak transmitral gradient of >16 mm Hg (per the modified Bernoulli equation, $P = 4v^2$), consistent with advanced MS. In addition, the valve area may be estimated using the pressure-half time, which is based on the correlation between the size of the mitral orifice and the time required for peak pressure to reach half its initial level. Finally, Doppler interrogation of the tricuspid regurgitant jet can help estimate the degree of elevated pulmonary artery pressure.

REFERENCE

Chandrashekhar Y, Westaby S, Narula J: Mitral stenosis. Lancet 374:1271, 2009.

ANSWER TO QUESTION 496

D (Braunwald, pp. 1666-1667; see also Answer 473)

This case illustrates a patient infected with human immunodeficiency virus (HIV) presenting with tuberculous pericarditis during the effusive stage of the illness. Whereas the incidence of tuberculous pericarditis has decreased in industrialized nations in recent decades, the disorder remains an important problem in immunosuppressed patients, including those with HIV disease. It is also a major cause of pericarditis among populations in developing regions, especially in sub-Saharan Africa.

Among Africans with HIV infection, tuberculosis is the most common cause of pericardial disease.

Tuberculous pericarditis usually manifests in the effusive stage as in this case or late in its course, following the development of constrictive pericarditis. The disease usually arises slowly and is marked by nonspecific systemic findings, including fever, night sweats, dyspnea, and fatigue. The acute onset of severe pericardial pain, which is seen frequently in viral or idiopathic pericarditis, is *uncommon* in tuberculous pericarditis. Abnormalities on physical examination may include fever, tachycardia, and a pericardial friction rub, as well as jugular venous distention, ascites, and hepatomegaly.

The chest radiograph in this case displays common features of effusive tuberculous pericarditis. These include an enlarged cardiac silhouette with accompanying mediastinal widening suggestive of a pericardial effusion, normal lung hila and apices, and a small pleural effusion. Patients may also present with chronic constrictive pericarditis with symptoms and signs consistent with severe systemic venous congestion. The diagnosis of tuberculous pericarditis requires a high index of suspicion and is best confirmed by obtaining both pericardial fluid and a pericardial biopsy specimen during the early effusive stage. The measurement of a high level of adenosine deaminase activity (>40 U/L) is also supportive of the diagnosis with a sensitivity of 88% and a specificity of 83%. In addition, polymerase chain reaction to detect *Mycobacterium tuberculosis* from small amounts of fluid or pericardial tissue can accelerate the diagnosis. Without antituberculous therapy, the disease is fatal, with an early mortality >80%. The effectiveness of corticosteroids in tuberculous pericarditis remains unclear, but some trials suggest that the addition of steroid therapy to standard antituberculous agents may shorten the time to resolution of symptoms.

REFERENCE

Syed FF, Mayosi BM: A modern approach to tuberculous pericarditis. Prog Cardiovasc Dis 50:218, 2007.

ANSWER TO QUESTION 497

A (Braunwald, pp. 1428-1430)

Atrioventricular (AV) septal defects include malformations characterized by varying degrees of incomplete development of the atrial septum, the inflow portion of the ventricular septum, and the AV valves. These anomalies are also known as endocardial cushion defects or AV canal defects.

An ostium primum atrial septal defect (ASD), a type of AV septal defect, occurs immediately adjacent to the AV valves, either of which may be deformed or incompetent. Most commonly it is only the anterior leaflet of the mitral valve that is displaced and "cleft"; the posterior leaflet of the mitral valve and the tricuspid valve are generally not involved. Ostium primum ASDs lead to prominent left-to-right transatrial shunting and have clinical features that resemble those of ostium secundum defects. In addition to similar findings on physical examination, imaging typically reveals right atrial and right ventricular prominence and increased pulmonary vascular markings. Echocardiography has supplanted invasive imaging in the diagnosis of this condition. If cardiac catheterization is undertaken, left ventriculography may show a pathognomonic "gooseneck" deformity that results from a narrowed and elongated left ventricular outflow tract.

When a ventricular septal defect accompanies an ostium primum septal defect (and a common AV orifice is therefore present) the malformation is known as a *complete AV canal defect.* Approximately 35% of patients with common AV canal have accompanying cardiovascular abnormalities, including tetralogy of Fallot, double-outlet right ventricle, transposition of the great arteries, total anomalous pulmonary venous connections, left ventricular outflow tract obstruction, pulmonic stenosis, and persistent left superior vena cava. In addition, common AV canal is often present in patients with trisomy 21.

REFERENCE

Warnes CA, Williams, RG, Bashore TM, et al: ACC/AHA 2008 Guidelines for the Management of Adults With Congenital Heart Disease: A Report of the American College of Cardiology/American Heart Association Task Force on Practice Guidelines (Writing Committee to Develop Guidelines on the Management of Adults With Congenital Heart Disease) Developed in Collaboration With the American Society of Echocardiography, Heart Rhythm Society, International Society for Adult Congenital Heart Disease, Society for Cardiovascular Angiography and Interventions, and Society of Thoracic Surgeons. J Am Coll Cardiol 52:143, 2008.

ANSWER TO QUESTION 498

D (Braunwald, pp. 1506-1508)

Once the decision is made to operate on a patient with mitral regurgitation, mitral valve repair is preferred to valve replacement. Excellent results are obtained with reconstructive procedures that employ a rigid or semirigid prosthetic annulus such as the Carpentier ring. Direct suture repair of the valve and replacement, reimplantation, elongation, or shortening of the chordae tendineae as necessary to make the valve competent are usually performed. The advantage of a repair as opposed to a replacement of the mitral valve is that the hazards of chronic anticoagulation and thromboembolism that accompany the use of a mechanical prosthesis can be avoided, as can the concern of late structural failure of a bioprosthesis. This procedure can be performed in a wide range of patients, including those with ruptured chordae tendineae, annular dilatation, and even active endocarditis.

Mitral valve repair is less likely to be successful in elderly patients with advanced calcification and/or scarred, deformed rheumatic leaflets. Mitral valve replacement is often the superior option in these patients.

REFERENCES

Amirak E, Chan KM, Zakkar M, et al: Current status of surgery for degenerative mitral valve disease. Prog Cardiovasc Dis 51:454, 2009.

Carabello BA: The current therapy for mitral regurgitation. J Am Coll Cardiol 52:319, 2008.

ANSWER TO QUESTION 499

D (Braunwald, pp. 1508-1509)

The optimal timing of mitral valve repair or replacement in patients with chronic asymptomatic mitral regurgitation (MR) is often a difficult clinical decision. The goal is to operate, even in asymptomatic individuals, before irreversible left ventricular (LV) dilatation and dysfunction have developed. If congestive heart failure or ventricular dysfunction develops, surgery should be performed as soon as possible to prevent further dysfunction. Thus, serial evaluation of the LV ejection fraction can be helpful in deciding when to intervene. The ejection fraction should be supranormal in patients with advanced MR. Once it falls below 60%, early systolic dysfunction is likely and the risk of postoperative LV dysfunction increases.[1] The LV end-systolic diameter (LVESD) is also helpful in timing surgical intervention. Patients should be referred for surgery before the LVESD exceeds 45 mm, to minimize the risk of postoperative LV dysfunction. Early pulmonary hypertension is considered a relative indication for mitral valve surgery, because patients with this complication, especially if it is accompanied by right ventricular dysfunction, have a worse prognosis.[2] Although they may reduce the regurgitant fraction and improve forward cardiac output, neither angiotensin-converting enzyme inhibitors nor other vasodilators have been shown to delay the need for surgery or improve long-term outcomes in patients with chronic MR.[3]

REFERENCES

1. Rosenhek R, Maurer G: Management of valvular mitral regurgitation: The importance of risk stratification. J Cardiol 56:255, 2010.
2. Adams DH, Rosenhek R, Falk V: Degenerative mitral valve regurgitation: Best practice revolution. Eur Heart J 31:1958, 2010.
3. Bonow RO, Carabello B, Chatterjee K, et al: 2008 Focused Update Incorporated Into the ACC/AHA 2006 Guidelines for the Management of Patients With Valvular Heart Disease: A Report of the American College of Cardiology/American Heart Association Task Force on Practice Guidelines (Writing Committee to Revise the 1998 Guidelines for the Management of Patients With Valvular Heart Disease) Endorsed by the Society of Cardiovascular Anesthesiologists, Society for Cardiovascular Angiography and Interventions, and Society of Thoracic Surgeons. J Am Coll Cardiol 52:e1, 2008.

ANSWER TO QUESTION 500

B (Braunwald, pp. 1435-1437)

This patient has tetralogy of Fallot, the components of which are (1) an outlet VSD, (2) obstruction to right ventricular (RV) outflow, (3) overriding of the aorta, and (4) RV hypertrophy. In general, total correction of tetralogy of Fallot is advised for almost all patients, even in infancy.[1] Successful early correction appears to prevent the consequences of progressive infundibular obstruction and acquired pulmonary atresia, delayed growth and development, and the complications secondary to hypoxemia and polycythemia. The size of the pulmonary arteries is most important in determining candidacy for primary repair of tetralogy of Fallot, as opposed to the age or size of the infant or child. Marked hypoplasia of the pulmonary arteries is a relative contraindication to a total corrective operation. If this is present, a palliative procedure designed to increase pulmonary blood flow is generally recommended, such as balloon valvuloplasty of the right ventricular outflow tract and pulmonary arteries. Total correction of the tetralogy may then be carried out later in childhood or adolescence at lower risk.

The postoperative period after palliative or corrective surgery is susceptible to several common complications. A sudden increase in pulmonary venous return may lead to *left* ventricular decompensation, whereas varying degrees of pulmonic valvular regurgitation may increase right ventricular cavity size. In addition, bleeding difficulties may be seen, especially in older polycythemic patients. Complete right bundle branch block or left anterior hemiblock is often observed postoperatively.[2] The greatest cause of early and late mortality and poor surgical results is restriction of pulmonary arterial flow owing to persistent right-sided outflow tract obstruction.[3] Most often, surgical repair leads to relief of symptoms of hypoxemia and severe exercise intolerance that mark the preoperative period.

REFERENCES

1. Apitz C, Webb GD, Redington AN: Tetralogy of Fallot. Lancet 374:1462, 2009.
2. Brickner ME, Hillis LD, Lange RA. Congenital heart disease in adults: II. N Engl J Med 342:334, 2000.
3. Therrien J, Marx GR, Gatzoulis MA: Late problems in tetralogy of Fallot: Recognition, management, and prevention. Cardiol Clin 20:395, 2002.

ANSWER TO QUESTION 501

A (Braunwald, pp. 1684-1686)

The high-resolution contrast-enhanced chest CT shows large thromboemboli in the right and left main pulmonary arteries (arrows in figure). The approach to the diagnosis of pulmonary embolism (PE) has been revolutionized by modern imaging technologies and, in particular, by intravenous contrast-enhanced chest CT. High-resolution chest CT has replaced pulmonary radionuclide perfusion scintigraphy ($\dot{V}/\dot{Q}$ scanning) as the primary imaging test in patients with suspected PE. Chest CT offers a number of advantages over other modalities, including direct visualization of thrombus within the pulmonary arteries, the ability to concurrently identify thrombi in the proximal veins in the legs, and imaging of the lung parenchyma to identify alternative diagnoses. Whereas first-generation CT scanners could image the proximal pulmonary arteries, newer generation multidetector CT scanners allow high-resolution imaging of even subsegmental pulmonary arteries.[1] Although invasive pulmonary angiography has historically been the gold standard in the diagnosis of PE, CT now provides images of excellent quality such that angiography is rarely necessary.

Echocardiography is very helpful in risk stratification in patients with large PE. The presence of right ventricular dysfunction portends a higher risk of complications and may warrant consideration of more aggressive treatment such as thrombolysis or suction catheter embolectomy.[2]

In patients with suspected PE, the identification of deep vein thrombosis (DVT) of the lower extremities by venous ultrasonography can provide circumstantial evidence of PE disease. The absence of DVT in such patients, however, does not exclude pulmonary embolism because the majority of patients with PE do not have imaging evidence of DVT elsewhere.[3]

REFERENCES

1. Hunsaker AR, Lu MT, Goldhaber SZ, et al: Imaging in acute pulmonary embolism with special clinical scenarios. Circ Cardiovasc Imaging 3:491, 2010.
2. Sanchez O, Trinquart L, Caille V, et al: Prognostic factors for pulmonary embolism: The PREP study, a prospective multicenter cohort study. Am J Respir Crit Care Med 181:168, 2010.
3. Righini M, Le Gal G, Aujesky D, et al: Complete venous ultrasound in outpatients with suspected pulmonary embolism. J Thromb Haemost 7:406, 2009.

ANSWER TO QUESTION 502

A (Braunwald, pp. 1655-1656; 1663-1664)

Each of the listed conditions results in elevated right-sided heart pressures. The diastolic "dip-and-plateau" pattern shown in the figure, also known as a "square root sign," is produced when early rapid diastolic inflow into the ventricle commences but is then abruptly halted by an opposing force. In the case of constrictive pericarditis, early diastolic inflow is terminated as ventricular filling reaches the volume limit imposed by the surrounding rigid pericardium. In restrictive cardiomyopathy, the myocardium is abnormally "stiff" and impaired relaxation accounts for a ventricular filling pattern that mimics pericardial constriction. Other conditions with similar right-sided hemodynamics as pericardial constriction include acute right ventricular infarction and massive pulmonary embolism. In these entities, filling of the acutely strained and dilated right ventricle is limited by an unprepared and relatively noncompliant pericardium.

In cardiac tamponade, the surrounding elevated pericardial pressure equalizes the diastolic pressures of the cardiac chambers. Because even early diastolic ventricular filling is impaired (manifest by blunting of the *y* descent on right atrial tracing), there is no dip-and-plateau configuration.

REFERENCE

Sorajja P: Invasive hemodynamics of constrictive pericarditis, restrictive cardiomyopathy, and cardiac tamponade. Cardiol Clin 29:191, 2011.

ANSWER TO QUESTION 503

E (Braunwald, pp. 1645-1648)

Primary cardiac tumors are much less common than metastatic cardiac lesions. Approximately 25% of primary cardiac tumors display malignant characteristics, and up to 75% of these are sarcomas. Primary cardiac lymphomas are the next most common group. The sites of cardiac malignancies, in decreasing order of frequency, are the right atrium, the left atrium, the right ventricle, and the left ventricle.

Tumors limited to the myocardium without intracavitary involvement may be asymptomatic or cause arrhythmias or conduction disturbances. Other typical presentations of cardiac malignancies include precordial pain, heart failure, pericardial effusion, tamponade, conduction system disorders, and/or vena caval obstruction. Tumors that involve the right-sided heart chambers may predominantly cause right-sided heart failure. The prognosis of cardiac malignancies is poor, with common survival times of a few weeks to 2 years after diagnosis. Historically, 75% of patients with cardiac sarcoma had evidence of distant metastases at the time of death, but more recent series have shown that only 25% to 50% of patients have metastatic disease at the time of diagnosis, likely owing to earlier detection with improvements in noninvasive diagnostic capabilities.

REFERENCE

Bruce CJ: Cardiac tumours: Diagnosis and management. Heart 97:151, 2011.

ANSWER TO QUESTION 504

C (Braunwald, pp. 1661-1665)

This patient has constrictive pericarditis. Because of the progressive nature of this condition, the majority of patients become symptomatic and come to medical attention because of weakness, peripheral edema, or ascites. The treatment of constrictive pericarditis is complete resection of the pericardium, including excision from the anterior and inferior surfaces of the right ventricle and the diaphragmatic and anterolateral surfaces of the left ventricle. This procedure has been performed more successfully via median sternotomy than by left thoracotomy because the former allows greater mobility of the heart. In recent series, the average operative mortality has ranged between 5% and 15%, with a clear correlation between the degree of the functional disability before the operation and survival after repair. Thus, it is generally recommended that patients undergo pericardiectomy soon after the development of symptoms. Between 14% and 28% of patients display a low-output syndrome in the immediate postoperative period, possibly related to rapid dilatation of the heart after release of the restraining pericardium.

Predictors of late survival include preoperative New York Heart Association class, age, renal function, pulmonary artery pressure, and history of radiotherapy exposure to the heart. Symptomatic improvement occurs in approximately 80% of survivors of pericardiectomy, although the time course for such recovery varies. Some patients experience an immediate decrease in symptoms, whereas others may have a delayed or partial response that requires weeks or months for resolution of elevated jugular venous pressure and abnormal filling pressures. The 5-year postoperative survival is approximately 75%.

REFERENCES

Imazio M, Brucato A, Mayosi BM, et al: Medical therapy of pericardial diseases: II. Noninfectious pericarditis, pericardial effusion and constrictive pericarditis. J Cardiovasc Med (Hagerstown) 11:785, 2010.

Schwefer M, Aschenbach R, Heidemann J, et al: Constrictive pericarditis, still a diagnostic challenge: Comprehensive review of clinical management. Eur J Cardiothorac Surg 36:502, 2009.

ANSWER TO QUESTION 505

B (Braunwald, p. 1598)

Lyme disease is a tickborne illness caused by the spirochete *Borrelia burgdorferi*. Patients who contract this condition typically develop a rash (erythema chronicum migrans) at the site of the tick bite. Weeks to months later, if the condition is treated, patients may develop complications involving the joints, central nervous system, and cardiovascular system.[1] Approximately 10% of patients develop cardiac complications, the most frequent manifestation of which is transient atrioventricular (AV) nodal block, including complete heart block.[2] Although some patients require temporary pacing, the AV conduction block usually improves and a permanent pacemaker is rarely needed. Lyme disease can also result in myocarditis, which is usually mild and self-limited. Manifestations include nonspecific ST-segment and T wave abnormalities on the ECG; only rarely do such patients develop symptoms of heart failure. The efficacy of antibiotics for Lyme carditis has not been established,[3] although they are routinely prescribed.

REFERENCES

1. Bratton RL, Whiteside JW, Hovan MJ, et al: Diagnosis and treatment of Lyme disease. Mayo Clin Proc 83:566, 2008.
2. Stanek G, Strle F: Lyme borreliosis. Lancet 362:1639, 2003.
3. Fish AE, Pride YB, Pinto DS: Lyme carditis. Infect Dis Clin North Am 22:275, 2008.

ANSWER TO QUESTION 506

C (Braunwald, pp. 1706-1707)

The National Institutes of Health (NIH) Registry of Primary Pulmonary Hypertension (PPH) provides the most extensive study to date on the natural history of this disorder. In this registry, 63% of the patients are female, with a mean age of 36 years at the time of diagnosis. The most common initial symptoms were dyspnea (80%), fatigue (19%), syncope (13%), and Raynaud phenomenon (10%). Patients may describe chest pain, but it is not a very common symptom. In the NIH Registry the most common physical finding was a loud pulmonic component of the second heart sound (P_2). Tricuspid regurgitation was found in 40% and peripheral edema in 32%. Eighty-seven percent of patients had electrocardiographic evidence of right ventricular hypertrophy.

The most common cause of death of patients in the NIH Registry was progressive right-sided heart failure (47%). Sudden cardiac death occurred in 26% and was limited to patients with severe (Class IV) symptoms.

REFERENCE

McLaughlin VV, McGoon MD: Pulmonary arterial hypertension. Circulation 114:1417, 2006.

ANSWER TO QUESTION 507

D (Braunwald, pp. 1468-1474)

The valve depicted is a calcified, stenotic aortic valve with three cusps. This is an acquired type of aortic stenosis (AS), and the thickened leaflets and nodular calcification are typical of the degenerative form seen in elderly patients. If the valve were bicuspid, it would reflect congenital AS. Historically, degenerative calcific AS has been assumed to be due to long-standing mechanical stress on the valve, but recent studies suggest that chronic inflammation with lipid accumulation is also evident, a process that may be similar to the cause of coronary atherosclerosis. It is therefore salient that diabetes mellitus, hypercholesterolemia (elevated low-density lipoprotein), smoking, and hypertension appear to increase the risk of aortic valve calcification.

The most likely murmur in this case would be crescendo-decrescendo during systole, loudest at the upper right sternal border and radiating toward the neck. Because apposition of the valve leaflets is otherwise intact, it is unlikely that this individual had significant aortic regurgitation.

REFERENCES

Carabello BA, Paulus WJ: Aortic stenosis. Lancet 373:956, 2009.
Vahanian A, Otto CM: Risk stratification of patients with aortic stenosis. Eur Heart J 31:416, 2010.

ANSWER TO QUESTION 508

C (Braunwald, pp. 1664-1665)

It is clinically important to differentiate constrictive pericarditis from restrictive cardiomyopathy, because the former is typically a treatable condition, whereas therapeutic options for the latter are very limited. Both conditions have similar hemodynamic findings during heart catheterization: all of the intracardiac diastolic pressures are elevated and the ventricular pressure tracings usually demonstrate a "dip-and-plateau" configuration. There are, however, several hemodynamic features that can help differentiate these two entities. Because restrictive cardiomyopathy tends to cause some left ventricular (LV) systolic dysfunction as well as the diastolic abnormality, pulmonary hypertension and elevated right ventricular (RV) systolic pressure are frequently also present. Therefore, the ratio of RV systolic pressure to RV end-diastolic pressure (RVEDP) is usually >3, whereas in constrictive pericarditis it is typically <3. Similarly, an RV systolic pressure >50 mm Hg is more consistent with restrictive cardiomyopathy than with pericardial constriction.

Close inspection of simultaneous RV and LV pressure tracings can also help discern which of these conditions is present. The pathophysiology of ventricular interdependence mandated by constrictive pericarditis leads to a discordance of LV and RV systolic pressures during respiration. In contrast to the normal situation, simultaneous LV and RV pressure measurements reveal that, during inspiration, RV systolic pressure rises as LV pressure falls. Furthermore, in constriction, the LV end-diastolic pressure (LVEDP) and RVEDP are equal, whereas in restriction, disproportionate LV involvement often causes the LVEDP to be more than 5 mm Hg greater than the RVEDP. In restriction (but not constriction), an intravenous volume challenge in the cardiac catheterization laboratory can help accentuate this difference.

In practice, other techniques are often used to distinguish constriction from restrictive cardiomyopathy. A transvenous endomyocardial biopsy would likely be normal in constriction but abnormal in myocardial restrictive disease. Conversely, a chest computed tomographic or magnetic resonance study most often demonstrates a thickened pericardium in constriction but not in pure restrictive disease.

REFERENCE

Sorajja P: Invasive hemodynamics of constrictive pericarditis, restrictive cardiomyopathy, and cardiac tamponade. Cardiol Clin 29:191, 2011.

ANSWER TO QUESTION 509

A (Braunwald, p. 1493)

Because the left ventricle is not subjected to excess volume or pressure load in pure mitral stenosis (MS), left ventricular (LV) dimensions are normal or even small. The mitral valve area can be measured by direct planimetry in the two-dimensional short-axis image of the valve and even more readily by Doppler techniques. The velocity of blood flow through the mitral valve in diastole can be measured by Doppler imaging in the apical views. The time interval required for the peak diastolic pressure across the mitral valve to fall to one half of its initial level (known as the pressure half-time, or $t_{1/2}$) is directly related to the severity of the mitral valve obstruction. Using the pressure half-time determination, the mitral valve area (MVA, in cm^2) is calculated as follows:

$$MVA = \frac{220}{t_{1/2}}$$

in which $t_{1/2}$ is measured in milliseconds and 220 is an empirically derived constant.

M-mode tracings of the mitral valve in MS show marked reduction ("flattening") of the diastolic slope of the EF segment, which indicates a persistent pressure gradient between the left atrium and left ventricle during diastole. Reduced excursion of the mitral leaflets occurs in MS but can also be observed in patients with low forward cardiac output owing to limited flow across the valve. However, echocardiographic features are diagnostic and include thickened, calcified leaflets, a thickened subvalvular apparatus, fusion and retraction of the chordae tendineae, and "doming" of the anterior and posterior valve leaflets during diastole. The latter pattern indicates that the tips of the leaflets (the commissures) are fused, a characteristic finding of rheumatic deformity, the most common cause of MS.

REFERENCE

Baumgartner H, Hung J, Bermejo J, et al: Echocardiographic assessment of valve stenosis: EAE/ ASE recommendations for clinical practice. Eur J Echocardiogr 10:1, 2009.

ANSWER TO QUESTION 510

D (Braunwald, p. 1669)

This patient has a malignant pericardial effusion. The most common tumors that invade the pericardium are, in order of decreasing frequency, lung, breast, and lymphoma.[1] Malignant pericardial effusions may result from direct extension of tumor into the pericardium or from hematogenous or lymphatic spread. In patients who develop malignant pericardial effusions, the prognosis is poor: In a recent study of patients with malignant pericardial effusion, the mean survival was 15.1 weeks.[2] After initial drainage of a large malignant pericardial effusion, a repeat echocardiographic study should be obtained within 72 hours to assess the rate of reaccumulation and to ensure the absence of tamponade physiology. If the fluid reaccumulates at a rapid rate, repeat pericardiocentesis followed by more aggressive therapy is warranted. Intrapericardial instillation of a sclerosing agent, such as tetracycline, during catheter drainage has been advocated as a means of controlling recurrences, although complications such as fever, chest pain, and constriction may be troublesome and prognosis of the underlying condition is not significantly improved by this technique.[3] Surgical pericardiectomy is not usually advocated in this situation because of the high operative mortality and the poor prognosis related to the underlying condition. Rather, more limited subxiphoid pericardiostomy ("pericardial window") or video-assisted thoracoscopic pericardiectomy is appropriate for symptomatic palliation.

REFERENCES

1. Bussani R, De-Giorgio F, Abbate A, et al: Cardiac metastases. J Clin Pathol 60:27, 2007.
2. Gornik HL, Gerhard-Herman M, Beckman JA: Abnormal cytology predicts poor prognosis in cancer patients with pericardial effusion. J Clin Oncol 23:5211, 2005.

3. Maisch B, Seferovic PM, Ristic AD, et al: Guidelines on the diagnosis and management of pericardial diseases: Executive summary. The Task Force on the Diagnosis and Management of Pericardial Diseases of the European Society of Cardiology. Eur Heart J 25:587, 2004.

ANSWER TO QUESTION 511

B (Braunwald, p. 1653; Fig. 75-2)

Acute pericarditis is believed to cause an actual current of injury owing to epicardial inflammation, which leads to electrocardiographic alterations that are diagnostically useful. Four stages of abnormalities of the ST segments and T waves may be distinguished. *Stage I* includes ST-segment elevation, in which the segment is concave upward; this elevation typically occurs in all leads *except* aVR and V_1. The T waves during this stage are usually upright. PR-segment depression occurs in this stage in approximately 80% of patients. The return of ST segments to baseline, accompanied by T wave flattening, comprises *stage II* of this process. The *third stage* is characterized by inversion of the T waves, such that the T wave vector is directed opposite to that of the ST segment. This should be contrasted to early inversion of the T wave in acute ST-segment elevation myocardial infarction, which occurs *before* the return of ST segments to baseline. *Stage IV* represents reversion of the T wave to normal and may not occur for weeks to months after the acute event.

Whereas all four stages are detected in approximately half of patients with acute pericarditis, about 90% of patients will demonstrate some electrocardiographic abnormalities that allow characterization of an acute chest pain episode as pericarditis.

Stage I changes of pericarditis must be differentiated from the electrocardiographic presentation of early repolarization. An ST-segment/T wave ratio > 0.25 in lead V_6 is more consistent with acute pericarditis, whereas a ratio < 0.25 is more suggestive of early repolarization.

REFERENCE

Khandaker M, Espinoza R, Nishimura R, et al: Pericardial disease: Diagnosis and management. Mayo Clin Proc 85:772, 2010.

ANSWER TO QUESTION 512

B (Braunwald, pp. 1468-1472)

The most serious symptoms of aortic stenosis (AS) in adults are angina pectoris, syncope, and heart failure. When symptoms become manifest, the prognosis for untreated AS is poor. Natural history survival curves show that the interval from the onset of symptoms to the time of death is approximately 5 years in patients with angina, 3 years in those with syncope, and 2 years in patients with heart failure (Fig. 4-34). Angina is present in approximately two thirds of patients with critical AS and is associated with coronary artery disease in approximately 50%. In AS, angina results from the combination of increased oxygen demand and the reduction of oxygen delivery.

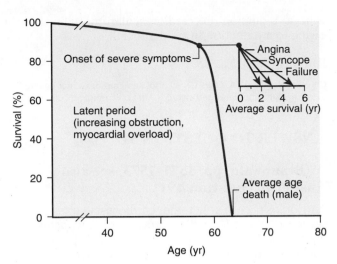

FIGURE 4-34 From Ross J Jr, Braunwald E: Aortic stenosis. Circulation 38(Suppl V):61, 1968.

Chagas disease is the most common cause of myocarditis in Central and South America. It is a late manifestation of infection by the protozoan *Trypanosoma cruzi*. After inoculation, the parasite migrates throughout the body, including to the myocardium. An immunologic response to the parasite leads to the myocarditis, and ventricular tachyarrhythmias are a common complicating feature.[3] Ventricular tachyarrhythmias are also an important cause of sudden cardiac death in patients with idiopathic dilated cardiomyopathy.

Hyperthyroidism commonly causes sinus tachycardia and atrial fibrillation, but serious ventricular tachyarrhythmias are rare.

REFERENCES

1. Pierre-Louis B, Prasad A, Frishman WH: Cardiac manifestations of sarcoidosis and therapeutic options. Cardiol Rev 17:153, 2009.
2. Cooper LT Jr: Giant cell and granulomatous myocarditis. Heart Fail Clin 1:431, 2005.
3. Rassi A Jr, Rassi A, Marin-Neto JA: Chagas disease. Lancet 375:1388, 2010.

Syncope in AS occurs most commonly after exertion. It is related to reduced cerebral perfusion caused by systemic vasodilatation during exercise in the presence of a fixed cardiac output. Sudden death occurs with increased frequency in patients with critical AS but almost invariably in those who have had previous symptoms.

Symptoms of AS may become exacerbated by the development of atrial fibrillation. Because of the decreased diastolic compliance of the hypertrophied ventricle, patients with AS are highly dependent on atrial contraction to deliver preload and maintain cardiac output. Thus when atrial fibrillation develops, significant hemodynamic deterioration may follow.

REFERENCE

Bonow RO, Carabello B, Chatterjee K, et al: 2008 Focused Update Incorporated Into the ACC/AHA 2006 Guidelines for the Management of Patients With Valvular Heart Disease: A Report of the American College of Cardiology/American Heart Association Task Force on Practice Guidelines (Writing Committee to Revise the 1998 Guidelines for the Management of Patients With Valvular Heart Disease) Endorsed by the Society of Cardiovascular Anesthesiologists, Society for Cardiovascular Angiography and Interventions, and Society of Thoracic Surgeons. J Am Coll Cardiol 52:e1, 2008.

ANSWER TO QUESTION 513

E (Braunwald, pp. 1565-1568, 1575-1576, 1602, 1611-1616)

Sudden cardiac death due to ventricular arrhythmias can complicate any cardiomyopathy, but for several causes this problem is particularly common. Ventricular dysrhythmias are among the more common cardiac manifestations of sarcoidosis because granuloma formation within the myocardium provides a substrate for electrical instability.[1] Giant cell myocarditis is another granulomatous disorder of the heart in which ventricular tachyarrhythmias are a prominent feature.[2]

ANSWER TO QUESTION 514

C (Braunwald, pp. 1672-1674)

Penetrating cardiac trauma is most commonly due to stab wounds and gunshot injuries. The consequences of such injury depend on the nature of the penetrating object, the size of the wound, the entering location, and the structures that are impacted. The site of cardiac injury can be predicted by the location of entry on the chest wall. Because of its anterior location, the *right* ventricle is at greatest risk of penetrating chest trauma. Of note, survival is higher in patients who suffer penetrating injuries to the ventricles than the atria, because the former are thicker walled structures more likely to seal the laceration site.

Patients who suffer penetrating injuries to the chest wall are at high risk of cardiac tamponade because of bleeding into the pericardial sac. If this complication develops, patients usually have muffled heart sounds, jugular venous distention, and hypotension with a narrowed pulse pressure; pulsus paradoxus is often present. Many trauma surgeons discourage pericardiocentesis for suspected tamponade after acute trauma because clots form quickly and often cannot be drained successfully through a needle and a negative pericardiocentesis does not rule out tamponade. Furthermore, if there is continued bleeding from cardiac perforation, any beneficial effect of pericardiocentesis would be short lived. Therefore, patients with penetrating chest injuries, significant bleeding, and a clinical picture that raises concern of tamponade should proceed directly to thoracotomy. Rupture of the interventricular septum has been described as a potential late complication in patients who have experienced penetrating chest trauma.

REFERENCE

Kang N, Hsee L, Rizoli S, Alison P: Penetrating cardiac injury: overcoming the limits set by nature. Injury 40:919, 2009.

ANSWER TO QUESTION 515

C (Braunwald, pp. 1432-1433)

The presentation of persistent PDA in adults depends on the degree of left-to-right shunting. Small *silent* shunts (i.e., those without murmurs) are almost always asymptomatic and are incidental findings during echocardiography. The risk of endarteritis is negligible in such patients. However, small *audible* shunts may occasionally present because of a superimposed endovascular infection.

Moderate shunts impose a volume load on the left ventricle and left atrium, resulting in left ventricular dysfunction and atrial fibrillation. Such patients typically present with either dyspnea or palpitations. On physical examination, a loud continuous "machinery" murmur is best appreciated in the first or second left intercostal space. The pulse pressure is usually *wide* owing to aortic diastolic runoff into the pulmonary trunk.

Large shunts initially cause left-sided volume overload but subsequently lead to irreversible pulmonary hypertension and Eisenmenger physiology. Chest radiology at that stage reveals enlarged central pulmonary arteries with peripheral pruning. Closure of a clinically detectable PDA is recommended except when it is accompanied by irreversible pulmonary hypertension. A multicenter trial of the Amplatzer occluder device indicates that transcatheter closure can achieve a success rate of 99% for complete ductal closure at 1 year.[1]

REFERENCE

1. Pass RH, Hijazi Z, Hsu DT, et al: Multicenter USA Amplatzer patent ductus arteriosus occlusion device trial: Initial and one-year results. J Am Coll Cardiol 44:513, 2004.

ANSWER TO QUESTION 516

C (Braunwald, pp. 1628-1630)

Chronic heavy consumption of alcohol is associated with systolic and diastolic ventricular dysfunction, systemic hypertension, arrhythmias, and sudden death. Alcohol abuse is the leading cause of nonischemic dilated cardiomyopathy in industrialized countries. The likelihood of developing alcohol-induced dilated cardiomyopathy correlates with the amount of alcohol consumed over a lifetime. Most men with this condition have consumed more than 80 grams of ethanol daily for over 5 years. Women appear to be more susceptible to the development of dilated cardiomyopathy at the same level of alcohol consumption as men. With abstinence from alcohol, LV systolic and diastolic function typically improve, often dramatically. Most of the improvement occurs in the first 6 months of abstinence, but systolic function may continue to normalize over a more prolonged time. The prognosis of patients who continue to drink heavily is poor.

Alcohol consumption at *moderate* levels in those without known coronary artery disease is associated with a reduction in cardiovascular mortality, largely owing to a reduction in sudden death.

REFERENCE

O'Keefe JH, Bybee KA, Lavie CJ: Alcohol and cardiovascular health: The razor-sharp double-edged sword. J Am Coll Cardiol 50:1009, 2007.

ANSWER TO QUESTION 517

A (Braunwald, pp. 1571-1573; see also Answer to Question 491)

Amyloidosis can afflict the cardiovascular system in several different ways. Restrictive cardiomyopathy with diastolic dysfunction is the most common presentation and is due to myocardial infiltration by amyloid protein.[1] In this situation, right-sided heart failure symptoms often predominate, with peripheral edema, hepatic congestion, and elevated jugular venous pressure. A second common presentation is biventricular heart failure due to systolic dysfunction. In some patients, congestive symptoms may be exacerbated by amyloid deposition in the atria with loss of effective atrial transport, despite the presence of sinus rhythm. Orthostatic hypotension occurs in 10% of patients with amyloidosis and results from infiltration of the autonomic nervous system. Other cardiovascular presentations include rhythm disturbances (especially atrial fibrillation) and conduction system disease. Small pericardial effusions are often observed by echocardiography in cardiac amyloidosis; however, significant pericardial disease is rare and cardiac tamponade and pericardial constriction are not common complications.

REFERENCE

1. Selvanayagam JB, Hawkins PN, Paul B, et al: Evaluation and management of the cardiac amyloidosis. J Am Coll Cardiol 50:2101, 2007.

ANSWER TO QUESTION 518

E (Braunwald, pp. 1544-1552)

Staphylococcus aureus is one of the most aggressive organisms in infective endocarditis, and infection with this bacterium results in rapid destruction of heart valves and surrounding tissues. *S. aureus* has a propensity to cause metastatic infections, including in the central nervous system, which is affected in 30% to 50% of patients.[1] Central nervous complications include cerebral embolism, meningitis, and cerebral and subarachnoid hemorrhage due to rupture of mycotic aneurysms. Patients with right-sided endocarditis (i.e., tricuspid valve involvement) due to *S. aureus* have a better prognosis than those with left-sided infections, with mortality rates of 2% to 4%.

Because *S. aureus* endocarditis is so destructive, it requires prompt and aggressive therapy. Although some experts have advocated early surgical intervention for native valve endocarditis due to this organism, there is a risk of infecting the new prosthetic valve if surgery is performed before adequate sterilization of the blood. Therefore, initial aggressive antibiotic therapy should be undertaken, with surgery reserved for those who fail to respond or for those who develop complications such as intractable heart failure. In contrast, prosthetic valve endocarditis caused by *S. aureus* carries an extremely high mortality rate, approaching 50% in patients treated medically,[2] and early surgical therapy should be advocated.

The historic cornerstone of medical therapy for *S. aureus* endocarditis has been a semisynthetic penicillinase-resistant penicillin (e.g., nafcillin or oxacillin) or cephalosporin. However, methicillin-resistant *S. aureus* (MRSA) is now a common cause of both nosocomial and community-acquired infections, such that empirical therapy for suspected *S. aureus* endocarditis should begin with an agent that is usually effective against MRSA, such as vancomycin.

REFERENCES

1. Johnson MD, Johnson CD: Neurologic presentations of infective endocarditis. Neurol Clin 28:311, 2010.
2. Nataloni M, Pergolini M, Rescigno G, et al: Prosthetic valve endocarditis. J Cardiovasc Med 11:869, 2010.

ANSWER TO QUESTION 519

B (Braunwald, pp. 1450-1452)

Anomalies that are associated with Ebstein anomaly include atrial septal defects (or patent foramen ovale) in 50% of patients, accessory conduction pathways (usually right sided) in 25%, and less commonly pulmonic stenosis or atresia, ventricular septal defects, aortic coarctation, and patent ductus arteriosus.

The usual clinical manifestations of Ebstein anomaly with severe tricuspid deformity in infancy are cyanosis, failure to thrive, and congestive heart failure. However, patients with less advanced disease may be asymptomatic until early adulthood, when symptoms include exertional dyspnea and fatigue, palpitations, and cyanosis due to right-to-left shunting. Cardiac examination typically shows wide splitting of S_1, a widely split S_2 (due to right bundle branch block [RBBB]), a right-sided S_3, and the murmur of tricuspid regurgitation.

The ECG may be normal, but common findings include right atrial enlargement, a prolonged PR interval, and RBBB. Accessory conduction pathways are present in up to 25% of patients, in which case the ECG may show signs of preexcitation with a shortened PR interval and a delta wave.

The diagnosis of Ebstein anomaly can usually be confirmed by echocardiography, with the finding of apical displacement of the septal leaflet of the tricuspid valve, combined with an elongated anterior leaflet.

REFERENCE

Attenhofer Jost CH, Connolly HM, Dearani JA, et al: Ebstein's anomaly. Circulation 115:277, 2007.

ANSWER TO QUESTION 520

C (Braunwald, p. 1576)

Löffler endocarditis is a cardiac syndrome associated with eosinophilia that occurs in temperate climates. The typical patient with this condition is a male in his fourth decade with a persistent eosinophilia count >1500/mm³ for at least 6 months and evidence of organ involvement.[1] Cardiac manifestations are seen in approximately 75% of patients. The cause of eosinophilia in most patients with this syndrome is unknown. On occasion, it may be reactive (e.g., associated with an allergic or parasitic disorder) or associated with leukemia. The combination of hypereosinophilia and cardiac involvement is also part of the Churg-Strauss syndrome, which can be differentiated from Löffler endocarditis by the coexisting presence of asthma, nasal polyposis, and necrotizing vasculitis.

The pathology of Löffler endocarditis involves mural endocardial thickening of the inflow and apical portions of both ventricles. Histologic findings include (1) an acute inflammatory eosinophilic myocarditis, (2) thrombosis and inflammation of intramural coronary vessels, (3) mural thrombosis, and (4) fibrotic thickening of the ventricular wall.

Clinically, patients present with weight loss, fever, cough, rash, and congestive heart failure. Cardiomegaly is present early in the course, even in the absence of congestive heart failure, and the murmur of mitral regurgitation is common. Systemic embolism is frequent and may lead to neurologic and renal dysfunction.

Laboratory findings include an elevated erythrocyte sedimentation rate and an increased eosinophil count. The echocardiogram frequently demonstrates localized thickening of the posterobasal left ventricular wall with absent or reduced motion of the posterior leaflet of the mitral valve. The apex may be filled with thrombus. Systolic ventricular function is usually normal. The hemodynamic consequences of the dense endocardial scarring are those of a restrictive cardiomyopathy (RCM) with abnormal diastolic filling. Findings at cardiac catheterization are consistent with RCM, including elevated ventricular filling pressures with an early diastolic "dip-and-plateau" ("square root sign") configuration.

Medical treatment of Löffler endocarditis is moderately effective. Administration of steroids and hydroxyurea can improve survival.

REFERENCE

1. Horenstein MS, Humes R, Epstein ML, Draper D: Loffler's endocarditis presenting in 2 children as fever with eosinophilia. Pediatrics 110:1014, 2002.

ANSWER TO QUESTION 521

D (Braunwald, pp. 1416-1417)

Cyanosis, which refers to a bluish discoloration of skin and mucous membranes, is due to augmented levels of reduced hemoglobin, in excess of 3 g/dL. Two forms of cyanosis are distinguished: peripheral and central. *Peripheral* cyanosis is due to increased oxygen extraction from normally saturated arterial blood as a result of cutaneous vasoconstriction. *Central* cyanosis results from arterial blood desaturation in conditions in which systemic venous blood is shunted to the arterial circulation. The degree of central cyanosis relates not only to the degree of arterial desaturation but also to the absolute amount of reduced hemoglobin and the oxyhemoglobin saturation of venous blood, which are in turn dependent on the extent of oxygen extraction by tissue metabolism. Thus, cyanosis may appear or worsen with physical exertion because of decreased venous oxygen saturation.

Differential cyanosis is characterized by the presence of normal oxygen saturation in the upper portions of the body but cyanosis in the lower parts. It may appear, for example, in patients with aortic coarctation who have *right-to-left* shunting across a patent ductus arteriosus.

Patients with cyanotic heart disease (e.g., tetralogy of Fallot) may be seen to assume the squatting position to relieve shortness of breath. Squatting decreases cyanosis and improves arterial oxygen saturation by increasing the systemic arterial resistance, which reduces the right-to-left shunt. Squatting also tends to pool desaturated venous blood in the lower extremities.

Hemostatic abnormalities, and bleeding tendencies in particular, are observed in up to 20% of cyanotic patients with secondary erythrocytosis. Potential explanations include abnormalities in the coagulation cascade (decreased factors V, VII, VIII, and IX) as well as platelet function or number. The clinical manifestations can range from mild and superficial bleeding to major, life-threatening hemorrhage.

ANSWER TO QUESTION 522

C (Braunwald, pp. 1520-1521)

This woman has rheumatic heart disease. She has mitral stenosis (MS) based on the loud S_1 and apical opening snap. Many patients with advanced MS have an early blowing diastolic murmur along the left sternal border and a normal systemic pulse pressure. In the majority of these patients the murmur is due to aortic regurgitation (AR) and it is usually of little clinical importance. However, approximately 10% of patients with MS have severe rheumatic AR. This can usually be recognized by peripheral signs of AR, such as a widened pulse pressure and signs of left ventricular (LV) enlargement by ECG and chest radiograph, with confirmation by echocardiography.

In patients with multivalvular disease, a proximal valve lesion may mask the presence of a more distal abnormality. Thus, significant AR may not be easily auscultated in patients with severe MS. The widened pulse pressure, in particular, may be absent in the presence of severe MS. Furthermore, the apical diastolic Austin Flint murmur associated with AR may be mistaken for the rumbling murmur of MS. These two murmurs may be distinguished during auscultation by means of bedside maneuvers. Isometric handgrip and squatting augment the diastolic murmur of AR (and the associated Austin Flint murmur) but have little effect on the murmur of MS. In this patient, the response to handgrip is consistent with the presence of an Austin Flint murmur.

The fact that the ECG of this patient shows LV hypertrophy in addition to left atrial enlargement is inconsistent with simple MS and suggests that the degree of superimposed AR is significant. There is no evidence on examination of tricuspid stenosis or mitral regurgitation. Pulmonic regurgitation due to pulmonary hypertension in patients with MS can also cause an early diastolic murmur along the left sternal border. However, such a murmur would be associated with a loud pulmonic component of S_2 and would not intensify with handgrip.

ANSWER TO QUESTION 523

E (Braunwald, p. 1495)

Diuretics and negative chronotropic agents are the mainstays of medical therapy for patients with symptomatic mitral stenosis (MS). The high left atrial pressure in this condition elevates pulmonary vascular pressures, resulting in dyspnea due to transudation of fluid into the alveolar spaces and stimulation of pulmonary J fibers. Diuretics reduce intravascular volume and left atrial pressure and therefore improve dyspnea. Maintaining a controlled, relatively slow heart rate prolongs diastole, maximizes the time for left atrial emptying, and reduces left atrial pressure. Thus, negative chronotropic agents such as beta blockers improve exercise capacity in MS patients, even in individuals in sinus rhythm.

Because left ventricular contractile function is normal in pure MS, digitalis glycosides have no beneficial hemodynamic effect and are useful only as agents for ventricular rate control if atrial fibrillation supervenes. There is insufficient evidence to support the routine use of anticoagulants to reduce the risk of thromboembolic events in patients with MS in the absence of atrial fibrillation, a history of thromboembolism, or extreme left atrial enlargement.

As reviewed in the Answer to Question 464, endocarditis prophylaxis before dental procedures is no longer recommended for native valve abnormalities such as MS.

REFERENCE

Bonow RO, Carabello B, Chatterjee K, et al: 2008 Focused Update Incorporated Into the ACC/AHA 2006 Guidelines for the Management of Patients With Valvular Heart Disease: A Report of the American College of Cardiology/American Heart Association Task Force on Practice Guidelines (Writing Committee to Revise the 1998 Guidelines for the Management of Patients With Valvular Heart Disease) Endorsed by the Society of Cardiovascular Anesthesiologists, Society for Cardiovascular Angiography and Interventions, and Society of Thoracic Surgeons. J Am Coll Cardiol 52:e1, 2008.

ANSWER TO QUESTION 524

D (Braunwald, pp. 1666-1667; Table 75-1)

Most cases of infectious acute pericarditis are caused by a virus. The most commonly implicated viruses are the enteroviruses and adenovirus. In contrast, the incidence of nontuberculous bacterial pericarditis is low, approximately 5% of cases, and it develops most often as a complication of pneumonia, mediastinitis, or infective endocarditis. The most commonly involved organisms are streptococcal and staphylococcal species. The overall survival in bacterial pericarditis is quite poor, averaging 30%.

Tuberculosis was once the leading cause of constrictive pericarditis worldwide. However, with effective screening and treatment programs, the incidence of this condition is now rare in Western nations, and it is seen mostly in immunocompromised hosts and in developing societies.

Pericarditis associated with fungal disease is most often caused by *Histoplasma*. It occurs in otherwise healthy young individuals and is thought to be a noninfectious inflammatory effusion secondary to fungal infection in nearby mediastinal lymph nodes. This process should be considered in patients with suspected pericarditis who live where the fungus is endemic—the Ohio and Mississippi River valleys. It is generally a self-limited disease, and treatment typically consists of nonsteroidal anti-inflammatory agents without antifungal therapy. Antifungal therapy is necessary only when there is evidence of disseminated histoplasmosis.

REFERENCES

Imazio M, Brucato A, Mayosi BM, et al: Medical therapy of pericardial diseases: I. Idiopathic and infectious pericarditis. J Cardiovasc Med 11:712, 2010.

ANSWER TO QUESTION 525

D (Braunwald, pp. 1611-1616)

Chagas disease is caused by the protozoan *Trypanosoma cruzi*. The major cardiovascular findings are extensive myocarditis with congestive heart failure. Typically, the disease becomes evident 20 to 30 years after the initial infection. Chagas disease is prevalent in Central and South America, where 10 to 20 million people are infected.

The disease is characterized by three phases: acute, latent, and chronic. During the acute phase, the disease is transmitted to humans by the bite of a reduviid bug, commonly called the kissing bug. After inoculation, protozoa multiply and migrate widely through the body. Clinical manifestations during the acute phase may include fever, muscle pains, hepatosplenomegaly, myocarditis, and meningoencephalitis. The disease then enters an asymptomatic latent phase for many years. Interestingly, although 30% of infected individuals develop symptoms of chronic Chagas disease, many individuals with high parasite burdens do not. There is poor correlation between the level of parasitemia and the severity of disease later.

Clinical manifestations of chronic Chagas disease include progressive heart failure, predominantly *right* sided. There is usually severe cardiomegaly, with the most common electrocardiographic abnormalities being right bundle branch block and left anterior fascicular block. Ventricular arrhythmias are a prominent feature of chronic Chagas disease. ST-segment and T wave abnormalities are common; atrioventricular block occurs less frequently. Echocardiography in advanced cases shows dilated cardiomyopathy, often with apical thinning and bulging that resembles an aneurysm.

The diagnosis of Chagas disease is confirmed using a complement-fixation test (Machado-Guerreiro test). At this time, no curative treatment is available; standard heart failure and antiarrhythmic approaches are often useful. Prevention of the disease using vector control methods is an important approach. Future immunoprophylaxis to prevent the disease appears promising, but a clinically useful vaccine is not yet available.

REFERENCE

Rassi A Jr, Rassi A, Marin-Neto JA: Chagas disease. Lancet 375:1388, 2010.

ANSWER TO QUESTION 526

C (Braunwald, pp. 1426-428, 1571-1573, 1640-1644)

The echocardiogram demonstrates prominent echogenicity along both surfaces of the interatrial septum (see arrow in Fig. 4-35), consistent with normal deployment of a transcatheter atrial septal defect (ASD) closure device. Indications for this method are the same as for surgical closure of an ASD, but strict structural criteria must be met. Successful closure can be accomplished in the majority of patients, and complications, such as device embolization or atrial perforation, are rare.

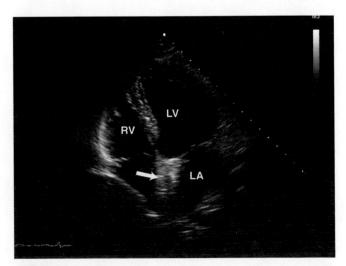

FIGURE 4-35

Atrial myxomas are the most common primary heart tumor. When attached to the interatrial septum, echocardiography most commonly demonstrates a mobile mass attached to the limbus of the fossa ovalis by a stalk. Lipomatous hypertrophy of the interatrial septum occurs most often in obese, elderly female patients. It represents a prominent fatty deposition at the interatrial septum that spares the fossa ovalis, creating a thick "dumbbell" appearance on echocardiography. This condition is associated with a high incidence of atrial arrhythmias. In cardiac amyloidosis, infiltration causes increased thickness of all cardiac chamber walls, not just the interatrial septum.

REFERENCES

Butera G, Carminati M, Chessa M, et al: Percutaneous versus surgical closure of secundum atrial septal defect: Comparison of early results and complications. Am Heart J 151:228, 2006.

Masura J, Gavora P, Podnar T: Long-term outcome of transcatheter secundum-type atrial septal defect closure using Amplatzer septal occluders. J Am Coll Cardiol 45:505, 2005.

ANSWER TO QUESTION 527

D (Braunwald, pp. 1490-1499; see also Answer to Question 522)

The parasternal long-axis view displays typical rheumatic deformity of the mitral valve with diastolic doming of the leaflets, with a "hockey-stick" appearance of the anterior leaflet (see arrow in Fig. 4-36). There is accompanying left atrial enlargement. The transmitral spectral Doppler in part B in Question 527 shows an increased early diastolic velocity with a slowed diastolic descent, indicative of a diastolic pressure gradient across the valve due to mitral stenosis (MS).

Atrial fibrillation (AF) is common in patients with MS, with an increasing prevalence with age. It tends to be poorly tolerated because of the lack of effective atrial contribution to filling and the shortened diastolic left ventricular filling time in patients with rapid ventricular rates. AF also predisposes to atrial thrombus formation

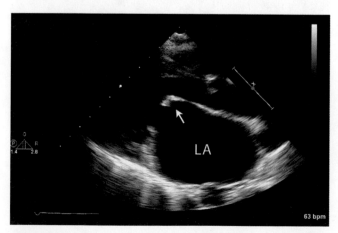

FIGURE 4-36

and embolization. The risk of systemic embolism in MS correlates directly with patient age and left atrial size and inversely with the cardiac output.

Infective endocarditis in MS tends to be more common in patients with milder forms of the disease, occurring less frequently on very thickened and calcified mitral valves.

Only about 15% of patients with isolated MS experience anginal type chest discomfort. This symptom may arise from right ventricular hypertension, concomitant atherosclerosis, or coronary obstruction due to embolization of left atrial thrombus.

REFERENCES

Carabello BA: Modern management of mitral stenosis. Circulation 112:432, 2005.

Iung B, Vahanian A: Rheumatic mitral valve disease. In Otto CM, Bonow RO (eds): Valvular Heart Disease: A Companion to Braunwald's Heart Disease. Philadelphia, Saunders/Elsevier, 2009, pp 221-242

Roberts WC, Ko JM: Clinical pathology of valvular heart disease. In Otto CM, Bonow RO (eds): Valvular Heart Disease: A Companion to Braunwald's Heart Disease. Philadelphia, Saunders/Elsevier, 2009, pp 19-38.

ANSWER TO QUESTION 528

A (Braunwald, pp. 1432-1434)

These findings are consistent with patent ductus arteriosus (PDA). In the majority of preterm infants weighing <1500 g, a patent ductus persists for a prolonged period, and in approximately one third of these infants a large shunt leads to significant cardiopulmonary deterioration. Noninvasive evaluation may reveal evidence of significant shunting before the appearance of physical findings of ductal patency. Physical examination may reveal bounding peripheral pulses, an infraclavicular and interscapular systolic murmur (occasionally heard as a continuous murmur), a hyperactive precordium, hepatomegaly, and recurrent episodes of apnea and bradycardia with or without respirator dependence. An increase in the cardiothoracic ratio is seen on sequential chest radiographs and may be accompanied by increased pulmonary arterial markings, perihilar edema, and ultimately generalized pulmonary edema. Echocardiography may demonstrate increased left ventricular end-diastolic and left atrial dimensions, and color Doppler confirms the presence of left-to-right shunting. Cardiac catheterization is rarely necessary.

Management of the premature infant with a PDA depends on the clinical presentation of the disorder. In an asymptomatic infant, intervention is usually unnecessary, because the PDA will almost always undergo spontaneous closure and will not require surgical ligation and division. Infants with respiratory distress syndrome and signs of a significant ductal shunt usually are unresponsive to medical measures to control congestive heart failure and require closure of the PDA for survival. This usually is accomplished pharmacologically, using indomethacin to inhibit prostaglandin synthesis and achieve constriction and closure. Approximately 10% of infants are unresponsive to indomethacin and require surgical ligation.

REFERENCE

Moore JW, Levi DS, Moore SD, et al: Interventional treatment of patent ductus arteriosus in 2004. Catheter Cardiovasc Interv 64:91, 2005.

ANSWER TO QUESTION 529

A (Braunwald, pp. 1582-1593)

The echocardiogram demonstrates hypertrophic cardiomyopathy (HCM) with asymmetric septal hypertrophy. The most common physiologic abnormality in HCM is not systolic but rather diastolic dysfunction. HCM is characterized by abnormal stiffness of the left ventricle, which results in impaired diastolic filling. The abnormal diastolic relaxation increases the left ventricular (LV) end-diastolic pressure with subsequent elevations of left atrial, pulmonary venous, and pulmonary capillary pressures.

Although the generation of a pressure gradient due to associated subaortic obstruction would imply that LV ejection is slowed or impeded during systole, there is actually *rapid* ventricular emptying and a normal, or even augmented, ejection fraction in such patients. Hemodynamic studies have confirmed that the majority of LV output is unusually rapid in patients with HCM and is completed earlier in systole than normal, regardless of whether an outflow gradient is present. Thus, the common symptom of dyspnea in this condition is largely due to impaired diastolic relaxation rather than compromised systolic ejection. Although there is a strong temporal and quantitative relationship between mitral valve systolic anterior motion and the development of subaortic obstruction, symptoms do not necessarily correlate with the magnitude of the generated gradient. Furthermore, there can be significant variations on a daily basis in both the extent of the obstruction (and associated murmur) and symptomatology.

Exertional syncope and angina occur in some patients with HCM, and these symptoms are likely related, at least in part, to systolic obstruction.

The echolucent space posterior to the left ventricle in the echocardiogram represents a tiny pericardial effusion.

REFERENCE

Maron BJ, Doerer JJ, Haas TS, et al: Sudden deaths in young competitive athletes: Analysis of 1866 deaths in the U.S., 1980-2006. Circulation 119:1085, 2009.

ANSWER TO QUESTION 530

D (Braunwald, pp. 1487-1489)

Acute aortic regurgitation (AR) is caused most often by infective endocarditis, aortic dissection, or trauma. Many of the physical findings typical of chronic AR are *not* present in patients with acute AR.[1] In acute AR the left ventricle has not had time to dilate and is relatively noncompliant, and its early diastolic pressure rises rapidly. If the left ventricular (LV) diastolic pressure exceeds the left atrial pressure, the mitral valve may close *prematurely* and can produce diastolic mitral regurgitation. Because the elevated LV diastolic pressure blunts runoff of blood from the aorta into the left ventricle, the aortic diastolic pressure does not decline as substantially as in chronic AR.[2] Therefore, the pulse pressure does not widen significantly, and physical findings typical of an increased pulse pressure, such as Corrigan pulse (abrupt upstroke, then quick collapse of the arterial pulse), are absent. Similarly, the duration of the diastolic murmur is shorter than in chronic AR.[3]

REFERENCES

1. Enriquez-Sarano M, Tajik AJ: Aortic regurgitation. N Engl J Med 351:1539, 2004.
2. Carabello B: Progress in mitral and aortic regurgitation. Prog Cardiovasc Dis 43:457, 2001.
3. Stout KK, Verrier ED: Acute valvular regurgitation. Circulation 119:3232, 2009.

ANSWER TO QUESTION 531

E (Braunwald, pp. 1435-1437)

Tetralogy of Fallot accounts for about 10% of all types of congenital heart disease and is one of the most common congenital cardiac defects associated with cyanosis after the first year of age.[1] As summarized in the Answer to Question 481, there are four anomalies that constitute this malformation: (1) ventricular septal defect (VSD), (2) right ventricular (RV) outflow obstruction, (3) overriding of the aorta, and (4) RV hypertrophy. The VSD is usually located high in the septum below the right aortic valve cusp. The aortic root may be displaced anteriorly and override the septal defect but, as in the normal heart, the aortic root is to the right of the origin of the pulmonary artery.

The clinical picture of tetralogy of Fallot depends on the degree of RV outflow obstruction. The obstruction can be infundibular, or it may coexist with valvular stenosis. When the obstruction is severe, pulmonary blood flow is markedly reduced and the degree of right-to-left shunting across the VSD is increased, resulting in cyanosis. Supravalvular and peripheral pulmonary artery stenosis can also be present in patients with tetralogy and may occur at single or multiple sites. Coronary anomalies occur in approximately 5% of patients.[2] The most common consists of an anterior descending artery that originates from the right coronary artery.

REFERENCES

1. Botto LD, Correa A, Erickson JD: Racial and temporal variations in the prevalence of heart defects. Pediatrics 107:E32, 2001.
2. Mawson JB: Congenital heart defects and coronary anatomy. Tex Heart Inst J 29:271, 2002.

ANSWER TO QUESTION 532

B (Braunwald, pp. 1713-1714)

The development of pulmonary hypertension in patients with chronic obstructive lung disease (COPD) arises from several factors including pulmonary vasoconstriction induced by alveolar hypoxemia, acidemia, the mechanical effects of the high lung volumes on the pulmonary vessels, and small-vessel loss in regions of emphysema.[1] Right ventricular (RV) hypertrophy and dilatation may develop over time (Fig. 4-37).

The only effective treatment for patients with COPD and pulmonary hypertension is supplemental oxygen,

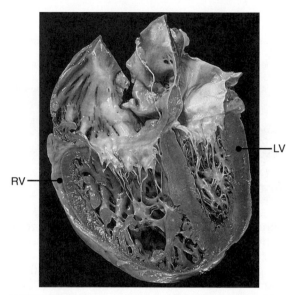

FIGURE 4-37 From Kumar V, Abbas AK, Fausto N (eds): Robbins and Cotran Pathologic Basis of Disease. 7th ed. Philadelphia, Elsevier, 2005, p 588.

with several studies showing an improvement in morbidity and mortality.[2] In a series of trials in the 1980s, continuous oxygen supplementation was more effective than nocturnal therapy alone. Thus, long-term oxygen therapy is recommended if the resting Pao_2 is < 55 mm Hg.

Although digoxin may improve the RV ejection fraction in some patients with RV dilation and dysfunction, it can also contribute to adverse pulmonary vasoconstriction and has not been shown to have a beneficial effect on survival. Furthermore, digitalis toxicity may be precipitated by the hypoxemia and acidemia often associated with COPD. Theophylline, beta agonists, hydralazine, and other vasodilators also have not been shown to improve survival of patients with pulmonary hypertension due to COPD.[3]

REFERENCES

1. Weitzenblum E: Chronic cor pulmonale. Heart 89:225, 2003.
2. Carbone R, Bossone E, Bottino G, et al: Secondary pulmonary hypertension: Diagnosis and management. Eur Rev Med Pharmacol Sci 9:331-342, 2005.
3. Stolz D, Rasch H, Linka A, et al: A randomised, controlled trial of bosentan in severe COPD. Eur Respir J 32:619, 2008.

ANSWER TO QUESTION 533

B (Braunwald, pp. 1452-1454)

Coarctation of the aorta (Fig. 4-38) occurs two to five times more commonly in males.[1] Most infants and children with coarctation are *asymptomatic*. In contrast, neonates with severe coarctation often develop overt heart failure due to the sudden rise in left ventricular (LV) afterload when the ductus arteriosus closes at birth. Coarctations discovered in the adult are associated with additional abnormalities, including bicuspid aortic valve (50% to 85%) and intracranial aneurysms.

Pathophysiologically, significant coarctation places a pressure load on the left ventricle, which leads to LV

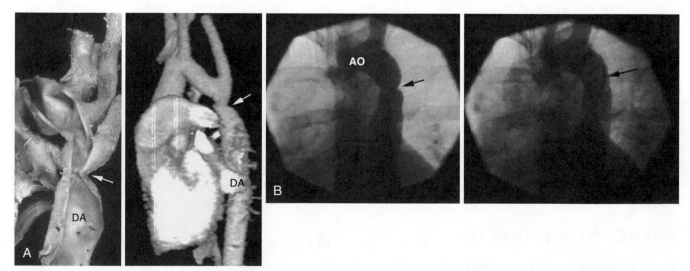

FIGURE 4-38 A, Montage of a coarctation of the aorta. The left image is a specimen that shows the site of the posterior shelf, as outlined by the arrow. the right image is from a CMR examination and shows the posterior shelf and some associated transverse arch hypoplasia. **B,** Angiogram of a coarctation of the aorta, before and after stenting. AO, aorta; DA, descending aorta.

hypertrophy and ultimately heart failure. On physical examination, findings include a differential systolic blood pressure (brachial artery pressure greater than popliteal artery pressure by > 10 mm Hg) and radial-femoral pulse delay. The mean survival time of patients with uncorrected coarctation is 35 years. Heart failure is the most common cause of death in adults, followed by bacterial endocarditis, intracranial hemorrhage, and aortic dissection. Surgical repair is associated with very low mortality. Outcomes are most influenced by the presence of other congenital anomalies or more complex variants of aortic coarctation involving the aortic arch, rather than the type of surgery performed.

Recoarctation and true aneurysm formation at the site of repair can occur.[2] The reported incidence of these complications varies widely in the surgical literature, ranging from 6% to 60%. Prior hypertension resolves in up to 50% of patients but may recur later in life.[2]

REFERENCES

1. Abbruzzese PA, Aidala E: Aortic coarctation: an overview. J Cardiovasc Med 8:123-128, 2007.
2. Bouchart F, Dubar A, Tabley A, et al: Coarctation of the aorta in adults: Surgical results and long term follow-up. Ann Thorac Surg 70:1483, 2000.

ANSWER TO QUESTION 534

B (Braunwald, pp. 1640-1643)

The apical four-chamber views demonstrate a large left atrial myxoma, which in diastole prolapses across the orifice of the mitral valve. Echocardiography is especially helpful in differentiating between left atrial thrombus and myxoma. Thrombus usually produces a layered appearance and tends to localize to the more posterior segments of the atrium. In contrast, left atrial myxoma is often mottled in appearance and typically attaches along the limbus of the fossa ovalis of the interatrial septum. In some atrial myxomas, including the one demonstrated here, echolucent areas are seen within the tumor mass that correspond pathologically to regions of hemorrhage within the tumor.

Eighty-three percent of cardiac myxomas appear in the left atrium and 12.7% in the right atrium; the remainder are biatrial or located in one of the ventricles. Signs and symptoms may be similar to those of mitral valve disease owing to interference of the mass with normal mitral valvular function. Physical examination may demonstrate pulmonary congestion and an intensified S_1. It is believed that the loud S_1 occurs because of late onset of mitral valve closure as a consequence of tumor prolapse through the valvular orifice. An early diastolic sound (tumor "plop") may be present, although this is often positional and may be confused with an opening snap or an S_3 unless the diagnosis of myxoma is suspected. Cardiac myxoma may also produce a variety of constitutional symptoms and extracardiac findings, including fever, weight loss, arthralgias, rash, and clubbing. The constitutional symptoms associated with cardiac myxoma are attributed to the tumor's production of interleukin-6. Several abnormal laboratory findings may be present, including an elevated erythrocyte sedimentation rate, polycythemia, leukocytosis, and anemia.

Approximately 10% of myxomas are familial. In such cases, patients typically present at a younger age and are more likely to have multiple myxomas in noncardiac locations. They often have associated dermatologic and endocrine abnormalities and may have a form of multiple endocrine neoplasia termed the *Carney complex*.

The treatment of symptomatic cardiac myxoma is prompt surgical resection of the tumor with the patient placed on cardiopulmonary bypass. Complete excision is the goal, although this may not be possible in all instances. Recurrent myxomas appear in approximately 3% of patients, with a higher incidence in those with familial myxomas.

REFERENCE

Ipek G, Erentug V, Bozbuga N, et al: Surgical management of cardiac myxoma. J Card Surg 20:300, 2005.

ANSWER TO QUESTION 535

D (Braunwald, pp. 1681-1682; Table 77-12)

Diagnostic approaches for pulmonary embolism (PE) have become increasingly reliable and streamlined. The most useful approach is the clinical assessment of likelihood, based on presenting symptoms and signs, in conjunction with judicious diagnostic testing (Fig. 4-39).

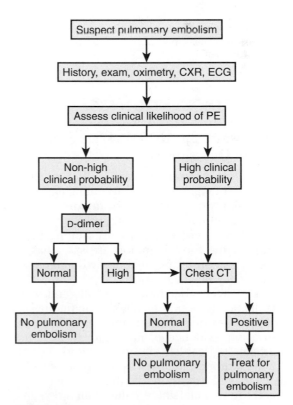

FIGURE 4-39

When PE is highly suspected, chest CT angiography is the superior imaging test.[1] This technique has the capability to visualize even subsegmental pulmonary emboli. When the clinical probability of PE is not high, a normal plasma D-dimer assay usually suffices to rule out this condition.[2] The D-dimer assay is >90% sensitive for the presence of PE but has low specificity because elevations also occur in sepsis, recent surgery or trauma, malignancies, and other systemic illnesses. The negative predictive value of a normal D-dimer assay is excellent at 95% (i.e., a patient with a normal D-dimer is 95% likely to *not* have PE).

Arterial blood gas determinations are generally not helpful in the diagnosis of PE. In the Prospective Investigation of Pulmonary Embolism Diagnosis (PIOPED) study, the Pao_2 did not differentiate between individuals with and without PE. In patients with large PE, electrocardiographic signs of right-sided heart strain may be present but such findings are generally absent when small PEs are present. The most common electrocardiographic abnormality in PE is sinus tachycardia; a normal tracing does not exclude this condition.

Ventilation-perfusion lung scanning results are often ambiguous. Although PE is very unlikely to be present with a completely normal scan, and very likely when the test is "high probability," scans frequently fall between these two extremes ("intermediate probability") and do not provide definitive results. This test is now generally used for diagnosis of acute PE only in certain circumstances (e.g., a history of anaphylaxis to IV contrast agents, renal insufficiency, or pregnancy).

REFERENCES

1. Schoepf UJ, Goldhaber SZ, Costello P: Spiral CT for acute pulmonary embolism. Circulation 109:2160, 2004.
2. Dunn KL, Wolf JP, Dorfman DM, et al: Normal d-dimer levels in emergency department patients suspected of acute pulmonary embolism. J Am Coll Cardiol 40:1475, 2002.

ANSWER TO QUESTION 536

D (Braunwald, pp. 1639-1647; see also Answer to Question 503)

Primary tumors of the heart are rare (0.2% of all cardiac tumors), with benign tumors representing approximately 75%. The majority of benign cardiac tumors are myxomas, followed in frequency by lipomas, papillary fibroelastomas, rhabdomyomas, and fibromas. Among the malignant tumors, the most common are sarcomas, and of these, angiosarcoma and rhabdomyosarcoma are the most frequently occurring forms.

Although it can be difficult to differentiate benign from malignant tumors clinically, certain findings may be helpful. The presence of distant metastases, local mediastinal invasion, evidence of rapid growth in tumor size, hemorrhagic pericardial effusion, precordial pain, location of the tumor on the *right* as opposed to the left side of the heart, and extension into the pulmonary veins are all suggestive of a malignant rather than a benign tumor. Furthermore, infiltration of the myocardium is much more common in malignant than benign tumors. Benign

tumors are more likely to occur on the left side of the interatrial septum and to grow slowly.

Cardiac symptoms caused by tumors are primarily determined by mechanical interferences. Myxomas that are located on the left side are more likely to produce mitral valve symptoms, whereas malignant tumors more commonly found on the right side of the heart tend to produce signs of right-sided failure.

REFERENCE

Ekmektzoglou KA, Samelis GF, Xanthos T: Heart and tumors: Location, metastasis, clinical manifestations, diagnostic approaches and therapeutic considerations. J Cardiovasc Med 9:769, 2008.

ANSWER TO QUESTION 537

C (Braunwald, pp. 1655-1660)

Echocardiography is the most useful noninvasive test to evaluate for cardiac tamponade. Findings most suggestive of tamponade physiology include (1) a large pericardial effusion, (2) right atrial and right ventricular (RV) diastolic collapse, (3) an exaggerated inspiratory increase in transtricuspid flow velocities with concurrent reduction of transmitral flow velocities, and (4) inferior vena caval dilatation with absence of normal inspiratory collapse.[1]

RV diastolic collapse is the most predictive sign of tamponade.[2] It is more specific than right atrial collapse and more sensitive and specific than pulsus paradoxus in detecting increased pericardial pressure. However, diastolic RV collapse may not be evident in patients with elevated intrapericardial pressure who also have pulmonary hypertension, because RV pressures are higher than normal in that case.

A small pericardial effusion makes tamponade less likely but does not exclude the diagnosis, especially if the pericardial fluid has accumulated rapidly. In addition, small pericardial effusions can be associated with "low-pressure" tamponade in patients with intravascular volume depletion. Small loculated effusions (e.g., after cardiac surgery) can also result in tamponade physiology because of localized chamber compression.

REFERENCES

1. Spodick DH: Acute cardiac tamponade. N Engl J Med 349:684, 2003.
2. Little WC, Freeman GL: Pericardial disease. Circulation 113:1622, 2006.

ANSWER TO QUESTION 538

D (Braunwald, pp. 1661-1663)

The lateral chest radiograph shows calcification of the pericardium, suggestive of constrictive pericarditis. Pericardial calcification is now seen only in the minority of patients with constriction and appears primarily in those with tuberculosis. In this patient's case, prior radiation therapy is the likely cause.

The clinical presentation of patients with chronic constrictive pericarditis (CP) is predominantly that of right-sided heart failure. In early stages, signs include jugular venous distention (with a rapidly collapsing *y* descent) and Kussmaul sign, which represents inspiratory augmentation of the jugular venous pressure, peripheral edema, and vague abdominal discomfort due to passive hepatic congestion and hepatomegaly. As the disease progresses, ascites, jaundice, and anasarca may ensue.

The most notable auscultatory finding observed in patients with advanced CP is the pericardial knock, an early diastolic sound heard best at the left sternal border or apex that corresponds to the sudden cessation of ventricular filling imposed by the rigid, constricting pericardium. The pericardial knock occurs earlier and is of higher frequency than an S_3 gallop sound and may be confused with the opening snap of mitral stenosis.

Heart catheterization in patients with CP is notable for elevation and equalization of the intracardiac diastolic pressures and a diastolic "dip-and-plateau" configuration of the ventricular pressure tracings. Intravascular volume depletion can mask these typical hemodynamic findings, but they can be uncovered with an intravenous fluid challenge in the catheterization laboratory. One important way to distinguish CP from restrictive cardiomyopathy (CMP) during catheterization is to observe the variation in simultaneously recorded right and left ventricular systolic pressures. In contrast to normal individuals or those with restrictive CMP, in CP there is usually a striking discordance between these pressures during respiration: with inspiration, the left ventricular systolic pressure falls while that of the right ventricle increases. This finding reflects the exaggerated ventricular interdependence that results from pericardial constraint.

REFERENCE

Talreja DR, Nishimura RA, Oh JK, Holmes DR: Constrictive pericarditis in the modern era: Novel criteria for diagnosis in the cardiac catheterization laboratory. J Am Coll Cardiol 22:315, 2008.

ANSWER TO QUESTION 539

D (Braunwald, pp. 1468-1469, 1489; see also Answer to Question 507)

The three primary causes of valvular aortic stenosis (AS) are (1) a congenitally bicuspid valve that becomes calcified, (2) calcification of a structurally normal trileaflet valve, and (3) rheumatic disease (Fig. 4-40). Age-related calcification of a congenitally bicuspid or normal trileaflet valve is now the most common cause of AS in adults.[1] In one U.S. series of 933 patients who underwent surgical valve replacement for AS, a bicuspid valve was found in >50%, including two thirds of those <70 years and 40% of those >70.[2]

Although calcific aortic valve disease was once considered to result from years of mechanical stress on a normal valve, it actually appears to represent proliferative and inflammatory changes, with lipid accumulation and infiltration of macrophages and T lymphocytes, in a manner similar to vascular calcification. As in atherosclerosis, cigarette smoking, hyperlipidemia, and diabetes are risk factors for the development of this valvular process.

Rheumatic valvular disease has declined in frequency in industrialized countries but remains an important condition in developing nations. Rheumatic AS results from postinflammatory fusion and adhesion of the valve commissures and rarely develops in the absence of rheumatic mitral involvement.

REFERENCES

1. Freeman RV, Otto CM: Spectrum of calcific aortic valve disease: Pathogenesis, disease progression, and treatment strategies. Circulation 111:3316, 2005.
2. Roberts WC, Ko JM: Frequency by decades of unicuspid, bicuspid, and tricuspid aortic valves in adults having isolated aortic valve replacement for aortic stenosis, with or without associated aortic regurgitation. Circulation 111:920, 2005.

ANSWER TO QUESTION 540

C (Braunwald, pp. 1478-1487)

Appropriate timing for surgical intervention in chronic aortic regurgitation (AR) depends on the patient's symptoms and state of left ventricular (LV) contractile function. Regardless of the severity of AR, patients who are symptomatic and have reduced LV systolic function should be referred for surgery, unless an absolute contraindication exists.[1] Asymptomatic patients with advanced AR who have normal LV function and no evidence of ventricular dilatation (end-systolic diameter <50 mm) have an excellent prognosis and typically can be observed clinically and by echocardiography to assess for changes in LV size and function. In such individuals, the end-systolic diameter, serially measured by echocardiography, is valuable in predicting the postoperative outcome. An end-systolic diameter <40 mm predicts a low likelihood of postoperative instability or heart failure. However, an end-systolic diameter >55 mm, or a preoperative ejection fraction <50%, increases the risk of postoperative death from LV dysfunction.[1] Several vasodilators, including angiotensin-converting enzyme inhibitors, have been shown to provide beneficial hemodynamic effects in chronic AR. However, a 7-year randomized trial compared nifedipine, enalapril, and placebo in patients with chronic AR and did not demonstrate a benefit of either vasodilator regimen in reducing symptoms or LV dysfunction warranting valve replacement.[2]

REFERENCES

1. Enriquez-Sarano M, Tajik AJ: Aortic regurgitation. N Engl J Med 351:1539, 2004.
2. Evangelista A, Tornos P, Sambola A, et al: Long-term vasodilator therapy in patients with severe aortic regurgitation. N Engl J Med 353:1342, 2005.

ANSWER TO QUESTION 541

E (Braunwald, pp. 1618-1621)

Identification of cardiac complications of human immunodeficiency virus (HIV) infection has increased as

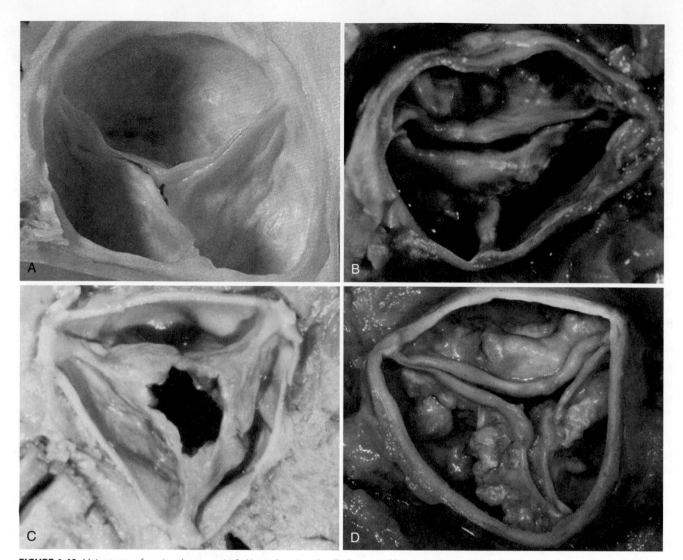

FIGURE 4-40 Major types of aortic valve stenosis. **A,** Normal aortic valve. **B,** Congenital bicuspid aortic stenosis. A false raphe is present at the 6-o'clock position. **C,** Rheumatic aortic stenosis. The commissures are fused with a fixed central orifice. **D,** Calcific degenerative aortic stenosis. **A,** from Manabe H, Yutani C (eds): Atlas of Valvular Heart Disease. Singapore, Churchill Livingstone, 1998, pp 6, 131; **B-D,** Courtesy of Dr. William C. Roberts, Baylor University Medical Center, Dallas, TX.

greater longevity has been achieved by highly effective antiretroviral therapies. Four to 28 percent of patients with HIV infection develop symptomatic heart failure over a 5-year period of observation.[1] Specifically, dilated cardiomyopathy afflicts 10% to 20% of HIV-infected patients and accounts for almost one third of HIV-related deaths.

The median survival of HIV-infected patients with left ventricular (LV) dysfunction is 101 days, compared with 472 days in those with normal LV function. Putative mechanisms for LV dysfunction include direct viral infection of myocytes, immune-mediated myocarditis, nutritional deficiencies, and direct toxicities of antiretroviral therapies.

Pericardial effusion is common in HIV disease, occurring in 7% to 10% of patients.[2] Typically such effusions are small and a large number resolve spontaneously. The effusion is most often "idiopathic" but can be related to opportunistic infections, drug toxicities, uremia, or malignancy. The presence of a pericardial effusion increases the mortality risk in HIV-infected patients.

There is a growing observational literature that HIV-infected patients are at increased risk of accelerated coronary artery disease, even in the absence of traditional risk factors. This may be related to direct HIV vasculopathy or coinfection with other viruses such as cytomegalovirus. Moreover, protease inhibitor therapy can lead to derangements in lipid metabolism and is associated with an increased risk of myocardial infarction.[3]

REFERENCES

1. Ho JE, Hsue PY: Cardiovascular manifestations of HIV infection. Heart 95:1193, 2009.
2. Barbaro G: Cardiovascular manifestations of HIV infection. Circulation 106:1420, 2002.

3. DAD Study Group: Class of antiretroviral drugs and the risk of myocardial infarction. N Engl J Med 356:1723, 2007.

ANSWER TO QUESTION 542

A (Braunwald, p. 1420)

Turner syndrome, also termed *gonadal dysgenesis,* occurs in 1 of every 2500 females. Clinical features include primary amenorrhea, short stature, and immature genital and breast development. The condition arises from defects of the X chromosome, including the 45,XO karyotype in about 50% of cases. Cardiovascular abnormalities are common, occurring in 20% to 50% of patients.[1] The most frequent manifestation is coarctation of the aorta, found in 50% to 70% of patients with Turner syndrome who have cardiovascular defects. Coarctation can occur alone or in combination with other aortic abnormalities, including bicuspid aortic valve and a dilated aortic root.

Patients with Turner syndrome are also at increased risk for aortic dissection independent of other aortic abnormalities. Histopathologic studies have shown abnormalities of the elastic media similar to those in patients with diseases of collagen formation. Partial anomalous pulmonary venous drainage is also found frequently in patients with this condition.

REFERENCE

1. Lin AE, Silberbach M: Focus on the heart and aorta in Turner syndrome. J Pediatr 150:572-574, 2007.

ANSWER TO QUESTION 543

B (Braunwald, pp. 1916-1919)

Duchenne muscular dystrophy (DMD) is an X-linked recessive disorder that arises from a mutation in the gene that encodes dystrophin. Most patients with DMD develop dilated cardiomyopathy, and specific mutations in the dystrophin gene are associated with the prevalence of left ventricular dysfunction.[1] Preclinical cardiac involvement is present in 25% by age 6. Up to 90% of patients with Duchenne muscular dystrophy who are 18 years of age or older will have developed echocardiographic evidence of dilated cardiomyopathy. There is a predilection for involvement of the inferobasal and lateral left ventricle, which likely accounts for the classically described electrocardiographic abnormalities: tall R waves and increased R/S amplitude in V_1 and deep narrow Q waves in the left precordial leads (Fig. 4-41). There does not appear to be an association between the presence of dilated cardiomyopathy and electrocardiographic abnormalities.[2]

Persistent or labile sinus tachycardia is the most common arrhythmia in DMD. Other atrial arrhythmias, including atrial fibrillation and atrial flutter, occur primarily as a preterminal rhythm. Ventricular arrhythmias occur on monitoring in 30%, primarily ventricular premature beats.

REFERENCES

1. Jefferies JL, Eidem BW, Belmont JW, et al: Genetic predictors and remodeling of dilated cardiomyopathy in muscular dystrophy. Circulation 112:2799, 2005.
2. Thrush PT, Allen HD, Viollet L, et al: Re-examination of the electrocardiogram in boys with Duchenne muscular dystrophy and correlation with its dilated cardiomyopathy. Am J Cardiol 103:262, 2009.

ANSWER TO QUESTION 544

C (Braunwald, p. 1901)

The anthracycline antineoplastic agents (doxorubicin, daunorubicin, and idarubicin) are widely recognized for their potential cardiac toxicity. Rarely, a single high dose of an anthracycline causes an acute cardiotoxic reaction manifested by atrial and ventricular arrhythmias and conduction disturbances. The more common effect is chronic cardiomyopathy after long-term exposure to these drugs.[1] The greatest risk factor for this complication is the cumulative dose. Retrospective analyses have suggested that the incidence of heart failure is 2.2% overall, but 7.5% in patients receiving a cumulative dose >550 mg/m[2] of doxorubicin. Thus, oncologists typically limit the total dose to no more than 450 to 500 mg/m[2]. Age at the time of exposure is another important risk

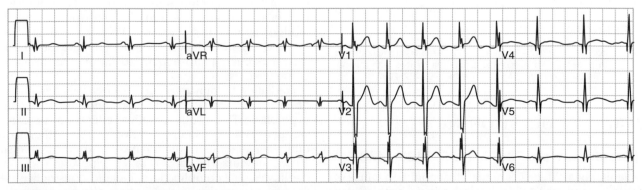

FIGURE 4-41 Dilated cardiomyopathy in a 19-year-old man with Duchenne muscular dystrophy. ECG shows a QRS complex that is typical of a Duchenne muscular dystrophy, with tall R waves in V[1] and deep narrow Q waves in leads I and aV[l].

factor, because the very young and the very old are particularly susceptible.[1] The incidence of anthracycline cardiotoxicity in children approaches 10% for cumulative doses of 550 mg/m².

Additional risk factors for anthracycline cardiotoxicity include prior mediastinal radiation, the concurrent administration of other cardiotoxic agents (e.g., cyclophosphamide or trastuzumab), and a history of cardiac disease.[2] For example, cardiotoxicity is more likely to arise when the baseline left ventricular ejection fraction is <50%.[3]

In randomized trials, the iron chelator dexrazoxane has demonstrated a protective effect against anthracycline cardiotoxicity. Because there has been concern that dexrazoxane may reduce anthracycline efficacy, its use is generally limited to patients who have received > 300 mg/m² of doxorubicin or its equivalent.

REFERENCES

1. Cremer LC, Huib C: Anthracycline cardiotoxicity in children. N Engl J Med 351:120, 2004.
2. Schimmel KJ, Richel DJ, van den Brink RB, Guchelaar HJ: Cardiotoxicity of cytotoxic drugs. Cancer Treat Rev 30:181, 2004.
3. Ng R, Better N, Green MD: Anticancer agents and cardiotoxicity. Semin Oncol 33:2, 2006.

ANSWER TO QUESTION 545

C (Braunwald, pp. 78-79, 1420, 1429-1430)

Vascular endothelial growth factor (VEGF) antagonists interfere with the vascular supply of tumors. The monoclonal antibody bevacizumab (Avastin) targets VEGF-A and, combined with chemotherapy, improves survival in patients with metastatic colorectal cancer and metastatic nonsquamous non–small cell lung cancer. Several adverse reactions may occur with this agent. Hypertension (not hypotension) is a common side effect and can be severe in 8% to 20% of patients. Bevacizumab is also associated with heart failure, and although the risk of precipitating left ventricular dysfunction is low, it is more likely to develop in patients who have also received anthracyclines or irradiation. There is an approximately twofold increase in arterial (but not venous) thromboembolic events with bevacizumab.[1]

Neither acute coronary syndromes nor hemorrhagic pericardial effusion is a common side effect of bevacizumab therapy.

REFERENCE

1. Scappaticci FA, Skillings JR, Holden SN, et al: Arterial thromboembolic events in patients with metastatic carcinoma treated with chemotherapy and bevacizumab. J Natl Cancer Inst 99:1232, 2007.

ANSWER TO QUESTION 546

B (Braunwald, pp. 78-79, 1420, 1429-1430)

Congenital heart defects are the most common cause of morbidity and mortality in individuals with Down syndrome. The most frequent abnormality is an endocardial cushion defect, including partial or complete atrioventricular septal defects. The typical presentation includes a history of poor weight gain and frequent respiratory infections in the first year of life. Cardiac auscultation findings depend on the degree of atrial and ventricular septal communications and whether there is atrioventricular valve involvement. In patients with the more common partial endocardial cushion defect, the examination findings are similar to those of an ostium primum atrial septal defect. There is a prominent midsystolic pulmonary flow murmur (because of increased flow into the pulmonary artery) followed by wide, fixed splitting of S_2. A mid-diastolic murmur is also common owing to increased flow through the tricuspid valve. When a cleft mitral valve is part of the partial endocardial cushion defect, a holosystolic murmur at the apex is present that frequently radiates toward the sternum, because the right atrium receives regurgitant flow in this condition. When an interventricular communication exists as part of the defect, a holosystolic murmur is usually present at the mid to lower left sternal edge.

A midsystolic click followed by a late systolic murmur at the apex describes the auscultatory findings of mitral valve prolapse. Mitral valve prolapse occurs more frequently in patients with Down syndrome than in typical individuals, but it generally does not become evident until later in life. Choice A describes rheumatic mitral stenosis, choice D is the murmur of aortic regurgitation, and choice E represents aortic stenosis. These entities do not occur at an increased frequency in patients with Down syndrome.

REFERENCE

Masuda M, Kado H, Tanoue Y, et al: Does Down syndrome affect the long-term results of complete atrioventricular septal defect when the defect is repaired during the first year of life? Eur J Cardiothorac Surg 27:405, 2005.

ANSWER TO QUESTION 547

E (Braunwald, pp. 1668-1669, 1901-1902)

Radiation therapy is used to treat several types of malignancies. Historically, the heart and vasculature have been subjected to high doses of radiation in patients with lymphoma and in those with cancers of the breast, lung, or esophagus. As a consequence, cardiovascular complications are leading causes of mortality among long-term cancer survivors treated with older radiation techniques. Modern approaches since the 1980s have limited and focused radiation delivery with less heart exposure, and there has been a subsequent decline in cardiovascular complications.

Radiation therapy may cause myocardial damage and fibrosis, endothelial dysfunction, and arterial intimal hyperplasia. The resulting clinical effects on the cardiovascular system usually do not manifest themselves until long after the irradiation has occurred, often arising 10 to 20 years (or longer) after exposure. These late cardiovascular complications include constrictive pericarditis, proximal coronary artery disease, conduction system disease, valvular disease (especially of the aortic valve), and heart failure due to myocardial fibrosis and restrictive cardiomyopathy.[1] In addition, long-term cancer survivors who have received head and neck irradiation have a two- to threefold increased risk of stroke and transient ischemic attacks.[2]

REFERENCES

1. Hull MC, Morris CG, Pepine CJ, Mendenhall NP: Valvular dysfunction and carotid, subclavian, and coronary artery disease in survivors of Hodgkin's lymphoma treated with radiation therapy. JAMA 290:2831, 2003.
2. De Bruin ML, Dorresteijn LD, van't Veer MB, et al: Increased risk of stroke and transient ischemic attack in 5-year survivors of Hodgkin lymphoma. J Natl Cancer Inst 101:928, 2009.

ANSWER TO QUESTION 548

D (Braunwald, pp. 1563-1569)

Dilated cardiomyopathy (DCM) is responsible for approximately one fourth of the cases of congestive heart failure in the United States. It is believed that up to 30% of patients with DCM have an inherited form of the disease that results from a genetic mutation. Most familial examples of DCM fit an autosomal *dominant* pattern of inheritance, although some autosomal recessive and X-linked examples have also been found. Familial DCM appears to result primarily from mutations in genes that code for cytoskeletal, nuclear membrane, or contractile proteins; mitochondrial DNA mutations have also been reported.

Like other forms of DCM, cardiac histologic examination typically demonstrates extensive areas of interstitial and perivascular fibrosis, particularly in the left ventricular subendocardium. There are currently no specific immunologic, histochemical, or ultrastructural markers that can differentiate a genetic cause from other causes of idiopathic DCM.

REFERENCES

Hershberger RE, Lindenfeld J, Mestroni L, et al: Genetic evaluation of cardiomyopathy: A Heart Failure Society of America practice guideline. J Card Fail 15:83, 2009.
Karkkainen S, Peuhkurinen K: Genetics of dilated cardiomyopathy. Ann Med 39:91, 2007.

ANSWER TO QUESTION 549

C (Braunwald, pp. 1681-1686; see also Answers to Questions 501 and 535)

The most common symptoms of pulmonary embolism (PE) are dyspnea and pleuritic chest pain. Physical examination findings may include tachycardia, tachypnea, and an increased pulmonic component of S_2. Although arterial blood gas studies may be useful in managing a patient's respiratory status, they do not provide value in the diagnosis of PE. Normal values of the alveolar-arterial oxygen gradient do not exclude PE.

The classic electrocardiographic manifestations of acute PE include an $S_1Q_3T_3$ pattern, right bundle branch block, P pulmonale, and right-axis deviation. However, the most common abnormality is simply sinus tachycardia.[1] Measurement of plasma D-dimer (a fibrin degradation product) is > 90% sensitive for detecting PE but is not specific for the diagnosis.[2] Importantly, this test can be elevated in many other medical illnesses and thus loses specificity in hospitalized or critically ill patients. The chest radiograph may provide some clues to the diagnosis of PE but is typically normal. In fact, a near-normal chest radiograph in the setting of marked respiratory compromise should prompt consideration of PE. Specific abnormalities may include focal oligemia (Westermark's sign) indicative of massive central embolic occlusion, or a peripheral, homogeneous, wedge-shaped density ("Hampton's hump") usually indicative of pulmonary infarction.

The first step in the recommended diagnostic strategy (see Fig. 4-39, p. 267) is a directed history and physical examination to assess the clinical likelihood of acute PE. If there is no high clinical probability of pulmonary embolism, then D-dimer testing should follow. A normal D-dimer assay essentially concludes the workup for PE and alternate diagnoses should be pursued. If the D-dimer *is* elevated, chest CT angiography usually provides definitive diagnosis or exclusion of PE. For patients in whom the clinical likelihood of PE is high, it is appropriate to proceed directly to chest CT without D-dimer assessment.

REFERENCES

1. Vanni S, Polidori G, Vergara R, et al: Prognostic value of ECG among patients with acute pulmonary embolism and normal blood pressure. Am J Med 122:257, 2009.
2. Goldhaber SZ: Pulmonary embolism. Lancet 363:1295, 2004.

ANSWERS TO QUESTIONS 550 TO 553

550−B, 551−A, 552−C, 553−D (Braunwald, pp. 1546-1548)

The classic peripheral manifestations of infective endocarditis (IE) are encountered only infrequently today. Janeway lesions are small, painless, nontender and macular lesions on the thenar and hypothenar eminences of the palms and soles. They appear less often on the tips of the fingers or plantar surfaces of the toes. Lesions on the hands and feet blanch with pressure and with elevation of the extremities. In cases of acute valvular infections, the lesions tend to be purple and hemorrhagic.

In contrast, Osler nodes are small raised, nodular, and tender lesions present most often in the pulp spaces of the terminal phalanges of the fingers. They may also be present on the backs of the toes, the soles, and the thenar and hypothenar eminences. The most characteristic feature of these lesions is their tenderness. Lesions may be fleeting in some cases, disappearing within a few hours after they have developed; however, they usually persist for 4 to 5 days. Although almost completely restricted to the subacute form of endocarditis, Osler nodes are occasionally present in acute valvular infection.

Subungual or splinter hemorrhages in IE are linear (or sometimes flame-shaped) dark red streaks in the proximal nailbed. Distal splinter hemorrhages at the nail tip are nondiagnostic and are frequently caused by trauma.

The ocular signs of endocarditis include retinal petechiae and Roth spots. The latter are located in the nerve layer of the retina and appear as hemorrhagic exudates. Histologically they consist of aggregations of cytoid bodies (perivascular accumulation of lymphocytes with or without surrounding hemorrhage).

Bracht-Wächter bodies represent embolic events to the myocardium in IE that cause a localized inflammatory reaction consisting of collections of lymphocytes and mononuclear cells.

REFERENCE

Paterick TE, Paterick TJ, Nishimura RA, et al: Complexity and subtlety of infective endocarditis. Mayo Clin Proc 82:615, 2007.

ANSWERS TO QUESTIONS 554 TO 558

554—C, 555—B, 556—E, 557—A, 558—B (Braunwald, pp. 1562, 1568, 1570-1572, 1598)

The ECG is often nonspecific in cardiomyopathic disorders, but certain features are common in each of the listed conditions. In chronic Chagas disease, the most common electrocardiographic findings are right bundle branch block, left anterior hemiblock, atrial fibrillation, and premature ventricular depolarizations. Sarcoidosis has a propensity to infiltrate the atrioventricular (AV) node and bundle of His, producing heart block. Ventricular tachyarrhythmias are also common in this disorder. Apical hypertrophic cardiomyopathy is associated with deeply inverted T waves in the precordial leads. Amyloidosis results in low QRS voltage due to myocardial infiltration by amyloid protein. Other electrocardiographic features in amyloidosis include a pseudoinfarct pattern in the inferior leads and the frequent presence of atrial fibrillation. Lyme carditis results in variable degrees of AV block. Diffuse ST-segment elevation is typical of acute myopericarditis.

ANSWERS TO QUESTIONS 559 TO 562

559—D, 560—C, 561—C, 562—B (Braunwald, pp. 1521-1523)

Artificial cardiac valves consist of mechanical prostheses and bioprosthetic (tissue) valves.[1] Mechanical prostheses are divided into three structural groups: caged-ball, bileaflet, and tilting-disc valves. The Starr-Edwards caged-ball valve was one of the earliest prostheses used and has a long record of predictable performance. However, it has a bulky design, which makes it unsuitable for patients with a small left ventricular cavity or a narrow aortic annulus. Furthermore, the flow characteristics and action of the ball in the cage can generate low-level hemolysis. Tilting-disc valves have replaced the caged-ball prostheses, primarily because they are less bulky and have a

lower profile. The Omniscience valve is a type of pivoting disc prosthesis. The bileaflet St. Jude valve has two semicircular discs that pivot between open and closed positions without need for supporting struts. It has a lower transvalvular gradient than either the caged-ball or tilting-disc types and has particularly favorable hemodynamic characteristics in the smaller sizes. Thrombogenicity of the St. Jude prosthesis may be the lowest of the mechanical valves, which makes it an excellent candidate for use in mitral valve replacement in adults.

All of the mechanical prosthetic valves are durable, but they are associated with a risk of thromboembolism, which is greatest in the first postoperative year. Without anticoagulation, the incidence of thromboembolism is three- to sixfold higher than in properly anticoagulated patients. Despite treatment with anticoagulants, the incidence of thromboembolic complications is still one to two nonfatal events per 100 patient-years. The incidence is significantly higher for prostheses in the mitral than in the aortic position. The thrombosis rate of mechanical prostheses in the tricuspid position is extremely high, and for this reason bioprostheses are preferred. Administration of warfarin also carries its own morbidity and mortality, estimated at 2.2 and 0.2 per 100 patient-years, respectively.

The high risk of thromboembolism inherent with the use of mechanical valves led to the development of bioprosthetic prostheses. Among the tissue valves that are currently available are the Hancock porcine heterograft and the Carpentier-Edwards bovine pericardial valve. Anticoagulation for such valves is generally desirable for the first 3 months postoperatively while the sewing ring endothelializes. Thereafter, anticoagulants are generally not required.

Selection of an artificial valve requires an assessment of the benefits versus the risks of durability, endocarditis, hemodynamic perturbations, and thromboembolism. In general, tissue valves are preferred over mechanical prostheses for patients in whom anticoagulation is difficult or especially hazardous because they are prone to hemorrhage or are noncompliant. The common recommendation is to employ mechanical prosthetic valves in patients < 65 to 70 years old who have no contraindications to anticoagulants. Bioprostheses are recommended for patients with coexisting disease that is likely to make them prone to hemorrhage, those who are noncompliant, those unable to take anticoagulants for other reasons, and those of advanced age.

REFERENCE

1. Pibarot P, Dumesnil JG: Prosthetic heart valves: Selection of the optimal prosthesis and long-term management. Circulation 119:1034, 2009.

ANSWERS TO QUESTIONS 563 TO 566

563—C, 564—A, 565—A, 566—B (Braunwald, pp. 1664-1665)

Clinical distinction between patients with constrictive pericarditis (CP) and those with restrictive cardiomyopathy (RCM) due to diseases such as amyloidosis, hemochromatosis, and the hypereosinophilic syndrome may be difficult. Both RCM and CP may show the electrocardiographic changes of atrial fibrillation, left atrial abnormality, diffuse low voltage, and T wave flattening. The presence of atrioventricular block and conduction disturbances may favor the diagnosis of RCM, especially infiltrative diseases such as amyloidosis.

In both conditions, right ventricular (RV) and left ventricular (LV) diastolic pressures are elevated, stroke volume and cardiac output are decreased, and LV end-diastolic volume is normal or decreased, with impaired diastolic filling. A diagnosis of RCM is more likely when marked RV systolic hypertension is present (pressure >60 mm Hg) and when LV and RV diastolic pressures at rest, or during exercise, differ by more than 5 mm Hg. Some patients with RCM may display hemodynamics that are indistinguishable from those seen with CP, including sustained and complete equilibration of RV and LV pressures, as well as the presence of a "dip-and-plateau" pattern in the ventricular waveform. Simultaneous RV and LV systolic pressure measurements may have greater predictive value in identification of CP. Owing to exaggerated interventricular dependence in CP, these patients often demonstrate marked discordance of RV and LV systolic pressure during inspiration.[1,2] Specifically, with the onset of inspiration, LV systolic pressure declines with a reciprocal increase in RV systolic pressure.

Echocardiography in restrictive cardiomyopathy may reveal abnormally thickened ventricular myocardium, often with a "sparkling" appearance if amyloidosis is present. Other useful differentiating features on echocardiography include a diastolic septal "bounce" in CP and an increased tissue Doppler E′ velocity in constriction, in distinction to a blunted value (<8 cm/sec) typical of patients with RCM. Chest computed tomography and magnetic resonance imaging are also helpful distinguishing these entities, demonstrating a thickened pericardium in > 80% of patients with constrictive pericarditis[3] but not in patients with restrictive cardiomyopathy.

REFERENCES

1. Talreja DR, Nishimura RA, Oh JK, Holmes DR: Constrictive pericarditis in the modern era: Novel criteria for diagnosis in the cardiac catheterization laboratory. J Am Coll Cardiol 22:315, 2008.
2. Sengupta PP, Krishnamoorthy VK, Abhayaratna WP, et al: Disparate patterns of left ventricular mechanics differentiate constrictive pericarditis from restrictive cardiomyopathy. J Am Coll Cardiol Cardiovasc Imaging 1:29, 2008.
3. Talreja DR, Edwards WD, Danielson GK, et al: Constrictive pericarditis in 26 patients with histologically normal pericardial thickness. Circulation 108:1852, 2003.

ANSWERS TO QUESTIONS 567 TO 571

567–A, 568–C, 569–C, 570–D, 571–B (Braunwald, pp. 1640-1644)

Cardiac myxomas and papillary fibroelastomas are two of the most common primary tumors of the heart. They are benign and do not undergo malignant transformation. Papillary fibroelastomas are the most common primary tumors found on cardiac valves. These lesions are usually small, frondlike structures that consist of a collagen core surrounded by elastic fibers and loose connective tissue. They are most often detected as an incidental finding on echocardiography or at postmortem examination. Most papillary fibroelastomas are clinically insignificant, although there is the potential for embolization or valve orifice obstruction if the tumor is large. Anticoagulation does not appear to protect against embolic risk. Surgical resection of these tumors is generally recommended, especially those in left-sided locations, to prevent thromboemboli. Resection can usually be performed with valve-sparing techniques. There is no known familial syndrome associated with papillary fibroelastomas.[1]

Conversely, approximately 10% of myxomas are familial, transmitted in an autosomal dominant pattern. Sporadic myxomas most commonly attach to the interatrial septum; valvular origins for myxoma are rare. Myxomas have a high risk of distal embolization due to the friable nature of the tumor. Surgical resection is recommended to avoid new or recurrent complications, including progressive constitutional symptoms, embolism, and valvular obstruction.[2]

REFERENCES

1. Sydow K, Willems S, Reichenspurner H, et al: Papillary fibroelastomas of the heart. Thorac Cardiovasc Surg 56:9, 2008.
2. Ipek G, Erentug V, Bozbuga N, et al: Surgical management of cardiac myxoma. J Card Surg 20:300, 2005.

ANSWERS TO QUESTIONS 572 TO 575

572–C, 573–B, 574–D, 575–A (Braunwald, pp. 1687-1691, 1857-1860, 1864-1865)

Unfractionated heparin has long been the traditional therapy for pulmonary embolism. It is a porcine- or bovine-derived glycosaminoglycan that acts by binding to antithrombin with subsequent inhibition of the procoagulant factors thrombin (IIa), Xa, IXa, XIa, and XIIa. Heparin prevents additional thrombus formation and promotes endogenous fibrinolysis; however, it does not directly dissolve formed clots. For patients at average bleeding risk, a weight-based IV bolus of 80 units/kg is begun, followed by 18 units/kg/hr by continuous infusion. The activated partial thromboplastin time should be maintained between 1.5 to 2.5 times the control value for effective treatment. A plasma heparin level (anti–factor Xa level) may be useful when the partial thromboplastin time (PTT) is elevated at baseline (e.g., in the presence of the lupus anticoagulant) or when monitoring patients with deep vein thrombosis (DVT) or pulmonary embolism (PE) who require large quantities of heparin. The major risk of heparin use is hemorrhage. Thrombocytopenia, osteopenia, and elevated liver enzymes may all complicate heparin therapy. Protamine may be used to reverse the anticoagulant effects of unfractionated heparin.

Low-molecular-weight heparins (LMWHs) are approved by the U.S. Food and Drug Administration for the outpatient treatment of DVT without PE and for the inpatient treatment of DVT with or without PE.[1] LMWH has greater bioavailability than unfractionated heparin, has a more predictable dose response, and does not require serial measurements of the aPTT. If needed, the effectiveness of LMWH can be monitored by measuring the plasma heparin (anti–factor Xa) level.

Both unfractionated heparin and LMWHs can inhibit the secretion of aldosterone, particularly with prolonged administration. This effect can result in hyperkalemia, especially in patients with renal failure or diabetes.

Fibrinolytic therapy (alteplase) physically dissolves anatomically obstructing pulmonary arterial thrombus and improves pulmonary capillary blood flow but is associated with a substantial risk of bleeding complications. High-risk subgroups who may benefit from fibrinolytic therapy include patients with massive pulmonary embolism who have moderate-to-severe right ventricular dysfunction and elevation of cardiac biomarkers. Unlike in acute ST-segment elevation myocardial infarction, fibrinolytic therapy for PE may be efficacious for up to 2 weeks after the onset of symptoms.[2]

REFERENCES

1. Kearon C, Kahn SR, Agnelli G, et al: Antithrombotic therapy for venous thromboembolic disease: American College of Chest Physicians Evidence-Based Clinical Practice Guidelines (8th edition). Chest 133:454S, 2008.
2. Todd JL, Tapson VF: Thrombolytic therapy for acute pulmonary embolism: A critical appraisal. Chest 135:1321, 2009.

ANSWERS TO QUESTIONS 576 TO 580

576—C, 577—A, 578—D, 579—A, 580—B (Braunwald, pp. 1571-1572, 1574-1575)

Hemochromatosis and amyloidosis are both infiltrative diseases. Hemochromatosis results in deposition of excessive iron within the myocardium and other organs, including the liver, pancreas, and gonads. It can occur in a familial pattern (transmitted in an autosomal recessive pattern), as an "idiopathic" disorder, or as a result of multiple blood transfusions. Certain forms of cardiac amyloidosis result in deposition of twisted beta-pleated sheet fibrils in the myocardium, formed from various proteins. Primary (AL) amyloidosis results from production of a protein derived from immunoglobulin light chains by plasma cells, usually in the setting of multiple myeloma. Myocardial involvement is less common in secondary (reactive) amyloidosis, in which nonimmunoglobulin AA protein deposits are smaller and less likely to cause myocardial dysfunction. A familial form of amyloidosis is inherited as an autosomal dominant trait with the abnormal production of the protein transthyretin. The senile form of amyloidosis is believed to be due to the production of an atrial natriuretic–like protein or transthyretin by older individuals.

Because of the infiltrative nature of these conditions, each initially leads to a "stiffened" myocardium and usually presents as a restrictive cardiomyopathy. In later stages, however, dilatation of the ventricles may ensue.

Although arrhythmias are common in both conditions, rhythm disorders are not usually prominent initial symptoms. The ECG in hemochromatosis usually shows diffuse ST-segment and T wave abnormalities as well as supraventricular arrhythmias. Abnormal rhythms, especially atrial fibrillation, are also common in amyloidosis, in addition to electrocardiographic findings of low-voltage QRS complexes and pseudoinfarction patterns.

If diagnosed early, the cardiomyopathy of hemochromatosis may be reversed with phlebotomy and chelating agents. Both computed tomography and cardiovascular magnetic resonance imaging have been used to detect early subclinical myocardial involvement at a time when therapy is most effective.[1] Cardiac involvement with amyloidosis carries a grim prognosis, and no therapy to date has been shown to consistently improve cardiac dysfunction. Cardiac transplantation has been performed for this condition; however, outcomes tend to be poor due to progression of amyloidosis in other organs or recurrence in the transplanted heart. Select patients with primary (AL) amyloidosis have been shown to benefit from chemotherapy with alkylating agents alone or in combination with autologous bone marrow stem cell transplantation.[2]

REFERENCES

1. Ptaszek LM, Price ET, Hu MY, et al: Early diagnosis of hemochromatosis-related cardiomyopathy with magnetic resonance imaging. J Cardiovasc Magn Reson 7:689, 2005.
2. Falk RH: Diagnosis and management of the cardiac amyloidoses. Circulation 112:2047, 2005.

ANSWERS TO QUESTIONS 581 TO 585

581—A, 582—B, 583—B, 584—A, 585—B (Braunwald, pp. 1514-1516, 1518-1521)

Tricuspid stenosis (TS) is most commonly rheumatic in origin. It almost never occurs as an isolated lesion but rather usually accompanies mitral valve disease. Typical findings include fatigue and right-sided heart failure, with hepatomegaly, abdominal swelling due to ascites, and anasarca. Auscultation usually reveals signs of mitral stenosis (MS), and these often overshadow those of TS. The diastolic murmur of TS is heard best along the lower left sternal border at the fourth intercostal space and is usually softer, higher pitched, and shorter in duration than the murmur of MS. The management of severe TS is surgical and requires valvulotomy or valve replacement when the orifice is < about 2 cm^2. In general, tissue valves are used preferentially in the tricuspid position because of the high risk of thrombosis with mechanical prostheses.

The most common form of pulmonic stenosis (PS) is congenital. A more rare form results from carcinoid plaques. The latter cause constriction of the pulmonic valve ring, retraction and fusion of the cusps, and PS with or without pulmonic regurgitation. Carcinoid heart disease can also involve the tricuspid valve but most commonly leads to tricuspid regurgitation.

Most adults with mild to moderate PS are asymptomatic, and it is only in the more severe forms that result in dyspnea and fatigue. Patients with advanced PS may develop secondary tricuspid regurgitation and frank right ventricular failure. The severity of PS is graded according to the peak systolic pressure gradient between the right ventricle and the pulmonary artery. Gradients of 50 to 79 mm Hg are considered "moderate," whereas those >80 mm Hg are "severe."

In the majority of patients, valvular PS is a stable or slowly progressive disease. Physical examination is notable for a systolic thrill along the left upper sternal border, a prominent systolic ejection murmur heard at the location of the thrill, and often an associated ejection click. In contrast to the inspiratory increase in most right-sided cardiac sounds, the intensity of the pulmonic click in PS decreases with inspiration. Echocardiography can define the lesion, and Doppler imaging allows accurate estimation of the gradient across the valve. In adults, percutaneous balloon valvuloplasty for typical valvular PS is safe and effective and is the treatment of choice.

REFERENCE

Bruce CJ, Connolly HM: Right-sided valve disease deserves a little more respect. Circulation 119:2726, 2009.

ANSWERS TO QUESTIONS 586 TO 589

586–C, 587–D, 588–B, 589–B (Braunwald, pp. 1707-1709)

Calcium channel blockers and prostacyclin are two forms of vasodilator therapy used in the chronic management of IPAH. They are prescribed to carefully selected patients with hemodynamic guidance. Up to 20% of patients with IPAH show a vasoreactive response and demonstrate a dramatic drop in pulmonary artery pressure and resistance with high-dose calcium channel blockers.[1] Such patients have improved quality of life and survival compared with control subjects and with those who do not demonstrate a dramatic hemodynamic response. Potential adverse effects of calcium channel blockers in IPAH include a right ventricular negative inotropic effect and reflex sympathetic stimulation with tachycardia, conditions that are detrimental to patients with IPAH.

Chronic intravenous epoprostenol (prostacyclin) administration has been shown to improve symptoms, quality of life, and survival in IPAH.[2] It also demonstrates antithrombotic effects that may be of benefit in the management of the thrombo-occlusive component of IPAH and may help to restore the integrity of the pulmonary vascular endothelium. Epoprostenol therapy is, however, cumbersome because it requires a surgically implanted central venous catheter and an infusion pump system. The prostacyclin analogs iloprost (by inhalation) and treprostinil (subcutaneously) improve symptoms and more easily administered, but evidence of survival benefit is lacking.

Additional agents that improve the quality of life in patients with pulmonary arterial hypertension have been approved for use. The phosphodiesterase type 5 inhibitors sildenafil and tadalafil reduce pulmonary arterial pressure, improve exertional capacity, and are well-tolerated. And a group of endothelin receptor blockers, including the nonselective antagonist bosentan, have been shown to improve hemodynamics, symptoms, and stamina in this condition.[3] Side effects of this group include peripheral edema and hepatic toxicity.

REFERENCES

1. Sitbon O, Humbert M, Jais X, et al: Long term response to calcium channel blockers in idiopathic pulmonary arterial hypertension. Circulation 111:3105, 2005.
2. Badesch DB, Abman SH, Simonneau G, et al: Medical therapy for pulmonary arterial hypertension. Chest 131:1917, 2007.
3. Dupuis J, Hoeper MM: Endothelin receptor antagonists in pulmonary arterial hypertension. Eur Respir J 31:407, 2008.

ANSWERS TO QUESTIONS 590 TO 593

590–C, 591–B, 592–A, 593–B (Braunwald, pp. 1663-1665; Table 75-6; see also Answers to Questions 563 to 566)

The clinical and hemodynamic features of restrictive heart disease such as those caused by cardiac amyloidosis may be very similar to those of chronic constrictive pericarditis. Endomyocardial biopsy, computed tomography, and magnetic resonance imaging may be useful in differentiating the two diseases. The typical hemodynamic feature present in both conditions is the deep and rapid early decline in ventricular pressure at the onset of diastole, with a rapid rise to a plateau in early diastole, referred to as the "square root" or "dip-and-plateau" sign. Patients with restrictive cardiomyopathy may have left ventricular filling pressures that exceed RV filling pressures by >5 mm Hg (whereas there is <5 mm Hg difference between them in pericardial constriction), and this difference can be accentuated by exercise. Furthermore, the pulmonary artery systolic pressure may be >60 mm Hg in patients with restrictive cardiomyopathy but is usually lower in constrictive pericarditis. As a result, the plateau of the RV diastolic pressure is usually greater than one third of the peak RV systolic pressure in patients with constrictive pericarditis while it is more commonly less than one third in patients with restrictive cardiomyopathy because of the elevated systolic pressure.

In the atrial tracings, the dip-and-plateau sign manifests as a prominent y descent followed by a rapid rise in pressure. The x descent may also be prominent, and the combination results in the characteristic M-shaped waveform in the atrial pressure tracing. Both systemic and pulmonary venous pressures are usually elevated.

REFERENCE

Talreja DR, Nishimura RA, Oh JK, Holmes DR: Constrictive pericarditis in the modern era: Novel criteria for diagnosis in the cardiac catheterization laboratory. J Am Coll Cardiol 22:315, 2008.

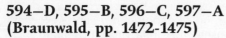

ANSWERS TO QUESTIONS 594 TO 597

594—D, 595—B, 596—C, 597—A
(Braunwald, pp. 1472-1475)

The natural history of aortic stenosis (AS) has been described in a cohort of patients who did not undergo aortic valve surgery. Patients whose only symptom of AS was angina had an average survival of 3 to 5 years. Those with syncope had a shorter average survival of 2 to 3 years. Those with signs and symptoms of congestive heart failure had the worst prognosis—an average survival of only 1.5 to 2 years. Because of such reduced longevity, patients with AS and any of these symptoms should be referred for surgical correction, especially if symptoms of heart failure are present. Palpitations are not a marker for adverse survival in patients with AS.

REFERENCES

Dal-Bianco JP, Khandheria BK, Mookadam F, et al: Management of asymptomatic severe aortic stenosis. J Am Coll Cardiol 52:1279, 2008.

Varadarajan P, Kapoor N, Bansal RC, et al: Clinical profile and natural history of 453 nonsurgically managed patients with severe aortic stenosis. Ann Thorac Surg 82:2111, 2006.

ANSWERS TO QUESTIONS 598 TO 601

598—A, 599—B, 600—C, 601—A
(Braunwald, pp. 1556-1559)

In 2007, the American Heart Association published an updated set of consensus recommendations for antibiotic prophylaxis for the prevention of infective endocarditis (IE).[1,2] This statement simplifies older guidelines and focuses on prophylaxis for patients at the highest risk for developing IE. High-risk patients are considered to be those with (1) prosthetic heart valves, (2) prior endocarditis, (3) specific types of congenital heart disease (unrepaired cyanotic lesions, repaired congenital lesions with residual defects, or during the first 6 months after repair with prosthetic material or device), and (4) cardiac transplant recipients with valvulopathy. Routine gastrointestinal or genitourinary tract procedures are no longer an indication for antibiotic prophylaxis unless there is an active gastrointestinal or genitourinary tract infection in a patient with one of these high-risk cardiac conditions.

The first patient in this question is at high risk owing to the prosthetic mitral valve, but prophylaxis is not recommended for routine gastrointestinal procedures such as colonoscopy. The second and third patients are at high risk owing to the prosthetic valves and prophylaxis is recommended. The third patient is penicillin allergic so an alternative regimen such as clindamycin should be administered instead. The fourth patient is not high risk, and prophylaxis for gastrointestinal procedures is not recommended unless there is active infection.

REFERENCES

1. Nishmura RA, Carabello BA, Faxon DP, et al: ACC/AHA 2008 Guideline Update on Valvular Heart Disease: Focused Update on Infective Endocarditis: A Report of the American College of Cardiology/American Heart Association Task Force on Practice Guidelines: Endorsed by the Society of Cardiovascular Anesthesiologists, Society for Cardiovascular Angiography and Interventions, and Society of Thoracic Surgeons. Circulation 118:887, 2008.

2. Wilson W, Taubert KA, Gewitz M, et al: Prevention of infective endocarditis. Guidelines from the American Heart Association: A Guideline from the American Heart Association Rheumatic Fever, Endocarditis, and Kawasaki Disease Committee, Council on Cardiovascular Disease in the Young, and the Council on Clinical Cardiology, Council on Cardiovascular Surgery and Anesthesia, and the Quality of Care and Outcomes Research Interdisciplinary Working Group. Circulation 115:1656, 2007.

ANSWERS TO QUESTIONS 602 TO 606

602—B, 603—B, 604—C, 605—A, 606—D
(Braunwald, pp. 1428-1430, 1444-1447)

Complete atrioventricular canal defects (also known as endocardial cushion defects) comprise a group of abnormalities in which the common features are (1) absence of the muscular atrioventricular septum (causing the atrioventricular (AV) valves to appear at the same level on echocardiography), (2) inlet/outlet disproportion resulting in an elongated left ventricular outflow tract (producing a "goose-neck" deformity on angiography), (3) lateral rotation of the posteromedial papillary muscle, and (4) abnormal configuration of the AV valves (e.g., the left AV valve is trileaflet with a "cleft" appearance). Ostium primum interatrial and interventricular septal defects are common.[1] Infants usually present in the first year of life with a history of poor weight gain and frequent respiratory infections, and heart failure is common. On physical examination, several murmurs may be present, including a holosystolic murmur along the lower left sternal border due to the VSD, a holosystolic murmur at the apex due to mitral regurgitation, and a right ventricular (RV) outflow tract systolic murmur. Because the direction of intracardiac shunting is left to right, cyanosis is not typical. Typical electrocardiographic findings include left-axis deviation due to left anterior hemiblock and incomplete right bundle branch block. Echocardiography is usually diagnostic for this condition.

In complete transposition of the great arteries (TGA), the aorta arises from the morphologic right ventricle and the pulmonary artery arises from the morphologic left ventricle. This anatomic arrangement results in two separate and parallel circulations. Some communication between the pulmonary and systemic circulations must exist after birth to sustain life. Almost all patients have an interatrial communication, two thirds have a patent ductus arteriosus (PDA), and one third have an associated VSD. The typical clinical manifestations are dyspnea and cyanosis, progressive hypoxemia, and congestive heart failure. Cardiac murmurs are absent or insignificant in 30% to 50% of patients with TGA and an intact ventricular septum. In infants with TGA and a large PDA, fewer than half have the typical continuous murmur of the aortopulmonary connection. Electrocardiographic findings include right-axis deviation, right atrial enlargement, and RV hypertrophy. Echocardiography is usually diagnostic for identifying the abnormal great-vessel relationship and accompanying abnormalities. An arterial switch operation is the treatment of choice.[2]

REFERENCES

1. Dunlop KA, Mulholland HC, Casey F, et al: A ten year review of atrioventricular defects. Cardiol Young 14:15-23, 2004.
2. Bove T, De Meulder F, Vandenplas G, et al: Midterm assessment of the reconstructed arteries after the arterial switch operation. Ann Thorac Surg 85:823, 2008.

ANSWERS TO QUESTIONS 607 TO 611

607–D, 608–C, 609–C, 610–A, 611–B (Braunwald, pp. 78-79, 1420)

Noonan syndrome is a relatively common (1 per 1000) genetic disorder with an inheritance that is consistent with an autosomal dominant pattern.[1] About one half of patients have mutations in the *PTPN11* gene on chromosome 12. This syndrome is characterized phenotypically by short stature, a unique facial appearance, mild mental retardation, webbing of the neck, cryptorchidism, and renal anomalies. Approximately half of all patients with Noonan syndrome have congenital heart disease, the most common lesion of which is valvular pulmonic stenosis. The ECG commonly displays left anterior fascicular block. Approximately 20% of patients with Noonan syndrome have an accompanying atrial septal defect or hypertrophic cardiomyopathy.

The *LEOPARD* syndrome is a rare, single-gene complex of congenital malformations. The acronym LEOPARD symbolizes the main components of the syndrome: L, lentigines; E, electrocardiographic conduction defects; O, ocular hypertelorism; P, pulmonic valve stenosis; A, abnormalities of the genitals; R, retardation of growth; and D, deafness. Eighty percent of patients display lentigines, whereas deafness and abnormalities of the genitals occur in about 20% of patients. The most common structural cardiac feature is pulmonic stenosis, which may exist as an isolated anomaly or in combination with aortic stenosis. The most common electrocardiographic conduction defects are PR-segment prolongation, QRS complex widening, left anterior fascicular block, and complete heart block. The most striking physical feature of the syndrome is the presence of small, dark lentigines, which are concentrated over the neck and upper extremities. LEOPARD syndrome is transmitted in an autosomal dominant fashion, with cardiovascular abnormalities in at least 95% of affected patients.

Kartagener syndrome is an autosomal recessive disorder, the primary defect of which has been elucidated by electron microscopic investigation of cilia from affected individuals' bronchial mucosa or sperm. Dynein arms, which are protein structures that normally form crossbridges between adjacent microtubules in cilia and sperm tails, are abnormal in this disorder. Several different mutations capable of producing the syndrome are recognized, and in each case, the mutant gene disrupts the synthesis either of the dynein protein itself or of a protein that binds dynein to the microtubules. Clinically, the syndrome consists of the triad of sinusitis, bronchiectasis, and situs inversus with dextrocardia. Cases of Kartagener syndrome usually come to attention in infancy due to recurrent upper respiratory infections or pneumonia, and development of classic sinusitis and chronic bronchiectasis occurs as childhood progresses. The majority of individuals with Kartagener syndrome have dextrocardia as the only cardiac manifestation, which leads to an abnormal 12-lead ECG but has no other clinical consequences. On rare occasions associated cardiac anomalies may be present, including transposition of the great vessels.

Holt-Oram syndrome is a rare autosomal dominant disorder. The classic clinical manifestation is the simultaneous occurrence of congenital heart disease and an upper limb deformity. The most common cardiovascular abnormality is an atrial septal defect of the secundum type, with ventricular septal defect being next most common. Electrocardiographic abnormalities are frequently present as well and may include first-degree atrioventricular block, right bundle branch block, and bradycardia. Deformities of the forearm and hand are the most apparent features of the Holt-Oram syndrome (e.g., hypoplasia or triphalangeal abnormalities of the thumbs). The most specific upper extremity finding, an abnormal scaphoid bone or accessory carpal bones or both, may be detected by wrist radiography. One form of Holt-Oram syndrome has been linked to mutations in the *TBX5* gene located on chromosome 12. *TBX5* is a member of the T-box family of transcription factors that critically regulate morphogenesis in the developing embryo.[2]

REFERENCES

1. Jongmans M, Otten B, Noordam K, van der Burgt I: Genetics and variation in phenotype in Noonan syndrome. Horm Res 62(Suppl 3):56, 2004.
2. Heinritz W, Moschik A, Kujat A, et al: Identification of new mutations in the *TBX5* gene in patients with Holt-Oram syndrome. Heart 91:383-384, 2005.

ANSWERS TO QUESTIONS 612 TO 615

612–C, 613–A, 614–B, 615–D (Braunwald, pp. 1546-1548, 1571-1573, 1887-1888)

Dermatologic manifestations of systemic disorders that have major cardiac involvement may provide important clues to the underlying diagnosis. One example is infective endocarditis, in which specific lesions may appear in the skin, its appendages, and the eyes. In the skin, these include petechiae, Osler nodes, Janeway lesions, Roth spots, subungual ("splinter") hemorrhages, and embolic infarcts of the digits, as may occur with *Staphylococcus aureus* infection of the left-sided valves; the last are illustrated in part A in the figure. Osler nodes are small, raised, nodular, and painful red to purple lesions that appear in the pulp spaces of the terminal phalanges of the fingers. Janeway lesions are small, irregular, flat and nontender macules occurring most often on thev thenar and hypothenar eminences of the hands and soles. Roth spots on the retina have the appearance on funduscopic examination of a "cotton wool" exudate and consist of aggregations of cytoid bodies. All of these peripheral stigmata of infective endocarditis have become rare in the antibiotic era.

Amyloidosis is a systemic illness in which unique protein-derived fibrils are deposited in a variety of organs. Cardiac involvement is common in primary (AL) amyloidosis (often a consequence of multiple myeloma) and in familial amyloidosis (an autosomal dominant condition that results from the production of the protein transthyretin).[1] Cardiac sequelae include restrictive cardiomyopathy with diastolic dysfunction, conduction abnormalities, systolic dysfunction, and orthostatic hypotension. Dermatologic findings include small papules on the face, scalp, neck fold, or intertriginous folds. In addition, small, smooth and yellowish papules may be seen in the area around the eyes and be mistaken for xanthomas. Amyloid infiltration can result in macroglossia, as shown in part B.

Fabry disease is a sex-linked disorder that is due to a deficiency of the enzyme alpha-galactosidase A. The disorder is characterized by the accumulation of glycosphingolipid within the myocardium, skin, and kidneys. Systemic hypertension, mitral valve prolapse, renovascular hypotension, and congestive heart failure are all common clinical manifestations of the disease. Fabry disease may also cause restrictive cardiomyopathy. Ocular signs in the disorder are common. Approximately 90% of patients have corneal opacities, whereas two thirds of patients have conjunctival vessel tortuosity as illustrated in part C of the figure.[2] Hypertensive cardiovascular disease, renal failure, and cerebrovascular disease are the major causes of death in this disorder. Purified human alpha-galactosidase A is available as an intravenous therapeutic option, which reduces tissue storage of the offending glycosphingolipid.

Progressive systemic sclerosis, or scleroderma, presents as tightening and thickening of the skin, with Raynaud's phenomenon occurring in almost all patients. Cardiac involvement is common and is a frequent cause of death, second only to involvement of the kidneys as a factor shortening survival.[3] Scleroderma heart disease is primarily a myocardial process, leading to vascular insufficiency and fibrosis in the small vessels of the heart, which produces cardiomyopathy with congestive heart failure and conduction system abnormalities and/or ventricular dysrhythmias. Pericardial involvement with fibrinous pericarditis is common, as is the development of pulmonary hypertension due to intrinsic pulmonary vascular disease or interstitial fibrosis. The CREST variant of this syndrome includes patients with calcinosis, Raynaud phenomenon, esophageal dysmotility, sclerodactyly, and telangiectasia. Recurrent painful ulcerations of the fingertips, which may become infected, are a common problem in this disorder and are illustrated in part D.

REFERENCES

1. Rapezzi C, Merlini G, Quarta CC, et al: Systemic cardiac amyloidoses: Disease profiles and clinical courses of the 3 main types. Circulation 120:1203, 2009.
2. Samiy N: Ocular features of Fabry disease: Diagnosis of a treatable life-threatening disorder. Surv Ophthalmol 53:416-423, 2008.
3. Kahan A, Coghlan G, McLaughlin V: Cardiac complications of systemic sclerosis. Rheumatology 48(Suppl 3):iii45, 2009.

ANSWERS TO QUESTIONS 616 TO 619

616–A, 617–B, 618–B, 619–C (Braunwald, pp. 78-79, 1420; see also Answers to Questions 607 to 611)

The Turner and Noonan syndromes share several superficial features, including shortness of stature, webbing of the neck, skeletal anomalies, renal abnormalities, and congenital heart disease. Because of these clinical similarities, Noonan syndrome is frequently referred to as male Turner syndrome or as Turner phenotype with normal chromosomes. However, there are several striking genetic and clinical differences that can readily distinguish these two disorders. The Turner syndrome occurs exclusively in females. In about 50% of patients, the karyotype is 45,XO. The remaining patients are mosaics with various other X chromosome abnormalities. Most fetuses with the 45,XO form of Turner syndrome die in utero. Of those that survive, cardiovascular abnormalities occur in 35% to 50%. Coarctation of the aorta is the most common cardiovascular lesion. Other abnormalities include bicuspid aortic valve, hypertrophic cardiomyopathy, atrial septal defect, mitral valve prolapse, and dextrocardia. Stenosis of the pulmonic valve is rarely seen in Turner syndrome, in contrast to Noonan syndrome.

Noonan syndrome appears physically similar to Turner syndrome; however, as indicated in Answers to Questions 607 to 611, affected patients have a unique facial appearance, with hypertelorism, strabismus, small chin, and low-set ears. It is inherited as an autosomal dominant trait and, in contrast to Turner syndrome, both males and females are susceptible to this condition; the karyotype in both sexes is normal. In many families, the genetic abnormality maps to chromosome 12q24; about half have a mutation in the *PTPN11* gene in that region. Approximately 50% of patients with Noonan syndrome have congenital heart disease; the most common lesion is valvular pulmonary stenosis, occurring in about 60% of patients. Characteristically, the annulus of the pulmonary valve is normal, but the leaflets are thickened and immobile. Other findings include atrial septal defect and hypertrophic cardiomyopathy.

ANSWERS TO QUESTIONS 620 TO 624

620–C, 621–A, 622–B, 623–A, 624–A (Braunwald, pp. 1435-1437)

The two-dimensional echocardiogram in part A of the figure displays an apical, four-chamber view of tricuspid atresia, demonstrating a dense band in the tricuspid annulus and an enlarged left ventricle. This anomaly is marked by the absence of the tricuspid orifice with an atrial septal defect, typically with hypoplasia of the right ventricle, and communication between the ventricles, typically via a ventricular septal defect. In 60% to 70% of patients with this condition, the great arteries have normal relationships; the remainder have d-transposition of these vessels. In addition, pulmonic stenosis or atresia may be present. Clinically, the marked diminution in pulmonary blood flow usually leads to severe cyanosis. In those infants in whom transposition coexists with a ventricular septal defect and an unobstructed pulmonary outflow tract, torrential pulmonary blood flow will occur, leading to heart failure rather than cyanosis as the predominant problem. The majority of infants with tricuspid atresia have pulmonary hypoperfusion and the clinical picture of cyanosis, with electrocardiographic findings of left ventricular hypertrophy, left-axis deviation, and right atrial enlargement.[1]

Echocardiographic examination in this disorder is usually diagnostic. At cardiac catheterization, the right ventricle cannot be entered from the right atrium. When the great arteries are normally related, pulmonary blood flow is maintained via a ventricular septal defect or patent ductus arteriosus. However, in complete transposition, the pulmonary artery blood flow is derived directly from the left ventricle. Functional correction of tricuspid atresia has been accomplished by the Fontan procedure, which consists of construction of a prosthetic conduit between the right atrium and pulmonary artery and closure of the intra-atrial communication.

The two-dimensional echocardiogram in part B is a parasternal long-axis view of tetralogy of Fallot, which demonstrates (1) the aorta overriding the interventricular septum and (2) a ventricular septal defect. The two other components that comprise this malformation are (1) right ventricular (RV) outflow obstruction and (2) RV hypertrophy.[2] The clinical presentation in tetralogy of Fallot is determined principally by the degree of obstruction to pulmonary blood flow. Infants with tetralogy of Fallot become symptomatic and cyanotic before the age of 1 year. There is a direct correlation between the time of onset of symptoms and the severity of pulmonary outflow tract obstruction. Intense cyanotic spells related to sudden increases in venoarterial shunting and simultaneous decreases in pulmonary blood flow occur between 2 and 9 months of age and may be life threatening.

Physical examination of infants with tetralogy of Fallot usually reveals varying degrees of underdevelopment and cyanosis, commonly with clubbing of the terminal digits within the first year of life. An RV impulse and systolic thrill may often be appreciated along the left sternal border. A systolic flow murmur across the pulmonic valve is often present, and the intensity and duration of this murmur vary inversely with the severity of the pulmonic outflow tract obstruction. The ECG usually shows RV hypertrophy. On chest radiography, a normal-sized boot-shaped heart with prominence of the right ventricle and a concavity in the region of the underdeveloped RV outflow tract is typical. Echocardiographic examination with Doppler interrogation is diagnostic. Cardiac catheterization is used to delineate the course of the pulmonary arteries and collateral channels when patients have pulmonary atresia as part of the syndrome and to document the coronary artery anatomy before surgical repair. Coronary variations in this disorder include the abnormal origin of the anterior descending artery from the right coronary artery or a single right or

left coronary artery giving rise to the remaining coronary vessels.

The management of tetralogy of Fallot consists of total correction of the anomaly, with early definitive repair being advocated in most centers, often during the first 6 months. Pulmonary arterial size is the single most important determinant in evaluating a patient for primary repair. For those in whom marked hypoplasia of the pulmonary arteries is present, balloon dilatation may be used in a palliative manner to allow the infant to survive until an older age, at which time total correction may be carried out at lower risk.

REFERENCES

1. Sittiwangkul R, Azakie A, Van Arsdell GS, et al: Outcomes of the tricuspid atresia in the Fontan era. Ann Thorac Surg 77:889, 2004.
2. Bashore TM: Adult congenital heart disease: Right ventricular outflow tract lesions. Circulation 115:1933-1947, 2007.

ANSWERS TO QUESTIONS 625 TO 629

625—A, 626—A, 627—B, 628—B, 629—D (Braunwald, pp. 1896-1901)

Radiation therapy and chemotherapeutic agents have potentially serious cardiac adverse effects.[1,2] Cardiac exposure may occur as a result of therapeutic irradiation of lung, breast, or esophageal cancers or mediastinal radiation for lymphomas. All cardiac structures are susceptible to radiation damage, especially the pericardium, but also the myocardium, coronary arteries, conduction system, and valves. The effects of radiation on the pericardium may be acute (e.g., hemorrhagic effusions) or delayed for several years (fibrosis with constrictive pericarditis). Radiation therapy is also a cause of premature coronary artery disease (CAD). Retrospective studies have demonstrated that children treated with radiation therapy for Hodgkin disease have a significantly increased risk of developing symptomatic CAD at an early age. Radiation-induced myocardial fibrosis is common and may lead to restrictive cardiomyopathy. Radiation effects on the conduction system may cause sinus node disease and atrioventricular block. Radiation exposure of the aortic valve and papillary muscles has been implicated as a cause of regurgitation of the aortic and mitral valves.

As described in the Answer to Question 544, the anthracycline chemotherapeutic agents can have an acute direct toxic effect on the myocardium, resulting in ventricular and supraventricular dysrhythmias as well as conduction system blocks. More commonly, cumulative exposure to anthracyclines results in a chronic cardiomyopathy, especially at a total cumulative dose >400 mg/m². Rare cases of acute myocarditis-pericarditis within 2 weeks of anthracycline therapy have been described.

Aortic dissection is not associated with these antineoplastic therapies.

REFERENCES

1. Ng R, Better N, Green MD: Anticancer agents and cardiotoxicity. Semin Oncol 33:2, 2006.
2. Heidenreich PA, Kapoor JR: Radiation induced heart disease: Systemic disorders in heart disease. Heart 95:252, 2009.

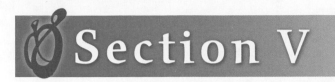

Section V
(Chapters 80-94)

CARDIOVASCULAR DISEASE IN SPECIAL POPULATIONS; CARDIOVASCULAR DISEASE AND DISORDERS OF OTHER ORGANS

DIRECTIONS: For each question below, select the ONE BEST response.

QUESTION 630

A 24-year-old man who is training for the Olympic decathlon team experiences a presyncopal event and is referred for evaluation. He has been training aggressively for the past 2 years and aside from occasional single palpitations has not noticed any prior lightheadedness, other cardiac symptoms, or physical limitations. He has no history of hypertension and his family history is free of premature coronary disease or sudden cardiac death. On physical examination his blood pressure and heart rate are normal. A grade II/VI rough crescendo-decrescendo systolic murmur is auscultated along the left sternal border, which becomes louder when the patient stands. The patient is anxious to return to his training regimen. Which of the following statements is TRUE?

A. Voltage criteria for left ventricular hypertrophy on this patient's ECG would establish the diagnosis of hypertrophic cardiomyopathy and should prohibit him from resuming competitive athletics
B. An echocardiographic end-diastolic septal wall thickness of 14 mm would be diagnostic of hypertrophic cardiomyopathy
C. Persistent left ventricular hypertrophy by echocardiography months after cessation of exercise is consistent with hypertrophic cardiomyopathy
D. A maximum oxygen uptake >45 mL/kg/min on cardiopulmonary exercise testing is more consistent with hypertrophic cardiomyopathy than "Athlete's Heart"
E. The most common cause of sudden cardiac death in athletes is anomalous origin of the left coronary artery

QUESTION 631

A 66-year-old man with chronic kidney disease (CKD) is referred for office evaluation after a recent admission for an acute coronary syndrome. Which of the following statements is TRUE concerning chronic kidney disease (CKD) and cardiovascular disease?

A. Patients with CKD are at increased risk of bleeding but decreased risk of thrombotic events when compared with normal individuals
B. The outcomes of patients with CKD who present with acute coronary syndromes are similar to those of patients with normal renal function
C. Renal dysfunction is the most significant independent predictor of mortality of patients in coronary care units
D. Patients with CKD who present to the hospital with chest pain comprise a relatively low-risk group of acute coronary syndromes, with a cardiac event rate of <5% at 30 days
E. Uremia is associated with enhanced platelet aggregation

QUESTION 632

A 20-year-old female student presents to the emergency department with recent malaise, myalgias, fevers, sweats, and claudication of the right lower extremity and left arm. On physical examination the blood pressure is 160/90 mm Hg in the right arm and 120/85 mm Hg in the left arm. The left radial and right femoral pulses are diminished and a left-sided subclavian bruit is auscultated. The erythrocyte sedimentation rate is markedly elevated. Which of the following statements about this condition is TRUE?

A. Arterial biopsy would reveal a polymorphonuclear infiltrate
B. Aortic aneurysm formation is more common than arterial stenoses
C. This condition is 10 times more common in women than men
D. Claudication occurs more commonly in the lower extremities than the upper extremities
E. Coronary vasculitis is not typical in this syndrome

QUESTION 633

A 58-year-old woman complains of a new-onset severe headache, jaw pain with chewing, and temporal artery tenderness. Laboratory examination shows an erythrocyte sedimentation rate (ESR) of 80 mm/hr. Which of the following is TRUE regarding treatment of this condition?

A. Corticosteroids should not be administered until biopsy evidence confirms the diagnosis
B. Clinical improvement with appropriate treatment generally occurs over several weeks
C. Anti-TNF therapies have been shown to be beneficial in this condition
D. In the absence of contraindications, low-dose aspirin should be prescribed for all patients with this condition
E. Normalization of the ESR is a reliable indicator of treatment response

QUESTION 634

A 35-year-old woman with hypertension is considering pregnancy. She is currently taking lisinopril 10 mg daily. Which of the following statements is TRUE?

A. She should remain on her current antihypertensive regimen before and during pregnancy
B. An angiotensin receptor blocker should be substituted
C. Labetalol is unsafe during pregnancy
D. Women with preexisting hypertension have a higher incidence of preeclampsia compared with those with new-onset hypertension during pregnancy
E. Antihypertensive therapy is effective in preventing preeclampsia during pregnancy

QUESTION 635

All of the following statements about heart disease in women are true EXCEPT:

A. Cardiovascular disease is the leading cause of death in women
B. In recent decades, age-adjusted cardiovascular mortality in the United States has increased in women while it has declined in men
C. Coronary heart disease presents approximately 10 years later in women than in men
D. Cardiovascular disease is twice as common in women with diabetes compared with nondiabetics
E. Hormone replacement therapy with estrogen does not reduce the risk of cardiac events in postmenopausal women

QUESTION 636

A 36-year-old woman with no prior history of cardiac disease develops exertional dyspnea and orthopnea 1 month after delivering a healthy full-term infant. Echocardiography demonstrates a dilated left ventricle with globally reduced contractile function. Each of the following statements about peripartum cardiomyopathy (PPCM) is correct EXCEPT:

A. Symptoms of PPCM arise during the last month of pregnancy or within 5 months of delivery

B. Clinical and hemodynamic findings in PPCM are indistinguishable from those of other forms of dilated cardiomyopathy
C. The incidence of PPCM is greatest in first pregnancies
D. Approximately 50% of PPCM patients show recovery within the first 6 months after delivery
E. Subsequent pregnancies in women with PPCM carry a 30% risk of relapse

QUESTION 637

A 67-year-old man with multivessel coronary disease is scheduled for coronary artery bypass graft surgery (CABG). Which of the following statements regarding CABG and perioperative complications is TRUE?

A. Perioperative myocardial infarction occurs, on average, in 5% to 10% of elective procedures
B. Early postoperative cognitive decline occurs in <10% of patients after CABG surgery
C. Atrial fibrillation appears in approximately 40% of patients after CABG surgery
D. Of patients who develop postoperative atrial fibrillation, only 20% will spontaneously revert to sinus rhythm within 24 hours
E. *N*-Acetylcysteine prevents renal dysfunction after CABG

QUESTION 638

The patient in Question 637 undergoes CABG without complication. At his first postoperative office visit he reports resolution of his anginal symptoms and he asks how long the benefit will last. Which of the following statements regarding coronary artery bypass grafts is TRUE?

A. Fewer than 2% of saphenous vein grafts become occluded in the early perioperative period
B. Internal mammary artery grafts typically develop intimal hyperplasia over time
C. Saphenous vein grafts have a 10-year patency rate of >75%
D. Radial artery grafts are less likely to develop vasospasm than internal mammary grafts
E. Patients who receive internal mammary artery grafts suffer fewer late deaths and myocardial infarctions than those who receive only saphenous vein grafts

QUESTION 639

A previously healthy 17-year-old high school athlete collapses during a basketball game. He is noted to have brief seizure-like activity and has no initial pulse but is immediately resuscitated by a brisk precordial thump. Assuming that this event represents sudden cardiac death (SCD), each of the following statements is true EXCEPT:

A. Arrhythmogenic right ventricular cardiomyopathy is responsible for approximately 30% of SCD in young athletes

B. Anomalous origin of the left main coronary artery from the right coronary cusp is the most common of the congenital coronary abnormalities that result in SCD in young athletes

C. His normal pretraining history and physical examination do not exclude the possibility of hypertrophic cardiomyopathy (HCM)

D. Patients who experience SCD due to HCM often have no history of prior cardiac symptoms

E. Congenital aortic stenosis is a cause of SCD in young athletes

QUESTION 640

A 68-year-old woman with a history of hypertension presents to the emergency department with the new onset of dyspnea and nausea. The ECG shows anterolateral ST-segment depressions, and the initial serum measurement of cardiac troponin T is elevated. Which of the following statements is TRUE regarding women who present with acute coronary syndromes (ACS)?

A. Most women presenting with an acute myocardial infarction do not describe chest pain

B. Women presenting with myocardial infarction are less likely than men to have accompanying cardiovascular comorbidities

C. Women with ACS are more likely to present earlier in the course of symptoms than men

D. Women who present with chest discomfort are more likely than men to have nonatherosclerotic causes of ischemia, such as vasospasm

E. Women are admitted to the hospital for the evaluation of chest pain less often than men

QUESTION 641

You are asked to evaluate a 72-year-old man who underwent coronary artery bypass graft (CABG) surgery 8 hours ago. He is hemodynamically stable. You review his laboratory studies and note a platelet count of 87,000/μL, a potassium level of 5.3 mg/dL, a normal phosphate level, and an elevated cardiac troponin T of 1.6 ng/mL. Which of the following statements regarding laboratory assessment after CABG is TRUE?

A. Platelet count <100,000/μL is rare

B. Potassium levels typically vary little and do not require frequent monitoring

C. The cardiac troponin concentration in the serum is often elevated but is not prognostically important

D. The cardiac troponin concentration is often elevated but is only prognostic in regard to short-term outcomes

E. Hypophosphatemia is common and is associated with prolonged mechanical ventilation

QUESTION 642

A 58-year-old postmenopausal women presents for a routine office visit. She was recently prescribed oral hormone replacement therapy by her gynecologist.

Which of the following statements is TRUE regarding the use of hormone replacement therapy and cardiovascular risk?

A. Current guidelines recommend hormone replacement therapy for postmenopausal women who do not have a history of coronary artery disease

B. The prospective Women's Health Initiative trial showed a reduced rate of coronary events in postmenopausal women randomized to estrogen-only treatment

C. The Women's Health Initiative showed no difference in the rate of stroke or pulmonary embolism in patients randomized to estrogen therapy

D. The American Heart Association guidelines assign a Class III recommendation to starting or continuing estrogen plus progestin therapy for primary or secondary prevention of cardiovascular disease

QUESTION 643

A 55-year-old overweight man with type 2 diabetes mellitus, coronary artery disease, and atrial fibrillation is scheduled for coronary artery bypass graft (CABG) surgery in 1 week. Which of the following conditions is associated with increased perioperative mortality in this patient?

A. Age
B. Timing of surgery
C. Diabetes mellitus
D. Atrial fibrillation
E. Obesity

QUESTION 644

A 38-year-old woman presents at the 37th week of pregnancy because of severe substernal chest pain over the past 30 minutes. An ECG demonstrates 4-mm ST-segment elevations in leads V_1 to V_4. Which of the following statements is true?

A. Coronary artery spasm is the most common cause of this finding during pregnancy

B. Coronary artery dissection is the most likely cause in the peripartum period

C. Pregnancy does not alter the risk of sustaining a myocardial infarction

D. Inferior wall myocardial infarction is more common than anterior wall myocardial infarction during pregnancy

E. Urgent angiography should be avoided in this setting

QUESTION 645

An 83-year-old man with hypertension and diabetes underwent a coronary artery bypass graft (CABG) operation 14 hours ago on an emergency basis. Preoperative angiography revealed severe stenoses of the left main and right coronary arteries. During the operation, the left internal mammary artery was grafted to the native left anterior descending artery and saphenous vein grafts were placed to the first obtuse marginal branch of the circumflex coronary artery and to the posterior descending artery. The surgeon consults you because he is concerned that the patient may have suffered a perioperative myocardial infarction (MI). Each of the following statements is true EXCEPT:

A. His age, the emergency nature of his procedure, and the presence of left main coronary artery disease put this patient at increased risk for perioperative MI
B. Chest pain is not a reliable sign of MI in the post-CABG patient
C. An elevation of the CK-MB isoenzyme > two times the upper limit of normal is considered diagnostic of MI in this setting
D. The finding of new Q waves on the ECG is a reliable sign of perioperative MI
E. Paradoxical motion of the interventricular septum on echocardiography is a common finding after cardiac surgical procedures and does not necessarily indicate MI

QUESTION 646

A 78-year-old man presents with chest pain and new 2-mm ST-segment elevations in leads V_1 to V_3. Which of the following statements is TRUE regarding the management of acute myocardial infarction (MI) in elderly patients?

A. Mortality rates associated with acute MI are higher in older men than in older women
B. Fibrin-specific fibrinolytic agents are not associated with heightened intracerebral bleeding rates in patients >75 years
C. Antiplatelet therapy with prasugrel leads to superior outcomes compared with clopidogrel in patients >75 years of age who undergo percutaneous intervention
D. Angiotensin-converting enzyme inhibitors have been shown to reduce fatal and nonfatal events after MI in elderly patients
E. Elderly patients are less likely than younger patients to benefit from beta blockade for secondary prevention

QUESTION 647

Preoperative factors that portend an increased risk of cardiac complications after major noncardiac surgery in patients >40 years of age include which of the following?

A. Presence of an S_3 gallop
B. Active cigarette smoking
C. Remote myocardial infarction without active angina
D. Mitral stenosis with calculated valve area of 2.0 cm^2
E. Controlled hypertension

QUESTION 648

A 69-year-old woman presents for a routine office visit. She has a history of hypertension and her blood pressure today is 145/90 mm Hg. Her only medication is metoprolol succinate 25 mg daily. Which of the following statements regarding hypertension in the elderly is TRUE?

A. Clinical studies have not established the effectiveness of therapy for mild diastolic hypertension in the elderly
B. Therapy for isolated systolic hypertension in the elderly does not reduce the incidence of future cardiac events
C. Clinical trials have shown that beta blockers offer less cardiovascular protection than diuretic therapy
D. The presence of left ventricular hypertrophy in hypertensive patients >age 65 is not an independent risk factor for adverse cardiovascular outcomes
E. Hypertensive hypertrophic cardiomyopathy of the elderly is more common in men

QUESTION 649

Each of the following statements regarding hemodynamic changes during normal pregnancy is correct EXCEPT:

A. Total blood volume increases
B. Cardiac output increases
C. Stroke volume increases
D. Heart rate increases
E. Systemic vascular resistance increases

QUESTION 650

A 64-year-old woman presents to the emergency department with nausea and vomiting. Her ECG shows ST-segment depressions in the inferior leads and the serum troponin T is elevated. Each of the following statements regarding acute coronary syndromes (ACS) in women is true EXCEPT:

A. Women are more likely to develop symptoms of angina than to present initially with a myocardial infarction (MI)
B. Women tend to be older than men at the time of presentation
C. In the setting of an MI, women are more likely than men are to present with nausea, palpitations, shortness of breath, and neck, jaw, and back pain
D. Women have a higher prevalence of vasospastic and microvascular angina than men
E. Women <50 years of age have lower mortality rates during ACS than men of the same age

QUESTION 651

A 60-year-old woman with a history of hypertension and diabetes mellitus is admitted to the hospital because of an acute severe headache, nausea, and vomiting. Physical examination demonstrates a blood pressure of 180/90 mm Hg, normal jugular venous pressure, bibasilar rales, no cardiac gallops or murmurs, and no focal neurologic signs. The troponin I is elevated at 0.62 ng/dL (normal: <0.10 ng/dL). Computed tomography of the brain demonstrates an acute subarachnoid hemorrhage. The patient's ECG is shown in Figure 5-1. Which of the following statements is TRUE?

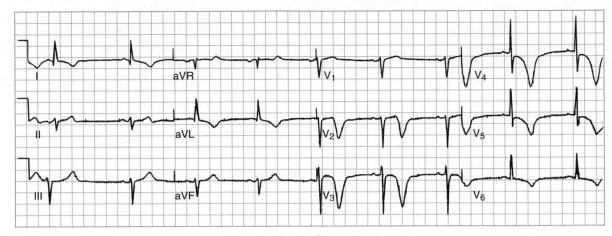

FIGURE 5-1 Courtesy of Dr. Charles Fisch, Indiana University School of Medicine, Indianapolis.

A. A ruptured coronary plaque with partially occlusive thrombus is likely present
B. QT interval prolongation is uncommon in this setting
C. All of the cardiac abnormalities can be attributed to autonomic dysfunction in the setting of acute brain injury
D. Beta blockers are not effective at controlling ventricular tachycardia and fibrillation in this situation
E. The magnitude of electrocardiographic abnormalities in such a patient correlates with a poor cardiovascular outcome

QUESTION 652

A 68-year-old man with a history of myocardial infarction is scheduled for elective hernia repair. Which of the following statements regarding perioperative medication use in coronary disease patients undergoing noncardiac surgery is TRUE?
A. Cardiac adverse event rates are reduced when high-dose beta-blocker therapy is initiated immediately before surgery
B. Nitrates decrease intraoperative myocardial ischemia and reduce rates of adverse cardiac outcomes
C. Most cardiac medications should be discontinued 2 to 3 days before surgery and resumed as soon as the patient can tolerate oral intake
D. Statin therapy has been associated with reduced perioperative cardiovascular event rates in high-risk patients

QUESTION 653

True statements regarding alterations in cardiovascular function with aging include each of the following EXCEPT:
A. Endothelial production of nitric oxide decreases with age
B. Left ventricular myocardial cells typically develop moderate hypertrophy
C. There is a fall in stroke volume and ejection fraction due to a decrease in peak contractile force

D. Heart rate during exercise increases less in older, compared with younger, individuals
E. The resting ejection fraction tends to remain constant with age in the absence of cardiac disease

QUESTION 654

A 58-year-old diabetic man develops fever and tenderness at the sternal wound site 12 days after coronary artery bypass graft surgery. All of the following have been associated with the development of deep sternal wound infection after cardiac surgery EXCEPT:
A. Prolonged cardiopulmonary bypass time
B. Use of both internal mammary arteries as bypass vessels
C. Diabetes
D. History of cigarette smoking prior to surgery
E. Preoperative atrial fibrillation

QUESTION 655

A 27-year-old woman undergoes right-sided heart catheterization for the assessment of suspected pulmonary arterial hypertension. The mean pulmonary artery pressure (PAP) is 44 mm Hg, and the pulmonary capillary wedge pressure (PCWP) is 11 mm Hg. Infusion of epoprostenol reduces the mean PAP to 31 mm Hg with no significant change in systemic blood pressure or PCWP. Each of the following statements is true EXCEPT:
A. Both intravenous adenosine and inhaled nitric oxide are alternative useful agents to assess vasoreactivity
B. The observed drop in mean PAP is predictive of a favorable response to oral calcium channel blockers
C. The failure of the systemic blood pressure to decline suggests that the vasodilator challenge was ineffective
D. Very high doses of chronic calcium channel blocker therapy would likely be necessary to realize full clinical benefit
E. A rise in PCWP in response to vasodilator therapy would be of concern for impending left ventricular failure

QUESTION 656

Which of the following interventions has been shown to reduce the incidence of contrast nephropathy after coronary angiography in patients with chronic renal insufficiency?
A. Infusion of 20% mannitol before angiography
B. Administration of atrial natriuretic peptide
C. Normal saline administration before and after angiography
D. Intravenous furosemide administration before angiography
E. Low-dose dopamine infusion

QUESTION 657

A 42-year-old woman presents to her primary care physician with recent fatigue and weight gain. Laboratory evaluation reveals a markedly elevated thyroid-stimulating hormone level. Common cardiac findings in patients with hypothyroidism include all of the following EXCEPT:
A. Hypotension
B. Decreased heart rate
C. Pericardial effusion
D. Decreased cardiac output
E. Prolonged QT interval on the ECG

QUESTION 658

A 28-year-old woman with Marfan syndrome presents for an office visit. Her echocardiogram shows mitral valve prolapse, an aortic root diameter of 4.5 cm, and mild aortic regurgitation. Each of the following statements regarding cardiovascular disease in patients with Marfan syndrome is true EXCEPT:
A. Sixty to 80 percent of patients with Marfan syndrome have mitral valve prolapse on echocardiography
B. The development of aortic regurgitation correlates with the aortic root diameter
C. Patients with Marfan syndrome should be considered for elective aortic root replacement once the aortic root diameter exceeds 6 cm
D. Beta blockers should be administered to all patients with Marfan syndrome unless a contraindication exists
E. The risk of aortic dissection during pregnancy in patients with Marfan syndrome is increased if the diameter of the aortic root exceeds 4 cm

QUESTION 659

A 54-year-old man was admitted to the hospital because of acute pulmonary embolism. Intravenous administration of heparin was begun. On admission, the platelet count was 223,000/μL. Four days later it had fallen to 16,000/μL, although the patient remained asymptomatic. Which of the following statements regarding this patient's condition is TRUE?
A. Low-molecular-weight heparin can be safely substituted for intravenous unfractionated heparin

B. A direct thrombin inhibitor, such as lepirudin, could be safely substituted for heparin
C. Intravenous heparin should be continued, because the low platelet count represents a laboratory artifact without clinical significance
D. Antibodies directed against the platelet glycoprotein IIb/IIIa receptor participate in this disorder
E. This is a transient reaction to heparin and does not preclude future heparin treatment for this patient

QUESTION 660

A 64-year-old man is brought to the emergency department because of confusion over the past 12 hours. Two weeks earlier he had undergone cardiac catheterization and a drug-eluting stent was placed in the right coronary artery. His medications include captopril, metoprolol, atorvastatin, aspirin, and clopidogrel. In the emergency department, he is febrile (101.3°F) and has a diffuse petechial rash. The remainder of his physical examination is unremarkable. Laboratory studies are notable for a new elevation in serum creatinine (3 mg/dL), a fall in the hematocrit to 22%, and the platelet count is reduced at 52,000/μL. Which medication is likely responsible for this patient's illness?
A. Captopril
B. Metoprolol
C. Atorvastatin
D. Clopidogrel
E. Aspirin

QUESTION 661

Which of the following statements regarding metastatic disease involving the heart is TRUE?
A. Tumor metastases frequently involve the cardiac valves
B. The most common primary tumor producing cardiac metastases is renal cell carcinoma
C. A chylous pericardial effusion is characteristic of metastatic breast carcinoma
D. More than 40% of patients with malignant melanoma have cardiac metastases
E. A solitary cardiac mass is more likely to be malignant than benign

QUESTION 662

While on rotation at a medical clinic in rural India you are asked to examine a 12-year-old girl who presents with fever, migratory polyarthritis, and an erythematous rash on her trunk that forms a snakelike ring with central clearing. Her cardiac examination is notable for a soft, blowing, high-pitched pansystolic murmur at the apex. She recalls a prolonged painful pharyngitis a few weeks ago. Two older family members are known to have mitral stenosis. In addition to the "major manifestations" considered diagnostic of this patient's likely condition, other

supporting evidence would include all of the following EXCEPT:
A. Prolonged QT interval
B. Fever
C. Elevated C-reactive protein
D. Normochromic, normocytic anemia
E. Rising streptococcal antibody titers

QUESTION 663

A 42-year-old woman with rheumatoid arthritis (RA) presents with exertional dyspnea. An echocardiogram shows a small circumferential pericardial effusion without evidence of hemodynamic compromise. Each of the following statements regarding cardiovascular involvement in rheumatoid arthritis is correct EXCEPT:
A. The pericardium is the most common site of cardiovascular involvement in RA
B. Conduction system disease in RA is associated with rheumatoid nodules impinging on the conduction pathways
C. Myocarditis is rare in RA
D. Epicardial coronary arteritis is seen in over half of patients with RA
E. Symptomatic involvement of the aorta and heart valves is rare

QUESTION 664

A 76-year-old man with hypertension and dyslipidemia is found to have atrial fibrillation for the first time on a routine office ECG. He has no history of cardiac symptoms, and an echocardiogram shows normal left ventricular contractile function and no valvular disease or pericardial effusion. His physician initiates dabigatran etexilate for long-term anticoagulation. Which of the following statements is TRUE?
A. Anticoagulation for this patient is not warranted because his risk of thromboembolism is low
B. Dabigatran etexilate is an oral factor Xa inhibitor
C. The risk of stroke or systemic embolism with dabigatran 150 mg twice daily is lower than that with warfarin anticoagulation and a target international normalized ratio (INR) of 2.0 to 3.0
D. Dabigatran 150 mg twice daily is associated with a higher rate of hemorrhagic stroke than warfarin anticoagulation
E. Hepatotoxicity is the major gastrointestinal side effect of dabigatran

QUESTION 665

A 66-year-old man with a history of atrial fibrillation successfully suppressed by amiodarone presents with tremors and recent weight loss. His physician suspects amiodarone-induced thyroid dysfunction. Each of the following statements about amiodarone and thyroid function is correct EXCEPT:
A. Amiodarone inhibits the peripheral conversion of thyroxine (T_4) to triiodothyronine (T_3)

B. During initial therapy, amiodarone decreases thyroid-stimulating hormone (TSH) levels
C. Amiodarone contains 30% iodine by weight
D. Amiodarone's iodine content inhibits synthesis and release of T_4 from the thyroid gland
E. Glucocorticoid therapy is beneficial for patients with amiodarone-induced hyperthyroidism who have elevated circulating levels of interleukin-6

QUESTION 666

A 54-year-old man presents for evaluation of excessive daytime sleepiness. His wife has observed his prominent snoring and gasping at night. Each of the following statements regarding sleep-related breathing disorders and cardiovascular disease is true EXCEPT:
A. Individuals with obstructive sleep apnea exhibit persistently increased sympathetic activity, even during daytime wakefulness
B. Obstructive sleep apnea is associated with drug-resistant hypertension, automatic tachycardias, and nocturnal bradycardias
C. Positive airway pressure therapy in obstructive sleep apnea is associated with reduced cardiovascular morbidity
D. Unlike obstructive sleep apnea, central sleep apnea is not associated with cardiovascular disease
E. Positive airway pressure benefits central sleep apnea as well as obstructive sleep apnea

QUESTION 667

A 65-year-old man is evaluated by the cardiology consult team 28 hours after completion of coronary artery bypass graft (CABG) surgery because the ECG demonstrates new Q waves in the anterior precordial leads. Which of the following statements about perioperative myocardial infarction (MI) in coronary artery bypass graft (CABG) surgery is TRUE?
A. Perioperative MI occurs in 5% to 10% of patients who undergo CABG surgery
B. Serum creatine kinase levels are rarely elevated after cardiac surgery in the absence of MI
C. Off-pump CABG is associated with lower serum concentrations of cardiac biomarkers and reduced mortality than conventional CABG
D. The presence of new Q waves after CABG is unreliable for the diagnosis of myocardial infarction
E. A prolonged pump time and older age are associated with perioperative MI

QUESTION 668

All of the following statements regarding perioperative cardiac risk in patients undergoing noncardiac surgery are true EXCEPT:
A. Emergency surgery carries a 2.5- to 4-fold increased risk of postoperative myocardial infarction (MI) and cardiac death compared with an elective operation

B. Insulin-dependent diabetes mellitus is a risk factor for postoperative adverse cardiac outcomes
C. Transurethral prostate surgery is considered a low-risk procedure with respect to cardiac complications
D. There is a 20% risk of reinfarction if surgery is performed 6 months after an acute MI
E. Most surgical procedures are well tolerated by patients with a history of angina who can carry groceries up one flight of stairs without stopping

QUESTION 669

A previously healthy 36-year-old woman presents to her primary care physician 3 weeks after the delivery of her second child because of new dyspnea, orthopnea, and peripheral edema. On examination, she appears fatigued. The blood pressure is 100/70 mm Hg and the heart rate is 120 beats/min. The jugular venous pressure is 12 cm H_2O. There are basilar rales, a prominent apical S_3 gallop, hepatomegaly, and bilateral lower extremity edema. An echocardiogram shows four-chamber cardiac enlargement and severe, global reduction of biventricular systolic function, compared with a normal study before pregnancy. Each of the following statements regarding this patient's condition is true EXCEPT:
A. The incidence of this disorder is greater with twin pregnancies
B. Approximately half of the patients with this disorder will completely recover normal cardiac function
C. Subsequent pregnancies are usually well tolerated
D. This condition becomes symptomatic in most patients during the last trimester of gestation or in the early postpartum period
E. The incidence of this disorder is higher among African-American women than among whites

DIRECTIONS: Each group of questions below consists of lettered headings followed by a set of numbered questions. For each question, select the ONE lettered heading with which it is most closely associated. Each lettered heading may be used once, more than once, or not at all.

QUESTIONS 670 TO 674

For each description listed below, match the appropriate diagnosis:
A. Behçet syndrome
B. Systemic sclerosis
C. Ankylosing spondylitis
D. Reiter syndrome
E. Giant cell arteritis

670. Granuloma formation in the coronary arteries
671. Aortitis, uveitis, and urethritis
672. Myocardial fibrosis and contraction band necrosis
673. Histologically similar to syphilitic aortitis
674. Occlusion of the subclavian artery and aneurysms of the common carotid artery

QUESTIONS 675 TO 678

Match the cardiac medication with the potential hematologic adverse effect:
A. Heparin
B. Alpha-methyldopa
C. Procainamide
D. Nitroglycerin

675. Erythematous rash, leukopenia
676. Coombs-positive hemolysis
677. Chocolate-brown blood, normal P_{O_2}
678. Thrombocytopenia

QUESTIONS 679 TO 683

Match the description with the associated disease:
A. Takayasu arteritis
B. Giant cell arteritis
C. Both
D. Neither

679. Occurrence is predominantly in women
680. Onset is typically during teenage years
681. Jaw muscle claudication suggests the diagnosis
682. Fever is almost always present
683. Steroid therapy is a cornerstone of management

QUESTIONS 684 TO 688

Match the chemotherapeutic agent with the likely cardiac complication:
A. Myocardial infarction
B. Acute myopericarditis
C. Capillary leak syndrome
D. Arrhythmias (acutely) and dilated cardiomyopathy (chronically)
E. Hypertension

684. Interleukin-2
685. 5-Fluorouracil
686. Cyclophosphamide
687. Doxorubicin
688. Sunitinib

QUESTIONS 689 TO 693

Match the cardiac finding with the most likely endocrine abnormality:
A. Hyperparathyroidism
B. Hypothyroidism
C. Hyperaldosteronism
D. Cushing syndrome
E. Hyperthyroidism

689. U waves on the ECG
690. Cardiac myxoma
691. Means-Lerman scratch

692. Shortened QT interval
693. Pericardial effusion

QUESTIONS 694 TO 697

Match the description to the associated fibrinolytic agent:
A. Streptokinase
B. Tissue-type plasminogen activator
C. Urokinase
D. Tenecteplase

694. Both single- and two-chain forms demonstrate proteolytic activity
695. Synthesized in renal tubular epithelial cells and endothelial cells
696. Prolonged half-life allows administration as a single bolus
697. Must form complex with plasminogen to exhibit enzymatic activity

QUESTIONS 698 TO 702

Match the finding to the associated anticoagulant:
A. Unfractionated heparin
B. Low-molecular-weight heparin

C. Both
D. Neither

698. Hyperkalemia
699. Bioavailability after subcutaneous injection is >90%
700. Inactivates clot-bound thrombus
701. Thrombocytopenia
702. Increases vascular permeability

QUESTIONS 703 TO 706

Match the following complications with the associated rheumatologic disorder:
A. Aortitis and headaches
B. Libman-Sacks endocarditis
C. Pulmonary hypertension
D. Aneurysmal dilatation of the subclavian and carotid arteries

703. Behçet syndrome
704. Systemic lupus erythematosus
705. Giant cell arteritis
706. Scleroderma

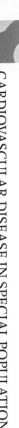

CARDIOVASCULAR DISEASE IN SPECIAL POPULATIONS; CARDIOVASCULAR DISEASE AND DISORDERS OF OTHER ORGANS

ANSWER TO QUESTION 630

C (Braunwald, pp. 1588-1590, 1785-1790)

In the United States, standard screening of young athletes typically consists only of history-taking and physical examination. This approach has a limited capability of detecting serious forms of cardiac disease that could lead to sudden cardiac death (SCD) during training, such as hypertrophic cardiomyopathy, anomalous origin of the coronary arteries, arrhythmogenic right ventricular cardiomyopathy, and inherited arrhythmia syndromes (e.g., long QT syndromes or Brugada syndrome). Patients with a family history of SCD or premature heart disease, those with cardiac symptoms (including inordinate exertional dyspnea, chest pain, syncope, or near-syncope) or a heart murmur that augments with standing or Valsalva maneuver warrant a more complete evaluation, usually including electrocardiography and echocardiography. This issue is particularly relevant since implantation of automatic defibrillators can prevent SCD in patients with predisposing conditions.

The most common cause of SCD in athletes in the United States is hypertrophic cardiomyopathy (HCM), accounting for 26.4% of episodes. This diagnosis can be difficult to distinguish from the physiologic hypertrophy ("athlete's heart") observed in individuals who participate in chronic endurance or isometric activities, in whom left ventricular (LV) wall thicknesses of 13 to 15 mm can be observed, (Fig. 5-2). Thus, voltage criteria for LV hypertrophy do not establish the diagnosis of hypertrophic or hypertensive cardiomyopathy in trained athletes. Echocardiographic findings more suggestive of *pathologic* hypertrophic hypertrophy include (1) LV wall thicknesses >15 mm, (2) prominent asymmetric LV hypertrophy, (3) LV end-diastolic cavity diameter < 45 mm, (4) marked left atrial enlargement, (5) abnormal LV Doppler filling patterns, and (6) lack of regression of hypertrophy after a period of deconditioning. A distinguishing feature during cardiopulmonary exercise testing is that conditioned athletes with physiologic hypertrophy can achieve maximum oxygen uptakes >45 mL/kg/min (>110% predicted), whereas those with HCM typically cannot. Patients in whom cardiac assessment reveals hypertrophic cardiomyopathy should be restricted from competitive athletics.

Anomalous origin of the coronary arteries is the second most common cause of SCD in athletes, accounting for 13.7% of episodes. Evaluation for this diagnosis includes coronary angiography or computed tomographic angiography.

REFERENCES

Baggish AL, Wood MJ: Athlete's heart and cardiovascular care of the athlete: Scientific and clinical update. Circulation 123:2723, 2011.
Maron BJ, Douglas PS, Graham TP, et al: Task Force 1: Preparticipation screening and diagnosis of cardiovascular disease in athletes. J Am Coll Cardiol 45:1322, 2005.

ANSWER TO QUESTION 631

C (Braunwald, pp. 1934, 1942)

Chronic kidney disease (CKD) identifies a patient population at high risk for cardiovascular events.[1] Up to 40% of patients with CKD who present to the hospital with chest pain have a cardiac event within 30 days. Moreover, retrospective studies of patients in coronary care units have identified renal dysfunction as the most significant prognostic factor for long-term adverse outcomes: patients with end-stage renal disease have the highest mortality after acute myocardial infarction of any population studied. Contributors to poor outcomes after acute coronary syndromes in patients with CKD include (1) frequently occurring comorbidities, including diabetes mellitus and heart failure, (2) reduced use of effective therapeutics due to fear of worsening renal dysfunction, (3) therapeutic toxicities, and (4) vascular dysfunction that is exacerbated by renal failure including a procoagulant and proinflammatory state. Whereas the latter contributes to increased rates of coronary thrombosis, uremia is also associated with impaired platelet aggregation, so patients with CKD can display increased bleeding risk at the same time.

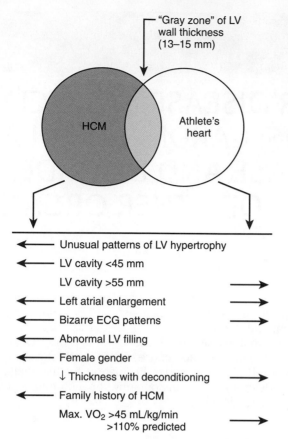

Unusual patterns of LV hypertrophy ←

LV cavity <45 mm ←

LV cavity >55 mm →

Left atrial enlargement ← →

Bizarre ECG patterns ← →

Abnormal LV filling ←

Female gender ←

↓ Thickness with deconditioning →

Family history of HCM ←

Max. VO$_2$ >45 mL/kg/min
>110% predicted →

FIGURE 5-2 Modified from Maron BJ, Pelliccia A: The heart trained athletes: Cardiac remodeling and the risks of sports including sudden death. Circulation 114;1633, 2006. Reproduced with permission of the American Heart Association.

REFERENCE

1. McCullough PA, Jurkovitz CT, Pergola PE, et al: Independent components of chronic kidney disease as a cardiovascular risk state: Results from the Kidney Early Evaluation Program (KEEP). Arch Intern Med 167:1122, 2007.

ANSWER TO QUESTION 632

C (Braunwald, pp. 1876-1878)

This patient has signs and symptoms of Takayasu arteritis (TA), an idiopathic large-vessel vasculitis that usually affects the aorta and its branches.[1] TA is 10 times more likely to affect women than men, and the median age at onset is 25 years old. This disease occurs worldwide with a prevalence of 2.6 per million in the United States and 1.26 per million in northern Europe. The cause of TA is unknown, but histopathologic analysis of acute lesions reveals mononuclear cell infiltrates consisting of macrophages, T lymphocytes, and natural killer lymphocytes.

Clinically, arterial stenoses occur three to four times more often than aneurysms. Thus, claudication (more common in the upper than lower extremities) is the major symptom; on physical examination, bruits and pulse asymmetries are the most frequent findings. When aneurysms occur, the aortic root is the most common location, which can lead to aortic regurgitation. Hypertension is common and is often caused by renal artery stenosis. Coronary arterial vasculitis most often affects the ostia of the vessels, leading to myocardial ischemia. In addition, myocarditis occurs in about 18% of patients.

Treatment involves high-dose corticosteroids, but relapses are common. Patients with resistant or relapsing symptoms may respond to cyclophosphamide or methotrexate. Recent data suggest pharmacologic blockade of tumor necrosis factor may decrease disease activity in patients who have experienced relapse on standard regimens.[2] Anatomic bypass of clinically significant stenosis may be necessary. Involvement of the aortic root may necessitate aortic repair, with or without valve replacement.

REFERENCES

1. Maksimowicz-McKinnon K, Clark TM, Hoffman GS: Takayasu's arteritis: Limitations of therapy and guarded prognosis in an American cohort. Arthritis Rheum 56:1000-1009, 2007.
2. Molloy ES, Langford CA, Clark TM, et al: Anti-tumour necrosis factor therapy in patients with refractory Takayasu arteritis: Long-term follow-up. Ann Rheum Dis 67:1567, 2008.

ANSWER TO QUESTION 633

D (Braunwald, pp. 1878-1879)

This patient has characteristic features of giant cell arteritis (GCA), which typically include the new onset of headache, scalp and temporal artery tenderness, polymyalgia rheumatica, acute visual abnormalities, and claudication of the jaw (Table 5-1). Such symptoms, in the presence of an increased erythrocyte sedimentation rate (ESR), support the diagnosis of GCA and mandate treatment, even without proof of diagnosis from a temporal artery biopsy. Corticosteroid treatment is the most effective therapy for GCA, and dramatic clinical improvement typically follows within 24 to 72 hours. The ESR itself does not always normalize with effective therapy, and it should not be relied on as the main measure of disease activity.

Cytotoxic and other immunosuppressive agents, including anti-TNF agents, have not proved effective in GCA in controlled trials.[1] Two retrospective studies have demonstrated that the use of low-dose aspirin reduces cerebral ischemic events (e.g., stroke) threefold to fourfold compared with patients who had not received such therapy. Therefore, most patients with GCA should receive low-dose daily aspirin.[2]

REFERENCES

1. Hoffman GS, Cid MC, Rendt-Zagar KE, et al: Infliximab-GCA Study Group: Infliximab for maintenance of glucocorticosteroid-induced remission of giant cell arteritis: A randomized trial. Ann Intern Med 146:621, 2007.
2. Lee MS, Smith SD, Galor A, et al: Antiplatelet and anticoagulant therapy in patients with giant cell arteritis. Arthritis Rheum 54:3306, 2006.

TABLE 5-1 Clinical Profile of Giant Cell Arteritis

ABNORMALITY	FREQUENCY (%)
Atypical headache	60-90
Tender temporal artery	40-70
Systemic symptoms not attributable to other diseases	20-50
Fever	20-50
Polymyalgia rheumatica	30-50
Acute visual abnormalities	12-40
Transient ischemic attack or stroke	5-10
Claudication Jaw Extremity	30-70 5-15
Aortic aneurysm	15-20
Dramatic response to corticosteroid therapy	~100
Positive temporal artery biopsy	~50-80

TABLE 5-2 Classification of Hypertension in Pregnancy

Chronic hypertension	Hypertension (blood pressure ≥140 mm Hg systolic or ≥90 mm Hg diastolic) present before pregnancy or that is diagnosed before the 20th week of gestation
Gestational hypertension	New hypertension with a blood pressure of 140/90 mm Hg on two separate occasions, without proteinuria, arising de novo after the 20th week of pregnancy. Blood pressure normalizes by 12 weeks postpartum.
Preeclampsia superimposed on chronic hypertension	Increased blood pressure above the patient's baseline, a change in proteinuria, or evidence of end-organ dysfunction
Preeclampsia-eclampsia	Proteinuria (>0.3 g during 24 hours or ++ in two urine samples) in addition to new hypertension. Edema is no longer included in the diagnosis because of poor specificity. When proteinuria is absent, suspect the disease when increased blood pressure is associated with headache, blurred vision, abdominal pain, low platelets, or abnormal liver enzymes.

From Gifford RW, August PA, Cunningham G, et al: Report of the National High Blood Pressure Education Program Working Group on High Blood Pressure in Pregnancy. Am J Obstet Gynecol 183:S1, 2000.

ANSWER TO QUESTION 634

D (Braunwald, pp. 1777-1778)

Hypertension during pregnancy is associated with increased maternal mortality and morbidity and consists of three forms (Table 5-2): (1) chronic hypertension (hypertension that precedes pregnancy); (2) gestational hypertension (hypertension that develops after 20 weeks of gestation and resolves by the 12th postpartum week); and (3) preeclampsia/eclampsia. *Preeclampsia* is identified by the new onset of hypertension after the 20th week of gestation with proteinuria. It is more likely to occur in primigravid patients, in twin pregnancies, and in those with preexisting hypertension. It can be accompanied by headache, blurred vision, a low platelet count, and/or abnormal liver enzyme levels. Preeclampsia is reversible and is treated with bed rest, salt restriction, and often magnesium sulfate to prevent eclamptic seizures; urgently delivering the fetus is usually necessary, after which blood pressure quickly normalizes. *Eclampsia* is present when findings of preeclampsia are accompanied by neurologic complications, including seizures.

Pharmacologic therapies that have been used successfully to lower blood pressure during pregnancy include methyldopa, beta blockers (particularly labetalol), calcium channel blockers, hydralazine, and hydrochlorothiazide. Although these medications are effective in treating chronic hypertension that has worsened during pregnancy, they are not effective in preventing preeclampsia.

Angiotensin-converting enzyme inhibitors and angiotensin receptor blockers can induce congenital malformations and neonatal renal failure and should *not* be used in pregnancy.

REFERENCE

Gifford RW, August PA, Cunningham G, et al: Report of the National High Blood Pressure Education Program Working Group on high blood pressure in pregnancy. Am J Obstet Gynecol 183:S1, 2000.

ANSWER TO QUESTION 635

B (Braunwald, pp. 1757-1761)

Cardiovascular disease is the number one cause of mortality for women in the United States, accounting for 1 in 3 deaths. Fortunately, statistical trends between 1980 and 2002 reveal that age-adjusted heart disease mortality has *declined* in both men (52%) and women (49%), attributed to beneficial risk factor modifications and the influence of evidence-based therapies in the treatment of coronary artery disease, acute coronary syndromes, and heart failure.[1,2]

Coronary heart disease first presents approximately 10 years later in women than in men, most commonly after menopause, and the INTERHEART study demonstrated that this pattern holds widely around the globe. The age difference is likely contributed to by a protective effect of circulating estrogen before menopause. Nonetheless, pharmacologic replacement of estrogen after menopause does not prevent clinical cardiovascular events.[3]

As in men, hyperlipidemia, hypertension, tobacco use, diabetes mellitus, obesity, and a sedentary lifestyle are all important modifiable risk factors for the development of heart disease in women. In the United States, nearly 32% of women >age 20 have a low density lipoprotein cholesterol level ≥130 mg/dL and more than 35 million women are hypertensive, a 15% higher prevalence than men. There are >9.5 million women with diabetes mellitus, a population in which cardiovascular disease is twice as common compared with nondiabetics.

REFERENCES

1. Lloyd-Jones D, Adams R, Carnethon M, et al: Heart disease and stroke statistics—2009 update: A report from the American Heart Association Statistics Committee and Stroke Statistics Subcommittee. Circulation 119:e21, 2009.
2. Ford ES, Ajani UA, Croft JB, et al: Explaining the decrease in U.S. deaths from coronary disease, 1980-2000. N Engl J Med 356:2388, 2007.
3. Ouyang P, Michos ED, Karas RH: Hormone replacement therapy and the cardiovascular system: Lessons learned and unanswered questions. J Am Coll Cardiol 47:1741, 2006.

ANSWER TO QUESTION 636

C (Braunwald, pp. 1776-1777)

Peripartum cardiomyopathy (PPCM) is a form of dilated cardiomyopathy that occurs for the first time in the antepartum or postpartum period and is clinically indistinguishable from other types of dilated cardiomyopathy.[1] It is generally defined by four criteria: (1) the development of cardiac failure in the last month of pregnancy or within 5 months of delivery, (2) absence of an identifiable cause for the cardiac failure, (3) absence of recognizable heart disease before the last month of pregnancy, and (4) left ventricular systolic dysfunction demonstrated by classic imaging criteria.

The incidence of PPCM is approximately 1 in 3000 pregnancies, and risk factors for its occurrence include multiparity, being black, older maternal age, and pre-eclampsia. In one retrospective study, 43% of patients had a history of hypertension, and twin pregnancies were present in 13%.[1]

Approximately 50% of patients with PPCM show complete or near-complete recovery during the first 6 months after delivery, whereas the remainder demonstrates either continued deterioration or persistent left ventricular dysfunction and chronic heart failure symptomatology. Subsequent pregnancies in patients with PPCM with persistent cardiac dysfunction should be discouraged because of the high likelihood of relapse. Even patients who have recovered from an episode of PPCM have a 30% risk of experiencing relapse during subsequent pregnancies.[2]

REFERENCES

1. Elkayam U, Akhter MW, Singh H, et al: Pregnancy-associated cardiomyopathy: Clinical characteristics and a comparison between early and late presentation. Circulation 111:2050, 2005.
2. Sliwa K, Fett J, Elkayam U: Peripartum cardiomyopathy. Lancet 368:687, 2006.

ANSWER TO QUESTION 637

C (Braunwald, pp. 1241, 1800-1808)

The frequency of perioperative complications in coronary artery bypass graft surgery (CABG) has increased because of the greater percentage of high-risk patients who undergo the operation. The rate of major morbidity (e.g., death, stroke, renal failure, reoperation, prolonged ventilation, sternal infection) within 30 days was 13.4% in the Society of Thoracic Surgeons (STS) database of CABG-only procedures between 1997 and 1999.[1] The reported incidence of perioperative myocardial infarction (MI) varies widely. The STS database reported an incidence of 1.1% in 2005, based on strict diagnostic criteria.

Neurologic complications can occur after cardiac surgery by mechanisms that include atherosclerotic cerebral emboli from the aorta, emboli related to the cardiopulmonary bypass machine, and intraoperative hypotension. Prospective studies reveal a postcardiac surgical incidence of stroke ranging from 1.5% to 5.0%.[2] Short-term cognitive decline has been reported in 33% to 83% of patients.

Atrial fibrillation (AF) is one of the most frequent complications of bypass surgery, developing in approximately 40% of patients within 3 days after surgery, and it is associated with a twofold to threefold increase in postoperative stroke. Up to 80% of patients spontaneously revert to sinus rhythm within 24 hours without treatment other than rate control agents. Prophylactic beta-blocker or amiodarone therapy reduces the incidence of postoperative AF.

The incidence of renal failure requiring dialysis after CABG is low (0.5% to 1.0%) but is associated with greater morbidity and mortality when it occurs. Predictors of postoperative renal dysfunction include advanced age, diabetes, pre-existing renal dysfunction, and heart failure. In a randomized trial, N-acetylcysteine did not prevent renal dysfunction after CABG.[3]

REFERENCES

1. Ferguson TB Jr, Hammill BG, Peterson ED, et al for the STS National Database Committee: A decade of change—risk profiles and outcomes for isolated coronary artery bypass grafting procedures, 1990-1999: A report from the STS National Database Committee and the Duke Clinical Research Institute. Society of Thoracic Surgeons. Ann Thorac Surg 73:480, 2002.
2. Dacey LJ, Likosky DS, Leavitt BJ, et al: Perioperative stroke and long-term survival after coronary bypass graft surgery. Ann Thorac Surg 79:532, 2005.
3. Burns KE, Chu MW, Novick RJ, et al: Perioperative N-acetylcysteine to prevent renal dysfunction in high-risk patients undergoing CABG surgery: A randomized controlled trial. JAMA 294:342, 2005.

ANSWER TO QUESTION 638

E (Braunwald, p. 1240)

A variety of conduit options are available for coronary artery bypass graft surgery. Saphenous vein grafts are relatively easy to harvest, but they suffer from several drawbacks. Approximately 8% to 12% of saphenous vein grafts become occluded during the early perioperative period. By 1 year, 15% to 30% of vein grafts occlude. Some of these occlusions may be due to endothelial denuding during surgical preparation, thereby predisposing the graft to early thrombosis. Intimal hyperplasia and accelerated atherosclerosis in vein grafts are common, and by 10 years after surgery, the patency rate of saphenous vein conduits is <50%.

In contrast, internal mammary artery (IMA) grafts, although more difficult to harvest, do not develop intimal hyperplasia and have 10-year patency rates of > 80%. Possible explanations for the superiority of IMA grafts include (1) the medial layer of arterial grafts may derive additional nourishment from the vasa vasorum, (2) the endothelium of the IMA produces high levels of endogenous vasodilators, and (3) the diameter of the IMA is closer to that of the recipient coronary artery than is the diameter of the saphenous vein. Compared with patients with saphenous vein grafts, patients who receive IMA conduits have a decreased risk of death, myocardial infarction, and reoperation. Other arterial conduits, such as the radial artery, are used less often. Although more likely to develop vasospasm than IMA grafts, radial artery grafts are also effective conduits with high long-term patency rates.

REFERENCES

Baskett RJ, Cafferty FH, Powell SJ, et al: Total arterial revascularization is safe: Multicenter ten-year analysis of 71,470 coronary procedures. Ann Thorac Surg 81:1243, 2006.

Nishida H, Tomizawa Y, Endo M, et al: Survival benefit of exclusive use of in situ arterial conduits over combined use of arterial and vein grafts for multiple coronary artery bypass grafting. Circulation 112(9 Suppl):1299, 2005.

ANSWER TO QUESTION 639

A (Braunwald, pp. 1786, 1790-1791; see also Answer 630)

Sudden cardiac death (SCD) in young athletes is a rare, tragic event. The most commonly identified abnormality in this situation is hypertrophic cardiomyopathy (HCM). A recent review confirmed that HCM accounts for one third of cases of SCD in which a cause is identified. It is not uncommon for such persons to have been asymptomatic throughout their lives, and even routine history and physical examination before undertaking competitive sports will miss many cases (Table 5-3).

The second most common etiology of SCD identified in young athletes is anomalous origin of a coronary artery, accounting for approximately 20% of cases. The most frequent form is anomalous origin of the left main coronary artery from the right coronary cusp. The opposite configuration, anomalous origin of the right coronary artery from the left aortic sinus, has also been identified as a cause of SCD. Myocardial ischemia in individuals with anomalous coronaries may relate to a kinked takeoff of the artery or compression of the vessel between the aorta and pulmonary trunk during exercise. Like HCM, coronary anomalies are very difficult to identify by routine screening.

Much less common causes of SCD in young athletes include atherosclerotic coronary disease, myocarditis, aortic dissection, congenital valvular aortic stenosis, and arrhythmogenic right ventricular cardiomyopathy.

TABLE 5-3 Cardiovascular Causes of Sudden Death in Young Athletes (N = 690)

CAUSE	PROPORTION OF ALL CAUSES (%)
Hypertrophic cardiomyopathy	36
Coronary artery anomalies	17
Possible hypertrophic cardiomyopathy*	8
Myocarditis	6
Arrhythmogenic right ventricular cardiomyopathy	4
Ion channel disease	4
Mitral valve prolapse	3
Bridged left anterior descending coronary artery	3
Atherosclerotic coronary artery disease	3
Aortic rupture	3
Aortic stenosis	2
Dilated cardiomyopathy	2
Wolff-Parkinson-White syndrome	2
Other	5

*Findings suggestive but not diagnostic of hypertrophic cardiomyopathy.
Data from Maron BJ, Doerer JJ, Haas TS, et al: Sudden death in young competitive athletes: Analysis of 1866 deaths in the United States, 1980-2006. Circulation 119:1085, 2009.

REFERENCE

Maron BJ, Doerer JJ, Haas TS, et al: Sudden death in young competitive athletes: Analysis of 1866 deaths in the United States, 1980-2006. Circulation 119:1085, 2009.

ANSWER TO QUESTION 640

D (Braunwald, p. 1760)

Compared with men, women experiencing an acute coronary syndrome more frequently describe milder symptoms and are more likely to express nonspecific prodromal symptoms such as fatigue.[1] Among all patients in emergency departments with symptoms of CAD other than chest pain, women more often than men describe dyspnea, nausea, indigestion, and arm or shoulder discomforts on presentation. However, the Myocardial Infarction Triage and Intervention (MITI) Project investigators demonstrated that chest pain was present in almost all women (99.6%) and men (99%) who experienced a documented acute myocardial infarction. In addition, women with myocardial infarction typically have more comorbidities, including hypertension, and present later in the course of symptoms and more frequently with high-risk clinical findings such as heart failure.[2]

Women are hospitalized more frequently than men each year for the evaluation of chest pain, but women who present with chest discomfort are more likely than men to have a noncardiac cause or other nonatherosclerotic causes, such as vasospasm.

CARDIOVASCULAR DISEASE IN SPECIAL POPULATIONS; CARDIOVASCULAR DISEASE AND DISORDERS OF OTHER ORGANS

REFERENCES

1. Kyker KA, Limacher MC: Gender differences in presentation and symptoms of coronary artery disease. Curr Womens Health Rep 2:115, 2002.
2. Shaw LJ, Bairey Merz CN, Pepine CJ, et al: Insights from the NHLBI-sponsored Women's Ischemia Syndrome Evaluation (WISE) Study: I. Gender differences in traditional and novel risk factors, symptom evaluation, and gender-optimized diagnostic strategies. J Am Coll Cardiol 47:4S, 2006.

ANSWER TO QUESTION 641

E (Braunwald, pp. 1798-1799)

Several abnormal laboratory findings are typical in the hours after cardiac surgery and cardiopulmonary bypass. Postoperative hematocrit levels are usually in the low 30s most often related to hemodilution and blood loss. A platelet count <100,000/µL is common, but thrombocytopenia <50,000/µL should be investigated for pathologic causes. Mild metabolic acidosis (serum bicarbonate levels of 18 to 26 mEq/liter and pH ≥7.3) may be present and resolves with rewarming and improvement in cardiac output. Potassium levels can change rapidly and require frequent surveillance. Calcium levels <7.0 mg/dL occur because of hemodilution and rarely require treatment. Phosphate levels should be routinely measured immediately after surgery and appropriate replacement instituted because significant hypophosphatemia is common (34.3%) and is associated with prolonged mechanical ventilation.[1]

Cardiac troponin T (cTnT) elevation is present in nearly all patients, with a median serum concentration of 1.08 ng/mL. A linear association has been noted between cTnT levels and length of stay in the intensive care unit and hospital and postoperative ventilator hours.[2] In addition, cTnT is independently prognostic for death, death or heart failure, death or need for vasopressors, and the composite of all three. Serum cTnT levels measured 24 hours after cardiac surgery predict short-, medium-, and long-term mortality.

REFERENCES

1. Cohen J, Kogan A, Sahar G, et al: Hypophosphatemia after open heart surgery: Incidence and consequences. Eur J Cardiothorac Surg 26:306, 2004.
2. Mohammed AA, Agnihotri AK, van Kimmenade RRJ, et al: Prospective, comprehensive assessment of cardiac troponin T testing after coronary artery bypass graft surgery. Circulation 120:843, 2009.

ANSWER TO QUESTION 642

D (Braunwald, pp. 1761-1763)

Past observational studies had suggested a benefit of postmenopausal hormone replacement therapy in primary and secondary prevention of coronary artery disease events. However, more recent large randomized prospective trials have shown that hormone replacement therapy fails to reduce coronary heart disease events. In the Women's Health Initiative estrogen-only trial, 10,739 postmenopausal women were randomized to placebo or 0.625 mg of oral conjugated equine estrogens daily. The trial was stopped early because there was no significant benefit of estrogen on the primary composite endpoint of death or nonfatal MI, but the risk of stroke and pulmonary embolism *increased* in the estrogen arm of the study. Current American Heart Association guidelines assign a Class III recommendation to the use of estrogen plus progestin for primary and secondary prevention (i.e., risk is greater than benefit and should not be used).

REFERENCES

Ouyang P, Michos ED, Karas RH: Hormone replacement therapy and the cardiovascular system: Lessons learned and unanswered questions. J Am Coll Cardiol 47:1741, 2006.
Women's Health Initiative Steering Committee: Effects of conjugated equine estrogen in postmenopausal women with hysterectomy: The Women's Health Initiative randomized controlled trial. JAMA 291:1701, 2004.

ANSWER TO QUESTION 643

D (Braunwald, pp. 1796-1798)

The factors that most significantly increase mortality with CABG include increasing age, emergency or urgent surgery, prior cardiac surgery, dialysis dependency or serum creatinine >2 mg/dL, female gender, left ventricular ejection fraction <40%, peripheral vascular disease, and chronic obstructive lung disease. With the exception of chronic obstructive lung disease and female gender, these variables are also predictors of cerebrovascular accidents in the perioperative period. A simple scoring system (EuroSCORE) can be used to assess the risk of adverse outcomes in individual patients.[1] Interestingly, diabetes and obesity have not been shown to be independent predictors of mortality or cerebrovascular accidents after CABG. These characteristics are, however, significant independent predictors for the development of postoperative mediastinitis.

Although not included in the EuroSCORE, preoperative atrial fibrillation is also associated with increased perioperative mortality and morbidity in patients undergoing cardiac surgery.[2]

REFERENCES

1. Ranucci M, Castelvecchio S, Menicanti L, et al: An adjusted EuroSCORE model for high-risk cardiac patients. Eur J Cardiothorac Surg 36:791, 2009.
2. Ad N, Barnett SD, Haan CK, et al: Does preoperative atrial fibrillation increase the risk for mortality and morbidity after coronary artery bypass grafting? J Thorac Cardiovasc Surg 137:901, 2009.

ANSWER TO QUESTION 644

B (Braunwald, pp. 1777-1778)

Acute myocardial infarction (AMI) is rare in women of childbearing age, but pregnancy increases the risk threefold to fourfold.[1] AMI can occur during any stage of pregnancy and is more frequent in multigravida women. Most events occur in women >age 30 and the majority of the time the location is the anterior wall. Although atherosclerotic disease is typically uncommon in young women, there is a relatively high incidence of traditional risk factors among those who experience AMI during pregnancy, including cigarette smoking, hyperlipidemia, hypertension, and diabetes.[1] The most common findings at coronary angiography in pregnant women with AMI are atherosclerotic disease (with or without intracoronary thrombus) or coronary artery dissection, the latter being the most common cause of AMI in the peripartum period.[1] Coronary spasm or embolism are much rarer. Even during pregnancy, acute management of ST-segment elevation AMI warrants urgent coronary angiography, with percutaneous coronary intervention and stenting if appropriate. The safety of drug-eluting stents and their required prolonged dual antiplatelet therapy is unknown in pregnancy, and most experience to date has been with bare metal stents.

REFERENCE

1. Roth A, Elkayam U: Acute myocardial infarction associated with pregnancy. J Am Coll Cardiol 52:171, 2008.

ANSWER TO QUESTION 645

C (Braunwald, pp. 1241, 1802)

Perioperative myocardial infarction (MI) in association with CABG has an adverse effect on early and late prognosis. The reported incidence of this complication is variable because of heterogeneous diagnostic criteria, with an approximate risk of 1.1% in the Society of Thoracic Surgeons (STS) database. The diagnosis of MI immediately after CABG can be difficult because usual criteria are not often applicable. For example, symptoms are not reliable because most patients are sedated and may not sense ischemic pain. Conversely, any chest discomfort described by the patient may be difficult to distinguish from sternal or pericardial sensations. The ECG may not be diagnostic because ST-segment abnormalities are very common after CABG. If new ST-segment *elevations* are observed, however, there should be concern for acute graft failure or spasm, which must be differentiated from the changes of postoperative pericardial inflammation. The most reliable electrocardiographic finding of a post-CABG MI is new and persistent Q waves. Echocardiography may aid in the diagnosis of postoperative MI. If a preoperative study is available, new wall motion abnormalities support the diagnosis of myocardial injury. Abnormal septal motion, however, is not specific because most patients who undergo cardiac surgery have paradoxical septal movement for at least several months after cardiac surgery. Serum markers of myocardial necrosis are also difficult to interpret in the post-CABG setting. Total creatine kinase elevations are almost universally observed because of damage to skeletal muscle in the chest wall. The myocardial-specific CK-MB isoenzyme and cardiac troponins are frequently detected in the serum as a result of myocardial incisions made during the institution of cardiopulmonary bypass. As a result, a higher than usual threshold for significant CK-MB elevation (more than *five* times the upper limit of normal) is required for the diagnosis of peri-CABG MI.

Clinical risk factors for peri-CABG MI include older age, longer pump time, elevated left-ventricular end-diastolic pressure, preoperative unstable angina, and significant left main coronary artery disease.

REFERENCES

Mangano DT, Miao Y, Tudor IC, et al: Post-reperfusion myocardial infarction: Long-term survival improvement using adenosine regulation with acadesine. J Am Coll Cardiol 48:206, 2006.

Ramsay J, Shernan S, Fitch J, et al: Increased creatine kinase MB level predicts postoperative mortality after cardiac surgery independent of new Q waves. J Thorac Cardiovasc Surg 129:300, 2005.

ANSWER TO QUESTION 646

D (Braunwald, pp. 1740-1742)

Older patients (>65 years of age) comprise 60% of hospital admissions for acute myocardial infarction (MI). According to a review of Medicare beneficiaries, elderly patients who present with an acute MI are more likely to have comorbid illnesses and exhibit higher rates of congestive heart failure, ventricular rupture, and mortality compared with younger individuals. Like younger age groups, there is a significant survival benefit from reperfusion therapies (percutaneous coronary intervention [PCI] or fibrinolysis) in acute ST-segment elevation MI in older patients, although few individuals >age 75 years have been included in pertinent clinical trials. For persons up to the age of 75 years, most trials show that fibrinolytic, antiplatelet, and antithrombin therapy is associated with a survival advantage, although bleeding and transfusion rates are higher in older patients. Even fibrin-specific fibrinolytic agents are associated with increased stroke risk due to intracerebral hemorrhage in those > age 75 years. In patients who undergo PCI, antiplatelet therapy with prasugrel is associated with an increased risk of fatal bleeding events compared with clopidogrel in patients >75 years and should be avoided in that population.

Ventricular remodeling after infarction may differ in the elderly because of alterations in the inflammatory response, decreased ability of the myocardium to hypertrophy, and increased collagen content of cardiac tissue. However, elderly patients benefit as much as younger individuals from beta-blocker therapy for secondary prevention. In addition, in patients >65 years of age who have sustained an MI with residual left ventricular ejection fraction <40%, angiotensin-converting enzyme inhibitors reduce fatal and nonfatal events just as they do for younger individuals.

REFERENCES

Antman E, Hand M, Armstrong P, et al: 2007 Focused Update of the ACC/AHA 2004 Guidelines for the Management of Patients with ST-Elevation Myocardial Infarction: A report of the American College of Cardiology/American Heart Association Task Force on Practice Guidelines: Developed in collaboration with the Canadian Cardiovascular Society endorsed by the American Academy of Family Physicians: 2007 Writing Group to Review New Evidence and Update the ACC/AHA 2004

Guidelines for the Management of Patients With ST-Elevation Myocardial Infarction, Writing on Behalf of the 2004 Writing Committee. Circulation 117:296, 2008.

Bardají A, Bueno H, Fernández-Ortiz A, et al: Type of treatment and short-term outcome in elderly patients with acute myocardial infarction admitted to hospitals with a primary coronary angioplasty facility. The TRIANA (TRatamiento del Infarto Agudo de miocardio eN Ancianos) Registry. Rev Esp Cardiol 58:351, 2005.

Mehta RH, Granger CB, Alexander KP, et al: Reperfusion strategies for acute myocardial infarction in the elderly: Benefits and risks. J Am Coll Cardiol 45:471, 2005.

ANSWER TO QUESTION 647

A (Braunwald, pp. 1811-1813)

Many patients >age 40 are likely to have coronary artery disease or other cardiac conditions that may influence the safety of noncardiac surgery. By recently accepted criteria, six independent predictors of complications have been identified: high-risk type of surgery, history of ischemic heart disease, history of congestive heart failure (e.g., the S_3 gallop described in the vignette for this question), history of cerebrovascular disease, preoperative treatment with insulin, and a preoperative serum creatinine >2 mg/dL. The greater the number of these factors, the more likely is a perioperative cardiovascular complication.

Notably, statistically nonsignificant risk factors include smoking, hyperlipidemia, and mild to moderate hypertension. And while preoperative unstable symptoms of angina portend a complicated postoperative course, that is not the case for patients with stable class I to II angina or remote MI without active angina. A history of supraventricular arrhythmias such as atrial fibrillation should alert the clinician to the possible development of similar rhythm disturbances postoperatively. Nonsustained ventricular tachycardia has not been associated with poor postoperative outcomes.

REFERENCES

Fleisher LA, Beckman JA, Brown KA, et al: 2009 ACCF/AHA focused update on perioperative beta blockade incorporated into the ACC/AHA 2007 guidelines on perioperative cardiovascular evaluation and care for noncardiac surgery: A report of the American College of Cardiology Foundation/American Heart Association Task Force on Practice Guidelines. Circulation 120:e169, 2009.

Poldermans D, Bax JJ, Boersma E, et al: Guidelines for pre-operative cardiac risk assessment and perioperative cardiac management in non-cardiac surgery: The Task Force for Preoperative Cardiac Risk Assessment and Perioperative Cardiac Management in Non-cardiac Surgery of the European Society of Cardiology (ESC) and endorsed by the European Society of Anaesthesiology (ESA). Eur Heart J 30:2769, 2009.

ANSWER TO QUESTION 648

C (Braunwald, pp. 935-937, 1735-1737)

Data from several major trials indicate that effective therapy for even mild diastolic hypertension leads to a reduction in mortality and cardiovascular events. Similar results have also been published on the effectiveness of therapy for isolated systolic hypertension (ISH) in older populations. In the SHEP study in the elderly, treatment of ISH was shown to reduce the incidence of both stroke and major cardiovascular events.

Several studies, including the ALLHAT trial, have demonstrated that thiazide diuretics are efficacious and generally should be the preferred first-line antihypertensive agent in the elderly. Additionally, in large clinical trials, beta blockers have resulted in less cardiovascular protection than diuretics as first-line therapy.

Data from the Framingham Study have proved the importance of left ventricular hypertrophy as an independent risk factor for adverse cardiac outcomes in older, hypertensive subjects. Hypertensive hypertrophic cardiomyopathy in the elderly tends to be more common in women, and the presenting symptom is usually dyspnea or chest pain.

REFERENCE

Beckett NS, Peters R, Fletcher AE, et al: Treatment of hypertension in patients 80 years of age or older. N Engl J Med 358:887, 2008.

ANSWER TO QUESTION 649

E (Braunwald, pp. 1770-1771)

Several hemodynamic alterations occur during normal pregnancy. Blood volume increases substantially, beginning during the second month, then rises to an average volume expansion of 50% by late pregnancy. The increase in blood volume occurs more quickly than the increase in hemoglobin, so anemia is common. The increased blood volume augments ventricular preload and stroke volume. The heart rate also rises steadily, usually by 10 to 20 beats/min by the third trimester. The augmented heart rate and stroke volume lead to a rise in cardiac output throughout pregnancy. Systemic vascular resistance begins to fall during the first trimester, reaches its lowest level in midpregnancy, then returns to the pre-pregnancy level before delivery. The drop in systemic vascular resistance likely represents a combination of circulating gestational hormones, vasodilating prostaglandins, atrial natriuretic peptides, and nitric oxide, as well as the low-resistance circulation of the gravid uterus.

ANSWER TO QUESTION 650

E (Braunwald, pp. 1760-1761)

It had long been thought that men and women had similar clinical presentations of coronary artery disease, but evidence now shows otherwise. Women are more likely to develop angina as the first manifestation of heart disease and less likely to present with an acute myocardial infarction (MI) than men. Women also tend to be, on average, 5 to 10 years older than men at the time of symptom onset. Compared with men, women presenting with an MI are more likely to experience nausea, shortness of breath, palpitations, and neck, jaw, and back pain and are less likely to experience diaphoresis.

It is not clear what accounts for these differences. Perhaps the age at presentation results in a higher incidence of comorbid conditions such as diabetes, hypertension, and congestive heart failure. Angiographic findings are similar, but women have a higher prevalence of vasospastic and microvascular angina.

Mortality rates appear to differ between men and women as well, with women <50 years of age having a twofold *greater* mortality in association with acute MI. The gender differences in mortality diminish with age.

REFERENCE

Gierach GL, Johnson BD, Bairey Merz CN, et al: Hypertension, menopause, and coronary artery disease risk in the Women's Ischemia Syndrome Evaluation (WISE) Study. J Am Coll Cardiol 47:S50, 2006.

ANSWER TO QUESTION 651

C (Braunwald, pp. 1930-1932)

This patient presents with an acute subarachnoid hemorrhage and a markedly abnormal ECG. Electrocardiographic abnormalities are present in approximately 70% of patients with subarachnoid hemorrhage and can include ST-segment elevation or depression, deep symmetric T wave inversions as in this patient, and a prolonged QT interval that can lead to torsades de pointes ventricular tachycardia.[1] The mechanism of cardiac and electrocardiographic abnormalities in acute brain injury likely relates to autonomic nervous system dysfunction and excessive myocardial catecholamine release.[2] In this setting, myocardial damage can occur with release of cardiac biomarkers, without primary acute coronary plaque rupture or thrombus formation. The magnitude of peak troponin elevation, but not the degree of electrocardiographic abnormality, is predictive of an adverse cardiac outcome. Beta blockers appear useful in minimizing myocardial damage and controlling arrhythmias in patients with subarachnoid hemorrhage.

REFERENCES

1. Naidech AM, Kreiter KT, Janjua N, et al: Cardiac troponin elevation, cardiovascular morbidity, and outcome after subarachnoid hemorrhage. Circulation 112:2851, 2005.
2. Samuels MA: The brain-heart connection. Circulation 116:77, 2007.

ANSWER TO QUESTION 652

D (Braunwald, pp. 1820-1822)

It is generally safe and appropriate to continue most chronically administered cardiac medications up to the day of surgery and to resume them as soon as possible after the operation. This is true of beta blockers in patients with underlying coronary artery disease (or other indications for chronic beta-blocker use) and continuing this therapy perioperatively is a Class I American College of Cardiology/American Heart Association guideline intervention, with improved cardiovascular outcomes.[1] Class IIa indications for initiation of a beta blocker, titrated to

heart rate and blood pressure before and after surgery, include patients scheduled for vascular or other intermediate-risk surgery who have known coronary artery disease or multiple atherosclerotic risk factors. However, initiating a high-dose beta blocker without dose titration immediately before surgery can be *harmful*, has been associated with increased mortality, and should be avoided.[2]

Although nitrates reduce intraoperative ischemia, cardiac outcomes are not affected.

Statins have anti-inflammatory and plaque-stabilizing properties, and studies in patients undergoing vascular surgery have demonstrated reduced cardiac event rates in patients on such therapy perioperatively.[3]

REFERENCES

1. Fleisher LA, Beckman JA, Brown KA, et al: 2009 ACCF/AHA focused update on perioperative beta blockade incorporated into the ACC/AHA 2007 guidelines on perioperative cardiovascular evaluation and care for noncardiac surgery: A report of the American College of Cardiology Foundation/American Heart Association Task Force on Practice Guidelines. Circulation 120:e169, 2009.
2. Devereaux PJ, Yang H, Yusuf S, et al: Effects of extended-release metoprolol succinate in patients undergoing non-cardiac surgery (POISE trial): A randomised controlled trial. Lancet 371:1839, 2008.
3. Durazzo AE, Machado FS, Ikeoka DT, et al: Reduction in cardiovascular events after vascular surgery with atorvastatin: A randomized trial. J Vasc Surg 39:967, 2004.

ANSWER TO QUESTION 653

C (Braunwald, pp. 1727-1730)

Study of the normal aging process of the heart is difficult because of the high prevalence of cardiovascular disease in the American population. Studies in which coronary artery disease and other common cardiovascular diseases have been carefully excluded have revealed several interesting findings. First, there is moderate hypertrophy of left ventricular (LV) myocardial cells, probably in response to increased arterial stiffness and loss of cardiac myocyte number with age. Although myocardial cells are unable to proliferate or increase in number, they can increase in size; this appears to be an adaptive response. Careful studies have shown that, despite alterations in the contractile proteins leading to reductions in the velocity of contraction and lengthening of contraction and relaxation times, peak contractile force production is maintained at normal levels. However, there are changes in beta-adrenoceptor–mediated inotropic and chronotropic cardiovascular responses with aging that result from a generalized desensitization. Thus, maximal heart rate during exercise and other cardiovascular responses to exercises are blunted.

In general, there appear to be no changes in cardiac output, stroke volume, or ejection fraction at rest with aging. Preservation of these functions is due to adaptive responses in contraction time and calcium transients. These adaptations compensate for the increased LV stiffness consequent to hypertrophy and the loss of elasticity of the pericardium and other supporting structures.

Among the cellular and molecular changes that occur with aging, endothelial production of nitric oxide (NO) decreases, likely reflecting a combination of decreased endothelial cell mass (increased cell senescence and apoptosis) and increased NO utilization because of elevated vascular superoxide anion production in older subjects.

REFERENCES

Lakatta E, Wang M, Najjar S: Arterial aging and subclinical arterial disease are fundamentally intertwined at macroscopic and molecular levels. Med Clin North Am 93:583, 2009.

O'Rourke M, Hashimoto J: Mechanical factors in arterial aging: A clinical perspective. J Am Coll Cardiol 50:1, 2007.

ANSWER TO QUESTION 654

D (Braunwald, pp. 1796-1798, 1807-1808)

Deep sternal wound infection is among the most serious complications of cardiac surgery. Approximately 1.4% of patients undergoing median sternotomy experience this adverse outcome. Such patients present approximately 2 weeks after surgery with fever, leukocytosis, bacteremia, discharge, and erythema at the wound site. Risk factors for the development of mediastinal infection include a prolonged cardiopulmonary bypass time, excessive bleeding necessitating reexploration for hemostatic control, the use of both internal mammary arteries, and older age. Recently, atrial fibrillation and an elevated C-reactive protein level were also found to be predictors of mediastinitis in patients undergoing coronary artery bypass grafting.[1] Obesity is the most important risk factor for sternal dehiscence, whether or not infection is present.

The incidence of postoperative deep sternal wound infection appears to be decreasing.[2] A significant contribution to this reduction is that the rate among diabetics has fallen from about 3.2% to about 1.0% over the past decade, possibly related to the introduction of perioperative intravenous insulin.

About half of deep sternal wound infections are caused by *Staphylococcus* species, whereas gram-negative organisms account for about 40%. Confirmation of a sternal wound infection often requires surgical exploration and removal of material for Gram stain and culture. Imaging techniques, including computed tomography or magnetic resonance imaging are helpful. Intravenous antibiotics, along with possible débridement and irrigation, may be required for prolonged periods. Early diagnosis and initiation of treatment enhance the prognosis. Mediastinal infections do not seem to change patency rates of the bypass grafts themselves.

REFERENCES

1. Elenbaas TW, Soliman Hamad MA, Schönberger JP, et al: Preoperative atrial fibrillation and elevated C-reactive protein levels as predictors of mediastinitis after coronary artery bypass grafting. Ann Thorac Surg 89:704, 2010.
2. Matros E, Aranki SF, Bayer LR, et al: Reduction in incidence of deep sternal wound infections: Random or real? J Thorac Cardiovasc Surg 139:680, 2010.

ANSWER TO QUESTION 655

C (Braunwald, pp. 1702-1706, 1707-1710; Table 78-5)

For patients with suspected pulmonary arterial hypertension (PAH), cardiac catheterization plays an important role in confirming the diagnosis, establishing the severity of disease, and determining prognosis. Patients with PAH demonstrate a normal or low pulmonary capillary wedge pressure (PCWP), distinguishing PAH from pulmonary venous hypertension. A vasodilator-challenge during catheterization allows assessment of pulmonary vasoreactivity and helps to guide therapy. Such a challenge can be accomplished with intravenous adenosine, intravenous epoprostenol, or inhaled nitric oxide. A favorable acute effect of these vasodilators (i.e., >10 mm Hg decrease in mean PAP and/or >33% decrease in pulmonary vascular resistance) without adverse effects (e.g., a decline in cardiac output or systemic blood pressure, or a rise in PCWP) is predictive of a favorable response to oral calcium channel blockers. An increase in PCWP during vasodilator testing would be consistent with pulmonary veno-occlusive disease or impending left ventricular failure.

When oral calcium channel blockers are used to treat PAH, high doses are required to achieve full clinical benefit (e.g., amlodipine 20 to 30 mg/day, nifedipine 180 to 240 mg/day, or diltiazem 720 to 960 mg/day).

REFERENCE

Ghofrani HA, Wilkins MW, Rich S: Uncertainties in the diagnosis and treatment of pulmonary arterial hypertension. Circulation 118:1195, 2008.

ANSWER TO QUESTION 656

C (Braunwald, pp. 1937-1940)

Risk factors for radiocontrast-induced nephropathy include chronic renal insufficiency, diabetic nephropathy, intravascular volume depletion, renal artery stenosis, and concurrent use of agents that alter renal hemodynamics (e.g., angiotensin-converting enzyme inhibitors). The smallest possible volume of contrast agent should be used in patients with renal insufficiency, because the risk of nephrotoxicity is related to the amount injected.

At present, the only intervention that has been demonstrated to consistently reduce the incidence of this complication in patients at risk is normal saline hydration before and after the procedure. Several other agents have historically been evaluated for this purpose, including mannitol, calcium channel antagonists, dopamine, and atrial natriuretic peptide; however, none has been shown to reduce the risk of renal complications. It has been hypothesized that lower ionic strength contrast agents should reduce the incidence of contrast nephropathy. Although that has not been demonstrated in patients with normal baseline renal function, the risk of contrast-induced nephropathy is reduced in patients with baseline renal insufficiency (with or without diabetes) if nonionic low-osmolar contrast medium is used.

Several small studies have suggested that oral administration of acetylcysteine, an antioxidant, can reduce the risk of contrast-associated nephropathy; however, this has not been confirmed in other series. A small prospective study evaluated the use of sodium bicarbonate infusion to prevent contrast nephropathy in patients with chronic renal insufficiency. In comparison with the normal saline infusion group, patients who received bicarbonate before and after administration of a contrast agent sustained fewer instances of nephropathy.

REFERENCES

Pannu N, Wiebe N, Tonelli M, Alberta Kidney Disease Network: Prophylaxis strategies for contrast-induced nephropathy. JAMA 295:2765, 2006

Tepel M, Aspelin P, Lameire N: Contrast-induced nephropathy: A clinical and evidence-based approach. Circulation 113:1799, 2006.

ANSWER TO QUESTION 657

A (Braunwald, pp. 1838-1839)

The major cardiovascular changes that occur in hypothyroidism include a reduction in cardiac contractility, an increase in systemic vascular resistance, and a decrease in the heart rate. The decreased cardiac contractility and relative bradycardia lead to a fall in cardiac output. Thyroid hormone normally reduces smooth muscle tone, resulting in a decrease in peripheral vascular resistance. In the relative absence of thyroid hormone, peripheral vascular tone increases and is thought to be a contributor to hypertension, which is common in hypothyroid patients. Thyroid hormone deficiency results in electrical changes in myocardial depolarization that can lead to slower heart rates and prolongation of the QT interval. Hypothyroidism is also associated with increased vascular permeability and leakage of protein into interstitial spaces. Thus, pericardial effusions are common, developing in approximately one third of patients, although progression to cardiac tamponade is rare.

REFERENCE

Rodondi N, Bauer DC, Cappola AR: Subclinical thyroid dysfunction, cardiac function, and the risk of heart failure. The Cardiovascular Health study. J Am Coll Cardiol 52:1152, 2008.

ANSWER TO QUESTION 658

C (Braunwald, pp. 1314-1320, 1776)

Marfan syndrome, caused by mutations in the fibrillin gene (FBN1), is associated with significant morbidity and mortality from cardiovascular causes. The most life-threatening complication is aortic dissection. Patients with Marfan syndrome are predisposed to this complication because of aortic cystic medial degeneration, and such dissections usually commence just above the coronary ostia and can extend into the entire length of the aorta. Beta blockers limit aortic shear stress and are an important component of prevention. Prospective studies have confirmed a slowing of aortic dilatation and reduced risk of dissection in patients treated with atenolol or propranolol. The size of the proximal aorta can be followed serially by transthoracic echocardiography, computed tomography, or magnetic resonance imaging. Prophylactic aortic root replacement is recommended in Marfan syndrome patients once the diameter approaches 5 cm to prevent dissection and progressive aortic regurgitation.[1] Some groups recommend replacement even earlier, when the diameter is in the 4.5- to 5.0-cm range.

Aortic dissection is also an unfortunate potential complication of pregnancy in Marfan syndrome, occurring most commonly in the period between the third trimester and the first month postpartum. The risk of dissection in this setting is related to the size of the aortic root and appears to be low in patients with root diameters of $\leq$ 4 cm.[2]

Progressive valvular impairments are also common in patients with Marfan syndrome. The risk of severe aortic regurgitation increases as the diameter of the aortic root enlarges. Mitral valve prolapse, associated with elongated and redundant leaflets, is detected in 60% to 80% of patients by echocardiography.[3] Progression to severe mitral regurgitation occurs in up to 25% of patients.

REFERENCES

1. Braverman AC: Timing of aortic surgery in the Marfan syndrome. Curr Opin Cardiol 19:549, 2004.
2. Goland S, Elkayam U: Cardiovascular problems in pregnant women with Marfan syndrome. Circulation 119:619, 2009.
3. Weyman AE, Scherrer-Crosbie M: Marfan syndrome and mitral valve prolapse. J Clin Invest 114:1543, 2004.

ANSWER TO QUESTION 659

B (Braunwald, pp. 1856-1851)

This patient has heparin-induced thrombocytopenia (HIT), of which there are two forms. Type I HIT is the common, milder form that likely results from non–immune-mediated heparin-induced aggregation of platelets. Platelet counts usually drop within 2 days of therapy but rarely fall below 100,000/µL, and patients do not often develop bleeding complications. In the majority of such cases, heparin can be continued and the platelet count will improve.

Type II HIT, which has developed in the patient presented in this question, is the more dangerous form. It produces more severe thrombocytopenia, with levels often <50,000/µL. It develops when antibodies form against the heparin–platelet factor 4 (PF4) complex on the surface of platelets. These antibodies are recognized by platelet receptors, an action that stimulates platelet activation and thrombosis. The diagnosis can be confirmed by the measurement of anti-heparin/PF4 antibodies.

Type II HIT usually becomes manifest for the first time within 4 to 14 days of the initiation of heparin therapy. However, on subsequent exposure, it can present quickly after even small doses of heparin. Therefore, patients with a history of type II HIT should never receive any form of heparin.[1]

When Type II HIT develops, heparin should be stopped immediately. If further anticoagulation is needed, a direct thrombin inhibitor can be substituted.[2] For example, lepirudin (a recombinant form of the direct thrombin inhibitor hirudin) and argatroban (a small-molecule direct thrombin inhibitor) have been shown to be effective treatment strategies in such patients. Low-molecular-weight heparins (LMWHs) are associated with a lower incidence of HIT than is intravenous unfractionated heparin (UFH). However, antibodies to UFH cross-react with LMWHs, so once a diagnosis of type II HIT is made, both types of heparin should be avoided.

Fondaparinux, a synthetic pentasaccharide with anti–factor Xa activity, holds promise as another alternate anticoagulant that appears to be safe in patients who have experienced HIT.[3]

REFERENCES

1. Arepally GM, Ortel TL: Clinical practice: Heparin-induced thrombocytopenia. N Engl J Med 355:809, 2006.
2. Warkentin TE: Heparin-induced thrombocytopenia. Hematol Oncol Clin North Am 21:589, 2007.
3. Dager WE, Andersen J, Nutescu E: Special considerations with fondaparinux therapy: Heparin-induced thrombocytopenia and wound healing. Pharmacotherapy 24:88S, 2004.

ANSWER TO QUESTION 660

D (Braunwald, pp. 1854-1855)

This patient's findings are consistent with thrombotic thrombocytopenic purpura (TTP), a rare but serious complication of thienopyridine antiplatelet therapy. The thienopyridines (ticlopidine, clopidogrel, and prasugrel) inhibit the adenosine diphosphate–dependent pathway of platelet activation through irreversible blockade of the platelet $P2Y_{12}$ receptor. TTP has been described in 0.02% to 0.06% of patients who have taken ticlopidine after coronary stenting and even less commonly (extremely rarely) in patients on clopidogrel or prasugrel. When it occurs, TTP usually develops within the first few weeks after initiation of the drug and typical findings include fever, renal insufficiency, mental status changes, thrombocytopenia, and microangiopathic hemolytic anemia.

REFERENCE

Goodwin MM, Desilets AR, Willett KC. Thienopyridines in acute coronary syndrome. Ann Pharmacother 45:207, 2011.

ANSWER TO QUESTION 661

D (Braunwald, pp. 1893-1894)

Metastatic tumors to the heart or pericardium are much more common than are primary cardiac malignancies. Metastases within cardiac structures are present at autopsy in approximately 6% of patients with malignant disease, whereas primary cardiac tumors are found in fewer than 1%. The most common malignancy that metastasizes to the heart is carcinoma of the lung, followed in frequency by carcinoma of the breast, malignant melanoma, and lymphoma. Single metastases to the heart are rare, such that the finding of a solitary cardiac tumor is usually indicative of a benign process.

Cardiac metastases typically involve the pericardium and myocardium, with the valves and endocardium rarely affected. Many cardiac metastases are clinically silent. For example, in malignant melanoma, 46% to 71% of patients have metastases to the myocardium or pericardium, yet cardiac symptoms are rare. The most common clinical manifestations of metastatic disease are due to pericardial effusion (i.e., tamponade), tachyarrhythmias, conduction blocks, and congestive heart failure.

A chylous pericardial effusion is characteristic of lymphoma.

REFERENCE

Luna A, Ribes R, Caro P, et al: Evaluation of cardiac tumors with magnetic resonance imaging. Eur Radiol 15:1446, 2005.

ANSWER TO QUESTION 662

A (Braunwald, pp. 1869-1872)

This patient presents with acute rheumatic fever after probable streptococcal pharyngitis. The diagnosis of acute rheumatic fever is based on five major manifestations (the "Jones criteria"): pancarditis, polyarthritis, chorea, subcutaneous nodules, and erythema marginatum. In addition, several other symptoms, laboratory findings, and data are commonly observed in this condition and are considered "minor manifestations." Nonspecific arthralgias, especially of large joints, and fever may occur. Elevated acute-phase reactants are a result of tissue inflammation. In the acute phase of the disease, the erythrocyte sedimentation rate and C-reactive protein are commonly elevated. Electrocardiographic findings in acute rheumatic fever include prolongation of the PR interval (not the QT interval), tachycardia, and ST-segment and T wave abnormalities consistent with myocarditis. Patients often develop leukocytosis and a normochromic, normocytic anemia.

Only about 11% of patients have positive throat cultures for group A streptococci at the time of diagnosis of acute rheumatic fever. A positive throat culture does not distinguish between a recent infection and chronic oropharyngeal colonization. Therefore, rising antistreptococcal antibody levels may provide a more reliable method to confirm infection.

REFERENCE

Carapetis JR, McDonald M, Wilson NJ: Acute rheumatic fever. Lancet 366:155, 2005.

ANSWER TO QUESTION 663

D (Braunwald, pp. 1883-1884)

Rheumatoid arthritis (RA) is the most common systemic rheumatic disorder. Symptomatic cardiac complications are rare but include pericardial, myocardial, coronary, or conduction system disease. Pericarditis is the most frequent form of cardiac involvement, but asymptomatic pericardial effusions are more common than acute pericarditis. Rarely, cardiac tamponade or pericardial constriction can occur. Treatment is usually directed at the underlying arthritis with anti-inflammatory agents and immunosuppressive therapy.

Conduction system disease has been reported in up to 10% of patients with RA and is believed to be due to impingement on the conduction system by rheumatoid nodules. First-degree heart block is the most common finding. Myocarditis is not common in patients with RA and, when present, rarely results in significant ventricular dysfunction.

Patients with RA have an increased incidence of atherosclerotic coronary artery disease (CAD), symptoms of which may be masked by their limited physical mobility. In addition, coronary arteritis has been reported in up to 20% of patients in autopsy series; however, it only rarely results in coronary insufficiency syndromes. The epicardial arteries are generally spared, because arteritis is usually confined to smaller intramyocardial vessels.

Autopsy studies have demonstrated frequent rheumatoid involvement of the cardiac valves and aorta, but such involvement is only occasionally of clinical significance.

REFERENCE

Sarzi-Puttini P, Atzeni F, Shoenfeld Y, Ferraccioli G: TNF-alpha, rheumatoid arthritis, and heart failure: A rheumatological dilemma. Autoimmun Rev 4:153, 2005.

ANSWER TO QUESTION 664

C (Braunwald, pp. 828, 1863-1864)

A major goal of therapy in patients with atrial fibrillation (AF) is to prevent thromboembolic complications such as stroke. This patient is at increased risk for thromboembolism in the setting of AF because of his age and hypertension (CHADS$_2$ score = 2) and therefore he warrants chronic anticoagulation therapy.

Dabigatran etexilate is an oral *direct thrombin inhibitor* that was recently approved for use in the United States to reduce the risk of stroke and systemic embolism in patients with nonvalvular atrial fibrillation. In the RE-LY trial, dabigatran (at dosages of 110 and 150 mg twice daily) was compared prospectively with warfarin (dose adjusted to achieve an international normalized ratio [INR] between 2.0 and 3.0) for stroke and systemic embolism prevention in 18,113 patients with nonvalvular atrial fibrillation for a median of 2 years. The annual rate of stroke or systemic embolism was 1.7% with warfarin, 1.5% with the lower-dose dabigatran regimen, and 1.1% with the higher-dose regimen. Thus, the lower-dose dabigatran regimen was noninferior to warfarin, whereas the higher dose regimen was actually superior for stroke and embolism prevention. The annual rates of major bleeding were 3.4% with

warfarin compared with 2.7% and 3.1% with the lower-dose and higher-dose dabigatran regimens, respectively. That is, the lower-dose dabigatran regimen was associated with less major bleeding than warfarin, whereas the rates were similar in the higher-dose dabigatran and warfarin cohorts. Episodes of hemorrhagic stroke were significantly fewer with either dose of dabigatran compared with warfarin.

The most common gastrointestinal side effects of dabigatran are dyspepsia and gastritis; hepatotoxicity was not observed with dabigatran in the RE-LY trial.

The current labeling for dabigatran recommends a dose adjustment to 75 mg twice daily for patients with a reduced creatinine clearance between 15 and 30 mL/min. There is insufficient experience to recommend a dose for a creatinine clearance <15 mL/min.

REFERENCE

Connolly SJ, Ezekowitz MD, Yusuf S, et al: Dabigatran versus warfarin in patients with atrial fibrillation. N Engl J Med 361:1139, 2009.

ANSWER TO QUESTION 665

B (Braunwald, pp. 1839-1840)

Amiodarone, a potent Class III antiarrhythmic agent, has two primary effects on thyroid function. First, it inhibits the peripheral conversion of thyroxine (T$_4$) to triiodothyronine (T$_3$), causing a reduction of serum T$_3$ and a transient rise in thyroid-stimulating hormone (TSH). Within a short time, however, a compensatory increase in serum T$_4$ levels occurs and TSH returns to normal. Clinically, such patients are euthyroid, even though the T$_4$ levels are elevated. Amiodarone's second effect relates to its large content of iodine (30% by weight), which inhibits synthesis and release of T$_4$ from the thyroid gland, causing a more sustained rise in TSH. In some patients, especially those with underlying thyroid disease, clinical hypothyroidism and a marked rise in TSH result.

Amiodarone-induced hyperthyroidism is less common and may arise from two distinct mechanisms. Type I develops primarily in individuals with underlying thyroid disease, typically in iodine-deficient environments. Such patients display evidence of thyroid autoimmunity, including antithyroid antibodies. In contrast, type II is a form of thyroiditis that develops in a previously normal gland, presumably mediated by proinflammatory cytokines, marked by an elevation of circulating interleukin-6. This condition is a thyroid-destructive process, and hyperthyroidism results from release of preformed thyroid hormone, a situation that can persist for months. Unlike type I, this form of hyperthyroidism tends to respond to glucocorticoid therapy.

REFERENCE

Cohen-Lehman J, Dahl P, Danzi S, Klein I: Effects of amiodarone on thyroid function. Nat Rev Endocrinol 6:34, 2010.

ANSWER TO QUESTION 666

D (Braunwald, pp. 1719-1724; see also Answer to Question 486)

The two principal sleep disorders associated with cardiovascular disease are obstructive sleep apnea (OSA) and central sleep apnea (CSA). OSA is characterized by transient upper airway occlusion that results in partial or complete cessation in airflow leading to hypoxia, sympathetic activation, repeated arousal and wakefulness, and sleep fragmentation. Individuals with OSA demonstrate persistently heightened sympathetic activity, even during daytime wakefulness. This in turn leads to peripheral vasoconstriction and hypertension, as well as automatic tachycardias driven by the augmented sympathetic tone. In addition, reflex parasympathetic activity can lead to profound nocturnal bradycardias.

Positive airway pressure (PAP) is the cornerstone of OSA management. This therapy effectively splints open the airway, thus preventing airway collapse. PAP improves nocturnal hypoxia and reduces sympathetic activity, and long-term observational studies show that OSA patients who utilize PAP are at decreased risk of major cardiovascular events including myocardial infarction, stroke, and death.[1]

In contrast to OSA, CSA represents an instability of ventilatory control, resulting in oscillations in ventilation and periodic hyperpnea and apnea. When manifest as Cheyne-Stokes respirations, it is associated with advanced heart failure. PAP is effective in the management of CSA by improving the hemodynamics of heart failure. It is associated with decreased sympathetic drive, reduced ventricular afterload, and improvement in left ventricular ejection fraction. PAP has been shown to improve nocturnal oxygen saturation and 6-minute distance in patients with Class II to IV heart failure and CSA, although no improvement in mortality was observed.[2]

REFERENCES

1. Marin JM, Carrizo SJ, Vicente E, Agusti AG: Long-term cardiovascular outcomes in men with obstructive sleep apnoea-hypopnoea with or without treatment with continuous positive airway pressure: An observational study. Lancet 365:1046, 2005.
2. Bradley TD, Logan AG, Kimoff RJ, et al: Continuous positive airway pressure for central sleep apnea and heart failure. N Engl J Med 353:2025, 2005.

ANSWER TO QUESTION 667

E (Braunwald, p. 1802; see also Answer to Question 645)

The diagnosis of myocardial infarction (MI) after cardiac surgery can be difficult because of the routine postoperative elevation of creatine kinase (CK) and troponin levels and the frequent finding of nonspecific ST-segment/T wave abnormalities on the ECG. The most reliable electrocardiographic finding of a post–coronary artery bypass graft (CABG) MI is new and persistent Q waves. The Society of Thoracic Surgeons database reports the incidence of perioperative MI to be approximately 1.1% based on criteria that include serum CK-MB > five times the upper limit of normal <24 hours postoperatively or one or more of the following more than 24 hours postoperatively: evolutionary ST-segment elevation, new Q waves in two or more contiguous leads, new left bundle branch block, or CK-MB > three times the upper limit of normal.

Risk factors for perioperative MI include an older age, a longer pump time, an elevated left-ventricular end-diastolic pressure, preoperative unstable angina, and left main coronary artery disease.

Compared with conventional CABG, off-pump bypass grafting appears to be associated with less acute release of cardiac biomarkers but not reduced mortality at 1 year after surgery.

REFERENCE

Selvanayagam JB, Neubauer S, Taggart DP: Quantification of perioperative myocardial infarction after coronary artery bypass surgery. Eur Heart J 25:2171, 2004.

ANSWER TO QUESTION 668

D (Braunwald, pp. 1811-1816; Table 85-3)

Emergency surgery is associated with increased mortality in patients with cardiovascular disease. The risk of postoperative cardiac events, including myocardial infarction (MI) or death, is 2.5 to 4 times higher than with an elective operation. When surgery is elective, it is appropriate to estimate cardiac risk using multifactorial indices. In such evaluations, insulin-dependent diabetes mellitus is an independent risk factor for postoperative adverse cardiac outcomes.[1] Other major risk factors include a history of ischemic heart disease, heart failure, stroke, or a serum creatinine level > 2 mg/dL. The degree of cardiac risk is also influenced by the type of surgery being undertaken. The greatest number of cardiovascular complications is associated with abdominal aortic aneurysm surgery, whereas low-risk procedures include endoscopy, cataract surgery, superficial procedures and biopsies, and transurethral prostate surgery. Carotid endarterectomy poses an intermediate risk.

Ischemic heart disease is a major determinant of perioperative morbidity and mortality. Studies from the 1970s concluded that purely elective surgery should be delayed for 6 months after an MI to ensure that cardiovascular risk had returned to baseline. In those studies, the risk of reinfarction or death was approximately 30% when patients were operated on within 3 months of an MI, but only 5% when 6 months had elapsed before the operation. More recent studies, in the era of careful perioperative monitoring, have demonstrated much lower cardiac complication rates: about a 6% risk of reinfarction for operations performed within 3 months of an MI and a 2% risk for operations performed within 3 to 6 months.

If noncardiac surgery needs to be performed sooner than a full 6 months post MI, risk assessment can be established based on the patient's functional capacity and left ventricular function. In general, if a patient can carry grocery bags up one flight of stairs without stopping or experiencing anginal symptoms, most surgical procedures are well tolerated.[2]

REFERENCES

1. Cohn SL, Auerbach AD: Preoperative cardiac risk stratification 2007: Evolving evidence, evolving strategies. J Hosp Med 2:174, 2007.
2. ACC/AHA 2002 Guideline: Perioperative cardiovascular evaluation for noncardiac surgery. J Am Coll Cardiol 39:542, 2002.

ANSWER TO QUESTION 669

C (Braunwald, pp. 1776-1777; see also Answer to Question 636)

The presentation of this patient is most consistent with peripartum cardiomyopathy. This disorder is a form of dilated cardiomyopathy that manifests in the last trimester of pregnancy or in the early postpartum period.[1] The etiology is unknown, and there are no diagnostic tests to confirm the diagnosis. Its incidence is higher in women >the age of 30, in twin pregnancies, in multiparous women, and in African Americans.

The prognosis of this disorder is favorable compared with other forms of dilated cardiomyopathy, with 50% to 60% of patients showing marked improvement or complete recovery within 6 months postpartum. The remainder either stabilizes with reduced cardiac function or declines progressively, eventually requiring cardiac transplantation. The predictors for a poor outcome include older age, higher parity, severe left ventricular dilatation, and onset of symptoms later after delivery. There is a high risk of relapse of peripartum cardiomyopathy in subsequent pregnancies, and that risk appears to be greatest in women who have persistently impaired cardiac function.[2]

REFERENCES

1. Elkayam U, Akhter MW, Singh H, et al: Pregnancy-associated cardiomyopathy: Clinical characteristics and a comparison between early and late presentation. Circulation 111:2050, 2005.
2. Sliwa K, Fett J, Elkayam U: Peripartum cardiomyopathy. Lancet 368:687, 2006.

ANSWERS TO QUESTIONS 670 TO 674

670–E, 671–D, 672–B, 673–C, 674–A (Braunwald, pp. 1876-1879, 1884-1885, 1887-1888)

The spondyloarthropathies, including ankylosing spondylitis, Reiter syndrome, and psoriatic arthritis, have a predilection for arthritis of the sacroiliac and lumbosacral joints. These diseases are associated with the histocompatibility antigen HLA-B27 and predominantly occur in men. *Ankylosing spondylitis* is the most common of these syndromes to involve the heart and classically causes dilatation of the aortic valve ring with fibrous thickening and inflammation. The aorta in ankylosing spondylitis is histologically similar to that in syphilitic aortitis, including adventitial scarring, intimal proliferation, and narrowing of the vasa vasorum. Aortic regurgitation results from thickening of the valvular cusps and dilatation of the aortic root.[1] Conduction system disorders, due to fibrous infiltration in the atrioventricular node and the bundle of His, may be seen in ankylosing spondylitis as well.

Reiter syndrome is a form of nonpurulent, reactive arthritis that may follow enteric or urogenital infections. It is frequently associated with uveitis/conjunctivitis and nongonococcal urethritis. The cardiac complications of Reiter syndrome are similar to those of ankylosing spondylitis.

Cardiac pathologic abnormalities in patients with *progressive systemic sclerosis/scleroderma* may include myocardial fibrosis and contraction band necrosis. Symptomatic pericarditis may be present. Conduction defects and thickening of the mitral and aortic valves may also occur.[2]

Giant cell arteritis/large vessel arteritis predominantly causes inflammation of the aorta, its major branches, and coronary arteries. Weakening of the vessels may lead to dilatation, aneurysm formation, and valvular insufficiency. The vascular pathology often reveals granuloma formation.

Behçet syndrome is a multisystem disorder highlighted by recurrent oral and genital ulcers and uveitis. The ulcers are often painful and necrotic, and eye involvement occasionally progresses to blindness. The etiology of the disease is unclear but appears to involve endothelial activation as a mediator of vascular inflammation. Venous and arterial thrombosis may occur, as well as aneurysm formation of the large vessels. Diffuse aortitis in Behçet syndrome can lead to aortic root dilatation and valvular insufficiency.[3]

REFERENCES

1. Huffer LL, Furgerson JL: Aortic root dilatation with sinus of Valsalva and coronary artery aneurysms associated with ankylosing spondylitis. Tex Heart Inst J 33:70, 2006.
2. Steen V: The heart in systemic sclerosis. Curr Rheumatol Rep 6:137, 2004.
3. Tsui KL, Lee KW, Chan WK, et al: Behcet's aortitis and aortic regurgitation: A report of two cases. J Am Soc Echocardiogr 17:83, 2004.

ANSWERS TO QUESTIONS 675 TO 678

675–C, 676–B, 677–D, 678–A (Braunwald, pp. 716-717, 964, 1138-1139, 1687-1688)

Numerous cardiac medications can cause hematologic complications. Most often, discontinuation of the offending drug results in resolution of symptoms.

Heparin can result in thrombocytopenia by two main mechanisms as described in the Answer to Question 659.

A positive direct Coombs test is seen in up to 10% of patients who receive the antihypertensive agent alphamethyldopa. In these patients, the IgG antibody is directed against the Rh complex of red cells. Hemolysis may be severe but improves within several weeks after cessation of the medication.

Methemoglobinemia may result from exposure to a wide variety of agents, including nitroglycerin, sulfonamides, and lidocaine, all chemicals that can oxidize ferrous (Fe^{2+}) hemoglobin to the ferric (Fe^{3+}) state. Patients with methemoglobinemia have an oxygen dissociation curve that is shifted to the left, have normal Po_2 levels, and appear cyanotic because of the decreased oxygen-carrying capacity of the ferric hemoglobin. Patients with methemoglobinemia may complain of nonspecific symptoms such as dizziness, fatigue, and headache or may present with respiratory distress, seizures, and arrhythmias. Blood with high levels of methemoglobin is chocolate brown. The syndrome is usually corrected by discontinuation of the offending agent; however, exchange transfusions or methylene blue therapy may be necessary.

Procainamide may cause a syndrome resembling systemic lupus erythematosus (SLE). Symptoms consist of polyarthralgias, pleuritis, and photosensitive rashes. Unlike conventional SLE, nephritis and central nervous system complications are very rare. Patients with drug-induced lupus are antinuclear antibody (ANA) positive with antibodies to histones but rarely display hypocomplementemia or antibodies to DNA. Discontinuation of procainamide typically results in improvement of symptoms within a few days to weeks. However, ANA levels may remain elevated for years.

ANSWERS TO QUESTIONS 679 TO 683

679–C, 680–A, 681–B, 682–B, 683–C (Braunwald, pp. 1876-1881)

Takayasu arteritis, also termed *pulseless disease,* is of unknown etiology and is characterized by marked fibrous and degenerative scarring of the elastic fibers of the vascular media. It most commonly involves the aorta and carotid arteries. The disease is 10 times more common in women than in men, and in most patients onset occurs during the teen years.[1] Patients typically present with malaise, weight loss, night sweats, arthralgias, pleuritic pain, anorexia, and fatigue. Regardless of whether a patient goes through this initial phase, after a latent period symptoms and signs referable to the obliterative and inflammatory changes in affected blood vessels begin to appear. These include diminished or absent pulses with claudication (upper extremities > lower extremities), hypertension (related to renal artery stenosis or increased vessel rigidity), and aortic root aneurysms with aortic regurgitation. Common laboratory abnormalities include elevated sedimentation rate, low-grade leukocytosis, and normocytic anemia. Treatment of this disorder includes glucocorticoid therapy. Patients with refractory symptoms may respond to the addition of cyclophosphamide. Recent studies have shown beneficial effects of tumor necrosis factor antagonists.[2]

Giant cell arteritis is a disease of unknown etiology characterized by granulomatous inflammation of large- to medium-caliber arteries with a special predilection for the vessels of the head and neck.[3] The disease is also known as granulomatous arteritis and temporal arteritis and is seen primarily in elderly people with a female predominance. Clinically, the triad of severe headache, fever, and marked malaise characterizes the illness. The headaches are often severe and are typically localized over involved temporal arteries. Claudication of the jaw muscles during chewing is present in up to two thirds of patients. Involvement of the ophthalmic artery leads to visual symptoms and may result in irreversible blindness. The syndrome of polymyalgia rheumatica, consisting of diffuse muscular aching and stiffness, occurs in about 40% of patients with giant cell arteritis. In a minority of cases, involvement of the aorta or its major branches may lead to symptoms and signs similar to those of Takayasu arteritis, although interestingly, renal artery involvement is almost never seen in this disorder.

Patients with giant cell arteritis appear ill and almost always have fever. Affected vessels feel abnormal to palpation and are tender, allowing experienced examiners to make the diagnosis of temporal arteritis at the bedside by identifying an indurated, beaded, tender temporal artery. Laboratory tests often reveal a very high sedimentation rate, normochromic, normocytic anemia, and elevated acute-phase reactants. Biopsy of an involved temporal artery confirms the diagnosis.

Management of giant cell arteritis includes early intervention with high-dose steroid therapy (60 to 80 mg of prednisone per day) followed by a gradual taper to a maintenance dose, which is typically continued for 1 to 2 years. Early administration of steroid therapy is crucial to the prevention of involvement of the ophthalmic arteries and possible blindness.

REFERENCES

1. Sheikhzadeh A, Tettenborn I, Noohi F, et al: Occlusive thromboaortopathy (Takayasu disease): Clinical and angiographic features and a brief review of literature. Angiology 53:29, 2002.
2. Molloy ES, Langford CA, Clark TM, et al: Anti-tumour necrosis factor therapy in patients with refractory Takayasu arteritis: long-term follow-up. Ann Rheum Dis 67:1567, 2008.
3. Weyand CM, Goronzy JJ: Medium and large vessel vasculitis. N Engl J Med 349:160, 2003.

ANSWERS TO QUESTIONS 684 TO 688

684–C, 685–A, 686–B, 687–D, 688-E (Braunwald, pp. 1896-1901, Table 90-2)

Several chemotherapeutic agents have potential cardiovascular toxicities. The anthracyclines (e.g., doxorubicin, daunorubicin, and idarubicin) may cause acute cardiac effects (including atrial and ventricular arrhythmias and pericardial effusion) or more chronic impairment (dilated cardiomyopathy with congestive heart failure). As described in the Answer to Question 544, heart failure due to anthracycline therapy is dose related and develops more frequently when concurrent risk factors are present, including prior heart disease, radiation therapy exposure to the heart, and use of other cardiotoxic chemotherapeutic agents (e.g., trastuzumab, paclitaxel).

Patients receiving 5-fluorouracil may experience acute chest pain and myocardial infarction during or immediately after infusion. The mechanism of this adverse effect is unclear. Cyclophosphamide and ifosfamide are alkylating agents that can cause an acute hemorrhagic myopericarditis. Interleukins, which are potent modulators of the immune system, are associated with capillary leak syndrome, hypotension, noncardiogenic pulmonary edema, and nephrotoxicity.

Sunitinib (Sutent) is a tyrosine kinase inhibitor that targets vascular endothelial cell growth factor receptors (VEGFRs) and is used to inhibit cancer progression in renal cell carcinoma and gastrointestinal stromal tumors. Hypertension is a common side effect, with marked elevations in blood pressure elevation in 8% to 20% of patients.

REFERENCE

Chu T, Rupnick MA, Kerkela R, et al: Cardiotoxicity associated with the tyrosine kinase inhibitor sunitinib. Lancet 270:2011, 2007.

Schimmel KJ, Richel DJ, van den Brink RB, Guchelaar HJ: Cardiotoxicity of cytotoxic drugs. Cancer Treat Rev 30:181, 2004.

ANSWERS TO QUESTIONS 689 TO 693

689–C, 690–D, 691–E, 692–A, 693–B (Braunwald, pp. 1829-1839)

Endocrine disorders often have cardiovascular effects. Excess thyroid hormone levels result in tachycardia, palpitations, and hypertension, often with a widened pulse pressure.[1] Cardiac examination reveals a hyperdynamic impulse with an accentuated S_1. Systolic murmurs are common, and a *Means-Lerman scratch*, a grating systolic sound at the upper left sternal border, may be auscultated during expiration.

The cardiovascular manifestations of hypothyroidism include bradycardia, diastolic hypertension with a narrowed pulse pressure, cardiomegaly with a reduced ejection fraction, and pericardial effusion, which only rarely results in tamponade physiology.[1]

Cushing syndrome is associated with accelerated atherosclerosis, likely related to hypertension and hyperglycemia in this condition. *Carney complex* is a genetic syndrome that includes Cushing syndrome, cardiac myxomas, and pigmented dermal lesions. This autosomal dominant syndrome maps to a region of chromosome 17.[2]

Hyperaldosteronism is associated with excess aldosterone production from an adrenal or extra-adrenal source. Hypertension, hypokalemia, and metabolic alkalosis are common findings. Many of the cardiac findings are nonspecific and are a consequence of the metabolic and electrolyte abnormalities. For example, U waves and ventricular arrhythmias result from associated hypokalemia.

Parathyroid hormone has a direct inotropic and chronotropic effect on the heart, likely due to increased calcium entry into myocytes.[3] Hypercalcemia associated with hyperparathyroidism may result in excess calcium deposition in the heart, hypertension, and shortening of the QT interval.

REFERENCES

1. Klein I, Danzi S: Thyroid disease and the heart. Circulation 116:1725, 2007.
2. Bertherat J: Carney complex. Orphanet J Rare Dis 1:21, 2006.
3. Andersson P, Rydberg E, Willenheimer R: Primary hyperparathyroidism and heart disease: A review. Eur Heart J 25:1776, 2004.

ANSWERS TO QUESTIONS 694 TO 697

694–B, 695–C, 696–D, 697–A (Braunwald, pp. 1864-1865)

Tissue-type plasminogen activator (tPA), the major physiologic activator of plasminogen, is both synthesized naturally by endothelial cells and produced commercially by recombinant DNA technology for the purpose of therapeutic fibrinolysis. The protein is synthesized in a single-chain form, which is subsequently converted to a two-chain form by proteolytic cleavage of a single plasmin-sensitive site. Both the single-chain and the two-chain forms have endogenous proteolytic activity. The alpha chain of tPA is derived from the amino-terminal portion of single-chain tPA and contains a pair of finger-like structures referred to as "kringle" domains. Lysine binding sites located on these domains confer binding specifically for fibrin. As a result, tPA is a relatively fibrin-specific activator that converts plasminogen to plasmin two or three times more efficiently in the presence of fibrin. The protease domain of tPA contains a proteolytic site that converts plasminogen to plasmin. This portion is homologous with other serine proteases, such as urokinase and trypsin.

Urokinase is a two-chain serine protease that is synthesized in both renal tubular epithelial cells and endothelial cells. While urokinase converts plasminogen to plasmin by hydrolyzing the same bond as that acted on by tPA, the proteolytic activity of urokinase is not enhanced by the presence of fibrin. Therefore, urokinase may activate circulating plasminogen as effectively as plasminogen absorbed onto fibrin thrombi.

Streptokinase is a single polypeptide chain of 414 amino acids that is produced by a strain of hemolytic streptococci. Streptokinase does not cause thrombolysis by intrinsic enzymatic activity. Instead, it activates the fibrinolytic system by combining with plasminogen to form a plasminogen activator complex that is then capable of converting plasminogen to plasmin. Plasmin then degrades fibrin and other procoagulant proteins and assists in dissolving the thrombus. Many individuals have circulating antibodies to streptokinase as a result of previous streptococcal infections. Therefore, a large dose of streptokinase is administered to neutralize these antibodies. Antistreptococcal antibodies may remain high up to 6 months after administration.

Tenecteplase is a genetically engineered mutant of tPA that displays a prolonged half-life and increased fibrin specificity. Unlike tPA, which requires a continuous infusion, tenecteplase is injected as a single intravenous bolus, which facilitates administration.

REFERENCE

Longstaff C, William S, Thelwell C: Fibrin binding and the regulation of plasminogen activators during thrombolytic therapy. Cardiovasc Hematol Agents Med Chem 6:212, 2008.

ANSWERS TO QUESTIONS 698 TO 702

698–A, 699–B, 700–D, 701–C, 702–A (Braunwald, pp. 1856-1860)

Unfractionated heparin (UFH) is a naturally occurring compound that acts in vivo by combining with antithrombin (an inhibitor of thrombin and factors X, IX, and XI). The conformational change that occurs in antithrombin allows for an accelerated interaction with the activated clotting factors, limiting thrombin generation and fibrin formation. Commercial heparin is extracted from porcine intestinal mucosa and bovine lung and does not inactivate clot-bound thrombin or factor VII. Heparin is not absorbed by the gastrointestinal tract and is therefore administered in intravenous or subcutaneous forms. The bioavailability of subcutaneous injections of UFH is only 30%.

The activated partial thromboplastin time (aPTT) test is used to determine the inhibitory effect of UFH. For acute thrombosis or embolism, intravenous heparin is administered with a goal aPTT of 1.5 to 2 times the control value. Subcutaneous UFH is often used for patients who require a lower level of anticoagulation. Heparin therapy's major complication is bleeding. There is up to a 30% incidence of heparin-induced thrombocytopenia that may be associated with thromboembolic events and often resolves with discontinuation of the drug. In addition, heparin may cause osteoporosis, elevated liver enzymes, increased vascular permeability, alopecia, and hypoaldosteronism (and associated hyperkalemia).

Low-molecular-weight heparin (LMWH) also produces an anticoagulant effect by binding to antithrombin. However, in distinction to UFH, LMWH preferentially inhibits factor Xa more than thrombin. LMWH formulations bind less with platelet factor 4, plasma proteins, and endothelial cells, and therefore have >90% bioavailability when administered by subcutaneous injection. Other advantages of LMWH include a prolonged half-life and predictable anticoagulant responses.

Patients receiving LMWH do not require serial laboratory monitoring to monitor the anticoagulant effect, except those with renal failure, extreme obesity, or pregnancy. Heparin-induced thrombocytopenia can occur with LMWH but is less common than with UFH.

REFERENCE

Gross PL, Weitz JI: New antithrombotic drugs. Clin Pharmacol Ther 86:139, 2009.

ANSWERS TO QUESTIONS 703 TO 706

703–D, 704–B, 705–A, 706–C (Braunwald, pp. 1878-1879, 1884-1888; see also Answers to Questions 670 to 674)

Rheumatologic disorders often involve the cardiovascular system and can result in pericardial, myocardial, valvular, or arterial abnormalities. Aortic involvement is estimated to occur in 15% of patients with giant cell arteritis. Inflammation often involves the proximal aorta and aortic valve cusps, resulting in dilatation of the vessel and aortic regurgitation.[1] Other rheumatologic diseases that prominently involve the aorta include ankylosing spondylitis and psoriatic arthritis.

Valvular abnormalities are found by transesophageal echocardiography in 50% of patients with systemic lupus erythematosus.[2] The most common involvement, termed *Libman-Sacks endocarditis*, represents noninfectious valve thickening, usually on the atrial side of the mitral valve and the arterial side of the aortic valve. Over time, fibrosis may result in valvular insufficiency. Much less commonly, the vegetations may occlude the valve orifice, causing stenosis. Clinical manifestations of Libman-Sacks lesions, such as infective endocarditis or peripheral embolism, are rare.[2]

Although pulmonary hypertension can develop in many rheumatologic disorders, it is a particularly prominent feature of scleroderma and is one of the leading causes of morbidity and mortality in that condition.[3] Behçet disease typically results in inflammation of the thoracic aorta and branch vessels, leading to stenoses and aneurysmal dilatation of the subclavian and carotid arteries. Thoracic and abdominal aortic aneurysms may also result.

REFERENCES

1. Weyand CM, Goronzy JJ: Medium and large vessel vasculitis. N Engl J Med 349:160, 2003.
2. Perez-Villa F, Font J, Azqueta M, et al: Severe valvular regurgitation and antiphospholipid antibodies in systemic lupus erythematosus: A prospective, long-term follow-up study. Arthritis Rheum 53:460, 2005.
3. Kahan A, Coghlan G, McLaughlin V: Cardiac complications of systemic sclerosis. Rheumatology 48:iii45, 2009.